Diarrhea: A Clinical Guide

Diarrhea: A Clinical Guide

Edited by Jonathan Perry

hayle
medical

New York

Hayle Medical,
750 Third Avenue, 9th Floor,
New York, NY 10017, USA

Visit us on the World Wide Web at:
www.haylemedical.com

ISBN: 978-1-63241-845-6

Cataloging-in-Publication Data

Diarrhea : a clinical guide / edited by Jonathan Perry.
   p. cm.
Includes bibliographical references and index.
ISBN 978-1-63241-845-6
1. Diarrhea. 2. Diarrhea--Treatment. 3. Clinical medicine. I. Perry, Jonathan.
RA644.D9 D53 2020
616.342 7--dc23

Table of Contents

Preface

The world is advancing at a fast pace like never before. Therefore, the need is to keep up with the latest developments. This book was an idea that came to fruition when the specialists in the area realized the need to coordinate together and document essential themes in the subject. That's when I was requested to be the editor. Editing this book has been an honour as it brings together diverse authors researching on different streams of the field. The book collates essential materials contributed by veterans in the area which can be utilized by students and researchers alike.

Diarrhea is the condition characterized by atleast three liquid or loose bowel movements each day. It typically lasts for a few days and can result in dehydration owing to fluid loss. Diarrhea is of three types- short duration bloody diarrhea, short duration watery diarrhea and persistent diarrhea. Irritable behavior and loss of the normal stretchiness of the skin are common signs of the disease. If it becomes severe, it can result in decreased urination, fast heart rate, loss of skin color and decrease in responsiveness. The underlying cause of the disease can be attributed to an infection of the intestines. Lactose intolerance, non-celiac gluten sensitivity, irritable bowel syndrome, celiac disease, hyperthyroidism, bile acid diarrhea, etc. are other causes of diarrhea. Oral rehydration solution and zinc tablets are ideal treatment strategies for diarrhea. This book is a comprehensive clinical guide to diarrhea. The topics included herein are of utmost significance and bound to provide incredible insights to readers. This book is appropriate for students seeking detailed information on this medical condition as well as for experts.

Each chapter is a sole-standing publication that reflects each author's interpretation. Thus, the book displays a multi-facetted picture of our current understanding of application, resources and aspects of the field. I would like to thank the contributors of this book and my family for their endless support.

Editor

Molecular Characterization of Enterotoxigenic *Escherichia coli* Strains Isolated from Diarrheal Patients in Korea during 2003–2011

Kyung-Hwan Oh[1], Dong Wook Kim[2], Su-Mi Jung[1], Seung-Hak Cho[1]*

1 Division of Enteric Bacterial Infections, Center for Infectious Diseases, Korea National Institute of Health, Osong-eup, Chungcheongbuk-do, Republic of Korea,
2 Department of Pharmacy, College of Pharmacy, Hanyang University, Ansan, Kyeonggi-do, Republic of Korea

Abstract

Enterotoxigenic *Escherichia coli* (ETEC) is one of the major causes of infectious diarrhea in developing countries. In order to characterize the molecular features of human ETEC isolates from Korea, we investigated the profiles of enterotoxin and colonization factor (CF) genes by polymerase chain reaction (PCR) and performed multilocus sequence typing (MLST) with a total of 291 ETEC strains. The specimens comprised 258 domestic strains isolated from patients who had diarrhea and were from widely separated geographic regions in Korea and 33 inflow strains isolated from travelers visiting other Asian countries. Heat-stable toxin (STh)-possessing ETEC strains were more frequent than heat-labile toxin (LT)-possessing ETEC strains in the domestic isolates, while the detection rates of both enterotoxin genes were similar in the inflow isolates. The profile of CF genes of domestic isolates was similar to that of inflow isolates and the major CF types of the strains were CS3-CS21-CS1/PCF071 and CS2-CS3-CS21. Most of these 2 CF types were detected in ETEC strains that possess both *lt* and *sth* genes. The major MLSTST types of domestic isolates were ST171 and ST955. Moreover, the 2 major CF types were usually found concomitantly with the 2 major MLST STs, ST171 and ST955. In conclusion, our genotyping results may provide useful information for guiding the development of geographically specific vaccines against human ETEC isolates.

Editor: Jamunarani Vadivelu, University of Malaya, Malaysia

Funding: This study was supported by a grant from the Korean National Institute of Health, Seoul, Republic of Korea (KNIH4800-4845-300 to S.H.C.). The funders had no role in study design, data collection and analysis, decision to publish, or preparation of the manuscript.

Competing Interests: The authors have declared that no competing interests exist.

* E-mail: skcho38@korea.kr

Introduction

Enterotoxigenic *Escherichia coli* (ETEC) is a major cause of diarrhea and diarrheal deaths among young children and travelers in developing countries [1,2]. The major virulence factors of diarrhea-causing ETEC strains are enterotoxins, that is, a heat-labile toxin (LT) and a heat-stable toxin (ST), that induce the watery diarrhea. The LT is an AB5 toxin with similarities to cholera toxin; it binds to ADP ribosylates the guanyl-nucleotied alpha regulatory binding protein of the adenylcyclase system thereby causing increased cyclic AMP levels. The ST is a small peptide molecule that activates guanylylcyclase, leading to the production of increased intracellular levels of cyclic GMP. The presence of the LT and/or ST leads to alterations in cellular signaling pathways that ultimately trigger increased chloride secretion and watery diarrhea [3,4]. The LT toxin is encoded by *elt*AB, whereas the ST toxin is encoded by 2 different genes, *est*A and *st*1, which produce STh (originally isolated from ETEC in humans) and STp (originally from a pig isolate) [3–5]. Many ETEC strains also produce surface colonization factors (CFs), which mediate adherence to the small intestinal wall. To date, over 25 human ETEC CFs have been described and divided into 3 different families: (1) CFA/I-like group, including CFA/1, CS1, CS2, CS4, CS14, and CS17; (2) CS5-like group, including CS5, CS7, CS18, and CS20; and (3) another unique group, including CS3, CS6, and CS10 to CS12 [2,6].

Targeting virulence factors such as toxins and CFs are the most effective approaches for ETEC vaccine development strategy [7,8]. Human ETEC strains that originate from the same ETEC lineage may have inherited many of the same epidemiological and phenotypic traits. Therefore, defining these lineages could provide an additional basis on which to understand ETEC epidemiology and for identifying new vaccine antigens. Although several methods are available for performing lineage definition studies, multilocus sequence typing (MLST) is now widely adopted. MLST is a sequence-based typing system based on determination of short nucleotide sequences (approximately 500 bp) of 7 housekeeping genes and has recently become the method of choice for bacterial typing [9].

To identify ETEC lineages in the present study, we performed MLST and phylogenetic analyses on a collection of human ETEC strains isolated from diarrheal patients in Korea and travelers in different developing countries. We have reported the distribution of the genes that encode enterotoxins and their associated CF types, as well as the antibiotic susceptibility profile of ETEC isolates obtained from patients with diarrhea between 2003 and 2011 in Korea.

Table 1. Primer pairs of multiplex PCR for the detection of CFs.

Multiplex PCR group	SFs	Primer name	Sequence (5′ to 3′)	Product size (bp)	References
Group 1	CFAI	CFAI-F	TGAGTGCTTCWGCAGTAGAGA	204	20
		CFAI-R	CAGCAAGTTTAACAATTACTTTTTTAGT		
	CS6	CS6-F	GGAGTGGTAAATGCAGGAAACT	416	20
		CS6-R	GTACCAGACGAATATCCGCTATTA		
	CS4	CS4-F	TGAGTGCTTCWGCAGTAGAGA	300	20
		CS4-R	AAGTCACATCTGCGGTTGATAGAG		
	CS14	CS14-F	TGAGTGCTTCWGCAGTAGAGA	357	20
		CS14-R	TACTATTCGAAACACCTGCCG		
Group 2	CS3	CS3-F	GGTCTTTCACTGTCAGCTATGAGTT	136	20
		CS3-R	TAATGTTAAATTATCCTGAGGAGCC		
	CS5	CS5-F	GCGTGACACGTCAGCTAATATAAAC	235	20
		CS5-R	GGCATTCATATCAATAGAAATATGAGAC		
	CS7	CS7-F	TGCTCCCGTTACTAAAAATACG	418	20
		CS7-R	GGCATTCATATCAATAGAAATATGAGAC		
	CS15	CS15-F	ATGCGTAGTAAATTATCCATTCTT	364	20
		CS15-R	CTACTATGGGCGTCGTCAT		
	CS18	CS18-F	TTTGCTGCACTGCCTGCGAA	502	20
		CS18-R	TAACAGTACCAGCTTTAACCTGAC		
	CS12	CS12-F	TTACGTCTCTGATCATGGCTGTTA	562	20
		CS12-R	ATAGTCATTACTGCATTTGCATCAAC		
Group 3	CS2	CS2-F	TCTGCTCGTATCAATACCCAAGTT	140	20
		CS2-R	GTGCCAGCGAATGAAACCTCTAAA		
	CS17/19	CS17/19-F	ACTCTRTCGCATTAACCTATTCT	169	20
		CS17/19-R	GTCACTTTCATCGGAATTTGCGAG		
	CS8	CS8-F	TATGAGCCTKCTGGAAGTYATCAT	526	20
		CS8-R	TATTGTAGTATTATCAGTAGCAGCCA		
	CS21	CS21-F	TATGAGCCTKCTGGAAGTYATCAT	292	20
		CS21-R	GTTATTACGCACTTCGTCTGGT		
	CS1/PCF071R	CS1/PCF071R-F	ACTCTRTCGCATTAACCTATTCT	334	20
		CS1/PCF071R-R	CCCTGATATTGACCAGCTGTTAGT		
	CS22	CS22-F	ATGCGTAGTAAATTATCCATTCTT	442	20
		CS22-R	CATTTTTTTGGAAGGCTTTAATA		
Group 4	CS13	CS13-F	TTGATGTGATGGTTATCGCTT	212	20
		CS13-R	AAAATCCAGGGTGGCGATCTG		
	CS20	CS20-F	ATGATTATGCCCTTTTAACTATGG	413	20
		CS20-R	CAAGTTTTTGATCGCTTCCAATA		

Materials and Methods

Identification of Bacterial Isolates as ETEC

A total of 291 human clinical isolates were collected between the years 2003 to 2011 through a routine surveillance system, which performed laboratory examination to isolate clinical specimens from stools of diarrheal patients in Korea and positively identified as ETEC. To avoid any bias in data analysis, information related to the patients was blinded during the analysis of the isolates. Among these 291 isolates, 258 strains were isolated from patients with diarrhea in widely separated geographic regions in Korea (domestic isolates) and 33 ETEC strains were isolated from travelers visiting other Asian countries (1 from Mongolia, 3 from Vietnam, 1 from Egypt, 1 from China, 2 from Indonesia, 5 from

India, 3 from Cambodia, 6 from Thailand, 1 from Turkey, 9 from Philippines, and 1 from Hong Kong) between 2010 and 2011 (inflow isolates). Individual colonies from positive ETEC samples were analyzed using separate polymerase chain reaction (PCR) assays for the LT and STh genes. Bacteria were directly inoculated into 3 mL of Luria-Bertani broth for enrichment and incubated overnight at 37°C under shaking conditions. After incubation, the enriched broth culture was centrifuged at 13,000 rpm (Sorvall, Biofuge Pico, Germany) for 1 min, and the pellet was heated at 100°C for 10 min. After centrifugation of the lysate, 5 mL of the supernatant was used for PCR. The primers used for detection of the LT genes were LT-F (GTACTTCGATAGAGGAACT-CAAATGAATAT) and LT-R (ATTCTGGGTCTCCTCATTA-CAAGTATC), and those used for detection of STh genes were

Table 2. Primer epairs used for MLST.

Locus	Primer name	Sequence (5' to 3')	Product size (bp)
aspC	aspC-F4	GTTTCGTGCCGATGAACGTC	594
	aspC-R7	AAACCCTGGTAAGCGAAGTC	
clpX	clpX-F6	CTGGCGGTCGCGGTATACAA	672
	clpX-R1	GACAACCGGCAGACGACCAA	
fadD	fadD-F6	GCTGCCGCTGTATCACATTT	580
	fadD-R3	GCGCAGGAATCCTTCTTCAT	
icdA	icd-F2	CTGCGCCAGGAACTGGATCT	669
	icd-R2	ACCGTGGGTGGCTTCAAACA	
lysP	lysP-F1	CTTACGCCGTGAATTAAAGG	628
	lysP-R8	GGTTCCCTGGAAAGAGAAGC	
mdh	mdh-F3	GTCGATCTGAGCCATATCCCTAC	650
	mdh-R4	TACTGACCGTCGCCTTCAAC	
uidA	uidA-277F	CATTACGGCAAAGTGTGGGTCAAT	658
	uidA-277R	CCATCAGCACGTTATCGAATCCTT	

STh-F (TTCGCTCAGGATGCTAAACCA) and STh-R (TTAA-TAGCACCCGGTACAAGCAGG).

Detection of CF Genes

To detect CF genes, multiplex PCR assays were performed using the primers shown in Table 1. PCR assays were carried out in a 50 mL volume with 2U DNA Taq polymerase (Takara Ex Taq, Japan) in a thermal cycler (PTC-100; MJ Research, Watertown, MA, USA) under the following conditions: initial denaturation at 94°C for 5 min; 30 cycles each of 94°C for 1 min, 55°C for 1 min, 72°C for 1 min; and final cycle at 72°C for 5 min. The amplified PCR products were analyzed by gel electrophoresis in 2% agarose gels stained with ethidium bromide, visualized with ultraviolet illumination, and imaged with the Gel Doc 2000 documentation system (Bio-Rad, Hercules, CA, USA).

Multilocus Sequence Typing (MLST) Analysis

ETEC isolates were analyzed by MLST. The 7-gene (st7) MLST system of the EcMLST (www.Shigatox.net/mlst) was used for MLST. The MLST is based on the sequencing of internal fragments of the 7 housekeeping genes (aspC, clpX, fadD, icdA, lysP, mdh, and uidA). PCR products of the genes were amplified for each isolate using the primers whose sequences have been shown in Table 2. All PCR reactions were performed in 50-µL volumes using 10–100 ng of boiled bacterial DNA as the template. PCR products were purified using the QIAquick PCR Purification Kit

(Qiagen, Hilden, Germany) and were sequenced in both directions using the same primer as that used for PCR. The MLST sequence type (ST) for each combination of alleles from sequences of 7 housekeeping genes was acquired on the EcMLST website and new allele numbers and STs were submitted to the EcMLST website.

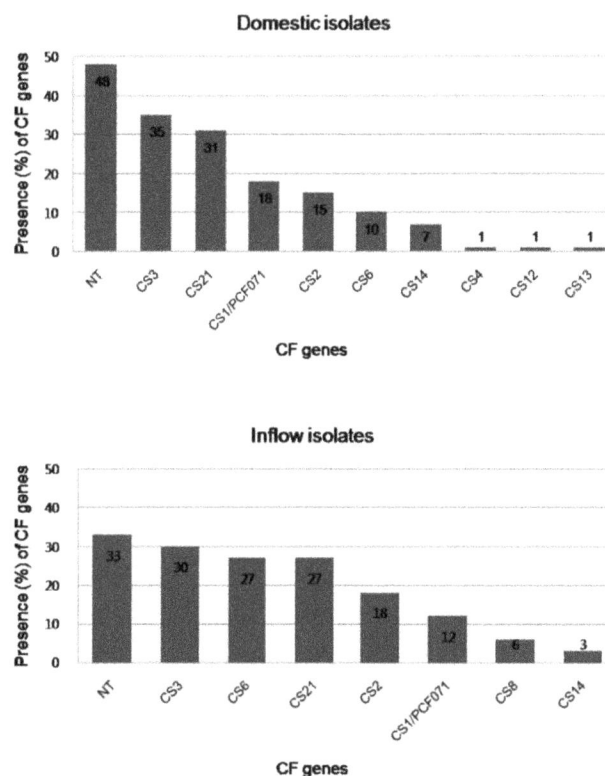

Figure 1. Profile of colonization factor (CF) genes in domestic and inflow isolates.

Table 3. Prevalence of enterotoxins of ETEC isolates.

Enterotoxin types	No. of Domestic isolates (n = 258)	No. of Inflow isolates (n = 33)	P value[a]
LT	42 (16.3%)	12 (36.4%)	0.008
STh	94 (36.4%)	11 (33.3%)	0.443
LT/STh	122 (47.3%)	10 (30.3)	0.047

[a]Data represent results of the Fisher exact test comparing toxin types in domestic isolates and inflow isolates.

Table 4. Prevalence of CFs and enterotoxins of ETEC isolates.

CF types	Domestic isolates				Inflow isolates			
	No. of CFs-type	No. of LT	No. of STh	No. of LT/STh	No. of CFs-type	No. of LT	No. of STh	No. of LT/STh
CS3-CS21-CS1/PCF071	38	0	2	36	4	0	0	4
CS2-CS3-CS21	31	0	0	31	1	0	0	1
CS6	22	11	7	4	6	6	0	0
CS14	15	2	9	4	0	0	0	0
CS2-CS3	5	1	0	4	5	0	1	4
CS3	6	0	0	6	0	0	0	0
CS3-CS21	6	0	0	6	0	0	0	0
CS21-CS1/PCF071	3	0	0	3	0	0	0	0
CS21	1	0	0	1	3	0	3	0
CS3-CS1/PCF071	3	0	0	3	0	0	0	0
CS6-CS8	0	0	0	0	2	1	0	1
CS3-CS4-CS1/PCF071	1	0	0	1	0	0	0	0
CS2	2	0	1	1	0	0	0	0
CS12	1	1	0	0	0	0	0	0
CS13	1	1	0	0	0	0	0	0
CS4-CS6	1	1	0	0	0	0	0	0
CS4-CS6-CS21	0	0	0	0	1	0	1	0
NT	122	25	75	22	11	5	6	10
Total	258	42	94	122	33	12	11	10

NT; non typable.

Domestic isolates

Inflow isolates

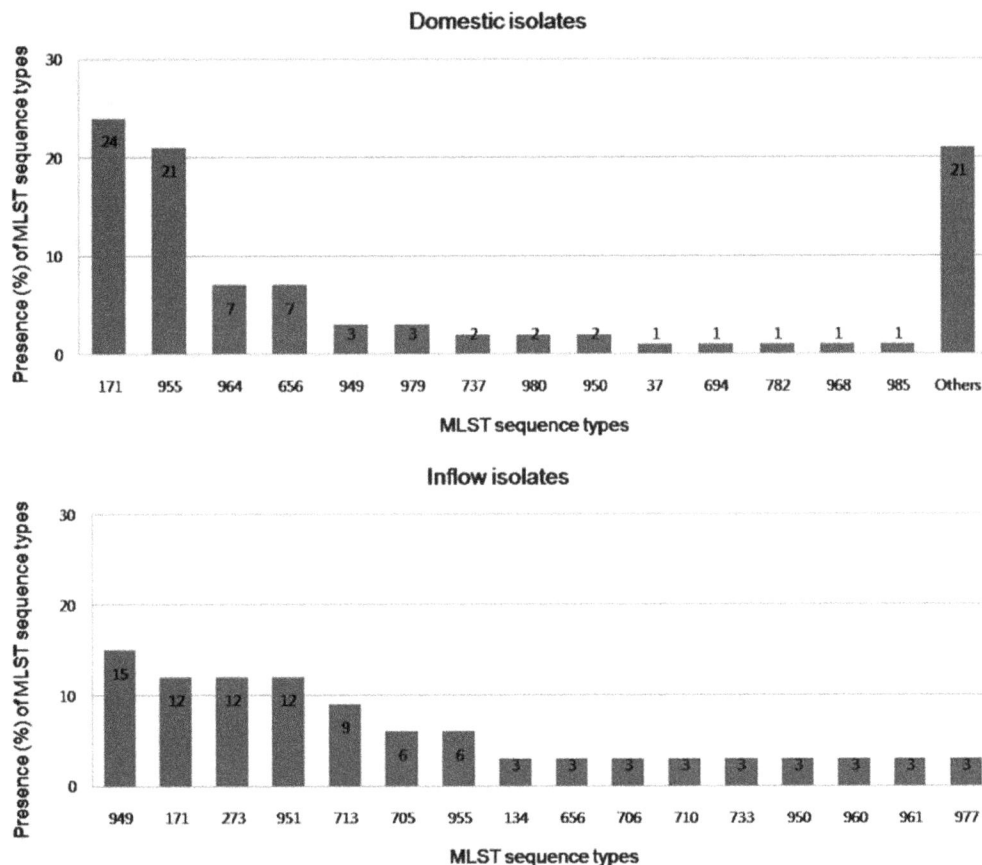

Figure 2. MLST sequence types in domestic and inflow isolates.

Phylogenetic Analysis

The MLST sequences were aligned using the ClustalW method, and the phylogenetic trees were generated using the maximum likelihood (ML) method implemented in the PAUP* (Phylogenetic Analysis Using Parsimony, 4.0 b10), RAxML Blackbox webserver. ML topologies were evaluated by bootstrap analysis of 100 ML iterations, implemented in the RAxML web server. Phylogenetic networks of MLST sequences were constructed by the median-joining algorithm using Network 4.6.

Antimicrobial Susceptibility

Antimicrobial susceptibility testing for *E. coli* isolates was determined with the VITEK 2 automated system using AST-N169 Card (bioMérieux, France) according to the guidelines of the Clinical and Laboratory Standards Institute (CLSI). The following antibiotics were tested: ampicillin, amoxicillin/clavalanic acid, ampicillin/sulbactam, cephalothin, cefotaxime, cefotetan, cefoxitin, cefazolin, ceftriaxone, imipenem, chloramphenicol, gentamicin, amikacin, nalidixic acid, ciprofloxacin, tetracycline, trimethoprim/sulfamethoxazole. *E. coli* ATCC 25922 was used for quality control.

Statistical Analysis

GraphPad Prism version 6 was used for statistical analysis. For comparisons of two variables, chi-square test or Fisher exact test was used. A P value <0.05 was considered statistically significant.

Results

Profile of Enterotoxin and CF Genes in Domestic and Inflow Isolates

The 291 human ETEC strains represented 3 different enterotoxin profiles: ETEC-LT strains, ETEC-STh strains and ETEC-LT/STh strains. The profile of enterotoxin genes of domestic isolates was somewhat different from that of inflow isolates. In the domestic isolates, ETEC-LT/STh strains constituted 47.3% of the isolates, while ETEC-LT and ETEC STh accounted for only 16.3% and 36.4%. As shown in Table 3, a greater number of STh-possessing ETEC (ETEC-STh and ETEC-LT/STh) strains were detected than LT-possessing ETEC (ETEC-LT and ETEC-LT/STh) strains (83.7% vs. 63.6%) in the domestic ETEC cases. The detection rates of the 3 enterotoxin types were similar in the inflow isolates: ETEC-LT (36.4%, 12 of 33 strains), ETEC-STh (33.3%, 11 of 33 strains), and ETEC-LT/STh (30.3%, 10 of 33 strains). The frequency of ETEC-LT/STh strains was significantly higher in the domestic isolates than in the inflow isolates (P value <0.05).

The CF gene profile of the domestic isolates was similar to that of inflow isolates. As shown in Figure 1, CS3 was predominantly isolated in both domestic and inflow human ETEC isolates (35% and 30%, respectively). In the domestic isolates, CS21, CS1/PCF071, CS2, CS6, and CS14 were frequently detected. In the inflow isolates, CS6, CS21, CS2, CS1/PCF071 and CS8 were frequently present. The proportion of CF-non typable strains was also high in both isolate groups (Figure 1 and Table S1, Table S2).

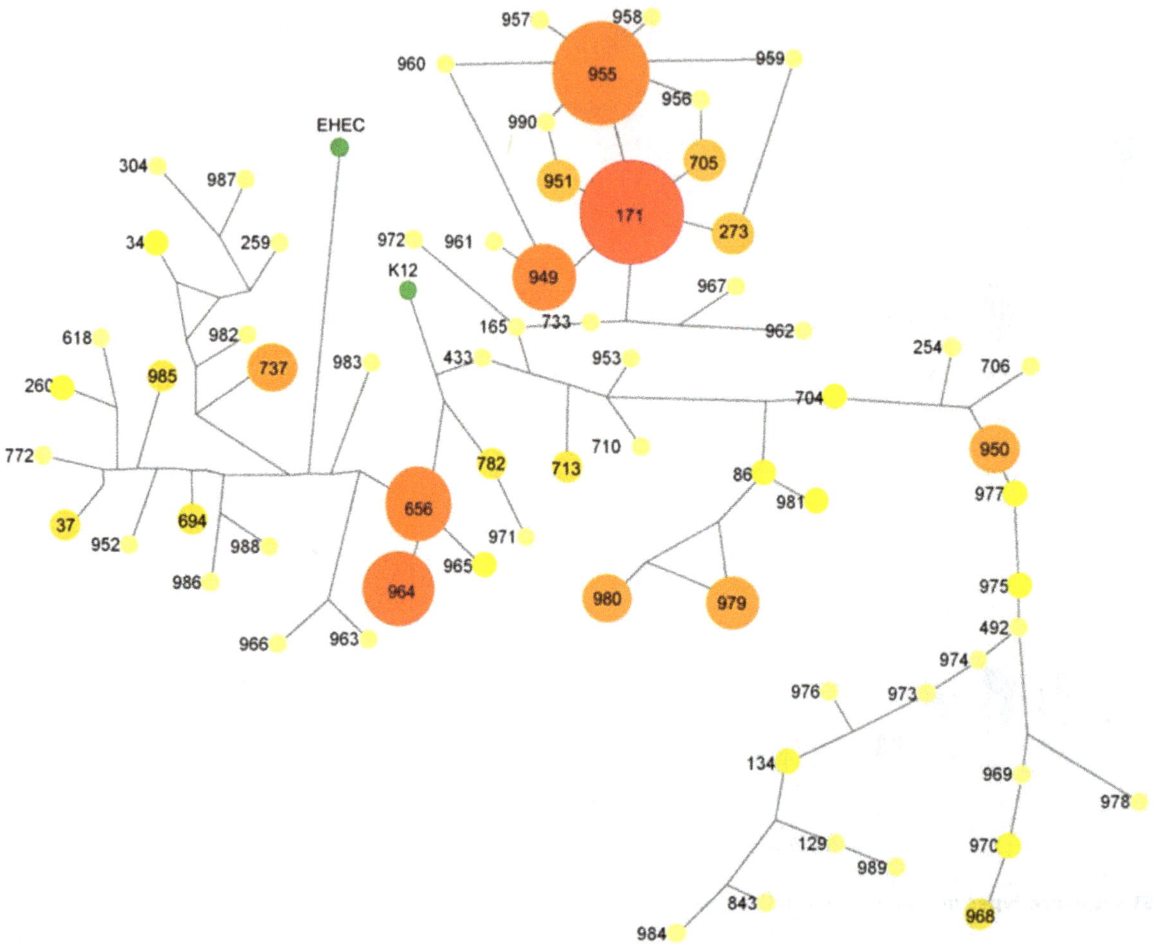

Figure 3. Phylogenetic networks of the isolates according to MLST STs. The sizes of the circles are proportional to the number of MLST STs. The major MLST STs such as ST171 and ST955 were 23% (66/291) and 19% (55/291).

Ten non-typable strains were directly examined by electron microscopy. Seven (70%) among the ten strains possessed fimbriae (data not shown). This result indicates that the seven strains express CFs, but the genes encoding the CFs do not react with the PCR primers used in this study. Moreover, one hundred strains of all were re-confirmed CFs using mono-PCR with primers described in Rodas et al., 2009 (data not shown).

The prevalent types of CF genes in the domestic isolates were CS3-CS21-CS1/PCF071, CS2-CS3-CS21, CS6, and CS14 and the major CF types of the inflow isolates were CS3-CS21-CS1/ PCF071, CS6, and CS2-CS3. Interestingly, most strains of the CS3-CS21-CS1/PCF071 and CS2-CS3-CS21 types were detected in ETEC-LT/STh strains. The CS6 type was found more often in LT-possessing ETEC strains, while the CS14 type was more frequent in STh-possessing ETEC strains (Table 4).

MLST Analyses of the Isolates

MLST of the 258 domestic human ETEC isolates represented 65 different MLST STs: 21 sequence types were known STs, and 44 new STs were recovered (Table S3). ST171 were the most common, with a frequency of 24% (62/258) and were constantly represented in each year between 2003 and 2011. The other predominant STs were ST955 (21%, 53/258) and ST964, ST656 (7%, 18/258) (Figure 2 and Table S1). Analysis of the 33 inflow isolates identified 16 different STs, which contained 7 new STs

(43.8%, Table S3). The most frequent ST type was ST949, that is, 15% (5/33), and this was followed by ST171, ST273, ST951 (12%, 4/33), ST713 (9%, 3/33) and ST705, ST955 (6%, 2/33) (Figure 2 and Table S2). Interestingly, 8 STs (ST273, ST706, ST710, ST713, ST733, ST951, ST960, and ST961) were found only in inflow ETEC isolates, and not in domestic isolates. ST171 strains represented various CF types, including 2 major CF types (CS3-CS21-CS1/PCF071 and CS2-CS3-CS21) and other CF types (CS6, CS3, CS21-CS1/PCF071, CS2-CS3, CS3-CS1/ PCF071, CS14, and CS12). ST955 strains also showed various CF types: CS3-CS21-CS1/PCF071, CS2-CS3-CS21, CS3-CS21, CS3-CS1/PCF071, CS2-CS3, CS6, and CS12. As shown in Table 5, 2 major CF types, CS3-CS21-CS1/PCF071 and CS2-CS3-CS21, were usually found in the 2 major domestic MLST STs, ST171 and ST955; 89% (34/38) of strains possessing the CS3-CS21-CS1/PCF071 type and 93% (29/31) of strains possessing the CS2-CS3-CS21 type were found in the 2 major MLST STs. However, there were more NT (not typeable) CF types in the strains of other MLST STs.

The phylogenetic trees of the STs analyzed above were generated and compared with those of 3 other reference strains (*E. coli* K12, EHEC EDL933, and ETEC H10407). Phylogenetic analysis showed that 7 STs (ST971, ST782, ST965, ST656, ST964, ST966, and ST963) were closely related to those of *E. coli* K12. EHEC EDL933 also has a close phylogenetic relationship

Table 5. Prevalence of MLST sequence types and CF types of domestic and inflow isolates.

Isolate groups	Major MLST sequence types (n)	No. of major – and oter CF types						
		CS3-CS21-CS1/PCF071	CS2-CS3-CS21	CS6	CS14	CS2-CS3	Etc.	NT
Domestic isolates	ST171 (62)	15	13	3	0	2	8	21
	ST955 (53)	19	16	1	0	2	7	8
	ST964 (18)	0	1	0	0	0	0	17
	ST656 (18)	0	0	1	0	0	0	17
	ST949 (8)	2	0	2	0	0	0	4
Inflow isolates	ST949 (5)	0	0	1	0	0	1	3
	ST171 (4)	0	1	0	0	0	0	3
	ST273 (4)	4	0	0	0	0	0	0
	ST951 (4)	0	0	0	0	4	0	0

etc.: Includes types present at lower incidence than the major types, NT; non typable.

with some STs such as ST988, ST737, ST985, ST986, ST982, and ST259. ETEC H10407 represented the ST171 type as similar as other many ETEC strains (Figure 3).

Antibiotic Resistance Analyses of the Isolates

Antibiotic resistance rates of domestic and inflow isolates are shown in Table 6. The isolates of both groups showed a higher resistance to ampicillin (30% and 49%, respectively), nalidixic acid (38% and 36%, respectively), and trimethoprim-sulfamethoxazole (26% and 27%, respectively) when compared with other antibiotics. Resistance to imipenem and amikacin was not found in any ETEC strains. The inflow isolates conferred a stronger resistance to antibiotics of the cephem class. However, no significant association was found between the ETEC genotype and antimicrobial susceptibility.

Discussion

ETEC is an important pathogen responsible for traveler's diarrhea and causes about 700,000 childhood deaths per year, mostly in young children [10]. A variety of strategies have been pursued in attempts to develop a vaccine against ETEC. The most promising vaccine candidate to date is a killed whole-cell vaccine comprising different ETEC strains that express the most prevalent enterotoxins and CFs [11,12].

The relative proportions of enterotoxin- and CF-possessing isolates seem to vary from 1 geographical area to another in both diarrhea and control patients with ETEC infection [2]. Our results also showed that the proportions of enterotoxins were different between the domestic and inflow isolates. The proportion of enterotoxin types of the domestic isolates identified here is similar to those for other studies conducted in Bangladesh [13] and Egypt [14], while other studies in Argentina [15], India [16], and Peru [17] reported that LT-producing ETEC were predominant. Clemens et al. [19] reported that ETEC strains that only express the LT are considered less important as pathogens. The identification of CFs is more important for epidemiological studies and for the development of CF-based vaccines against ETEC because ETEC organisms carrying more than 1 CF gene are common [20,21]. In this study, CS3 and CS21 were the most prevalent CFs detected in both domestic and inflow strains. In other studies, CFA/I was the most prevalent CF type [2,14,18], while strains possessing CFA/1 were rarely detected in this study. Interestingly, CS6 was found more in inflow strains (17%) than domestic strains (6%). Thus, variations in the prevalence of CF antigens may be related to location. Of strong interest, 2 major prevalent CF gene types were found in ETEC strains isolated in Korea. Moreover, we observed a strong correlation between some CF genes and enterotoxin types. In brief, we have demonstrated that STh and CS3/CS21 genes are the most prevalent enterotoxin and CF genes in the domestic ETEC isolates in Korea.

Resistance to common antibiotics such as ampicillin, tetracycline and trimethoprim-sulfamethoxazole was frequently detected in ETEC strains, consistent with reports from other authors [22–27]. High-level resistance to antibiotics has developed in part because of heavy clinical use of antibiotics, since these drugs are associated with excellent safety and have a low cost. Therefore, empirical use of these antibiotics should be limited. Moreover, among the cephems, high resistance to cephalothin underscores the importance of ongoing surveillance. However, we did not find any association between the genotypes and antibiotic susceptibility profiles of ETEC strains.

MLST is a very useful tool for determination of bacterial lineages [28–30]. Therefore, we used MLST to characterize

Table 6. Comparison of antibiotic resistance of domestic and inflow isolates.

Antibicrobial agents	Antibiotic resistances (%) of isolates	
	Domestic isolates	Inflow isolates
β-lactams		
Ampicillin (AM)	30	49
β-lactam/β-lactamase inhibitor combinations		
Ampicillin-sulbactam (SAM)	11	28
Amoxicillin/Clavulanic Acid (AMC)	3	3
Cephems		
Cephalothin (CF)	12	27
Cefazolin (CZ)	10	21
Ceftriaxone (CRO)	3	12
Cefotaxime (CTX)	3	12
Cefoxitin (FOX)	2	0
Carbapenems		
Imipenem (IPM)	0	0
Quinolones		
Nalidixic Acid (NA)	38	36
Ciprofloxacin (CIP)	2	0
Aminoglycosides		
Amikacin (AN)	0	0
Gentamicin (GM)	5	0
Tetracyclines		
Tetracycline (TE)	29	18
Phenicols		
Chloramphenicol (C)	3	0
Folate pathway inhibitors		
Trimethoprim-sulfamethoxazole (SXT)	26	27

ETEC lineages in association with the distribution of enterotoxin and CF genes. In general, we observed that different MLST STs were associated with different CFs. These genes appeared to be spread across several different lineages. Such genes have been reported to spread through horizontal transfer by transposable elements [31,32]. However, a strong association was found between the major CF types and MLST types. Two major CF types were usually found in 2 major MLST STs, that is, ST171 and ST955, in the domestic isolates.

Currently, there is no licensed vaccine for use against ETEC diarrhea. To our knowledge, this study is the first to report the distribution of enterotoxin and CF genes in ETEC strains from Korea. We have also provided information regarding ETEC lineages, obtained using MLST, and the antimicrobial susceptibility profile of the isolates. Our data on the frequency and geographic association of the various antigenic virulence factors will provide useful information for strategies to develop novel and effective anti-ETEC vaccines.

Supporting Information

Table S1 Profile of enterotoxin- and CF genes, MLST sequence types and antobiotic resistance of domestic ETEC isolates.

Table S2 Profile of enterotoxin- and CF genes, MLST sequence types and antobiotic resistance of inflow ETEC isolates.

Table S3 New MLST sequence types of domestic and inflow ETEC isolates.

Author Contributions

Conceived and designed the experiments: SHC DWK. Performed the experiments: KHO SMJ. Analyzed the data: SHC DWK. Contributed reagents/materials/analysis tools: SHC KHO. Wrote the paper: SHC DWK.

References

1. Wenneras C, Erling V (2004) Prevalence of enterotoxigenic *Escherichia coli*-associated diarrhoea and carrier state in the developing world. J Health Popul Nutr 22: 370–382.

2. Qadri F, Svennerholm AM, Faruque AS, Sack RB (2005) Enterotoxigenic *Escherichia coli* in developing countries: epidemiology, microbiology, clinical features, treatment, and prevention. Clin Microbiol Rev 18: 465–483.

3. Nataro JP, Kaper JB (1998) Diarrheagenic *Escherichia coli*. Clin Microbiol Rev 11: 142–201.

4. Kaper JB, Nataro JP, Mobley HL (2004) Pathogenic *Escherichia coli*. Nat Rev Microbiol 2: 123–140.

5. Lasaro MA, Rodrigues JF, Mathias-Santos C, Guth BE, Balan A, et al. (2008) Genetic diversity of heat-labile toxin expressed by enterotoxigenic *Escherichia coli* strains isolated from humans. J Bacteriol 190: 2400–2410.

6. Gaastra W, Svennerholm AM (1996) Colonization factors of human enterotoxigenic *Escherichia coli* (ETEC). Trends Microbiol 4: 444–452.

7. Levine MM (2006) Enteric infections and the vaccines to counter them; future directions. Vaccine 24: 3865–3873.

8. Walker RI, Steele D, Aguado T, Ad Hoc ETEC Technical Expert Committee (2007) Analysis of strategies to successfully vaccinate infants in developing countries against enterotoxigenic *E. coli* (ETEC) disease. Vaccine 25: 2545–2566.

9. Maiden MC, Bygraves JA, Feil E, Morelli G, Russell JE, et al. (1998) Multilocus sequence typing: a portable approach to the identification of clones within populations of pathogenic microorganisms. Proc Natl Acad Sci U S A 95: 3140–3145.

10. WHO (2006) Future directions for research on enterotoxigenic *Escherichia coli* vaccines for developing countries. Wkly Epidemiol Rec 81: 97.

11. Sizemore DR, Roland KL, Ryan US (2004) Enterotoxigenic *Escherichia coli* virulence factors and vaccine approaches. Expert Rev Vaccines 3: 585–595.

12. Svennerholm AM, Tobias J (2008) Vaccines against enterotoxigenic *Escherichia coli*. Expert Rev Vaccines 4: 795–804.

13. Qadri F, Saha A, Ahmed A, Al Tarique A, Begum YA, et al. (2007) Disease burden due to enterotoxigenic *Escherichia coli* in the first 2 years of life in an urban community in Bangladesh. Infect Immun 75: 3961–3968.

14. Shaheen HI, Abdel Messih IA, Klena JD, Mansour A, El-Wakkeel Z, et al. (2009) Phenotypic and genotypic analysis of enterotoxigenic *Escherichia coli* in samples obtained from Egyptian children presenting to referral hospitals. J Clin Microbiol 47: 189–197.

15. Viboud GI, Jouve MJ, Binsztein N, Vergara M, Rivas M, et al. (1999) Prospective cohort study of enterotoxigenic *Escherichia coli* infections in Argentinean children. J Clin Microbiol 37: 2829–2833.

16. Sommerfelt H, Steinsland H, Grewal HM, Viboud GI, Bhandari N, et al. (1996) Colonization factors of enterotoxigenic *Escherichia coli* isolated from children in north India. J Infect Dis 174: 768–776.

17. Rivera FP, Ochoa TJ, Maves RC, Bernal M, Medina AM, et al. (2010) Genotypic and Phenotypic Characterization of Enterotoxigenic *Escherichia coli* Strains Isolated from Peruvian Children. J Clin Microbiol 48: 3198–3203.

18. Nirdnoy W, Serichantalergs O, Cravioto A, LeBron C, Wolf M, et al. (1997) Distribution of colonization factor antigens among enterotoxigenic *Escherichia coli* strains isolated from patients with diarrhea in Nepal, Indonesia, Peru, and Thailand. J Clin Microbiol 35: 527–530.

19. Clemens J, Savarino S, Abu-Elyazeed R, Safwat M, Rao M, et al. (2004) Development of pathogenicity-driven definitions of outcomes for a field trial of a killed oral vaccine against enterotoxigenic *Escherichia coli* in Egypt: application of an evidence-based method. J Infect Dis 189: 2299–2307.

20. Nada RA, Shaheen HI, Touni I, Fahmy D, Armstrong AW, et al. (2010) Design and validation of a multiplex polymerase chain reaction for the identification of enterotoxigenic *Escherichia coli* and associated colonization factor antigens. Diagn Microbiol Infect Dis 67: 134–142.

21. Valvatne H, Steinsland H, Sommerfelt H (2002) Clonal clustering and colonization factors among thermolabile and porcine thermostable enterotoxin-producing *Escherichia coli*. APMIS 110: 665–672.

22. Binsztein N, Picandet AM, Notario R, Patrito E, De Lesa ME, et al. (1999) Antimicrobial resistance among species of *Salmonella*, *Shigella*, *Escherichia*, and *Aeromonas* isolated from children with diarrhea in 7 Argentinian centers. Rev Latinoam Microbiol 41: 121–126.

23. Estrada-García T, Cerna JF, Paheco-Gil L, Velázquez RF, Ochoa TJ, et al. (2005) Drug-resistant diarrheogenic *Escherichia coli*, Mexico. Emerg Infect Dis 11: 1306–1308.

24. Shaheen HI, Khalil SB, Rao MR, Abu Elyazeed R, Wierzba TF, et al. (2004) Phenotypic profiles of enterotoxigenic *Escherichia coli* associated with early childhood diarrhea in rural Egypt. J Clin Microbiol 42: 5588–5595.

25. Al-Gallas N, Abbassi SM, Hassan AB, Aissa RB (2007) Genotypic and phenotypic profiles of enterotoxigenic Escherichia coli associated with acute diarrhea in Tunis, Tunisia. Curr Microbiol 55: 47–55.

26. Cohen D, Tobias J, Spungin-Bialik A, Sela T, Kayouf R, et al. (2010) Phenotypic characteristics of enterotoxigenic *Escherichia coli* associated with acute diarrhea among Israeli young adults. Foodborne Pathog Dis 7: 1159–1164.

27. Ochoa TJ, Ecker L, Barletta F, Mispireta ML, Gil AI, et al. (2009) Age-related susceptibility to infection with diarrheagenic *Escherichia coli* among infants from periurban areas in Lima, Peru. Clin Infect Dis 49: 1694–1702.

28. Maiden MC, Bygraves JA, Feil E, Morelli G, Russell JE, et al. (1998) Multilocus sequence typing: a portable approach to the identification of clones within populations of pathogenic microorganisms. Proc Natl Acad Sci U S A 95: 3140–3145.

29. Nicklasson M, Klena J, Rodas C, Bourgeois AL, Torres O, et al. (2010) Enterotoxigenic *Escherichia coli* multilocus sequence types in Guatemala and Mexico. Emerg Infect Dis 16: 143–146.

30. Turner SM, Chaudhuri RR, Jiang ZD, DuPont H, Gyles C, et al. (2006) Phylogenetic comparisons reveal multiple acquisitions of the toxin genes by enterotoxigenic *Escherichia coli* strains of different evolutionary lineages. J Clin Microbiol 44: 4528–4536.

31. Gaastra W, Svennerholm AM (1996) Colonization factors of human enterotoxigenic *Escherichia coli* (ETEC). Trends Microbiol 4: 444–452.

32. Froehlich B, Parkhill J, Sanders M, Quail MA, Scott JR (2005) The pCoo plasmid of enterotoxigenic *Escherichia coli* is a mosaic cointegrate. J Bacteriol 187: 6509–6516.

2

MALDI-TOF Identification of the Human Gut Microbiome in People with and without Diarrhea in Senegal

Bissoume Samb-Ba[1,2], Catherine Mazenot[1], Amy Gassama-Sow[2], Grégory Dubourg[1], Hervé Richet[1], Perrine Hugon[1], Jean-Christophe Lagier[1], Didier Raoult[1], Florence Fenollar[1]*

1 Unité de Recherche sur les Maladies Infectieuses et Tropicales Emergentes (URMITE) UM63, CNRS 7278, IRD 198, INSERM 1095, Aix-Marseille Université, Marseille, France and Dakar, Senegal, 2 Unité de Bactériologie Expérimentale, Institut Pasteur de Dakar, Dakar, Senegal

Abstract

Background: In Africa, there are several problems with the specific identification of bacteria. Recently, MALDI-TOF mass spectrometry has become a powerful tool for the routine microbial identification in many clinical laboratories.

Methodology/Principal Findings: This study was conducted using feces from 347 individuals (162 with diarrhea and 185 without diarrhea) sampled in health centers in Dakar, Senegal. Feces were transported from Dakar to Marseille, France, where they were cultured using different culture conditions. The isolated colonies were identified using MALDI-TOF. If a colony was unidentified, 16S rRNA sequencing was performed. Overall, 2,753 isolates were tested, allowing for the identification of 189 bacteria from 5 phyla, including 2 previously unknown species, 11 species not previously reported in the human gut, 10 species not previously reported in humans, and 3 fungi. 2,718 bacterial isolates (98.8%) out of 2,750 yielded an accurate identification using mass spectrometry, as did the 3 *Candida albicans* isolates. Thirty-two bacterial isolates not identified by MALDI-TOF (1.2%) were identified by sequencing, allowing for the identification of 2 new species. The number of bacterial species per fecal sample was significantly higher among patients without diarrhea (8.6±3) than in those with diarrhea (7.3±3.4; $P = 0.0003$). A modification of the gut microbiota was observed between the two groups. In individuals with diarrhea, major commensal bacterial species such as *E. coli* were significantly decreased (85% versus 64%), as were several *Enterococcus* spp. (*E. faecium* and *E. casseliflavus*) and anaerobes, such as *Bacteroides* spp. (*B. uniformis* and *B. vulgatus*) and *Clostridium* spp. (*C. bifermentans, C. orbiscindens, C. perfringens,* and *C. symbosium*). Conversely, several *Bacillus* spp. (*B. licheniformis, B. mojavensis,* and *B. pumilus*) were significantly more frequent among patients with diarrhea.

Conclusions/Significance: MALDI-TOF is a potentially powerful tool for routine bacterial identification in Africa, allowing for a quick identification of bacterial species.

Editor: Dipshikha Chakravortty, Indian Institute of Science, India

Funding: This work was supported by the Institut Hospitalo-Universitaire Méditerranée-Infection. The funders had no role in study design, data collection and analysis, decision to publish, or preparation of the manuscript.

Competing Interests: The authors have declared that no competing interests exist.

* E-mail: florence.fenollar@univ-amu.fr

Introduction

There are several problems in the specific identification of bacterial infections in Africa. Currently, bacterial identification is based on phenotypic tests, including Gram staining, bacterial culture, culture growth characteristics, and biochemical profiles. Even if culture processes are available in major hospitals in Africa, there are limitations to the performance of biochemical identification methods. Such traditional methods require the possession of many API strips including API-20E, API-20NE, API Staph kits, and API Anaerobe kits and many unique reagents that should be stocked under specific conditions and have expiration dates. Biochemical methods are time consuming. They often required knowledge about the type of microorganism being tested, and fail to accurately identify several bacteria species [1,2].

Five years ago, a revolution occurred in bacteriology with the advent of the routine identification of bacteria by matrix-assisted laser desorption ionization time-of-flight mass spectrometry (MALDI-TOF) [1,3–5]. Currently, this technique allows accurate identification of bacteria without a priori knowledge of the type of microorganism. This technique is in widespread use in many clinical laboratories in Europe [1,3,4,6,7]. This method allows for the detection of bacteria in less than 1 hour and is cost effective. Thus, this technique has become a powerful tool for routine identification and could replace Gram staining and biochemical identification, but to this point, many studies using this technique have been mainly performed in Europe [2].

The bacterial repertoire is different depending on the environment from which the microorganisms are obtained [8,9]. For example, differences at the species level have been observed among the microbes in the human between Asian versus American people and European versus African people [10,11]. Another recently developed high-throughput method involves the combination of culturomics using a large panel of media incubated at several atmospheric conditions and MALDI-TOF mass spectrometry for the quick and accurate identification of a large number of colonies [12–14].

In this study, we evaluated the effectiveness of MALDI-TOF mass spectrometry on the identification of bacterial species isolated from feces from Senegalese patients with and without diarrhea by combining several culture conditions and rapid mass spectrometry identification.

Materials and Methods

Ethics Statement

All aspects of this study were approved by the National Ethical Committee (CNERS) of Senegal (SEN25/07). Written consent was obtained for all participants. For children, their parents or guardians provided also a written informed consent.

Patient Recruitment and Sample Management

This study was based on 347 individuals, adults and children, sampled from March 2009 to January 2010: 162 individuals with diarrhea and 185 without diarrhea (Table 1). Five health centers in Dakar, Senegal and its suburbs (Dominique-Pikine, Sicap Mbao, Roi Baudoin, Institut d'Hygiène Sociale, and Saint Martin) were included. Stool samples were collected from children and adults who attended these health centers. Control patients were hospitalized patients or outpatients without intestinal pathogens or recent treatment with antibiotics.

Stool specimens were collected in special sterile stool containers or with swabs for stool samples collected from infants. All stool samples were labeled and transported in cool boxes for examination within 24 hours of collection to Institut Pasteur de Dakar (Senegal). At the laboratory, macroscopic and microscopic analyses were performed on fresh stool samples to look for enteric pathogens including eggs, cysts, and trophozoites of intestinal parasites as well as enteric viruses. Stool samples were preserved in two Nunc tubes (Fisher Thermo Scientific, Denmark) and stored at $-20°C$. They were transported from Dakar to Marseille, France in ice packs.

Culturomics Methods

To enumerate the number of colony forming units (CFU) in the stool samples, 1 g of pasty stool was diluted in 9 ml of phosphate buffered saline (PBS), and 100 μl of watery stool was diluted in 900 μl of PBS. The diluted samples were introduced with a syringe for preincubation into aerobic and anaerobic blood culture bottles (BD Bactec Plus Lytic/10 Anaerobic, Aerobic, 39 Heidelberg, Germany) for 24 hours before being inoculated on agar plates as it has been previously reported that this strategy allowed the growth of bacterial species, mainly anaerobic, that were not detected by standard axenic culture, species [12,15]. Plates for anaerobic culture were pre-incubated for 24 h anaerobically. To identify the maximum number of bacterial species, stool samples were diluted from 10^{-1} to 10^{-10} and inoculated on agar plates using nine

different culture conditions that had been previously determined to be the most useful (Table 2) [12]. The microaerophilic and anaerobic incubations were carried out using microaerophilic bags (Oxoid, Basingstoke, England), anaerobic jars (Mitsubishi) and atmosphere generators (BD Diagnostics, Heidelberg, Germany). Each agar plate was carefully observed after 2 and 7 days of incubation. Any isolated colony was applied to mass spectrometry for identification.

Identification Using Mass Spectrometry

The isolated colonies were deposited on a MALDI-TOF target microflex (Bruker Daltonik, Wissembourg, France) and overlaid with matrix solution, a saturated solution of α- cyano-4-hydroxycinnamic acid in 50% acetonitrile and 2.5% trifluoroacetic acid, after air-drying at room temperature for 5 minutes. Each colony was picked from an Eppendorf tube containing the Trypticase-Casein-Soy (AES) culture medium stored at 37°C. Broth culture-specific thioglycollate (BD Diagnostics) was used for anaerobes. Two spots were examined for each colony. Each deposit was covered with 2 μl of the matrix solution. The Biotyper software was used to compare the protein profile of the bacteria obtained from a database (Bruker and the base of the Timone hospital) of protein profiles regularly updated based on the results of clinical diagnosis. This software takes into account a maximum of 100 mass peaks between 3,000 and 15,000 Da. A score >1.9 indicates a high-level identification of genus and species. A score > 1.7 indicates the identification of genus but not species, and a score lower than 1.7 indicates no identification of bacteria. If the species was still not accurately identified by MALDI-TOF after two attempts, the isolate was analyzed by 16S rRNA sequencing.

16S rRNA Amplification and Sequencing Identification

Bacterial DNA was extracted using the MagNA Pure LC kit DNA isolation kit III (Roche, France) with the MagNA Pure LC instrument, according to the manufacturer's instructions. The 16S rRNA gene was amplified by PCR using the universal primer pair *fd1* and *rp2* and an annealing temperature of 52°C, as described elsewhere [16]. PCR products were purified using the PCR kit Nucleofast 96 (Macherey-Nagel, Hoerdt, France). Sequencing reactions were performed with the sequencing kit Big Dye Terminator version 1.1 (Perkin-Elmer, Coignieres, France) with primers *536F, 536R, 800F, 800R, 1050F,* and *1050R* (Table 3). Products of the sequencing reactions were purified and the sequences analyzed on an ABI PRISM 3130X Genetic Analyzer (Applied Biosystems, California, USA). The obtained sequences were compared with the GenBank database using BLAST software. A threshold value of similarity ≥98.7% was used for identification at the species level. Below this value, sequences were repeated to confirm the first obtained results. A new species was

Table 1. Population description.

| Age (years) | Patients | | Controls | |
	Number	%	Number	%
[0–5]	71	43.8	9	4.9
[5–20]	35	21.6	46	24.9
[20	56	34.6	130	70.2
Total	**162**	**100.00**	**185**	**100.00**

Table 2. Culture media and conditionings used in this study.

Media	Culture conditions	Suppliers
Direct inoculation		
5% sheep blood agar	Aerobe, 37°C, 48 hours	Biomérieux, Marcy l'Etoile, France
5% sheep blood agar	Anaerobe, 37°C, 48 hours	Biomérieux
MacConkey	Aerobe, 37°C, 48 hours	Biomérieux
BCYE	Aerobe with 2.5% CO_2, 37°C, 5 days	Biomérieux
BCP	Aerobe, 37°C, 48 hours	Biomérieux
LAMVAB	Anaerobe, 37°C	Home-made*
Inoculation in a blood culture bottle for 24 h, followed by inoculation in		
Columbia	Aerobe, 37°C, 3 days	Biomérieux
MacConkey	Aerobe, 37°C, 1 day	Biomérieux
Columbia	Anaerobe, 37°C, 3 days	Biomérieux

BCYE: Buffered Charcoal Yeast Extract; BCP: Bromocresol Purple; LAMVAB: Lactobacillus Anaerobic MRS with Vancomycin and Bromocresol green. *from Hartemink *et al.* [15].

suspected when the similarity in the GenBank database with described bacteria was <98.7% [17,18].

Statistical Analyses

Statistical analyses were performed using EpiInfo6 software (http://www.cdc.gov/epiinfo/Epi6/EI6dnjp.htm). The results were concluded to be statistically significant when $P<0.05$. The corrected chi-squared test or Fisher's exact test was used where indicated.

Results

Culture

Overall, 2,753 isolates were tested, which allowed us to identify 189 bacterial species from 5 phyla, including an unknown species and 3 fungi (Table 4 and Figure 1) [19]. Two stool specimens from patients with diarrhea did not allow for the recovery of any bacteria. *Candida albicans* was detected from 3 patients with diarrhea (3/162 versus 0/185, $P=0.1$). A total of 1,175 bacterial isolates were detected among patients with diarrhea and 1,575 were detected among patients without diarrhea. The number of different bacterial species per stool sample was significantly higher among patients without diarrhea (mean of 8.6±3, range 1 to 18) than among those with diarrhea (mean of 7.3±3.4, range 0 to 22; $P=0.0003$). Finally, 59 out of the 153 bacterial species (38.6%)

identified among patients with diarrhea were specific for this group whereas 36 out of the 129 bacterial species (27.9%) identified among patients without diarrhea were specific for this group, although this difference is not significant ($P=0.059$).

MALDI-TOF Mass Spectrometry Identification

Of the 2,750 bacterial isolates analyzed, 2,718 (98.8%) yielded an accurate identification using MALDI-TOF mass spectrometry (Table 4).

16S rRNA Amplification and Sequencing Identification

Thirty-two isolates out of the 2,750 (1.2%) were not identified by MALDI-TOF mass spectrometry. Among these isolates, 11 were identified using 16S rRNA sequencing: *Bacteroides nordii*, *Bacillus clausii*, *Bacillus thuringiensis*, *Clostridium cadaveris*, *Clostridium neonatale*, *Paenibacillus polymyxa*, *Staphylococcus sciuri*, *Shigella boydii*, *Shigella sonnei*, and two new species were identified: a new clostridial species that was called *Clostridium dakarense* sp. nov. (GenBank accession number KC517358) and a new *Bacillus* species, *Bacillus casamencensis* sp. nov. (GenBank accession number AF519462.1). The 16S rRNA sequence of this *Bacillus* species has been already detected in rice soils in Senegal but no description of the bacterium has been yet reported. The full genome of *C. dakarense* has been recently sequenced and reported [20].

Table 3. Primers used for 16S rRNA PCR and sequencing.

Primers	Sequences (5′–3′)	Annealing temperature
FD1	AGAGTTTGATCCTGGCTCAG	52°C
RP2	ACGGCTACCTTGTTACGACTT	52°C
536F	CAGCAGCCGCGGTAATAC	50°C
536R	GTATTACCGCGGCTGCTG	50°C
800F	ATTAGATACCCTGGTAG	50°C
800R	CTACCAGGGTATCTAAT	50°C
1050F	TGTCGTCAGCTCGTG	50°C
1050R	CACGAGCTGACGACA	50°C

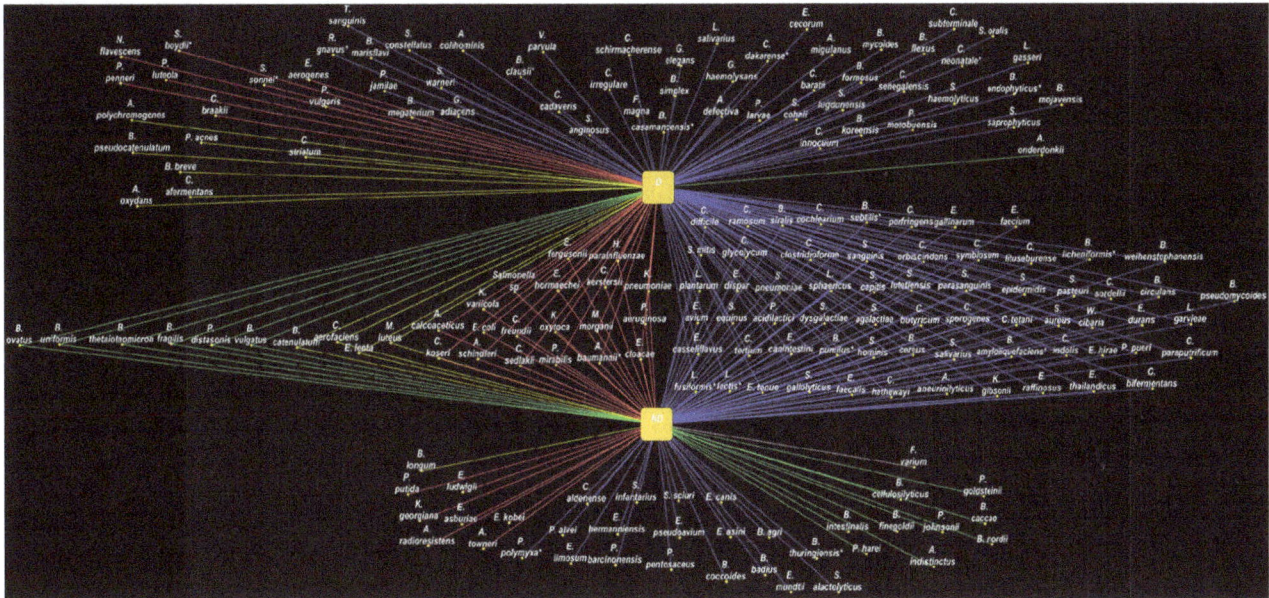

Figure 1. Isolates from individuals with diarrhea (D; top) and without diarrhea (ND; bottom). Each bacterial species corresponds to a node. The edge color represents the phylum (blue: *Firmicutes*; red: *Proteobacteria*; green: *Bacteroidetes*; yellow: *Actinobacteria*; pink: *Fusobacteria*). The common and specific bacteria detected from patients with diarrhea and those without are provided.

The other isolates identified by 16S rRNA sequence included 1 of 2 *Parabacteroides goldsteinii* isolates detected in the study, 1 of 2 *Aneurinibacillus migulanus* isolates, 2 (11%) of 18 *Bacillus amyloliquefaciens* isolates, 1 of 2 *Bacillus endophyticus* isolates, 1 (7.7%) of 13 *Bacillus licheniformis* isolates, 2 (7.7%) of 26 *Bacillus pumilus* isolates, 3 (8%) of 37 *Bacillus subtilis* isolates, 1 of 4 *Clostridium clostridioforme* isolates, 1 of 13 (7.7%) *Clostridium lituseburense* isolates, 1 of 13 (7.7%) *Kurthia gibsonii* isolates, 1 of 4 *Lactococcus lactis* isolates, 1 of 25 (4%) *Lysinibacillus fusiformis* isolates, 1 of 2 *Lysinibacillus sphaericus* isolates, 1 of 2 *Ruminococcus gnavus* isolates, 1 of 12 (8.3%) *Weissella cibaria* isolates, and 2 of 11 (18.2%) *Acinetobacter baumannii* isolates. When the spectra of the aforementioned isolates were added to the Bruker database, further identifications of these organisms by MALDI-TOF were accurate.

Common bacteria. Seven bacterial species (3.7%) were identified more than 100 times in fecal samples (261 *Escherichia coli* isolates, 256 *Enterococcus faecium* isolates, 159 *Clostridium bifermentans* isolates, 153 *Enterococcus faecalis* isolates, 152 *Clostridium perfringens* isolates, 137 *Bacillus cereus* isolates, and 106 *Enterococcus hirae* isolates). Surprisingly, several bacteria were more common in patients without diarrhea including *E. coli* than those without ($P \leq 10^{-3}$), *E. faecium* ($P \leq 10^{-3}$), *C. bifermentans* ($P = 0.002$), and *C. perfringens* ($P \leq 10^{-3}$), see Table 4 and Figure 2.

Thirty-nine bacterial species (20.6%) from 18 different genera were identified from between 10 and 100 fecal samples (Table 4 and Figure 2). Several were more common in patients with diarrhea than those without, such as *Bacillus licheniformis* ($P = 0.02$), *Bacillus pumilus* ($P = 0.002$), and *Staphylococcus aureus* ($P = 0.01$). In contrast, people without diarrhea had more commonly *Lysinibacillus fusiformis* ($P = 0.001$), *Clostridium orbiscindens* ($P = 0.01$), *Clostridium symbiosum* ($P = 0.03$), *Enterococcus casseliflavus* ($P = 0.03$), *Kurthia gibsonii* ($P = 0.02$), and *Collinsella aerofaciens* ($P = 0.01$), *Eggerthella lenta* ($P = 0.004$), *Bacteroides uniformis* ($P = 0.001$), and *Bacteroides vulgatus* ($P = 0.03$).

Rare bacterial species. Overall, 81 out of 189 bacterial species (43%) were identified from between 2 and 10 fecal samples

(Table 4). Among them, *Bifidobacterium breve*, *Propionibacterium acnes*, *Bacillus mojavensis*, *Finegoldia magna*, and *Streptococcus anginosus* were each detected in only 4 patients with diarrhea ($P = 0.047$). *Staphylococcus haemolyticus* was detected in only 5 patients with diarrhea ($P = 0.02$). *Staphylococcus epidermidis* was significantly more frequent among people with diarrhea (7/162) than among those without (1/185, $P = 0.02$). In contrast, *Eubacterium limosum* was identified only in 5 people without diarrhea ($P = 0.04$).

Bacterial species isolated only once. Overall, 51 bacterial species were identified only once (Table 4). Among them, 5 different bacterial species from the phylum *Actinobacteria*, 5 from the genera *Bacillus*, 4 from the genera *Clostridium*, and 2 from the genera *Shigella* were detected among patients with diarrhea. In contrast, several species of the genera *Bacteroides* (4) and *Enterococcus* (2) were detected only among patients without diarrhea.

Bacterial identification depending of the age range. The isolates obtained from people with and without diarrhea depending of the age range (less than 5 years, from 5 to 20 years, and more than 20 years) were compared. Only significant differences are presented (Table S1). For children from 0 to 5 year-old, 2 species of the genera *Clostridium* were significantly more frequent among those without diarrhea, including 1 species *C. glycolycum*, for which the data were not significant when the entire population was analyzed. For adult of more than 20 year-old, 6 species (*E. coli*, *E. faecium*, *B. uniformis*, *B. vulgatus*, *C. orbiscindens*, and *E. lenta*), as previously observed in the entire population, were significantly more observed in people without diarrhea. In contrast, those with diarrhea had more commonly *S. aureus*, *F. magna*, *B. pumilus*, as previously observed, as well as another *Bacillus* species, *B. subtilis*. For people from 5 to 20 year-old, *E. faecium*, *C. perfringens*, and *C. symbosium* were significantly more detected in people without diarrhea, as observed in the entire population. Finally, the comparison of the isolates from people with diarrhea between them depending of the age range did not yield statistically significant results.

Table 4. Comparison between the prevalence of 189 bacterial species identified among 2,750 isolates from fecal samples of 162 individuals with diarrhea and 185 without diarrhea.

Phyla	Bacteria	162 with diarrhea		185 without diarrhea		Total = 347		
		N° of isolate	%	N° of isolate	%	N° of isolate	%	P value
>100								
Proteobacteria	*Escherichia coli*	104	64.2	157	84.9	261	75.2	≤10⁻³
Firmicutes	*Enterococcus faecium*	102	63	154	83.2	256	73.8	≤10⁻³
Firmicutes	*Clostridium bifermentans*	60	37	99	53.5	159	45.8	0.002
Firmicutes	*Enterococcus faecalis*	76	46.9	77	41.6	153	44	ns
Firmicutes	*Clostridium perfringens*	53	32.7	99	53.5	152	43.8	≤10⁻³
Firmicutes	*Bacillus cereus*	57	35.2	80	43.2	137	39.5	ns
Firmicutes	*Enterococcus hirae*	48	29.7	58	31.3	106	30.5	ns
>10–100								
Firmicutes	*Enterococcus gallinarum*	34	21	52	28.1	86	24.8	ns
Proteobacteria	*Klebsiella pneumoniae*	33	20.4	51	27.6	84	24.2	ns
Firmicutes	*Clostridium sordellii*	29	17.9	48	25.9	77	22.2	ns
Firmicutes	*Lactococcus garvieae*	23	14.2	34	18.4	57	16.4	ns
Bacteroidetes	*Bacteroides fragilis*	20	12.5	35	18.9	55	15.8	ns
Firmicutes	*Enterococcus avium*	20	12.3	32	17.3	52	14.5	ns
Firmicutes	*Clostridium orbiscindens*	12	7.4	30	16.2	42	12.1	0.01
Proteobacteria	*Enterobacter cloacae*	23	14.2	18	9.7	41	11.8	ns
Bacteroidetes	*Bacteroides uniformis*	8	5	30	16.2	38	10.9	0.001
Firmicutes	*Bacillus subtilis*[1]	22	13.6	15	8.1	37	10.7	ns
Firmicutes	*Clostridium symbiosum*	10	6.2	25	13.5	35	10	0.03
Firmicutes	*Enterococcus casseliflavus*	10	6.2	25	13.5	35	10	0.03
Bacteroidetes	*Bacteroides thetaiotaomicron*	9	5.5	21	11.3	30	8.6	ns
Firmicutes	*Streptococcus equinus*	13	8	16	8.6	29	8.4	ns
Actinobacteria	*Collinsella aerofaciens*	6	3.7	20	10.8	26	7.5	0.01
Firmicutes	*Bacillus pumilus*[1]	19	11.7	7	3.8	26	7.5	0.002
Firmicutes	*Streptococcus lutetiensis*	16	9.9	10	5.4	26	7.5	ns
Firmicutes	*Lysinibacillus fusiformis*[1]	4	2.5	21	11.3	25	7.2	0.001
Bacteroidetes	*Bacteroides ovatus*	10	6	14	7.6	24	6.9	ns
Firmicutes	*Streptococcus gallolyticus*	16	9.9	8	4.3	24	6.9	ns
Proteobacteria	*Proteus mirabilis*	9	5.6	15	8.1	24	6.9	ns
Actinobacteria	*Eggerthella lenta*	4	2.5	19	10.3	23	6.6	0.004
Proteobacteria	*Comamonas kerstersii*	8	4.9	12	6.5	20	5.8	ns
Firmicutes	*Clostridium butyricum*	6	3.7	13	7	19	5.5	ns
Firmicutes	*Clostridium glycolycum*	5	3	14	7.6	19	5.5	ns
Bacteroidetes	*Bacteroides vulgatus*	2	1.2	16	8.7	18	5.2	≤10⁻³
Firmicutes	*Bacillus amyloliquefaciens*[1]	10	6.2	8	4.3	18	5.2	ns
Firmicutes	*Clostridium tertium*	11	6.8	7	3.8	18	5.2	ns
Firmicutes	*Clostridium cochlearium*	4	2.5	12	6.5	16	4.6	ns
Bacteroidetes	*Parabacteroides distasonis*	7	4.3	8	4.3	15	4.3	ns
Proteobacteria	*Morganella morganii*	6	3.7	9	4.9	15	4.3	ns
Firmicutes	*Bacillus licheniformis*[1]	10	6.2	3	1.6	13	3.7	0.02
Firmicutes	*Clostridium lituseburense*[1]	4	2.5	9	4.9	13	3.7	ns
Firmicutes	*Kurthia gibsonii*[1]	2	1.2	11	5.9	13	3.7	0.02
Firmicutes	*Clostridium ramosum*	5	3	7	3.8	12	3.5	ns
Firmicutes	*Staphylococcus aureus*	10	6.2	2	1	12	3.5	0.01
Firmicutes	*Weissella cibaria*[1]	4	2.5	8	4.3	12	3.5	ns

Table 4. Cont.

Phyla	Bacteria	162 with diarrhea N° of isolate	%	185 without diarrhea N° of isolate	%	Total = 347 N° of isolate	%	P value
Proteobacteria	*Acinetobacter baumannii[1]*	4	2.5	7	3.8	11	4	ns
Firmicutes	*Streptococcus parasanguinis*	8	4.9	3	1.6	11	3.2	ns
1–10 isolates								
Firmicutes	*Bacillus circulans*	5	3	5	2.7	10	2.9	ns
Firmicutes	*Bacillus weihenstephanensis*	5	3	4	2.2	9	2.6	ns
Firmicutes	*Enterococcus thailandicus[2]*	3	1.8	6	3.2	9	2.6	ns
Firmicutes	*Streptococcus pneumoniae*	5	3	4	2.2	9	2.6	ns
Firmicutes	*Enterococcus canintestini*	4	2.5	4	2.2	8	2.3	ns
Firmicutes	*Enterococcus durans*	6	3.7	2	1	8	2.3	ns
Firmicutes	*Staphylococcus epidermidis*	7	4.3	1	0.5	8	2.3	**0.02**
Actinobacteria	*Micrococcus luteus*	5	3	2	1	7	2	ns
Firmicutes	*Bacillus siralis*	3	1.8	4	2.2	7	2	ns
Firmicutes	*Enterococcus dispar*	4	2.5	3	1.6	7	2	ns
Firmicutes	*Enterococcus raffinosus[3]*	3	1.8	4	2.2	7	2	ns
Proteobacteria	*Enterobacter hormaechei*	5	3	2	1	7	2	ns
Firmicutes	*Aneurinibacillus aneurinilyticus*	2	1.2	4	2.2	6	1.7	ns
Firmicutes	*Clostridium sporogenes*	4	2.5	2	1	6	1.7	ns
Firmicutes	*Streptococcus agalactiae*	4	2.5	2	1	6	1.7	ns
Firmicutes	*Streptococcus dysgalactiae[3]*	5	3	1	0.5	6	1.7	ns
Proteobacteria	*Citrobacter freundii*	1	0.6	5	2.7	6	1.7	ns
Firmicutes	*Eubacterium limosum*	0	0	5	2.7	5	1.4	**0.04**
Firmicutes	*Paenibacillus pueri*	2	1.2	3	1.6	5	1.4	ns
Firmicutes	*Staphylococcus haemolyticus*	5	3	0	0	5	1.4	**0.02**
Firmicutes	*Streptococcus salivarius*	4	2.5	1	0.5	5	1.4	ns
Proteobacteria	*Acinetobacter calcoaceticus*	2	1.2	3	1.6	5	1.4	ns
Proteobacteria	*Escherichia fergusonii*	3	1.8	2	1	5	1.4	ns
Proteobacteria	*Klebsiella oxytoca*	2	1.2	3	1.6	5	1.4	ns
Actinobacteria	*Bifidobacterium breve*	4	2.5	0	0	4	1.1	**0.047**
Actinobacteria	*Propionibacterium acnes*	4	2.5	0	0	4	1.1	**0.047**
Firmicutes	*Bacillus mojavensis*	4	2.5	0	0	4	1.1	**0.047**
Firmicutes	*Clostridium clostridioforme[1]*	3	1.8	1	0.5	4	1.1	ns
Firmicutes	*Clostridium hathewayi*	3	1.8	1	0.5	4	1.1	ns
Firmicutes	*Clostridium paraputrificum*	3	1.8	1	0.5	4	1.1	ns
Firmicutes	*Enterococcus asini*	0	0	4	2.2	4	1.1	ns
Firmicutes	*Finegoldia magna*	4	2.5	0	0	4	1.1	**0.047**
Firmicutes	*Lactococcus lactis[1]*	1	0.6	3	1.6	4	1.1	ns
Firmicutes	*Streptococcus anginosus*	4	2.5	0	0	4	1.1	**0.047**
Proteobacteria	*Enterobacter asburiae*	0	0	4	2.2	4	1.1	ns
Proteobacteria	*Haemophilus parainfluenzae*	3	1.8	1	0.5	4	1.1	ns
Proteobacteria	*Pseudomonas aeruginosa*	2	1.2	2	1	4	1.1	ns
Proteobacteria	*Salmonella enterica*	3	1.8	1	0.5	4	1.1	ns
Firmicutes	*Lactobacillus gasseri*	3	1.8	0	0	3	0.9	ns
Firmicutes	*Lactobacillus plantarum*	1	0.6	2	1	3	0.9	ns
Firmicutes	*Paenibacillus jamilae[2]*	3	1.8	0	0	3	0.9	ns
Firmicutes	*Paenibacillus larvae[3]*	3	1.8	0	0	3	0.9	ns
Firmicutes	*Staphylococcus capitis*	2	1.2	1	0.5	3	0.9	ns
Firmicutes	*Staphylococcus hominis*	2	1.2	1	0.5	3	0.9	ns

Table 4. Cont.

Phyla	Bacteria	162 with diarrhea		185 without diarrhea		Total = 347		
		N° of isolate	%	N° of isolate	%	N° of isolate	%	P value
Firmicutes	*Staphylococcus lugdunensis*	3	1.8	0	0	3	0.9	ns
Firmicutes	*Staphylococcus pasteuri*	2	1.2	1	0.5	3	0.9	ns
Firmicutes	*Streptococcus alactolyticus*[3]	0	0	3	1.6	3	0.9	ns
Proteobacteria	*Enterobacter kobei*	0	0	3	1.6	3	0.9	ns
Proteobacteria	*Acinetobacter schindleri*	1	0.6	1	0.5	2	0.6	ns
Actinobacteria	*Bifidobacterium catenulatum*	1	0.6	1	0.5	2	0.6	ns
Actinobacteria	*Bifidobacterium longum*	0	0	2	1	2	0.6	ns
Bacteroidetes	*Parabacteroides goldsteinii*[1]	0	0	2	1	2	0.6	ns
Bacteroidetes	*Parabacteroides johnsonii*	0	0	2	1	2	0.6	ns
Firmicutes	*Aneurinibacillus migulanus*[1]	2	1.2	0	0	2	0.6	ns
Firmicutes	*Bacillus badius*	0	0	2	1	2	0.6	ns
Firmicutes	*Bacillus endophyticus*[1]	2	1.2	0	0	2	0.6	ns
Firmicutes	*Bacillus megaterium*	2	1.2	0	0	2	0.6	ns
Firmicutes	*Bacillus pseudomycoides*[2]	1	0.6	1	0.5	2	0.6	ns
Firmicutes	*Clostridium aldenense*	0	0	2	1	2	0.6	ns
Firmicutes	*Clostridium difficile*	1	0.6	1	0.5	2	0.6	ns
Firmicutes	*Clostridium indolis*	1	0.6	1	0.5	2	0.6	ns
Firmicutes	*Clostridium innocuum*	2	1.2	0	0	2	0.6	ns
Firmicutes	*Clostridium subterminale*[3]	2	1.2	0	0	2	0.6	ns
Firmicutes	*Clostridium tetani*[3]	1	0.6	1	0.5	2	0.6	ns
Firmicutes	*Enterococcus canis*[2]	0	0	2	1	2	0.6	ns
Firmicutes	*Enterococcus cecorum*	2	1.2	0	0	2	0.6	ns
Firmicutes	*Enterococcus pseudoavium*[3]	0	0	2	1	2	0.6	ns
Firmicutes	*Enterococcus tenue*	1	0.6	1	0.5	2	0.6	ns
Firmicutes	*Lysinibacillus sphaericus*[1]	1	0.6	1	0.5	2	0.6	ns
Firmicutes	*Paenibacillus alvei*	0	0	2	1	2	0.6	ns
Firmicutes	*Pediococcu acidilactici*	1	0.6	1	0.5	2	0.6	ns
Firmicutes	*Ruminocus gnavus*[1]	2	1.2	0	0	2	0.6	ns
Firmicutes	*Streptococcus infantarius*	0	0	2	1	2	0.6	ns
Firmicutes	*Streptococcus mitis*	1	0.6	1	0.5	2	0.6	ns
Firmicutes	*Streptococcus oralis*	2	1.2	0	0	2	0.6	ns
Firmicutes	*Streptococcus sanguinis*	1	0.6	1	0.5	2	0.6	ns
Proteobacteria	*Acinetobacter radioresistens*	0	0	2	1	2	0.6	ns
Proteobacteria	*Citrobacter koseri*	1	0.6	1	0.5	2	0.6	ns
Proteobacteria	*Citrobacter sedlakii*	1	0.6	1	0.5	2	0.6	ns
Proteobacteria	*Klebsiella variicola*	1	0.6	1	0.5	2	0.6	ns
Proteobacteria	*Proteus vulgaris*	2	1.2	0	0	2	0.6	ns
1 isolate								
Actinobacteria	*Arthrobacter polychromogenes*	1	0.6	0	0	1	0.3	ns
Actinobacteria	*Arthrobacter oxydans*	1	0.6	0	0	1	0.3	ns
Actinobacteria	*Bifidobacterium pseudocatenulatum*	1	0.6	0	0	1	0.3	ns
Actinobacteria	*Corynebacterium afermentans*	1	0.6	0	0	1	0.3	ns
Actinobacteria	*Corynebacterium striatum*	1	0.6	0	0	1	0.3	ns
Bacteroidetes	*Alistipes indistinctus*	0	0	1	0.5	1	0.3	ns
Bacteroidetes	*Alistipes onderdonkii*	1	0.6	0	0	1	0.3	ns
Bacteroidetes	*Bacteroides caccae*	0	0	1	0.5	1	0.3	ns
Bacteroidetes	*Bacteroides cellulosilyticus*	0	0	1	0.5	1	0.3	ns

Table 4. Cont.

Phyla	Bacteria	162 with diarrhea		185 without diarrhea		Total = 347		
		N° of isolate	%	N° of isolate	%	N° of isolate	%	P value
Bacteroidetes	*Bacteroides finegoldii*	0	0	1	0.5	1	0.3	ns
Bacteroidetes	*Bacteroides intestinalis*	0	0	1	0.5	1	0.3	ns
Bacteroidetes	*Bacteroides nordii*[1]	0	0	1	0.5	1	0.3	ns
Bacteroidetes	*Peptoniphilus harei*	0	0	1	0.5	1	0.3	ns
Firmicutes	*Abiotrophia defectiva*	1	0.6	0	0	1	0.3	ns
Firmicutes	*Anaerotruncus colihominis*	1	0.6	0	0	1	0.3	ns
Firmicutes	*Bacillus casamancensis*[1,4]	1	0.6	0	0	1	0.3	ns
Firmicutes	*Bacillus clausii*[1]	1	0.6	0	0	1	0.3	ns
Firmicutes	*Bacillus flexus*	1	0.6	0	0	1	0.3	ns
Firmicutes	*Bacillus koreensis*[2]	1	0.6	0	0	1	0.3	ns
Firmicutes	*Bacillus marisflavi*	1	0.6	0	0	1	0.3	ns
Firmicutes	*Bacillus mycoides*	1	0.6	0	0	1	0.3	ns
Firmicutes	*Bacillus simplex*	1	0.6	0	0	1	0.3	ns
Firmicutes	*Bacillus thuringiensis*[1]	0	0	1	0.5	1	0.3	ns
Firmicutes	*Bacillus coccoides*	0	0	1	0.5	1	0.3	ns
Firmicutes	*Bacillus agri*	0	0	1	0.5	1	0.3	ns
Firmicutes	*Bacillus formosus*[2]	1	0.6	0	0	1	0.3	ns
Firmicutes	*Clostridium baratii*	1	0.6	0	0	1	0.3	ns
Firmicutes	*Clostridium cadaveris*[1]	1	0.6	0	0	1	0.3	ns
Firmicutes	*Clostridium dakarense*[1,4]	1	0.6	0	0	1	0.3	ns
Firmicutes	*Clostridium irregulare*[3]	1	0.6	0	0	1	0.3	ns
Firmicutes	*Clostridium neonatale*[1]	1	0.6	0	0	1	0.3	ns
Firmicutes	*Clostridium schirmacherense*[2]	1	0.6	0	0	1	0.3	ns
Firmicutes	*Clostridium senegalense*	1	0.6	0	0	1	0.3	ns
Firmicutes	*Enterococcus hermanniensis*[2]	0	0	1	0.5	1	0.3	ns
Firmicutes	*Enterococcus mundtii*	0	0	1	0.5	1	0.3	ns
Firmicutes	*Gemella haemolysans*	1	0.6	0	0	1	0.3	ns
Firmicutes	*Granulicatella adiacens*	1	0.6	0	0	1	0.3	ns
Firmicutes	*Granulicatella elegans*	1	0.6	0	0	1	0.3	ns
Firmicutes	*Lactobacillus salivarius*	1	0.6	0	0	1	0.3	ns
Firmicutes	*Paenibacillus barcinonensis*	0	0	1	0.5	1	0.3	ns
Firmicutes	*Paenibacillus motobuensis*[2]	1	0.6	0	0	1	0.3	ns
Firmicutes	*Paenibacillus polymyxa*[1,3]	0	0	1	0.5	1	0.3	ns
Firmicutes	*Pediococcus pentosaceus*	0	0	1	0.5	1	0.3	ns
Firmicutes	*Staphylococcus cohnii*	1	0.6	0	0	1	0.3	ns
Firmicutes	*Staphylococcus saprophyticus*	1	0.6	0	0	1	0.3	ns
Firmicutes	*Staphylococcus sciuri*[1]	0	0	1	0.5	1	0.3	ns
Firmicutes	*Staphylococcus warneri*	1	0.6	0	0	1	0.3	ns
Firmicutes	*Streptococcus constellatus*	1	0.6	0	0	1	0.3	ns
Firmicutes	*Turicibacter sanguinis*	1	0.6	0	0	1	0.3	ns
Firmicutes	*Veillonella parvula*	1	0.6	0	0	1	0.3	ns
Fusobacteria	*Fusobacterium varium*	0	0	1	0.5	1	0.3	ns
Proteobacteria	*Acinetobacter towneri*[2]	0	0	1	0.5	1	0.3	ns
Proteobacteria	*Citrobacter braakii*	1	0.6	0	0	1	0.3	ns
Proteobacteria	*Enterobacter aerogenes*	1	0.6	0	0	1	0.3	ns
Proteobacteria	*Enterobacter ludwigii*[3]	0	0	1	0.5	1	0.3	ns
Proteobacteria	*Kluyvera georgiana*[3]	0	0	1	0.5	1	0.3	ns

Table 4. Cont.

Phyla	Bacteria	162 with diarrhea		185 without diarrhea		Total = 347		
		N° of isolate	%	N° of isolate	%	N° of isolate	%	P value
Proteobacteria	*Neisseria flavescens*	1	0.6	0	0	1	0.3	ns
Proteobacteria	*Proteus penneri*	1	0.6	0	0	1	0.3	ns
Proteobacteria	*Pseudomonas luteola*	1	0.6	0	0	1	0.3	ns
Proteobacteria	*Pseudomonas putida*	0	0	1	0.5	1	0.3	ns
Proteobacteria	*Shigella boydii*[1]	1	0.6	0	0	1	0.3	ns
Proteobacteria	*Shigella sonnei*[1]	1	0.6	0	0	1	0.3	ns

P value is specified only when a significant difference was observed.
N° of isolate: Number of isolate; %: Percentage; ns: non significant value.
[1]Strains identified using a molecular analysis;
[2]Bacterial species that were never isolated in humans;
[3]Bacterial species isolated in humans but not in the human gut;
[4]New bacterial species.

Viral and Parasites Identification

Analyses in Dakar have allowed the detection of several viruses and parasites in feces. Ten rotaviruses (6.2%), 4 adenoviruses (2.7%), and 7 co-infections with both rotaviruses and adenoviruses (4.3%) were detected among diarrheic patients. Sixteen *Enterobius vermicularis* (9.9%), 6 *Trichomonas intestinalis* (3.7%), 5 *Cryptosporidium* spp. (3%), 5 cysts of *Entamoeba* spp. (3%), 4 *Schistosoma mansoni* (2.7%), and 1 *Microsporidium* spp. (0.6%) were detected among 37 diarrheic people. Thirty-six *Ascaris lumbricoides* (among 24 diarrheic people and 12 without diarrhea), 8 *Giardia duodenalis* (among 6 diarrheic people and 2 without diarrhea), and 4 *Trichuris trichiura* (among 1 diarrheic people and 3 without) were detected. Finally, 2 co-infections (*Cryptosporidium* spp. with *Ascaris lumbricoides* and *Microsporidium* spp. with *Ascaris lumbricoides*) were detected in patients with diarrhea and 1 co-infection (*Trichuris trichiura* with *Ascaris lumbricoides*) among a people without diarrhea.

Discussion

MALDI-TOF mass spectrometry coupled with culturomics has allowed for the identification of a large collection of bacterial species from specimens from Senegal and a preliminary comparison between the bacterial microbiota of people with and without diarrhea. This technique has allowed for the accurate identification of a large panel of anaerobes that are usually poorly identified by current phenotypic methods, which lack specificity and result in ambiguous or even erroneous identification [21,22]. For several bacterial species, their identification by MALDI-TOF failed because either the corresponding species missed in the database or either the number of spectra of the species was insufficient. Indeed, the continuous increases of the entries in database with the addition of our new spectra solved these problems and improved bacterial identification. In addition, the use of MALDI-TOF mass spectrometry detects the presence of previously rare bacteria that were difficult to identify using phenotypic methods [6,23–27].

Overall, the percentage of isolates from Senegal that were correctly identified at the genus and species level by mass spectrometry (98.2%) is nearly the same than the percentage (95.4%) observed in the first large scale experiment that used mass spectrometry in Marseille, France [1]. Both studies were performed using the same database. This study has allowed us to test a large collection of isolated strains from Senegalese people. Only 3 bacterial species, *Clostridium senegalense*, *Bacillus casamancensis*, and *Clostridium dakarense*, have been currently identified in Senegal. This confirms the high potential for culturomics approaches to result in the detection of new bacterial species associated with humans [28–39]. The increases in the database by the addition of more bacteria have allowed for improved bacterial identification by MALDI-TOF mass spectrometry. Thus, the current database seems accurate for the identification of bacteria in Senegal. This work allowed for the identification of 166 bacterial species already found in the human gut, 11 species previously detected in humans but not in the gut, 10 species detected in humans for the first time, and 2 unknown species.

The composition of the gut microbiota is complex [40]. A recent culturomics experiment using many culture conditions was performed on fecal samples from 2 healthy Senegalese individuals, 1 obese person, 1 person with resistant tuberculosis, and a patient with anorexia nervosa. This allowed the identification of 99, 219, 192, 39, and 133 different bacterial species per fecal sample, respectively [12–14]. Although the storage and transport conditions of the fecal samples were not optimal and many fewer culture conditions were used, this study demonstrates a modification of gut microbiota with several significant differences between the bacterial species identified among people with diarrhea and those without diarrhea. In people with diarrhea, major commensal bacterial species such as *E. coli* were significantly decreased, as were several *Enterococcus* spp. (*E. faecium* and *E. casseliflavus*); anaerobes, such as *Bacteroides* spp. (*B. uniformis* and *B. vulgatus*); and *Clostridium* spp. (*C. bifermentans*, *C. orbiscindens*, *C. perfringens*, *C. symbosium*, and *C. glycolycum*). Conversely, several *Bacillus* spp. (*B. licheniformis*, *B. mojavensis*, *B. pumilus*, and *B. subtilis*) were significantly more frequent among patients with diarrhea. In addition, the diversity of *Bacillus* species identified in patients with diarrhea is higher (19) than among those without diarrhea (11), but this difference was not significant ($P=0.055$). Overall, a decrease of anaerobes in the gut flora, particularly Bacteroidetes, has already been reported during gastroenteritis using both culture and molecular methods [41,42]. Our data shows the occurrence of an imbalance of natural bacterial flora among patients with diarrhea.

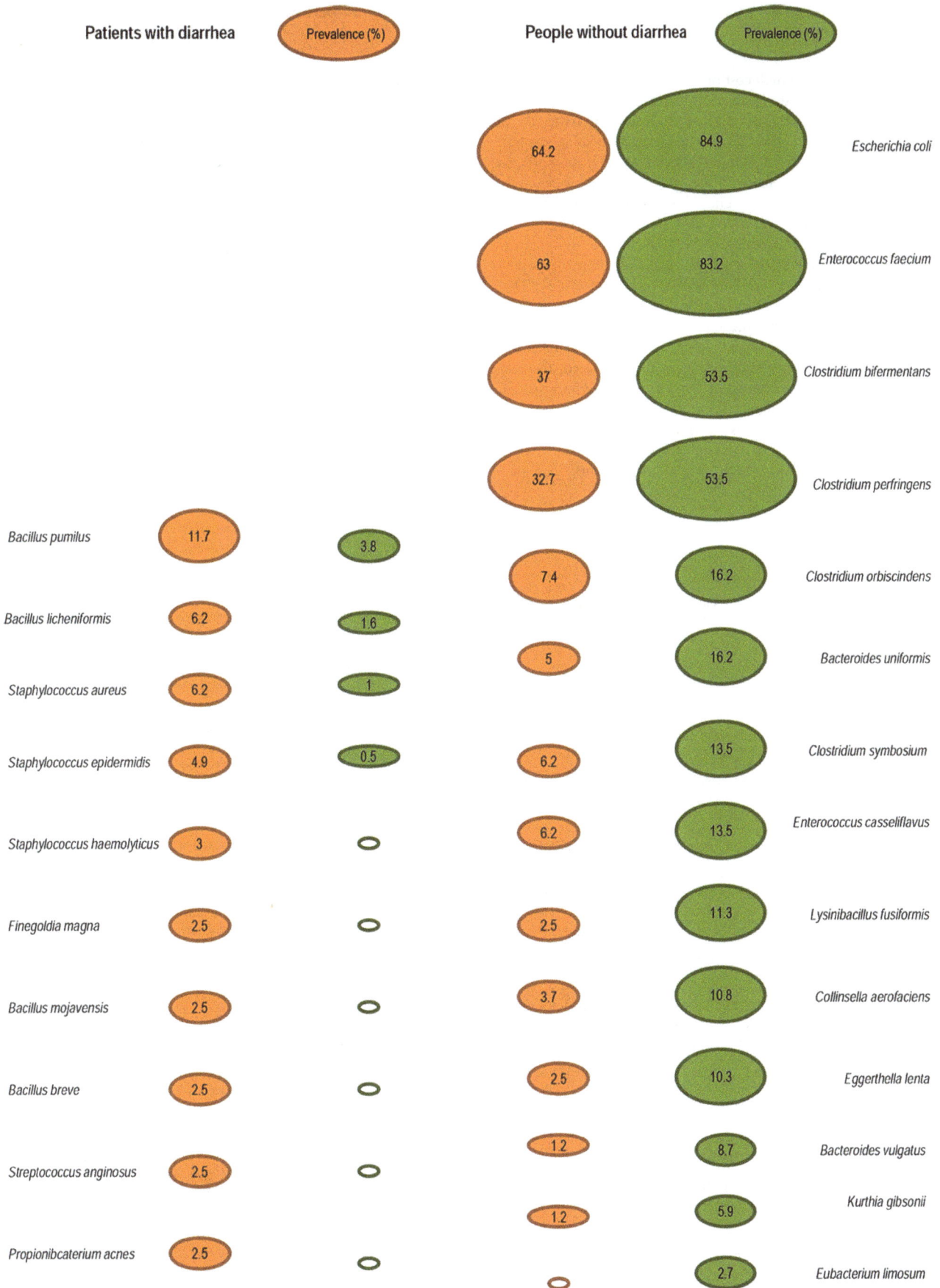

Patients with diarrhea — Prevalence (%)

People without diarrhea — Prevalence (%)

	Patients with diarrhea	People without diarrhea	
Escherichia coli	64.2	84.9	
Enterococcus faecium	63	83.2	
Clostridium bifermentans	37	53.5	
Clostridium perfringens	32.7	53.5	
Bacillus pumilus	11.7	3.8	
Clostridium orbiscindens	7.4	16.2	
Bacillus licheniformis	6.2	1.6	
Bacteroides uniformis	5	16.2	
Staphylococcus aureus	6.2	1	
Clostridium symbosium	6.2	13.5	
Staphylococcus epidermidis	4.9	0.5	
Enterococcus casseliflavus	6.2	13.5	
Staphylococcus haemolyticus	3		
Lysinibacillus fusiformis	2.5	11.3	
Finegoldia magna	2.5		
Collinsella aerofaciens	3.7	10.8	
Bacillus mojavensis	2.5		
Eggerthella lenta	2.5	10.3	
Bacillus breve	2.5		
Bacteroides vulgatus	1.2	8.7	
Streptococcus anginosus	2.5		
Kurthia gibsonii	1.2	5.9	
Propionibcaterium acnes	2.5		
Eubacterium limosum		2.7	

Figure 2. Bacterial species for which significant differences have been observed between individuals with diarrhea and those without diarrhea.

For a long time, the high cost of a MALDI-TOF apparatus and the lack of specific reagent have limited the development of this technology. The expense of using MALDI-TOF mass spectrometry for identification now lies in the acquisition of a machine, which costs between €100,000 and €200,000 [21]. Recently, the cost per sample was calculated to be 1.35 euros for the Microflex system from Bruker [21]. The time required for bacterial identification has been improved to 1 minute 46 seconds using the Microflex system. In addition, MALDI-TOF mass spectrometry also has the potential for identification at the serotype level and antibiotic resistance profiling within minutes [43–51]. Thus, the rapid and accurate identification of routinely encountered bacterial species can be performed to improve the care of patients with infectious diseases. This technique will be a promising alternative for bacterial identification in Africa. Indeed, the main cost is based on the investment of purchasing the apparatus. The used reagents do not expire, do not require specific storage conditions, and are not expensive [1,6]. Finally, the protocol that involves directly deposited bacterial colonies onto the MALDI-TOF mass spectrometry plate regardless of the agar-based

medium and without any subculture or colony preparation is very simple and can be widely used.

Overall, MALDI-TOF mass spectrometry is a potentially powerful tool for routine bacterial identification in Africa, as it allows for the rapid identification of bacterial species, including those that are rare and difficult to identify using phenotypic methods. The next step will be to install MALDI-TOF mass spectrometers in African hospitals.

Acknowledgments
We thank Denis Piak for his help.

Author Contributions
Conceived and designed the experiments: AGS FF DR. Performed the experiments: BSB JCL PH GD. Analyzed the data: CM HR FF DR. Contributed reagents/materials/analysis tools: BSB GD PH HR FF. Wrote the paper: FF JCL DR.

References

1. Seng P, Drancourt M, Gouriet F, La Scola B, Fournier PE, et al (2009) Ongoing revolution in bacteriology: routine identification of bacteria by matrix-assisted laser desorption ionization time-of-flight mass spectrometry. Clin Infect Dis 49: 543–551.
2. Patel R (2013) Matrix-Assisted Laser Desorption Ionization-Time of Flight Mass Spectrometry in Clinical Microbiology. Clin Infect Dis 57: 564–572.
3. van Veen SQ, Claas EC, Kuijper EJ (2010) High-throughput identification of bacteria and yeast by matrix-assisted laser desorption ionization-time of flight mass spectrometry in conventional medical microbiology laboratories. J Clin Microbiol 48: 900–907.
4. Cherkaoui A, Hibbs J, Emonet S, Tangomo M, Girard M, et al (2010) Comparison of two matrix-assisted laser desorption ionization-time of flight mass spectrometry methods with conventional phenotypic identification for routine identification of bacteria to the species level. J Clin Microbiol 48: 1169–1175.
5. Stevenson LG, Drake SK, Shea YR, Zelazny AM, Murray PR (2010) Evaluation of matrix-assisted laser desorption ionization-time of flight mass spectrometry for identification of clinically important yeast species. J Clin Microbiol 48: 3482–3486.
6. Seng P, Abat C, Rolain JM, Colson P, Gouriet F, et al (2013) Emergence of rare pathogenic bacteria in a clinical microbiology laboratory: impact of MALDI-TOF mass spectrometry. J Clin Microbiol 51: 2182–2194.
7. Bizzini A, Durussel C, Bille J, Greub G, Prod'hom G (2010) Performance of matrix-assisted laser desorption ionization-time of flight mass spectrometry for identification of bacterial strains routinely isolated in a clinical microbiology laboratory. J Clin Microbiol 48: 1549–1554.
8. Lagier JC, Million M, Hugon P, Armougom F, Raoult D (2012) Human gut microbiota: repertoire and variations. Front Cell Infect Microbiol 2: 136.
9. Lozupone CA, Stombaugh JI, Gordon JI, Jansson JK, Knight R (2012) Diversity, stability and resilience of the human gut microbiota. Nature 489: 220–230.
10. De Filippo C, Cavalieri D, Di Paola M, Ramazzotti M, Poullet JB, et al (2010) Impact of diet in shaping gut microbiota revealed by a comparative study in children from Europe and rural Africa. Proc Natl Acad Sci U S A 107: 14691–14696.
11. Lee S, Sung J, Lee J, Ko G (2011) Comparison of the gut microbiotas of healthy adult twins living in South Korea and the United States. Appl Environ Microbiol 77: 7433–7437.
12. Lagier JC, Armougom F, Million M, Hugon P, Pagnier I, et al (2012) Microbial culturomics: paradigm shift in the human gut microbiome study. Clin Microbiol Infect 18: 1185–1193.
13. Dubourg G, Lagier JC, Armougom F, Robert C, Hamad I, et al (2013) The gut microbiota of a patient with resistant tuberculosis is more comprehensively studied by culturomics than by metagenomics. Eur J Clin Microbiol Infect Dis 32: 637–645.
14. Pfleiderer A, Lagier JC, Armougom F, Robert C, Vialettes B, et al (2013) Culturomics identified 11 new bacterial species from a single anorexia nervosa stool sample. Eur J Clin Microbiol Infect Dis 32: 1471–1481.
15. Hartemink R, Domenech VR, Rombouts FM (1997) LAMVAB–A new selective medium for the isolation of lactobacilli from faeces. J Microbiol Methods 29: 77–84.
16. Drancourt M, Berger P, Raoult D (2004) Systematic 16S rRNA gene sequencing of atypical clinical isolates indentified 27 new bacterial species associated with humans. J Clin Microbiol 42: 2197–2202.
17. Stackebrandt E, Frederiksen W, Garrity GM, Grimont PA, Kampfer P, et al (2002) Report of the ad hoc committee for the re-evaluation of the species definition in bacteriology. Int J Syst Evol Microbiol 52: 1043–1047.
18. Weisburg WG, Barns SM, Pelletier DA, Lane DJ (1991) 16S ribosomal DNA amplification for phylogenetic study. J Bacteriol 173: 697–703.
19. Shannon P, Markiel A, Ozier O, Baliga NS, Wang JT, et al (2003) Cytoscape: a software environment for integrated models of biomolecular interaction networks. Genome Res 13: 2498–2504. 1.
20. Lo CI, Mishra AK, Padhmanabhan R, Samb-Ba B, Gassama-Sow A, et al (2013) Non-contiguous finished genome sequence and description of Clostridium dakarense sp. nov. Stand Genomic Sci 9: 14–27.
21. Seng P, Rolain JM, Fournier PE, La Scola B, Drancourt M, et al (2010) MALDI-TOF-mass spectrometry applications in clinical microbiology. Future Microbiol 5: 1733–1754.
22. La Scola B, Fournier PE, Raoult D (2011) Burden of emerging anaerobes in the MALDI-TOF and 16S rRNA gene sequencing era. Anaerobe 17: 106–112.
23. Tani A, Sahin N, Matsuyama Y, Enomoto T, Nishimura N, et al (2012) High-throughput identification and screening of novel Methylobacterium species using whole-cell MALDI-TOF/MS analysis. PLoS ONE 7: e40784.
24. Chan JF, Lau SK, Curreem SO, To KK, Leung SS, et al (2012) First report of spontaneous intrapartum Atopobium vaginae bacteremia. J Clin Microbiol 50: 2525–2528.
25. Gouriet F, Million M, Henri M, Fournier PE, Raoult D (2012) Lactobacillus rhamnosus bacteremia: an emerging clinical entity. Eur J Clin Microbiol Infect Dis 31: 2469–2480.
26. Dridi B, Raoult D, Drancourt M (2012) Matrix-assisted laser desorption/ionization time-of-flight mass spectrometry identification of Archaea: towards the universal identification of living organisms. APMIS 120: 85–91.
27. Fernandez-Olmos A, Morosini MI, Lamas A, Garcia-Castillo M, Garcia-Garcia L, et al (2012) Clinical and microbiological features of a cystic fibrosis patient chronically colonized with Pandoraea sputorum identified by combining 16S rRNA

sequencing and matrix-assisted laser desorption ionization-time of flight mass spectrometry. J Clin Microbiol 50: 1096–1098.

28. Lagier JC, El Karkouri K, Nguyen TT, Armougom F, Raoult D, et al (2012) Non-contiguous finished genome sequence and description of *Anaerococcus senegalensis* sp. nov. Stand Genomic Sci 6: 116–125.

29. Kokcha S, Mishra AK, Lagier JC, Million M, Leroy Q, et al (2012) Non contiguous-finished genome sequence and description of *Bacillus timonensis* sp. nov. Stand Genomic Sci 6: 346–355.

30. Mishra AK, Lagier JC, Rivet R, Raoult D, Fournier PE (2012) Non-contiguous finished genome sequence and description of *Paenibacillus senegalensis* sp. nov. Stand Genomic Sci 7: 70–81.

31. Mishra AK, Lagier JC, Robert C, Raoult D, Fournier PE (2012) Non contiguous-finished genome sequence and description of *Peptoniphilus timonensis* sp. nov. Stand Genomic Sci 7: 1–11.

32. Kokcha S, Ramasamy D, Lagier JC, Robert C, Raoult D, et al (2012) Non-contiguous finished genome sequence and description of *Brevibacterium senegalense* sp. nov. Stand Genomic Sci 7: 233–245.

33. Lagier JC, Ramasamy D, Rivet R, Raoult D, Fournier PE (2012) Non contiguous-finished genome sequence and description of *Cellulomonas massiliensis* sp. nov. Stand Genomic Sci 7: 258–270.

34. Mishra AK, Lagier JC, Robert C, Raoult D, Fournier PE (2012) Non-contiguous finished genome sequence and description of *Clostridium senegalense* sp. nov. Stand Genomic Sci 6: 386–395.

35. Ramasamy D, Kokcha S, Lagier JC, Nguyen TT, Raoult D, et al (2012) Genome sequence and description of *Aeromicrobium massiliense* sp. nov. Stand Genomic Sci 7: 246–257.

36. Lagier JC, Armougom F, Mishra AK, Nguyen TT, Raoult D, et al (2012) Non-contiguous finished genome sequence and description of *Alistipes timonensis* sp. nov. Stand Genomic Sci 6: 315–324.

37. Kokcha S, Mishra AK, Lagier JC, Million M, Leroy Q, et al (2012) Non contiguous-finished genome sequence and description of *Bacillus timonensis* sp. nov. Stand Genomic Sci 6: 346–355.

38. Mishra AK, Hugon P, Robert C, Raoult D, Fournier PE (2012) Non contiguous-finished genome sequence and description of *Peptoniphilus grossensis* sp. nov. Stand Genomic Sci 7: 320–330.

39. Lagier JC, Gimenez G, Robert C, Raoult D, Fournier PE (2012) Non-contiguous finished genome sequence and description of *Herbaspirillum massiliense* sp. nov. Stand Genomic Sci 7: 200–209.

40. Gill SR, Pop M, Deboy RT, Eckburg PB, Turnbaugh PJ, et al (2006) Metagenomic analysis of the human distal gut microbiome. Science 312: 1355–1359.

41. Albert MJ, Bhat P, Rajan D, Maiya PP, Pereira SM, et al (1978) Faecal flora of South Indian infants and young children in health and with acute gastroenteritis. J Med Microbiol 11: 137–143.

42. Balamurugan R, Janardhan HP, George S, Raghava MV, Muliyil J, et al (2008) Molecular studies of fecal anaerobic commensal bacteria in acute diarrhea in children. J Pediatr Gastroenterol Nutr 46: 514–519.

43. Hrabak J, Walkova R, Studentova V, Chudackova E, Bergerova T (2011) Carbapenemase activity detection by matrix-assisted laser desorption ionization-time of flight mass spectrometry. J Clin Microbiol 49: 3222–3227.

44. Kempf M, Bakour S, Flaudrops C, Berrazeg M, Brunel JM, et al (2012) Rapid detection of carbapenem resistance in *Acinetobacter baumannii* using matrix-assisted laser desorption ionization-time of flight mass spectrometry. PLoS ONE 7: e31676.

45. Edwards-Jones V, Claydon MA, Evason DJ, Walker J, Fox AJ, et al (2000) Rapid discrimination between methicillin-sensitive and methicillin-resistant *Staphylococcus aureus* by intact cell mass spectrometry. J Med Microbiol 49: 295–300.

46. Walker J, Fox AJ, Edwards-Jones V, Gordon DB (2002) Intact cell mass spectrometry (ICMS) used to type methicillin-resistant *Staphylococcus aureus*: media effects and inter-laboratory reproducibility. J Microbiol Methods 48: 117–126.

47. Jackson KA, Edwards-Jones V, Sutton CW, Fox AJ (2005) Optimisation of intact cell MALDI method for fingerprinting of methicillin-resistant *Staphylococcus aureus*. J Microbiol Methods 62: 273–284.

48. Du Z, Yang R, Guo Z, Song Y, Wang J (2002) Identification of *Staphylococcus aureus* and determination of its methicillin resistance by matrix-assisted laser desorption/ionization time-of-flight mass spectrometry. Anal Chem 74: 5487–5491.

49. Majcherczyk PA, McKenna T, Moreillon P, Vaudaux P (2006) The discriminatory power of MALDI-TOF mass spectrometry to differentiate between isogenic teicoplanin-susceptible and teicoplanin-resistant strains of methicillin-resistant *Staphylococcus aureus*. FEMS Microbiol Lett 255: 233–239.

50. Camara JE, Hays FA (2007) Discrimination between wild-type and ampicillin-resistant *Escherichia coli* by matrix-assisted laser desorption/ionization time-of-flight mass spectrometry. Anal Bioanal Chem 389: 1633–1638.

51. Sparbier K, Schubert S, Weller U, Boogen C, Kostrzewa M (2012) Matrix-assisted laser desorption ionization-time of flight mass spectrometry-based functional assay for rapid detection of resistance against beta-lactam antibiotics. J Clin Microbiol 50: 927–937.

3

Quantifying Bias in Randomized Controlled Trials in Child Health

Lisa Hartling[1]*, Michele P. Hamm[1], Ricardo M. Fernandes[2,3], Donna M. Dryden[1], Ben Vandermeer[1]

1 Alberta Research Centre for Health Evidence, Department of Pediatrics, University of Alberta, Edmonton, Alberta, Canada, 2 Clinical Pharmacology Unit, Faculty of Medicine, Instituto de Medicina Molecular, University of Lisbon, Lisbon, Portugal, 3 Department of Pediatrics, Santa Maria Hospital, Lisbon, Portugal

Abstract

Objective: To quantify bias related to specific methodological characteristics in child-relevant randomized controlled trials (RCTs).

Design: Meta-epidemiological study.

Data Extraction: Two reviewers independently assessed RCTs using items in the Cochrane Risk of Bias tool and other study factors. We used meta-epidemiological methods to assess for differences in effect estimates between studies classified as high/unclear vs. low risk of bias.

Results: We included 287 RCTs from 17 meta-analyses. The proportion of studies at high/unclear risk of bias was: 79% sequence generation, 83% allocation concealment, 67% blinding of participants, 47% blinding of outcome assessment, 49% incomplete outcome data, 32% selective outcome reporting, 44% other sources of bias, 97% overall risk of bias, 56% funding, 35% baseline imbalance, 13% blocked randomization in unblinded trials, and 1% early stopping for benefit. We found no significant differences in effect estimates for studies that were high/unclear vs. low risk of bias for any of the risk of bias domains, overall risk of bias, or other study factors.

Conclusions: We found no differences in effect estimates between studies based on risk of bias. A potential explanation is the number of trials included, in particular the small number of studies with low risk of bias. Until further evidence is available, reviewers should not exclude RCTs from systematic reviews and meta-analyses based solely on risk of bias particularly in the area of child health.

Editor: Tammy Clifford, Canadian Agency for Drugs and Technologies in Health, Canada

Funding: This study was funded through the Canadian Institutes of Health Research (CIHR). Dr. Hartling holds a New Investigator Salary Award through CIHR. The funders had no role in the study design, data collection and analysis, decision to publish, or preparation of the manuscript.

* E-mail: hartling@ualberta.ca

Introduction

While randomized controlled trials (RCTs) are considered to be the gold standard for evidence on therapeutic interventions, [1] they are nonetheless susceptible to bias. [2] Bias, or the systematic over- or under-estimation of a treatment's effect, has important implications for decision-making. The implications stem from false positive and false negative results. In practice this may result in the implementation of interventions that are not efficacious and potentially harmful, or withholding of interventions that truly are efficacious. The types of bias that may occur in RCTs can generally be classified as selection, performance, detection, attrition, and reporting bias. [3] The extent to which these biases operate in a given trial may yield inaccuracies of varying magnitude and direction in the estimates of a treatment's effect.

There is a growing body of empirical evidence based on meta-epidemiological methods to quantify different biases in RCTs; however, there are some inconsistencies across studies and clinical areas. Biases may vary across different clinical areas and investigation within different areas is warranted. [4,5] Balk et al. found variation in the direction of effects across studies which "calls into question whether any of these associations could provide a general rule for evaluating RCTs across clinical areas." [4] Furthermore, the evidence to date has stemmed primarily from examination of trials involving adult participants; no meta-epidemiological studies have focused specifically on pediatric trials. Research in children presents specific methodological and practical challenges, such as generating adequate sample sizes, and use of surrogate outcomes or outcome tools that have not been validated for the pediatric population. [6,7] A meta-epidemiological study to quantify bias in a sample of pediatric trials would better inform the design, conduct, reporting, and interpretation of research in child health.

The goal of this project was to quantify the extent of bias related to specific methodological characteristics in child-relevant RCTs. This will allow for more informed appraisal and application of research findings to patient care, thus providing children with the most appropriate interventions to optimize health outcomes. Our specific objectives were to measure the association between pre-specified methodological characteristics and treatment effect estimates, and explore variations based on different analytic approaches and types of outcomes.

Methods

We conducted a meta-epidemiological study based on a sample of RCTs contributing to the meta-analyses identified within child-relevant systematic reviews (SRs).

Study Sample

The sampling frame was the Cochrane Database of Systematic Reviews (CDSR). As part of ongoing work through the Cochrane Child Health Field, child-relevant SRs in the CDSR are identified. A total of 793 child-relevant SRs were considered for eligibility in the present study. These reviews have been previously described. [8] The CDSR was chosen for the sampling frame because: 1) Cochrane reviews provide tabulated data from the component trials as well as detailed descriptions of key characteristics (e.g., study population); 2) Cochrane reviews provide a detailed list of references for all relevant trials; 3) Cochrane reviews have been reported to be of higher methodological quality[9–13] which may translate into more comprehensive searches, hence more variability with respect to methodological characteristics; 4) the CDSR offers a more homogeneous sample with respect to domains (i.e., therapeutic effectiveness) and study design (i.e., focus on RCTs).

SRs were included if they: 1) contained a minimum of five RCTs[5;14] involving only pediatric patients (ages 0 to 17 years), and a maximum of 40 RCTs, [15] that contribute to at least one meta-analysis; and 2) addressed a question of therapeutic effectiveness. Further, the RCTs in the SRs must have been: superiority studies with parallel designs involving at least two comparison groups; and, reported in "full-length". [16,17] Trials that appeared in more than one meta-analysis were retained in the meta-analysis that was randomly selected. From the full sample of child-relevant SRs, 424 (53%) had no meta-analysis and 302 (38%) had meta-analyses with fewer than five studies. From the remaining 68 systematic reviews, we selected those with the largest numbers of studies included in order to optimize the power to detect differences. In particular, we wanted to optimize the chances of having sufficient numbers of studies with low risk of bias as this was the reference category for the analyses. We know from previous work that the vast majority of pediatric trials are at high or unclear risk of bias. [18,19] We included meta-analyses until we met our intended sample size.

Data Extraction

Data from the meta-analysis that corresponded to the primary outcome in each SR were extracted. For binary outcomes, the numbers in each group with or without the event and the total number in each group were extracted. For continuous outcomes, the mean and standard deviation for each group was extracted. The outcomes were categorized as objective or subjective based on previously reported criteria. [20].

The following methodological characteristics were assessed for each trial: sequence generation; allocation concealment; blinding of study personnel/participants; blinding of outcome assessment; incomplete outcome reporting; selective outcome reporting;

baseline imbalance; trials stopped early for benefit; blocked randomization in unblinded trials; inappropriate influence of trial sponsors; and, sample size. Each methodological characteristic was assessed as high, unclear, or low risk of bias based on guidelines for applying the Cochrane Risk of Bias tool. [3] For selective outcome reporting, we compared the presented results with the outcomes mentioned in the methods section of the same article. [21,22] Sample size was categorized as large (low risk; minimum 200 patients across two groups[1,23,24]) and small (high risk; less than 200 patients).

In addition to the methodological characteristics of interest, the following study characteristics were extracted for each trial: year of publication; publication status; single versus multi-centre; type of intervention; [17] type of control; [4] completeness of outcome reporting; [21] and, source of funding.

A data extraction form and instruction manual were developed to capture study characteristics, methodological characteristics (i.e., risk of bias), and outcome data. The data extraction form was pilot tested by all members of the study team using five trials and revisions were made. One individual independently extracted data from each trial and a second individual checked for completeness and accuracy. Discrepancies were resolved through discussion.

Data Analysis

The RCTs were described in terms of the study characteristics and methodological characteristics listed above using frequencies and percentages.

For continuous data, a standardized mean difference (SMD) was computed for each study and pooled within each meta-analysis. Outcomes were coded such that higher results were undesirable, thus an SMD of less than zero suggests treatment is beneficial. For dichotomous data, endpoints were re-coded, as necessary, so that the outcome occurrence was undesired (e.g., death rather than survival); hence, an odds ratio of less than one suggests that the treatment is beneficial. For each trial, we calculated a log odds ratio and standard error of the odds ratio for the effect of treatment on the binary outcome of interest. [17] Within each meta-analysis results were pooled using a random effects method.

The pooled results of all the meta-analyses were then combined in a "meta-meta" analysis, using an inverse variance random effects method and subgrouped by the different risk of bias components. For dichotomous data, odds ratios were converted to SMDs using the methods proposed by Hasselblad and Hedges [25] in order to allow us to combine both dichotomous and continuous meta-analyses. A "difference of differences" was then computed between the two subgrouped categories (e.g. low versus unclear or high risk of bias) [26] in order to ascertain differences in results based on the various risk of bias components. A priori, we planned a sensitivity analysis comparing studies at low or unclear vs. high risk of bias. We also conducted meta-regression analyses for each risk of bias component with the individual risk of bias categories (high, unclear, low) as independent variables.

Analyses were performed using Review Manager version 5.0 (Nordic Cochrane Centre, The Cochrane Collaboration, Copenhagen) and Stata version 7.0 (Stata Corporation, College Station, Texas). The raw data used for these analyses are available from authors on request.

There are few precedents in the literature for calculating sample sizes in meta-epidemiological studies. [27] Two previous method-ological studies based their sample size on anticipated workload [15] and time constraints. [28] Sample size for another study was based on the sample size used in a previous similar study. [16] We used a pragmatic approach to sample size. The previous meta-epidemiological studies, exclusive of meta-meta-epidemiological

Table 1. Description of meta-analyses included in sample.

Topic area	Intervention type	Comparison type	Outcome	Outcome classification	Number of studies	Year of publication (range)	Single-centre/multi-centre*
Glucocorticoids for croup	Drug	Placebo	Clinical score	Subjective	12	1982–1999	10/2
Antibiotics for the prevention of acute and chronic suppurative otitis media in children	Drug	Placebo	Prevention of AOM or CSOM	Objective	14	1972–2008	6/8
Chemoprophylaxis and intermittent treatment for preventing malaria in children	Drug	Placebo	Clinical malaria	Objective	10	1993–2007	4/6
Immunostimulants for preventing respiratory tract infection in children	Drug	Placebo	Acute respiratory tract infections	Objective	26	1976–2004	10/7
Interventions for educating children who are at risk of asthma-related emergency department attendance	Non-drug	Mixed	ED visits	Objective	17	1986–2006	11/5
Oral versus intravenous rehydration for treating dehydration due to gastroenteritis in children	Non-drug	Active intervention	Failure to rehydrate	Objective	12	1982–1995	10/2
Oral zinc for treating diarrhoea in children	Drug	Mixed (mostly placebo)	Diarrhoea duration	Objective	13	1998–2010	8/5
Polymer-based oral rehydration solution for treating acute water diarrhoea	Non-drug	Active intervention	Diarrhoea duration	Objective	11	1982–2001	11/0
Probiotics for treating acute infectious diarrhoea	Non-drug	Mixed (mostly placebo)	Diarrhoea duration	Objective	33	1994–2009	26/6
Rotavirus vaccine for preventing diarrhoea	Non-drug	Placebo	Episodes of diarrhoea	Objective	19	1987–1997	11/8
School-based secondary prevention programmes for preventing violence	Non-drug	Mixed (mostly no intervention)	Aggression	Subjective	32	1977–2001	14/17
Alarm interventions for nocturnal enuresis in children	Non-drug	No intervention	Nights without bedwetting	Objective	13	1973–2002	12/1
Desmopressin for nocturnal enuresis in children	Drug	Placebo	Nights with bedwetting	Objective	10	1978–2001	1/6
Tricyclic drugs for depression in children and adolescents	Drug	Placebo	Depression	Subjective	12	1981–2001	9/3
Cognitive behavioural therapy for anxiety disorders in children and adolescents	Non-drug	No intervention	Anxiety	Subjective	12	1994–2003	8/4
Fluoride gels for preventing dental caries in children and adolescents	Non-drug	Mixed	D(M)FS increment	Subjective	12	1970–1999	1/9
Fluoride mouth rinses for preventing dental caries in children and adolescents	Non-drug	Mixed (mostly placebo)	D(M)FS increment	Subjective	29	1967–1998	3/23

* where totals do not equal number of studies, the balance of studies did not report this variable.

Table 2. Risk of bias assessments by domain (N = 287).

Domain	Risk of bias assessments – n (%)		
	High	**Unclear**	**Low**
Sequence generation	11 (3.8)	217 (75.6)	59 (20.6)
Allocation concealment	12 (4.2)	226 (78.8)	48 (16.7)
Blinding – participants/personnel	59 (20.6)	132 (46.0)	105 (36.6)
Blinding – outcome assessment	24 (8.4)	111 (38.7)	152 (53.0)
Incomplete data	37 (12.9)	103 (35.9)	141 (49.1)
Selective outcome reporting	40 (13.9)	53 (18.5)	194 (67.6)
Other sources of bias	32 (11.2)	93 (32.4)	162 (56.5)
Overall risk of bias	134 (46.7)	144 (50.2)	9 (3.1)
Funding	8 (2.8)	154 (53.7)	125 (43.6)
Baseline imbalance	13 (4.5)	88 (30.7)	186 (64.8)
Blocked randomization	20 (7.0)	16 (5.6)	22 (7.7)
Early stopping for benefit	2 (0.7)	1 (0.4)	2 (0.7)

research, had sample sizes ranging from 127 to 523 trials (median 220, inter-quartile range 158, 282) from 11 to 48 SRs (median 20, inter-quartile range 14, 32). [17] Therefore, we planned for a sample size of 300 trials.

Results

Meta-analyses from 17 SRs, comprising 287 studies, were included in the study sample (Table 1). The SRs covered a range of topics which included both drug (n = 7) and non-drug (n = 10) interventions. Comparisons also varied and included placebo or no intervention (n = 9), another active intervention (n = 2), or mixed comparators (n = 6). The outcomes were considered objective in 11 and subjective in 6 of the included meta-analyses. The number of studies included in the meta-analyses ranged from 10 to 32 with a median of 13. 155 RCTs were conducted at a single center, 112 were conducted at multiple centers, and in 20 trials the number of centers was not reported or was unclear. The majority of trials were published (97%) and year of publication ranged from 1965 to 2010 (median 1995). Sources of funding for the trials included: government (n = 73), pharmaceutical industry (n = 33), multiple sources (n = 29), other (n = 7), and unclear or not reported (n = 131).

The methodological quality or risk of bias of the included trials is described in Table 2. The majority of trials were unclear for sequence generation (76%) and allocation concealment (79%). Two-thirds of studies were high or unclear risk for blinding of participants and personnel; approximately half were high or unclear risk for blinding of outcome assessment. The majority of studies were considered low risk for incomplete outcome data, selective outcome reporting, and other sources of bias. Less than half of trials were low risk for source of funding. The majority of trials were low risk for bias associated with baseline imbalances. Among 58 trials that used blocked randomization, there was an equal distribution among high, unclear, and low risk of bias. Five trials reported stopping early for benefit and there was an equal distribution across risk of bias categories.

Table 3 summarizes the results of the meta-epidemiological analyses based on the combined data from all meta-analyses,

including dichotomous and continuous outcomes. No significant differences were observed between trials that were high or unclear versus low risk of bias for any of the domains examined. Results were consistent when examined by type of outcome (i.e., dichotomous and continuous). We conducted a sensitivity analysis examining trials grouped as high risk vs. unclear or low and no differences were found (Table S1 in Appendix S1). Post hoc, based on comments from a peer-reviewer, we conducted sensitivity analyses for high vs. low risk of bias and found no differences (Table S2 in Appendix S1). We conducted meta-regression using the three categories of bias as independent variables and again found no significant differences in effect estimates. Table S3 in Appendix S1 shows results for subgroup analyses based on type of intervention (drug vs. non-drug), type of comparison (placebo/standard care vs. another active intervention), and type of outcome (objective vs. subjective). There were no notable differences within the subgroups between studies at high or unclear versus low risk of bias. Specifically for subgrouping by objective and subjective outcomes, no differences were found between high/unclear and low risk of bias studies for any domain: sequence generation (-0.08 [95% CI -0.71, 0.43] vs. -0.07 [-0.32, 0.17]), allocation concealment (0.25 [-0.06, 0.56] vs. -0.16 [-0.39, 0.06]), blinding of participants/personnel (0.10 [-0.05, 0.24] vs. -0.06 [-0.17, 0.06]), blinding of outcome assessment (0.08 [-0.10, 0.25] vs. 0.07 [-0.18, 0.05]), incomplete outcome data (-0.07 [-0.30, 0.17] vs. -0.15 [-0.43, 0.13]), selective outcome reporting (-0.04 [-0.21, 0.12] vs. -0.08 [-0.20, 0.05]), other sources of bias (0.11 [-0.10, 0.32] vs. -0.08 [-0.32, 0.16]), baseline imbalance (-0.02 [-0.39, 0.35] vs. -0.07 [-0.31, 0.17]), and funding (0.02 [-0.20, 0.24] vs. 0.04 [-0.20, 0.29]).

Discussion

There is a growing body of empirical evidence that aims to quantify the association between different methodological characteristics of randomized trials and treatment effect estimates; however, differences have been found among studies. Some of this variation has been attributed to differences across clinical areas, while another explanation for lack of significant findings or inconsistent findings has been insufficient sample sizes to adequately detect differences. This is the first study to our knowledge that has attempted to quantify bias in a sample of pediatric-only trials. We found no differences in effect estimates based on any of the methodological characteristics that we examined.

The characteristics we examined form the basis for tools that are well-accepted for assessing methodological quality or risk of bias of randomized trials in SRs. However, there is variation in how SR authors handle risk of bias assessments; some may choose to exclude studies outright from a review or meta-analysis based on risk of bias. [29] Given that we did not find any significant differences in effect estimates, we would recommend that trials not be excluded from SRs and/or meta-analyses based on high or unclear risk of bias assessments. Rather, risk of bias should be explored as a potential source of heterogeneity where there is substantial variation observed in effect estimates across studies. Further, the body of evidence being reviewed should be discussed in light of potential methodological weaknesses; however, dismissing large bodies of evidence (for example, all trials without blinding) will severely limit our ability to make recommendations for pediatric care.

Our recommendation not to exclude studies from meta-analyses based on risk of bias is consistent with conclusions from a recently published study reporting on a combined analysis of meta-

Table 3. Results of meta-epidemiological analysis of bias items and treatment effect estimates.

Domain	Difference of standardized mean differences	95% CI
Sequence generation	−0.07	−0.22, 0.08
Allocation concealment	0.09	−0.15, 0.33
Blinding (participants/personnel)	0.00	−0.09, 0.09
Blinding (outcome assessment)	−0.00	−0.11, 0.11
Incomplete outcome data	−0.09	−0.26, 0.07
Selective outcome reporting	−0.06	−0.15, 0.04
Other sources of bias	0.05	−0.09, 0.20
Baseline imbalance	−0.07	−0.28, 0.14
Early stopping for benefit	−0.17	−0.49, 0.14
Blocked randomization in unblinded trials	−0.18	−0.47, 0.11
Funding	0.02	−0.13, 0.18

epidemiological studies. [26,30] The study examined the influence of sequence generation, allocation concealment, and double-blinding on effect estimates and between-trial heterogeneity based on 1,973 trials included in 234 meta-analyses. The authors found that the methodological characteristics examined were associated with exaggerated treatment effects and increased between-trial heterogeneity. Specifically, the study found exaggerated effect estimates in trials with inadequate or unclear sequence generation (ratio of odds ratio 0.89, 95% credible interval 0.82 to 0.96), allocation concealment (ROR 0.93, 95% CrI 0.87 to 0.99), and double-blinding (ROR 0.87, 95% CrI 0.79 to 0.96). However, when examined by type of outcome (subjective and objective), the results remained significant only for subjective outcomes suggesting an average exaggeration in treatment effect of 17% for sequence generation (CrI 0.74 to 0.94), 15% for allocation concealment (CrI 0.75 to 0.95), and 22% for double-blinding (CrI 0.65 to 0.92). The results were not statistically significant for mortality or other objective outcomes. The authors proposed down-weighting trials at high risk of bias in meta-analyses rather than excluding them completely which results in loss of precision.

Excluding trials completely from an analysis due to risk of bias could leave very little evidence for decision-making. Consistent with previous research, we found that a high proportion of our sample of trials was at high or unclear risk of bias for many domains. [18,19] Further, only 3% were considered low risk of bias overall which is similar to other reported samples of pediatric trials. [18] Other samples of adult only trials have also found the majority of studies to be at high or unclear risk of bias overall. [31] From an epidemiological perspective, there may be no difference in how typical biases (e.g., selection, performance, detection, attrition, reporting) operate in trials based on population characteristics. Moreover, a recent standard, developed by the international organization StaR Child Health, for minimizing risk of bias in pediatric trials could be equally applied to any trial. [32] Consistent with Savovic et al's findings, other features may be more salient in assessing possible bias such as choice of outcomes (subjective vs. objective).

There are several limitations to note with the present study. The RCTs included in this study were parallel, superiority design. This may limit the generalizability to other types of trials; however, superiority trials are most common in the scientific literature. The median year of publication in this sample was 1995. Results may differ with more recent trials; however, this does not invalidate the present findings. Newer studies may add to the number of trials assessed as low risk of bias and increase statistical power for the analyses. We based the sample size for the present study on other similar studies; however, this may have limited our ability to identify statistically significant differences. Moreover, Savovic et al. found significant associations primarily in the context of subjective outcomes which represented only a portion of our sample. [26,30] One of the driving factors for imprecision in the present study was the small number of studies in the low risk of bias (or reference) category. This problem is accentuated for blinding in studies with subjective outcomes.

In summary, we found no significant differences in effect estimates of pediatric randomized trials based on key methodological characteristics. Based on these findings, we recommend that trials not be excluded from SRs and/or meta-analyses based on risk of bias. Rather potential for bias due to methodological characteristics should be considered when exploring heterogeneity and interpreting results.

Supporting Information

Appendix S1   Includes Tables S1–S3. -Table S1. Results of meta-epidemiological analysis of bias items and treatment effect estimates based on sensitivity analyses comparing low/unclear versus high risk of bias. -Table S2. Results of meta-epidemiological analysis of bias items and treatment effect estimates based on sensitivity analyses comparing low versus high risk of bias. -Table S3. Results of meta-meta-analysis of bias items and treatment effect estimates, by sub-groups.

Acknowledgments

We thank Annabritt Chisholm, Dion Pasichnyk, Marta Oleszczuk, and Elizabeth Schellenberg-Sumamo for assisting with quality assessment and data extraction.

Author Contributions

Conceived and designed the experiments: LH MPH RMF DMD BV. Performed the experiments: LH MPH. Analyzed the data: LH BV. Wrote the paper: LH. Edited manuscript: MPH RMF DMD BV.

References

1. Schulz KF, Grimes DA (2002) Generation of allocation sequences in randomised trials: chance, not choice. Lancet 359: 515–519.
2. Sterne JA, Juni P, Schulz KF, Altman DG, Bartlett C, et al. (2002) Statistical methods for assessing the influence of study characteristics on treatment effects in 'meta-epidemiological' research. Stat Med 21: 1513–1524.
3. Higgins JPT, Green S (2008) Cochrane Handbook for Systematic Reviews of Interventions Version 5.0.0 [updated February 2008]. The Cochrane Collaboration.
4. Balk EM, Bonis PA, Moskowitz H, Schmid CH, Ioannidis JP, et al. (2002) Correlation of quality measures with estimates of treatment effect in meta-analyses of randomized controlled trials. JAMA 287: 2973–2982.
5. Egger M, Juni P, Bartlett C, Holenstein F, Sterne J (2003) How important are comprehensive literature searches and the assessment of trial quality in systematic reviews? Empirical study. Health Technol Assess 7: 1–76.
6. Klassen TP, Hartling L, Hamm M, van der Lee JH, Ursum J, et al. (2009) StaR Child Health: an initiative for RCTs in children. Lancet 374: 1310–1312.
7. Klassen TP, Hartling L, Craig JC, Offringa M (2008) Children are not just small adults: the urgent need for high-quality trial evidence in children. PLoS Med 5: e172.
8. Bow S, Klassen J, Chisholm A, Tjosvold L, Thomson D, et al. (2010) A descriptive analysis of child-relevant systematic reviews in the Cochrane Database of Systematic Reviews. BMC Pediatr;10: 34.
9. Moseley AM, Elkins MR, Herbert RD, Maher CG, Sherrington C (2009) Cochrane reviews used more rigorous methods than non-Cochrane reviews: survey of systematic reviews in physiotherapy. J Clin Epidemiol 62: 1021–1030.
10. Tricco AC, Tetzlaff J, Pham B, Brehaut J, Moher D (2009) Non-Cochrane vs. Cochrane reviews were twice as likely to have positive conclusion statements: cross-sectional study. J Clin Epidemiol 62: 380–386.
11. Sheikh L, Johnston S, Thangaratinam S, Kilby MD, Khan KS (2007) A review of the methodological features of systematic reviews in maternal medicine. BMC Med 5: 10.
12. Moher D, Tetzlaff J, Tricco AC, Sampson M, Altman DG (2007) Epidemiology and reporting characteristics of systematic reviews. PLoS Med 4: e78.
13. Collier A, Heilig L, Schilling L, Williams H, Dellavalle RP (2006) Cochrane Skin Group systematic reviews are more methodologically rigorous than other systematic reviews in dermatology. Br J Dermatol 155: 1230–1235.
14. Clarke M (2002) Commentary: searching for trials for systematic reviews: what difference does it make? Int J Epidemiol 31: 123–124.
15. Pildal J, Hrobjartsson A, Jorgensen KJ, Hilden J, Altman DG, et al (2007) Impact of allocation concealment on conclusions drawn from meta-analyses of randomized trials. Int J Epidemiol 36: 847–857.
16. Kjaergard LL, Villumsen J, Gluud C (2001) Reported methodologic quality and discrepancies between large and small randomized trials in meta-analyses. Ann Intern Med 135: 982–989.
17. Siersma V, ls-Nielsen B, Chen W, Hilden J, Gluud LL, et al. (2007) Multivariable modelling for meta-epidemiological assessment of the association between trial quality and treatment effects estimated in randomized clinical trials. Stat Med 26: 2745–2758.
18. Hartling L, Ospina M, Liang Y, Dryden DM, Hooton N, et al. (2009) Risk of bias versus quality assessment of randomised controlled trials: cross sectional study. BMJ 339: b4012.
19. Hamm MP, Hartling L, Milne A, Tjosvold L, Vandermeer B, et al. (2010) A descriptive analysis of a representative sample of pediatric randomized controlled trials published in 2007. BMC Pediatr 10: 96.
20. Wood L, Egger M, Gluud LL, Schulz KF, Juni P, et al. (2008) Empirical evidence of bias in treatment effect estimates in controlled trials with different interventions and outcomes: meta-epidemiological study. BMJ 336: 601–605.
21. Chan AW, Hrobjartsson A, Haahr MT, Gotzsche PC, Altman DG (2004) Empirical evidence for selective reporting of outcomes in randomized trials: comparison of protocols to published articles. JAMA 291: 2457–2465.
22. Chan AW, Altman DG (2005) Identifying outcome reporting bias in randomised trials on PubMed: review of publications and survey of authors. BMJ 330: 753.
23. Juni P, Nuesch E, Reichenbach S, Rutjes A, Scherrer M, et al. (2008) Overestimation of treatment effects associated with small sample size in osteoarthritis research. Z Evid Fortbild Qual Gesundhwes 102: 62.
24. Lachin JM (1988) Properties of simple randomization in clinical trials. Control Clin Trials 9: 312–326.
25. Hasselblad V, Hedges LV (1995) Meta-analysis of screening and diagnostic tests. Psychol Bull 117: 167–178.
26. Savovic J, Jones H, Altman D, Harris R, Juni P, et al. (2012) Influence of reported study design characteristics on intervention effect estimates from randomised controlled trials: combined analysis of meta-epidemiological studies. Health Technol Assess 16: 1–82.
27. Furukawa TA, Watanabe N, Omori IM, Montori VM, Guyatt GH (2007) Association between unreported outcomes and effect size estimates in Cochrane meta-analyses. JAMA 297: 468–470.
28. Marshall M, Lockwood A, Bradley C, Adams C, Joy C, et al. (2000) Unpublished rating scales: a major source of bias in randomised controlled trials of treatments for schizophrenia. Br J Psychiatry 176: 249–252.
29. McDonagh M, Peterson K, Raina P, Chang S, Shekelle P (2013) Avoiding bias in selecting studies. Methods Guide for Comparative Effectiveness Reviews. AHRQ Publication No. 13-EHC045-EF. Rockville, MD. Agency for Healthcare Research and Quality.
30. Savovic J, Jones HE, Altman DG, Harris RJ, Juni P, et al. (2012) Influence of reported study design characteristics on intervention effect estimates from randomized, controlled trials. Ann Intern Med 157: 429–38.
31. Hartling L, Hamm MP, Milne A, Vandermeer B, Santaguida PL, et al. (2013) Testing the risk of bias tool showed low reliability between individual reviewers and across consensus assessments of reviewer pairs. J Clin Epidemiol 66: 973–81.
32. Hartling L, Hamm M, Klassen T, Chan AW, Meremikwu M, et al. (2012) Standard 2: containing risk of bias. Pediatrics 129 Suppl 3: S124–S131.

4

Using Informatics and the Electronic Medical Record to Describe Antimicrobial use in the Clinical Management of Diarrhea Cases at 12 Companion Animal Practices

R. Michele Anholt[1]*, John Berezowski[2], Carl S. Ribble[1,3], Margaret L. Russell[4], Craig Stephen[1,3]

1 Faculty of Veterinary Medicine, University of Calgary, Calgary, Alberta, Canada, 2 Veterinary Public Health Institute, University of Bern, Bern, Switzerland, 3 Centre for Coastal Health, Nanaimo, British Columbia, Canada, 4 Community Health Sciences, University of Calgary, Calgary, Alberta, Canada

Abstract

Antimicrobial drugs may be used to treat diarrheal illness in companion animals. It is important to monitor antimicrobial use to better understand trends and patterns in antimicrobial resistance. There is no monitoring of antimicrobial use in companion animals in Canada. To explore how the use of electronic medical records could contribute to the ongoing, systematic collection of antimicrobial use data in companion animals, anonymized electronic medical records were extracted from 12 participating companion animal practices and warehoused at the University of Calgary. We used the pre-diagnostic, clinical features of diarrhea as the case definition in this study. Using text-mining technologies, cases of diarrhea were described by each of the following variables: diagnostic laboratory tests performed, the etiological diagnosis and antimicrobial therapies. The ability of the text miner to accurately describe the cases for each of the variables was evaluated. It could not reliably classify cases in terms of diagnostic tests or etiological diagnosis; a manual review of a random sample of 500 diarrhea cases determined that 88/500 (17.6%) of the target cases underwent diagnostic testing of which 36/88 (40.9%) had an etiological diagnosis. Text mining, compared to a human reviewer, could accurately identify cases that had been treated with antimicrobials with high sensitivity (92%, 95% confidence interval, 88.1%–95.4%) and specificity (85%, 95% confidence interval, 80.2%–89.1%). Overall, 7400/15,928 (46.5%) of pets presenting with diarrhea were treated with antimicrobials. Some temporal trends and patterns of the antimicrobial use are described. The results from this study suggest that informatics and the electronic medical records could be useful for monitoring trends in antimicrobial use.

Editor: Herman Tse, The University of Hong Kong, Hong Kong

Funding: This research was partially funded by the University of Calgary (www.ucalgary.ca) and The Centre for Coastal Health (www.centreforcoastalhealth.ca). The funders had no role in study design, data collection and analysis, decision to publish, or preparation of the manuscript.

Competing Interests: The authors have declared that no competing interests exist.

* Email: rmanholt@ucalgary.ca

Introduction

Diarrhea is a common clinical presentation in companion animals [1]. The pathophysiology of diarrhea is complex, poorly understood and can involve a wide array of infectious and non-infectious etiologies [2,3]. Clinical evaluation of ill animals directs the selection of diagnostic procedures such as parasite studies, microbiological examinations and/or toxin testing. Clinicians must weigh the cost of diagnostic procedures, the owner's willingness to pay for them and the time spent waiting for a result against the likelihood that the results of a diagnostic test will affect their therapeutic recommendations. This cost-benefit analysis often results in diarrhea in pets being managed by empirical therapy with antihelmintics and antimicrobials [4].

Infectious disease specialists advocate restricting antimicrobial use (AMU) to cases where there is evidence that AMU will result in improved clinical outcomes [3,5,6]. Warnings against indiscriminate AMU in animals are increasing because the consequences of AMU include antimicrobial resistance (AMR) with decreased efficacy of important antimicrobials against significant animal and human pathogens [7,8]. In their closely shared environment, pets may be a source of antimicrobial resistant enteric bacteria or resistance genes for their owners [9–11].

Understanding the clinical management of common veterinary problems and patterns of AMU may provide the necessary exposure information to help interpret AMR trends, identify potential problem areas in prescribing practices and provide evidence-based practice guidelines for practitioners [12–16]. Collecting clinical management and AMU data at the veterinary patient level has not been legislated in Canada and remains a challenge in veterinary medicine in Canada [11,17,18].

The uptake of the electronic medical record (EMR) by companion animal practitioners provides an opportunity for accessing case management and AMU data. Informatics is "the application of information and computer science technology to public health practice, research and learning" [19]. Informatics has been applied elsewhere to text-based clinical records to describe disease-drug associations by physicians [20]. In this paper we used the EMR's from a participating practice network and explored text mining for accessing and analyzing the textual orders for diagnostic testing and AMU in the medical records.

The objectives of this study were to:

1. Apply and evaluate text-mining technology of EMR's to characterize the clinical management of diarrhea cases by companion animal veterinarians in a network of participating veterinary practices.
2. Describe the diagnostic management of diarrhea in companion animals and the proportion of cases for which there was documented evidence of an infectious process.
3. Describe the use of antimicrobials in the management of diarrhea cases.
4. Describe the temporal patterns of the use for each antimicrobial class used in the treatment of diarrhea cases for a 4 year period (January 1, 2007 to December 31, 2010).

Materials and Methods

Study area and data

The study area included 6 communities in the province of Alberta, Canada including: Calgary, Cochrane, Airdrie, Chestermere, Strathmore and Okotoks. A survey of all of the companion animal practices in the study area identified the practices that had completely computerized medical records and the same veterinary practice management software. Twelve of the 20 eligible practices agreed to participate in this project; a sample of convenience. A data sharing agreement was signed by each of the practice's managing partners and the author (Anholt). Approval from the University of Calgary Conjoint Faculties Research Ethics Board did not require permission from the pet owners.

A custom-built data extraction program was used to extract the anonymized electronic medical records (n = 428,783) from the veterinary practice management programs from January 1, 2007 to December 31, 2010. All records were stored in a secure data warehouse at the University of Calgary. The appointment schedule, medical notes (history, clinical exam, interpretations of diagnostic tests, assessment, differential diagnoses, and treatment) and prescription data for each case were combined into one free-text variable named 'Note', in the data file. Data was stored and managed using Microsoft Office Excel 2007 (Microsoft Corporation, Redmond, Washington) and Konstanz Information Miner 2.2.2 (Knime, http://www.knime.org). The features of the participating practices, data extraction and management of the warehoused data have been described elsewhere [21].

Linguistics-based text-mining software (QDAMiner3.1/Word-Stat6, Provalis Research, Montreal, QC), was used in this study. Text, in the form of individual words or phrases was organized into categorization dictionaries which were used to identify and retrieve cases. A categorization dictionary was applied to the 'Note' variable in the warehoused records to identify and retrieve records that met the case definition of any companion animal species (dog, cat, small mammal, bird, reptile) with clinical diarrhea or a description of feces consistent with diarrhea (n = 18,827 records). The case definition and the development, optimization and validation of the text miner to identify and retrieve records of diarrhea is further described in Anholt et al.[22].

Each of the 18,827 records represented a uniquely identified patient classified as having diarrhea, seen at a participating practice on a recorded date. After the initial visit, animals may have been hospitalized, returned for re-examination or there may have been a telephone consultation with the owners for the same complaint. To minimize repeated counts of the same case of diarrhea, all records of veterinary utilization (consultations, hospitalizations, laboratory results) for the same animal within 14 days of the initial visit were combined to represent one diarrhea case. There were 15,928 diarrhea cases in this study.

Development of the categorization dictionary in the text miner

Text mining was used to identify and retrieve cases for which one or more of the following activities were recorded:

- diagnostic testing had been performed.
- an etiological diagnosis had been made.
- treatment with an antimicrobial had been initiated.

Case definitions were developed for diagnostic testing and etiological diagnoses to classify cases using the text miner and also by an external reviewer. For classification purposes a diagnostic test was a laboratory test that could either be performed in the practice by the animal health technologist or sent to an external veterinary laboratory. A case was classified as positive for diagnostic testing if any of the following diagnostic tests were recorded within the variable 'Note':

- Fecal flotations and fecal smears and using light microscopy that provided a morphological diagnosis of helminths, protozoa or bacteria.
- Enzyme-linked immunosorbent (ELISA) assays to identify canine parvovirus or *Giardia* spp. infections from fecal samples.
- Real time PCR tests were performed to screen fecal samples for canine distemper virus, canine coronavirus, canine parvovirus, *Clostridium perfringens* enterotoxin A, *Cryptosporidium* spp. *Giardia* spp., *Salmonella* spp., feline coronavirus, feline panleukopenia, *Toxoplasma gondii*, and *Tritrichomonas foetus*.
- Fecal bacteria culture was performed.

A case was classified as positive for etiologic diagnosis if a positive outcome for any of the diagnostic tests described above was recorded. The positive classification included imprecise morphological diagnoses of bacterial infections such as bacterial overgrowth and *Campylobacter*-type spp. as recorded by a veterinarian or technician.

Positive antimicrobial use cases were defined as those diarrhea cases that were administered, dispensed or prescribed antimicrobials for the management of the diarrhea signs.

To calculate the number of diarrhea cases required to assess the ability of the text miner to accurately classify the cases by each management activity (diagnostic testing, etiological diagnosis and antimicrobial treatment), the assumptions of the precision-based sample size calculation were: i) significance level, 0.05, ii) *a priori* estimate of the proportion, conservatively = 0.5, iii) precision = 0.1. The calculated number of cases positive for each activity required in the sample was 96. To reach the target of 96 positive cases in the sample required an estimate of the proportion of cases that would be positive for each activity. This was unknown and was expected to differ for each activity so a proportion of 0.20 was selected. The number of controls required was calculated using, $N_{controls} = N_{Cases}(1-Prev/Prev) = 384$ controls +96 cases = 480 [23]. A sample of 500 records was randomly selected from the entire file of 15,928 diarrhea cases.

An experienced veterinarian clinician, blinded to the results of the text miner, reviewed all of the information contained in the extracted EMR's for the sample of 500 cases. The clinician reviewer classified each case as positive or negative for each of: i) laboratory diagnostics performed; ii) etiological diagnosis made; and iii) antimicrobial treatment. This served as the external standard.

We cross-tabulated the dichotomous results from the text miner and the external standard. The results for each case definition were summarized as the sensitivity and the specificity of the text miner's ability to correctly classify cases. The 95% confidence intervals for the sensitivity and specificity were also calculated (Exact method, Stata/IC 10.0, StataCorp, College Station, Tx). The cases that were improperly classified (false positives and false negatives) were reviewed to determine why they had been misclassified and if there were any opportunities to improve the text-mining classifier.

The sample of 500 diarrhea positive cases was categorized into three categories: i) no diagnostic testing performed, ii) diagnostic testing performed with a negative result or no result recorded; and iii) diagnostic testing performed with a positive diagnosis. Within each of the 3 categories the proportion of patients that were managed with antimicrobials was determined. Odds ratios (OR) and their 95% confidence intervals (CI) were used to quantify the difference between the odds of cases within each category receiving antimicrobials.

Antimicrobial use trends

The text miner's categorization dictionary for antimicrobial use (described above) was then applied to all of the 15,928 diarrhea cases to classify cases that had been administered, dispensed or prescribed antimicrobials. Antimicrobial use was described by the class of antimicrobial used and by Health Canada's categorization of antimicrobial drugs based on importance to human medicine [24]. Co-occurrences of antimicrobial use were identified by the text miner and the antimicrobials used in combination were described.

We examined the temporal trends of the Category I (very high importance in human medicine) and Category II (high importance in human medicine) antimicrobials [24] for the 4 years of the study. For each month of the study, we determined the proportion of cases that had been treated with any antimicrobial and the proportions treated with each class of antimicrobial. The temporal trend for all antimicrobials combined and for each antimicrobial was examined by fitting a linear regression model to the data. The number of antimicrobial treated cases, normalized by the total number of diarrhea cases for each month, was the dependent variable and the month/year was the independent variable. If the antimicrobial use data fit the slope estimated by the linear regression (p<0.05), the proportions of cases treated with this antimicrobial were plotted as a function of time [25]. Further exploratory data analysis included data smoothing by: i) pooling

the number of cases treated with each class of antimicrobial in each quarter of each year; and ii) plotting the results in scatterplots with quadratic overlays (Stata/IC 10.0).

Results

Text mining

Estimates of the text miner's ability to distinguish between cases that had diagnostic testing performed (sensitivity = 70% and specificity = 85.1%) and which had an etiological diagnosis made (sensitivity = 72.4% and specificity = 97.4), were relatively low. There were wide confidence intervals around sensitivity which indicated poor precision of the estimate (Table 1, Table 2). The primary reason the text miner performed poorly when classifying these cases was that the context was relevant to the classification of the case. For example, the word "parvo" was associated with a diagnosis, a differential diagnosis, a past diagnosis, a diagnostic test, a serological titer, a vaccine, and a recommendation or a warning to owners. Despite repeated efforts, it was not possible to improve the performance of the text miner to classify cases by the diagnostic test performed or their etiological diagnosis, so the text miner was not used for these purposes.

In contrast, text mining classified cases that had been treated with an antimicrobial with high sensitivity (92.3%) and specificity (85%) when compared to a human reviewer (Table 3). The text miner misclassified cases if the name of the antimicrobial was not provided or improperly spelled, if the record contained information about past treatment or future considerations for treatment or if the pet was receiving antimicrobials but they were being used to treat a co-morbidity (not dispensed for diarrhea). Given the high sensitivity and specificity of the text miner for classifying cases with respect to antimicrobial use, it was used for the remainder of the analysis.

Diagnostic testing, diagnoses and antimicrobial use

As the text miner did not accurately classify cases that had laboratory testing performed or a diagnosis made, the results presented are from the manual review of the sample of 500 diarrhea positive cases only. The remaining diarrhea cases were not described by their diagnostic testing or etiological diagnosis. There were 88 cases (17.6%) in the sample of 500 diarrhea positive cases tested to identify an etiological diagnosis (Figure 1, Table 4). Fecal examinations (smears and/or floats) were performed in 56 of the 88 (63.6%) cases that underwent diagnostic testing; ELISA assays were run on 58 (65.9%) cases to identify canine parvovirus or *Giardia* spp.; multiple testing using a combination of fecal exams and ELISA tests was documented in 29 (33%) of those tested. Fecal cultures or PCR tests were each ordered in 1 (1.1%) and 3 (3.4%) of the cases respectively; all of which were negative. Thirty-six cases (40.9% of those tested, 7.2% of all cases) had a

Table 1. From a random sample of 500 companion animal cases of diarrhea, the accuracy of the text miner for classifying the cases as positive or negative for *'had diagnostic testing'* when compared to a manual review of the medical records serving as the external standard.

	External standard +	External standard -	Sum
Text miner +	63	61	124
Text miner -	27	349	376
Sum	90	410	500
	Sensitivity = 70.0% (95%CI, 59.4% - 79.2%)	Specificity = 85.1% (95%CI, 81.3% - 88.4%)	

Table 2. From a random sample of 500 companion animal cases of diarrhea, the accuracy of the text miner for classifying the cases as positive or negative for *'had an etiological diagnosis made'* when compared to a manual review of the medical records serving as the external standard.

	External standard +	External standard -	Sum
Text miner +	21	17	38
Text miner -	8	454	462
Sum	29	466	500
	Sensitivity = 72.4% (95%CI, 52.8%–87.3%)	Specificity = 97.4% (95%CI, 95.5%–98.7%)	

stated etiologic diagnosis in the EMR; all were prescribed an antihelmintic or antimicrobial medication. We inferred that given the management of cases with a positive result, that the veterinarians considered the findings to be relevant.

Patients that had diagnostic procedures performed had more antimicrobials administered, dispensed or prescribed (72.7%) than patients that had no diagnostic testing performed (41%) (OR = 3.8; 95% CI 2.2–6.7). There was little difference in the proportion of patients that were treated with antimicrobials and had a positive diagnostic test and those treated with antimicrobials and a negative diagnostic test (OR = 1.2, 95% CI 0.4–3.6) (Figure 1). Two hundred and thirty-three of the 500 diarrhea cases (46.6%) received antimicrobials; none of the cases receiving antimicrobials were culture positive for bacteria (Figure 1, Table 4).

Text mining of the diarrhea cases (n = 15,928) identified 7400 (46.5%) cases that were administered, dispensed or prescribed antimicrobials. There were 8041 occurrences of AMU in the 7400 cases. The distribution of the antimicrobial classes used in the management of diarrhea positive cases is summarized in Table 5. Category 1 (very high importance to human health) antimicrobials were prescribed in most (87.1%) of the antimicrobial-treated diarrhea cases. Veterinarians prescribed more than one antimicrobial in 641 (8.7%) of all cases treated with an antimicrobial. Nitroimidazole plus a penicillin was the most frequent treatment combination (n = 346) followed by nitroimidazole together with first and second generation cephalosporins (n = 79), penicillins with fluorquinolones (n = 67), and nitroimidazoles in combination with fluorquinolones (n = 66).

Antimicrobial use temporal trends

The linear regression analyses of 'all antimicrobials' (n = 7400), 'nitroimidazole' (n = 5814) and 'penicillin' (n = 808) were significant (p<0.05) and these variables were plotted against time (Figure 2). The graph and the slope coefficients (0.0002 to 0.0004) indicate a very small statistically significant, upward trend in the proportions of diarrhea cases treated with any antimicrobial and

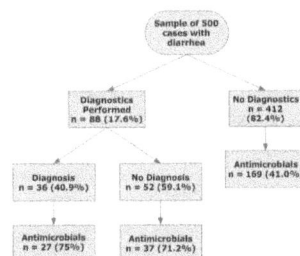

Figure 1. From a random sample of 500 companion animal cases with diarrhea, a flow diagram describing the proportion of cases that had laboratory diagnostics performed, had an etiological diagnosis made, and were administered, prescribed or dispensed antimicrobials.

treated with nitroimidazoles and penicillins. The regression analyses of the remaining antimicrobials were not statistically significant.

Smoothed scatterplots of the quarterly counts of cases treated with $3^{rd}/4^{th}$ generation cephalosporins and the penicillin β-lactamase inhibitor combinations showed patterns of antimicrobial use that were mirror images of each other (Figure 3). Scatterplots of the remaining antimicrobial class combinations did not show any recognizable patterns.

Discussion

Results of the text mining methods used in this study varied depending on the variable of interest. Text mining results for AMU were relatively accurate because the documentation of antimicrobial treatments by veterinarians was usually explicit and unambiguous; the meaning of the words did not depend upon the context in which they were used. However, the language used to

Table 3. From a random sample of 500 companion animal cases of diarrhea, the accuracy of the text miner for classifying the cases as positive or negative for *'had an antimicrobial administered, dispensed or prescribed'* when compared to a manual review of the medical records serving as the external standard.

	External standard +	External standard -	Sum
Text miner +	215	40	255
Text miner -	18	227	245
Sum	233	267	500
	Sensitivity = 92.3% (95%CI, 88.1%–95.4%)	Specificity = 85.0% (95%CI, 80.2%–89.1%)	

Table 4. Distribution of a sample of companion animal cases with diarrhea by the stated etiological diagnosis (n = 500).

Diagnosis	Number of cases (% of 500 cases)	% of diagnosed cases	Diagnostic test
All	36 (7.2)	-	
Helminths	1 (0.2)	2.7	Morphology
Coccidia	5 (1.0)	13.9	Morphology
Bacterial overgrowth	9 (1.8)	25	Morphology
Campylobacter-type	1 (0.2)	2.8	Morphology
Canine parvovirus	9 (1.8)	25.0	ELISA
Giardia spp.	11 (2.2)	30.6	Morphology or ELISA

record diagnostic procedures and diagnoses was highly context specific and the linguistic-based text mining approach used in this study was unable to discriminate between the various meanings. It is possible that trained or rule-based text-mining software could more accurately distinguish these cases and is an area for future study [26,27].

Most cases of acute (less than 14 days) diarrhea are mild and self-limiting and supportive treatment without a diagnosis is considered appropriate [2]. Therefore, it was not unexpected that less than 18% of the diarrhea cases in our study had diagnostic procedures performed. The recommended initial diagnostic approach to acute diarrhea is a fecal exam [28]. More than half of the diagnostic procedures in our study were fecal flotation and/ or fecal smears. In animals with severe disease (febrile, dehydrated, hemorrhagic or persistent diarrhea) further efforts at establishing an etiological diagnosis are warranted [2,28]. Animals in this study that were subjected to diagnostic laboratory testing were more likely to be given antimicrobials than those that were not tested regardless of the test results. This may indicate an assessment of more severe disease by the veterinarian although this judgment was not often explicitly stated in the medical record. Despite efforts

to identify an etiological agent, a positive diagnosis was established in less than half of the cases undergoing diagnostic testing.

Giardiasis was the most frequent diagnosis in this study and antimicrobial treatment is usually recommended in *Giardia*-positive diarrheic animals [29]. However, *Giardia* spp. is commonly misdiagnosed in veterinary practice and most cases are self-limiting [30]. Antimicrobials are also recommended in the management of diarrhea in companion animals if there is a positive diagnosis of secondary bacterial overgrowth associated with inflammatory bowel disease or culture-confirmed primary bacterial infections of *Salmonella*, *Campylobacter*, *Clostridium* and enterotoxigenic *E. coli* [2,4,5,29], if there is evidence of a breach in the mucosal integrity of the intestines (hemorrhagic diarrhea), or to manage the immunosuppressive effects of parvovirus [2,4,5,28,29]. Other authors argue that while antimicrobials are commonly used in cases with a confirmed culture or if there is evidence of hematochezia, there is little objective information as to whether they are needed in all cases [3,5].

Our findings indicated that veterinarians commonly prescribed antimicrobials for diarrhea without any documentation that the

Table 5. Distribution of antimicrobials used by the veterinary practices in the treatment of companion animal diarrhea cases (n = 15,928) in 2007, 2008, 2009 and 2010.

Health Canada Category [24]	Antibiotic class	Number of cases (% of 15,928 diarrhea cases)	% antimicrobial treated cases (n = 7400)
Category 1 (Very High Importance)	3rd/4th Generation Cephalosporins	124 (0.8)	1.7
	Fluorquinolones	200 (1.3)	2.7
	Nitroimidazoles	5814 (36.5)	78.6
	Penicillin β – lactam inhibitors	310 (1.9)	4.2
	Total for Category I	**6448 (40.5)**	**87.1**
Category II (High Importance)	1st/2nd Generation Cephalosporins	426 (2.7)	5.8
	Lincosamides	76 (0.5)	1.0
	Macrolides	124 (0.8)	1.7
	Penicillins	808 (5.1)	10.9
	Timethoprim-Sulpha	84 (0.5)	1.1
	Total for Category II	**1518 (9.5)**	**20.5**
Category III (Medium Importance)	Choramphenicol	5 (0.0)	0.1
	Sulphonamides	62 (0.4)	0.8
	Tetracycline	8 (0.1)	0.1
	Total for Category III	**75 (0.5)**	**1.0**

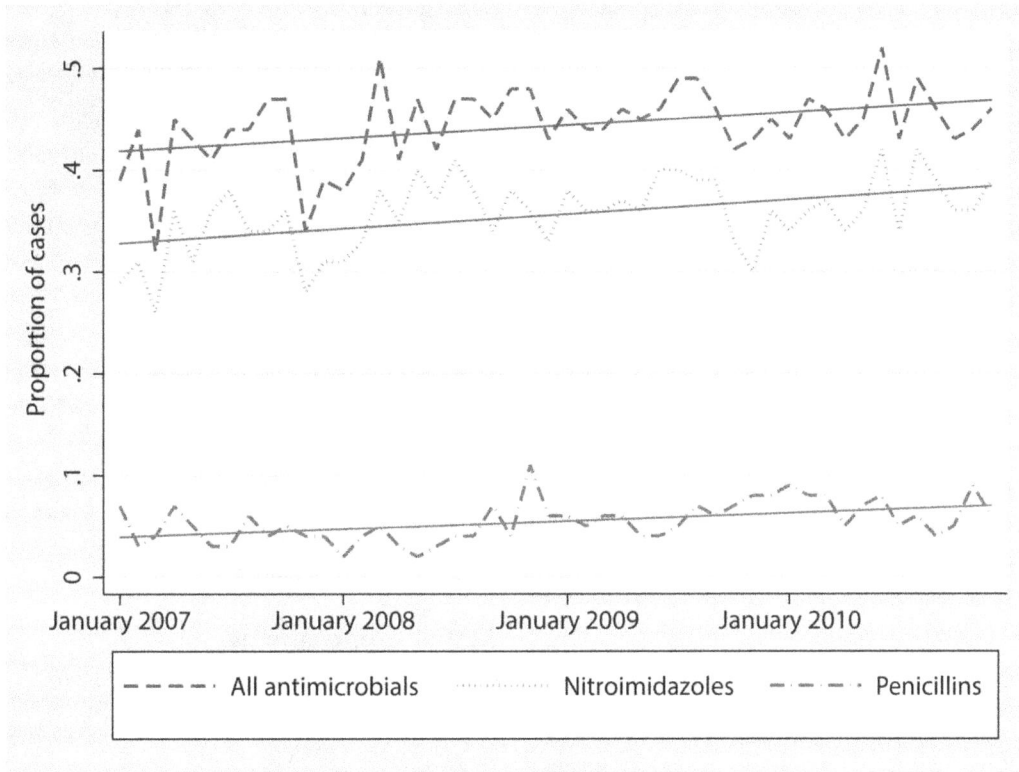

Figure 2. Changes in the proportion of companion animal diarrhea cases (n = 15,928) treated with any antimicrobial, nitroimidazole class and penicillin class from January 1, 2007 to December 31, 2010.

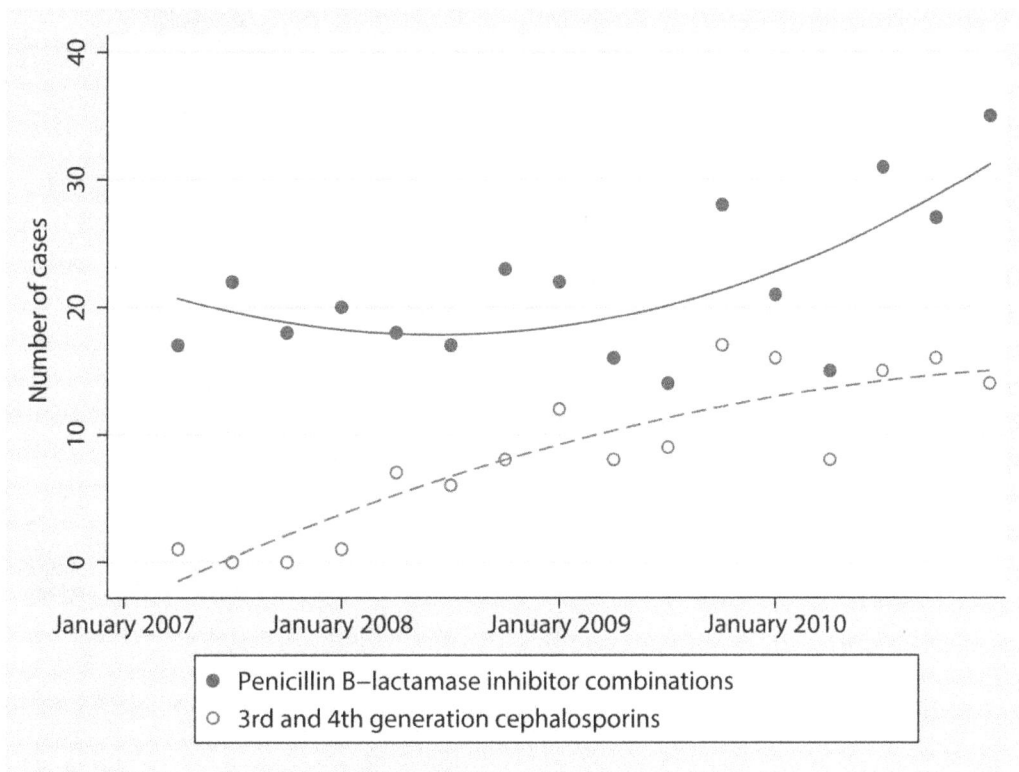

Figure 3. From 15,928 cases of companion animals with diarrhea, scattergrams of the counts of cases treated with B-lactam inhibitors and cephalosporins in each yearly quarter from January 1, 2007 to December 31, 2010.

animal's diarrhea had an infectious etiology. Empirical combinations of antimicrobial treatments was also common. Empirical antimicrobial use may lead to treatment failures and antimicrobial resistance [3,4,28,29]. We found no post-prescription, pharmacoepidemiological studies evaluating empirical antimicrobial management of diarrhea in pets in the refereed literature.

Using the data extracted from medical records it was possible to detect changing trends in AMU. Despite increased AMR concerns [4,6] there was evidence that nitroimidazole and penicillin use for the management of diarrhea in companion animals was increasing. Metronidazole (a drug of the Nitroimidazoles Class) was the most frequently prescribed antimicrobial and its use increased over the 4 years of the study. It is the drug of choice for anaerobic and microaerophilic bacteria (*Bacteroides* and *Clostridia*) and parasites (*Giardia* spp.) in animals [4]. In people it is important in the management of these pathogens and *Helicobacter pylori* [31,32]. There are few therapeutic alternatives for these infections in people and so it is classified as a Category I antimicrobial [24]. Sensitivity testing for anaerobes is not routinely performed but treatment failures have been documented [32,33] and the molecular basis for resistance has been established [31]. We found no papers documenting the transmission of metronidazole-resistant bacteria from pets to people.

The increase in the number of cases treated with 3rd and 4th generation cephalosporins in early 2008 coincided with the Canadian approval on May 30, 2007 and subsequent distribution of Convenia (Pfizer Animal Health, Kirkland, QC) later in 2007 [34]. Convenia is the trade name for cefovecin, a third generation cephalosporin. The increase in cefovecin use corresponded to a decrease in the use of penicillin β-lactamase inhibitor combinations. The indications for use are similar for the 2 classes of drugs so it is possible that one class was being used as an alternative to the other. Starting in the middle of 2009, the relationship appeared to be inverted and this trend continued until the end of 2010, the reason for which is unknown.

The results from this study suggest that informatics and EMR's could be useful for supporting evidence-based practice, and for monitoring trends in AMU and changes in veterinary prescription behavior following interventions to modify their use. Temporal trends and regional differences could prompt further investigations to explore why the observed trends were developing. Interventions such as confidential benchmarking by comparing AMU among veterinarians may serve to help veterinarians recognize problems and reduce AMU [35]. Analytical studies to see if there is an association between AMU in companion animals with diarrhea and the development of AMR in fecal microorganisms are indicated and informatics could provide the exposure data necessary to interpret AMR results.

Author Contributions

Conceived and designed the experiments: RMA JB CS. Performed the experiments: RMA. Analyzed the data: RMA. Contributed reagents/materials/analysis tools: RMA JB CR MR CS. Contributed to the writing of the manuscript: RMA JB CR MR CS.

References

1. Lidbury JA Turpin I, Suchodolski JS (2008) Gastrointestinal disease in a population of insured dogs and cats from the United Kingdome (2006–2007); 18th ECVIM-CA Congress; Ghent, Belgium. pp. 219.
2. Hall EJ, German AJ (2010) Diseases of the small intestine. In: Ettinger SJ, Feldman EC, editors. Textbook of Veterinary Internal Medicine, Diseases of the Dog and Cat. 7th ed. St. Lois, Missouri: Sanders Elsvier. pp. 1527–1572.
3. Weese JS (2011) Bacterial enteritis in dogs and cats: diagnosis, therapy, and zoonotic potential. Vet Clin North Am Small Anim Pract 41: 287.
4. Boothe DM (2012) Principles of antimicrobial therapy. In: Boothe DM, editor. Small Animal Clinical Pharmacology and Therapeutics. 2nd ed. St. Louis, Missouri: Elsevier Saunders.
5. Guerrant RL, Van Gilder T, Steiner TS, Thielman NM, Slutsker L, et al. (2001) Practice guidelines for the management of infectious diarrhea. Clin Infect Dis 32: 331–351.
6. Center for Disease Control Website. Interagency Task Force on Antimicrobial Resistance (2011) A public health action plan to combat antimicrobial resistance. Available: www.cdc.gov/./pdf/public-health-action-plan-combat-antimicrobial-resistance.pdf. Accessed 2013 February 2.
7. Morley PS, Apley MD, Besser TE, Burney DP, Fedorka-Cray PJ, et al. (2005) Antimicrobial drug use in veterinary medicine. J Vet Intern Med 19: 617–629.
8. Coffman JR (Chairman) National National Research Council (1999) The use of drugs in food animals: Benefits and risks. Washington, DC: Institute of Medicine.
9. Weese JS (2008) Antimicrobial resistance in companion animals. Anim Health Res Rev/Conf Res Workers Anim Dis 9: 169–176.
10. Guardabassi L, Schwarz S, Lloyd DH (2004) Pet animals as reservoirs of antimicrobial-resistant bacteria Review. J Antimicrob Chemother 54: 321–332.
11. Prescott JF, Hanna WJ, Reid-Smith R, Drost K (2002) Antimicrobial drug use and resistance in dogs. Can Vet J 43: 107–116.
12. Singer RS, Reid-Smith R, Sischo WM (2006) Stakeholder position paper: epidemiological perspectives on antibiotic use in animals. Prev Vet Med 73: 153–161.
13. Greco PJ, Eisenberg JM (1993) Changing physicians' practices. N Engl J Med 329: 1271–1274.
14. Meyer E, Schwab F, Jonas D, Rueden H, Gastmeier P, et al. (2004) Surveillance of antimicrobial use and antimicrobial resistance in intensive care units (SARI): 1. Antimicrobial use in German intensive care units. Intensive Care Med 30: 1089–1096.
15. Vlahović-Palc???evski V, Dumpis U, Mitt P, Gulbinovic J, Struwe J, et al. (2007) Benchmarking antimicrobial drug use at university hospitals in five European countries. Clin Microbiol Infect 13: 277–283.
16. Goossens H, Ferech M, Vander Stichele R, Elseviers M (2005) Outpatient antibiotic use in Europe and association with resistance: a cross-national database study. Lancet 365: 579–587.
17. Monnet D, López-Lozano JM, Campillos P, Burgos A, Yagüe A, et al. (2001) Making sense of antimicrobial use and resistance surveillance data: application of ARIMA and transfer function models. Clin Microbiol Infect 7: 29–36.
18. Public Health Agency of Canada website. Canadian Integrated Program for Antimicrobial Resistance Surveillance (2008) 2008 Annual Report. Available: http://www.phac-aspc.gc.ca/cipars-picra/2008/index-eng.php. Accessed 2012 November 29.
19. Friede A, Blum HL, McDonald M (1995) Public health informatics: how information-age technology can strengthen public health. Annu Rev Public Health 16: 239–252.
20. Chen ES, Hripcsak G, Xu H, Markatou M, Friedman C (2008) Automated acquisition of disease–drug knowledge from biomedical and clinical documents: an initial study. J Am Med Inform Assoc 15: 87–98.
21. Anholt RM, Berezowski J, MacLean K, Russel M, Jamal I, Stephen C (2014) The application of medical informatics to the veterinary management programs at companion animal practices in Alberta, Canada: A case study. Prev Vet Med 113: 165–174.
22. Anholt R, Berezowski J, Jamal I, Ribble C, Stephen C (2014) Mining free-text medical records for companion animal enteric syndrome surveillance. Prev Vet Med 113: 417–422.
23. Guyatt G SD, Haynes B. (2006) Evaluating diagnostic tests. In: Haynes BSD, Guyatt G., Tugwell P., editor. Clinical Epidemiology; How to do Clinical Practice Research. Third edition. Philadelphia: Lippincott William and Wilkins.
24. Health Canada website. Veterinary Drug Directorate (2009) Categorization of antimicrobial drugs based on importance to human medicine. Available: http://www.hc-sc.gc.ca/dhp-mps/vet/antimicrob/amr_ram_hum-med-rev-eng.php. Accessed 2012 November 29.
25. Jump RLP, Olds DM, Seifi N, Kypriotakis G, Jury LA, et al. (2012) Effective Antimicrobial Stewardship in a Long-Term Care Facility through an Infectious Disease Consultation Service: Keeping a LID on Antibiotic Use. Infect Control Hosp Epidemiol 33: 1185–1192.
26. Mooney RJ, Bunescu R (2005) Mining knowledge from text using information extraction. ACM SIGKDD Explorations newsl 7: 3–10.
27. Meystre SM, Savova GK, Kipper-Schuler KC, Hurdle JF (2008) Extracting information from textual documents in the electronic health record: a review of recent research. Yearbook Med Inform: 128–144.
28. Sherding RG, Johnson SE (2006) Diseases of the intestines. In: Birchard SJ, Sherding, RG, editor. Saunders Manual of Small Animal Practice. 3rd ed. St. Louis, Missouri: Saunders Elsevier.
29. Eddlestone SM (2002) Drug Therapies Used in Gastrointestinal Disease. Compendium: Small animal/exotics 24: 452–468.
30. Payne PA, Artzer M (2009) Biology and control of Giardia spp. and Tritrichomonas foetus. Vet Clin North Am Small Anim Pract 39: 993–1007.

31. Dhand A, Snydman DR (2009) Mechanism of Resistance in Metronidazole. Antimicrob Drug Resist: 223–227.

32. Megraud F, Lamouliatte H (2003) Review article: the treatment of refractory Helicobacter pylori infection. Aliment Pharmacol Ther 17: 1333–1343.

33. Fang H, Edlund C, Hedberg M, Nord CE (2002) New findings in beta-lactam and metronidazole resistant Bacteroides fragilis group. Int J Antimicrob Agents 19: 361.

34. Health Canada website. Veterinary Drug Directorate (2007) Notice of Compliance. Available: http://www.hc-sc.gc.ca/dhp-mps/prodpharma/notices-avis/index-eng.php. Accessed 2012 November 29.

35. Ibrahim OM, Polk RE (2012) Benchmarking antimicrobial drug use in hospitals. Expert Rev Anti Infect Ther 10: 445–457.

5

Modulatory Effects of Vasoactive Intestinal Peptide on Intestinal Mucosal Immunity and Microbial Community of Weaned Piglets Challenged by an Enterotoxigenic *Escherichia coli* (K88)

Chunlan Xu[1]*, **Youming Wang**[2], **Rui Sun**[1], **Xiangjin Qiao**[1], **Xiaoya Shang**[1], **Weining Niu**[1]

1 The Key Laboratory for Space Bioscience and Biotechnology, School of Life Sciences, Northwestern Polytechnical University, Xi'an, Shaanxi, China, 2 Institute of Feed Science, College of Animal Sciences, Zhejiang University, Hangzhou, PR China

Abstract

Toll-like receptors (TLRs) recognize microbial pathogens and trigger immune response, but their regulation by neuropeptide-vasoactive intestinal peptide (VIP) in weaned piglets infected by enterotoxigenic *Escherichia coli* (ETEC) K88 remains unexplored. Therefore, the study was conducted to investigate its role using a model of early weaned piglets infected by ETEC K88. Male Duroc×Landrace×Yorkshire piglets (n = 24) were randomly divided into control, ETEC K88, VIP, and ETEC K88+VIP groups. On the first three days, ETEC K88 and ETEC K88+VIP groups were orally administrated with ETEC K88, other two groups were given sterile medium. Then each piglet from VIP and ETEC K88+VIP group received 10 nmol VIP intraperitoneally (i.p.) once daily, on day four and six. On the seventh day, the piglets were sacrificed. The results indicated that administration of VIP improved the growth performance, reduced diarrhea incidence of ETEC K88 challenged pigs, and mitigated the histopathological changes of intestine. Serum levels of IL-2, IL-6, IL-12p40, IFN-γ and TNF-α in the ETEC K88+ VIP group were significantly reduced compared with those in the ETEC group. VIP significantly increased IL-4, IL-10, TGF-β and S-IgA production compared with the ETEC K88 group. Besides, VIP could inhibit the expression of TLR2, TLR4, MyD88, NF-κB p65 and the phosphorylation of IκB-α, p-ERK, p-JNK, and p-38 induced by ETEC K88. Moreover, VIP could upregulate the expression of occludin in the ileum mucosa compared with the ETEC K88 group. Colon and caecum content bacterial richness and diversity were lower for pigs in the ETEC group than the unchallenged groups. These results demonstrate that VIP is beneficial for the maturation of the intestinal mucosal immune system and elicited local immunomodulatory activities. The TLR2/4-MyD88 mediated NF-κB and MAPK signaling pathway may be critical to the mechanism underlying the modulatory effect of VIP on intestinal mucosal immune function and bacterial community.

Editor: Markus M. Heimesaat, Charité, Campus Benjamin Franklin, Germany

Funding: The research was supported by National Natural Science Foundation of China, No.31001012 and No.31101304; and Programs for Agricultural Science and Technology Development of Shanxi Province, China, No.2013K02-16. The funders had no role in study design, data collection and analysis, decision to publish, or preparation of the manuscript.

Competing Interests: The authors have declared that no competing interests exist.

* Email: clxu@nwpu.edu.cn

Introduction

Weaning is often stressful for piglets and accompanied by morphological, histological, microbial, and immunological changes along the digestive tract, which caused diarrhea and reduced growth [1,2]. Thus, weaned piglets are often subjected to myriad of enteric diseases, and these diseases are the leading cause of mortality and economic losses in the swine industry. The intestine is the major site of digestion, nutrient absorption and hydro-mineral exchange homeostasis, harbouring a complex microbiota and a highly evolved mucosal immune system. The mucosal immune system fulfils two functions, to mount active responses against pathogens and to mount tolerance against harmless food and commensal bacterial antigens [3,4]. Gut microbiota may play an important role in host health [5]. In the absence of the gut microbiota, normal immune development and function are impaired. The main challenge in a young animal is to obtain a balanced microbial population to prevent the establishment of pathogenic microorganisms [3]. Understanding the factors that influence the intestinal mucosal immunity and composition of the microbial community in the piglet infected by pathogens is crucial in regulating the intestinal immunity function and microflora, which will improve animal performance. Consequently, identification of the factors controlling the intestinal mucosal immunity, bacterial acquisition and community composition is of particular significance.

Under physiological and pathological conditions the enteric nervous system regulates intestinal mucosal function [6]. The small intestine possesses a net-work fiber that contains immunomodulating neuropeptides. VIP is an important signal molecule of the neuroendocrine-immune network [7], and a well characterized endogenous anti-inflammatory neuropeptide with therapeutic potential for a variety of immune disorders [8]. It is a member of the secretin-glucagon family and is involved in the modulation of numerous biological functions. It is known to affect the gastrointestinal, neuronal, and endocrine as well as the circulatory and immune systems [9]. A beneficial effect of VIP on experimental animal models of acute and chronic inflammation, such as acute pancreatitis [10], septic shock [11], arthritis [12], inflammatory bowel disease [13] and lipopolysaccharide (LPS)-induced acute inflammatory [14], has been demonstrated. Recently, VIP has been incorporated into the list of prospective immunotherapeutics for the treatment of inflammatory and autoimmune disorders. However, the possible protective effect of VIP achieved in the intestine mucosal immunity of piglets still remains obscure. Moreover, VIP displayed a direct antimicrobial activity against a variety of pathogens, including bacteria [15]. It was recently reported that VIP and its derivatives showed the strongest antimicrobial activities against E.coli strains that express complete O-antigen-containing LPS [16]. These antimicrobial activities add a further dimension to the immunomodulatory roles for VIP in the inflammatory and immune responses. Additionally, the recent discovery of Toll-like receptors (TLRs) has improved our understanding of the induction of both innate and adaptive immune responses against infection and injury. TLRs are implicated in protective immunity as well as in many inflammatory and autoimmune diseases; inhibitors of TLR signaling are being harnessed for a variety of therapeutic applications. Neuroendocrine mediators have been shown to play an important role in modulating both aspects of TLR regulation contributing to the endogenous control of homeostasis among the different players implicated in defense mechanisms [7]. However, the role of TLRs/nuclear factor-kappa-B (NF-κB) and (or) TLRs/mitogen-activated protein kinases (MAPK) in modulatory effects of VIP on intestinal mucosal immune function in early weaned piglets under infection is unclear. Moreover, in a preliminary in vitro study, VIP was shown to be effective against Enterotoxigenic Escherichia coli (ETEC), but this observation has not been confirmed in vivo.

Thus, in the present study, we used early weaned piglets infected by ETEC K88 as model to evaluate the morphologic alterations in the intestinal mucosa, and investigate the effect VIP on intestinal mucosal immunity and bacterial community, and the role of TLRs/myeloid differentiation factor 88 (MyD88)/NF-κB and (or) TLRs/MyD88/MAPK in modulatory effect of VIP on intestinal mucosal immune function under infection by ETEC K88. In addition, we investigated the involvement of paracellular pathway in the intestinal damage by evaluating the expression of the critical protein occludin. The information could provide valuable evidence for investigating the benefit effect of VIP on weaned piglet and explaining the mechanism of immune modulation by the porcine neuropeptide VIP.

Materials and Methods

Ethics Statement and experimental animals

This study was carried out in strict accordance with the recommendations in the Guide for the Care and Use of Laboratory Animals of the National Institutes of Health. The protocol was approved by the Committee on the Ethics of Animal Experiments of College of Animal Sciences, Zhejiang University (Permit Number: 2012072701) and the Committee on the Ethics of Animal Experiments of School of Life Sciences, Northwestern Polytechnical University (Permit Number: 12-015). All efforts were made to minimize suffering. Twenty four male Duroc×Landrace×Yorkshire piglets, 28 days of age and weighing 7.70 ± 0.71 kg had been weaned at 21 days after birth. The feeding trial was

carried out in the Swine Research and Teaching Farm at Zhejiang University. The disposal of experimental animals is strict comply with the management requirements of experimental animals.

Bacterial strain and reagents

The ETEC strain used in this study was kindly donated by Professor Yizhen Wang of Zhejiang University. The enterotoxigenic E.coli was confirmed by Polymerase Chain Reaction (PCR) genotyping as genes expressing K88 fimbrial antigen and primarily cultured in Luria broth (LB) medium. Bacteria growing at 37°C in LB broth to log stationary phase ($OD_{600 nm}$ of 0.8) was adjusted to a final concentration of 1×10^{10} CFU/ml before being used in the current experiment. Mainly Antibodies used in the experiment were as following: IκB-α (EPI), $Ser^{32/36}$-phosphorylated IκB-α (CST), NF-κB p65 (Santa), p44/42 MAPK (ERK1/2) (Bioworld), p-p44/42 (p-ERK1/2) (Bioworld), JNK/SAPK (Santa), p-JNK/SAPK(Santa), p38 MAPK (EPI), p-p38 MAPK(CST), TLR2(EPI), TLR4(Santa), MyD88(Abcam), occludin and β-actin (Santa). Other reagents were obtained from Sigma Chemical Co. (St. Louis, MO, USA) unless otherwise mentioned.

Establishment of the animal model

Twenty four 28-day male crossbred (Duroc×Landrace×Yorkshire) piglets weaned at 21 d were randomly divided into four groups of six piglets each: control, ETEC K88, ETEC K88+VIP, and VIP. Before infection, all the animals' fecal samples were confirmed as being free of ETEC K88 by PCR. All piglets were housed in stainless steel pens (1.5×1.0 m) (three piglets per pen) with plastic-coated and wood-expanded floors at 25°C and under constant light with ad libitum access to feed and water. Moreover, ETEC K88 challenged groups and none-ETEC K88 challenged groups were housed in different unit with same environment conditions to prevent cross infection in the process of experiment. All treatments received the same basal diets. Diets were formulated to meet requirements for all nutrients and did not contain any antibiotics or medicine. After an acclimation period of 7 days, twelve piglets from ETEC K88 and ETEC K88+VIP groups were infected orally with 1×10^{10} CFU/ml of ETEC K88 [17,18], whereas the control and VIP groups received sterile medium orally on the first 3 days. Then each piglet from VIP and ETEC K88+VIP groups were given 10 nmol VIP (GL Biochem (shanghai) Ltd, China) intraperitoneally (i.p.) once daily, on day four and six based on previous reports [19,20] and the preliminary experiment in our Lab. Following the same protocol, piglets from control and ETEC K88 groups were given the same volumes of normal saline.

Animal observation and sample collection

All the infected piglets were fecal-culture positive for ETEC K88 and developed similar clinical signs of gastrointestinal disease, including increased rectal temperature, diarrhea and lethargy. The Average daily gain (ADG), Average daily feed intake (ADFI), and Body weight gain efficiency (G:F) of each pig were monitored throughout the experimental period. The number of pigs with diarrhea was recorded daily, and the diarrhea ratio was calculated according to the following equation: diarrhea ratio = total number of pigs with diarrhea/(total number of experimental pigs×trail days)×100. On the sixth day after the first infection, all pigs were anesthetized with Zoletil (20 mg/kg, i.m.) and blood samples were drawn in collection tubes by venipuncture of the anterior vena cava of pigs. The pigs were euthanized with an overdose of the anesthetic. Serum was obtained after centrifugation at 3000 g for 15 min at 4°C and stored at −80°C until further use. Tissue sampling included collection of duodenal (5 cm distal of the pyloric sphincter), jejuna (35 cm distal of the pyloric sphincter), and ileum segments (10 cm proximal to the ileocecal junction). One 4 cm long piece segment from each region was divided into two pieces. One piece was fixed with 4% paraformaldehyde for histological analysis. Caecum and distal colon content were collected in sterile sample bags, snap-frozen in liquid nitrogen and stored at −80°C until used for microbial DNA extraction. After collection of intestinal contents, mucosal tissue was gently scraped from the other piece using a sterile scalpel, and then mixture of mucosal scrapings was flash frozen in liquid nitrogen and stored at −80°C for protein isolation.

Histological examination for the intestinal morphology

Partial intestine tissues (duodenum, jejuna and ileum) were fixed in 4% paraformaldehyde for 24 h, and then embedded in paraffin wax. Sections of 5 μm were cut and stained with hematoxylin and eosin (H&E). An independent pathologist blinded to the experimental group of the samples performed the histological analysis. Images were captured using a high-resolution Samsung camera coupled to a light Nikon E200 microscope and subsequently analyzed using AxioVision-Rel software (Zeiss). Total mucosal thickness (TMT), villous height (VH), and crypt depth (CD) were evaluated. The VH: CD (VCR) was calculated. Each variable was measured three times for all three portions of the intestine, so the final value of a given variable for one specimen is the mean of these nine measurements.

Enzyme linked-immuno sorbent assay (ELISA) for detection of serum levels of cytokines and Secretory IgA (S-IgA)

Piglets serum was collected as described previously. The serum levels of interleukin-2 (IL-2), interleukin-4 (IL-4), interleukin-6 (IL-6), interleukin-10 (IL-10), interleukin-12 p40 (IL-12 p40), tumor necrosis factor α (TNF-α), transforming growth factor β (TGF-β), interferon γ (IFN-γ) and S-IgA were measured using commercially available ELISA kits (R&D, USA) in strict accordance with the manufacturer's instructions. The color intensity was read using optical density (OD) at 450 nm with a tunable microplate reader (VersaMax, Molecular Devices, CA, USA) and the concentration of cytokine calculated from a standard curve.

Western blot for detection of TLRs, MAPK and NF-κB signaling molecules and occludin expression

Protein was isolated from 200 mg of ileal mucosal tissue using a total protein extraction kit and cytoplasmic and nuclear protein extraction kit (Beyotime Biotechnology, Haimen, China) according to the manufacturer's instructions. The BCA method was used to measure protein concentrations. Cytosolic occludin, IκB-α, p-IκB-α, p44/p42 (ERK1/2), p-p44/p42, p38, p-p38, JNK/SAPK, p-JNK/SAPK, TLR4, TLR2, MyD88, nuclear NF-κB p65 proteins and β-actin were detected. Cytosolic or nuclear proteins (35 μg) were loaded into 10% sodium dodecyl sulfate (SDS)-polyacrilamide gel electrophoresis (PAGE) and transferred to a 0.45 μm-pore polyvinylidene difluoride membrane (PVDF; Immuno-Blot, BioRad). The membranes were then incubated with blocking solution (150 mM NaCl, 20 mM Tris-HCl, 0.1% Tween 20, 5% skim milk, pH 7.4) for 1 h at room temperature (RT). After the blocking reaction, membranes were incubated with first antibodies against occludin (1:800), IκB-α (1:1000), p- IκB-α (1:1000), p44/p42 (ERK1/2) (1:1000), p-p44/p42 (1:1000), p38 (1:1000), p-p38 (1:1000), JNK/SAPK (1:500), p-JNK/SAPK (1:500), p65 (1:1000), TLR4 (1:500), TLR2 (1:1000), MyD88 (1:500) and β-actin (1:1000) for 90 min at RT, and then washed thrice with TBS-T (1% Tween 20 in Tris buffered saline) followed

by incubation with secondary antibody-horseradish peroxidase-conjugated goat anti-rabbit IgG (Santa Cruz Biotechnology, CA, USA) for 1 h at RT. An ECL agent was added for chemiluminescence imaging. The images were collected using the Gel EQ system (Bio-Rad, Inc.), and the built-in software was used to analyze the gray values of the bands. The relative expression levels of the proteins were expressed as the gray value of the target band over the gray value of β-actin in the same sample. Each sample had 3 replicates.

Composition and diversity of bacterial community through 454 pyrosequencing analysis

Before DNA extraction, equal masses of sub-samples (caecum or distal colon content) collected from each pigs in the same treatment group were pooled together and homogenized in a sterile Stomacher (Seward Laboratory, London, UK) at 4°C. Genomic DNA in caecum and colon contents was extracted using DNA Kit (Omega Bio-Tek) according to the manufacture's protocol with slight modification, then identified by 1% agarose gel electrophoresis. According to the specific sequence region (533R-27F) in the 16S rRNA gene that covering the V1–V3 region, the bar-coded primers 27F and 533R containing the A and B sequencing adaptors were synthesized and used to amplify this region. The forward primer (B-27F) was 5'-*CCTATCCC-CTGTGTGCCTTGGCAGTCTCAG*AGAGTTTGATCCTGGCT-CAG-3', where the sequence of the B adaptor is shown in italics and underlined. The reverse primer (A-533R) was 5'-*CCATCT-CATCCCTGCGTGTCTCCGACTCAG* NNNNNNNNNNTTA-CCGCGGCTGCTGGCAC-3', where the sequence of the A adaptor is shown in italics and underlined and the Ns represent an eight-base sample specific barcode sequence. The identified DNA was subjected to polymerase chain reaction (PCR) using TranS-tartFastpfu DNA Polymerase (MBI. Fermentas, USA) in a 20 μL volume containing 5 mM each of the primer, 10 ng of template DNA, and 5×FastPfu Buffer, 1 U of FastPfu DNA Polymerase. PCR was performed in a thermocycler (Gene Amp PCR System 9700, ABI, USA). The PCR profile included denaturation at 95°C for 2 min, followed by 25 cycles of denaturation at 95°C for 30 s, annealing at 55°C for 30 s, and extension at 72°C for 30 s, and a final extension at 72°C for 5 min. Triplicate PCR products of the same sample were mixed, and then detected by 2% agarose gels electrophoresis containing ethidium bromide. PCR products were recycled and purified with a AxyPreDNA gel extraction kit (Axygen, China) according to the manufacture's instruction. The recycled PCR products were visualized on agarose gels. Furthermore, the PCR products were quantitatively determined using QuantiFluor-ST Fluoremeter (Promega, USA) and PicoGreen dsDNA Quantitation Reagent (Invitrogen, Germany) Following quantitation, the amplification from each reaction mixture were pooled in equimolar ratios based on concentration and subjected to emulsion PCR (emPCR) using RocheGS FLX Titanium emPCR kits to generate amplification libraries. Amplification pyrosequencing was performed from the A-end using a 454/Roche A sequencing primer kit on a Roche Genome Sequencer GS FLX Titanium platform at Majorbio Bio-Pharm Technology Co., Ltd., Shanghai, China.

Statistical analysis

Statistical analyses were performed using SPSS 18.0 (Chicago, IL, USA). Independent sample t-test was adopted to determine significant differences, in which the data were expressed as mean ± standard error of mean (SEM), and differences were considered significant at $p < 0.05$. The pyrosequencing data were subjected to bioinformatic analysis. Prior to analyze, the original pyrosequencing data must be filtered and optimized to obtain the valid and trimmed sequences through Seqcln and Mothur (http://sourceforge.net/projects/seqclean/ & http://www.mothur.org/wiki/Main_Page). Then, these trimed sequences were analyzed from two aspects: operational taxonomic units (OTUs) cluster (97% similarity) and taxonomy which mainly performed on Mothur (http://www.mothur.org) and compared with the Bacterial SILVA database (http://www.arb-silva.de/), and by methods of kmer searching (http://www.mothur.org/wiki/Align.seqs) and UCHIME (http://drive5.com/uchime). Rarefaction analysis and Good's coverage for the nine libraries were determined. Community figure was generated using R tools according to the data from document "tax.phylum.xls". Heatmap figure were generated using Vegan-package (distance measure: Bray-Curtis; cluster analysis: complete).

Results

Growth performance and diarrhea ratio

The effect of administration with VIP on growth performance and diarrhea ratio are presented in Table 1. The ADG ($P<0.001$), ADFI ($P<0.001$), and G:F ($P<0.01$) of piglets in ETEC K88+ VIP group was higher than those of piglets in ETEC K88 group. The pigs in the VIP group presented a significantly higher ADG ($P<0.001$), ADFI ($P<0.001$), and G:F ($P<0.001$) compared with the pigs in the control group. Administration with VIP effectively alleviated the incidence of diarrhea in ETEC K88 challenged piglets. None of the piglets in group control and VIP showed any signs of diarrhea throughout the experiment.

Intestinal morphology

As shown in Figure 1 and Table 2, the histological analyses of the intestine showed that a significant decrease in VH (duodenum: $P<0.01$; jejunum: $P<0.01$; ileum: $P<0.05$), CD (duodenum: $P<0.001$) and TMT (duodenum: $P<0.001$; jejunum: $P<0.001$) in the ETEC K88 group when compared with the control group (). No differences ($P>0.05$) among treatments were observed in the VCR values. Compared with the ETEC K88 group, the reduction in TMT (duodenum: $P<0.001$; jejunum: $P<0.001$; ileum: $P<0.05$), VH (duodenum: $P<0.001$; jejunum: $P<0.001$; ileum: $P<0.01$), and CD (duodenum: $P<0.001$; jejunum: $P<0.001$) were lower in the ETEC K88+ VIP group. The intestinal morphology (VH, CD, and VCR) of piglets in the control group did not differ from those of piglets receiving VIP ($P>0.05$). These results indicated that VIP may have the positive regulation function on the intestinal tract, which may be related to the decline of diarrhea cause by ETEC K88.

Serum levels of cytokines and S-IgA

As shown in Figure 2, the serum concentrations of IL-2 ($P<0.001$), IL-6 ($P<0.05$), IL-12p40 ($P<0.001$), IFN-γ ($P<0.001$) and TNF-α ($P<0.01$) in the ETEC K88 group were significantly

higher than those in the control group, suggesting ETEC K88 induced inflammatory response. The concentrations of IL-4 ($P<0.001$), IL-10 ($P<0.001$), TGF-β ($P<0.001$) and S-IgA ($P<0.001$) in the serum of piglets from the ETEC K88 group were significantly lower than the concentrations in those from the control group. However, VIP-treatment significantly reduced the serum levels of IL-2 ($P<0.001$), IL-6 ($P<0.05$), IL-12p40 ($P<0.001$), IFN-γ ($P<0.001$) and TNF-α ($P<0.05$), increased the serum levels of IL-4 ($P<0.001$), IL-10 ($p<0.05$), TGF-β ($p<0.05$) and S-IgA ($p<0.05$) compared with the ETEC K88 group. These results suggested that VIP-treatment reversed ETEC K88-induced increase of inflammatory mediators.

TLRs, MAPK, NF-κB and occludin protein expression

Toll-like receptors (TLRs) are a family of pattern-recognition receptors that play a key role in the innate immune system. Western blot (Figure 3) analysis showed that the expression levels of TLR2 and TLR4 in the ETEC K88+VIP group were lower than that in the ETEC K88 group, and MyD88 levels in the ETEC K88+VIP group were lower than that in group ETEC K88. Activation of NF-κB and MAPKs, particularly the stimulation of ERK subgroup, has been demonstrated as the critical signals to trigger the cytokine production from immune-responsive cells. So we detected the phosphorylation of MAPKs and NF-κB pathways proteins by western blotting. Reduce phosphorylation of IκB-α was observed in the ETEC K88+VIP group. The expression levels of NF-κB p65 in the ETEC K88 group were higher than that in the control group. Administration of VIP significantly inhibited the expression of NF-κB p65, the phosphorylation of IκB-α compared with the ETEC K88 group. Since the activation of MAPK requires phosphorylation of threonine or tyrosine residues, antibodies against ERK, JNK, and p38 were used and their phospho-forms detected using western blot. The data show administration of VIP significantly inhibited the phosphorylation of p-38, ERK and JNK compared with the ETEC K88 group. In addition, we investigated the involvement of paracellular pathway in the intestinal damage by evaluating the expression of this critical protein occludin. As shown in Figure 3, group ETEC K88 showed significantly decreased expression of occludin compared to the control group. VIP administration rescued ETEC K88 induced reduction of occludin, as shown by increased occludin protein in the ETEC K88+VIP group.

Bacterial composition and diversity in the caecum and colon content

A total of 104,799 valid reads and 6,009 operational taxonomic units (OTUs) were obtained from the samples through 454 pyrosequencing analysis. 53 reads and 49 OTUs were eukaryotes and were therefore excluded in the subsequent analysis. Good's coverage estimations revealed that 89.7% to 98% of the species

Table 1. Effect of VIP on growth performance and diarrhea incidence of piglets challenged with ETEC K88.

Item	Control	ETEC K88	ETEC K88+ VIP	VIP
ADG, g/d	200.00±4.24	98.33±4.37###	136.7±5.34***	251.7±5.08###
ADFI, g/d	284.38±4.88	189.08±5.84###	238.65±4.17***	315.67±2.36###
G:F	0.70±0.00	0.52±0.01###	0.57±0.01**	0.80±0.01###
Diarrhea incidence, %	0	32.58±2.06###	12.72±0.95***	0

Note: ###$P<0.001$ compared to Control; **$P<0.01$, ***$P<0.001$ compared to ETEC K88. Values are expressed as mean ± SEM. ADG, ADFI, G:F represents average daily gain, average daily feed intake, and feed conversion efficiency (G:F), respectively.

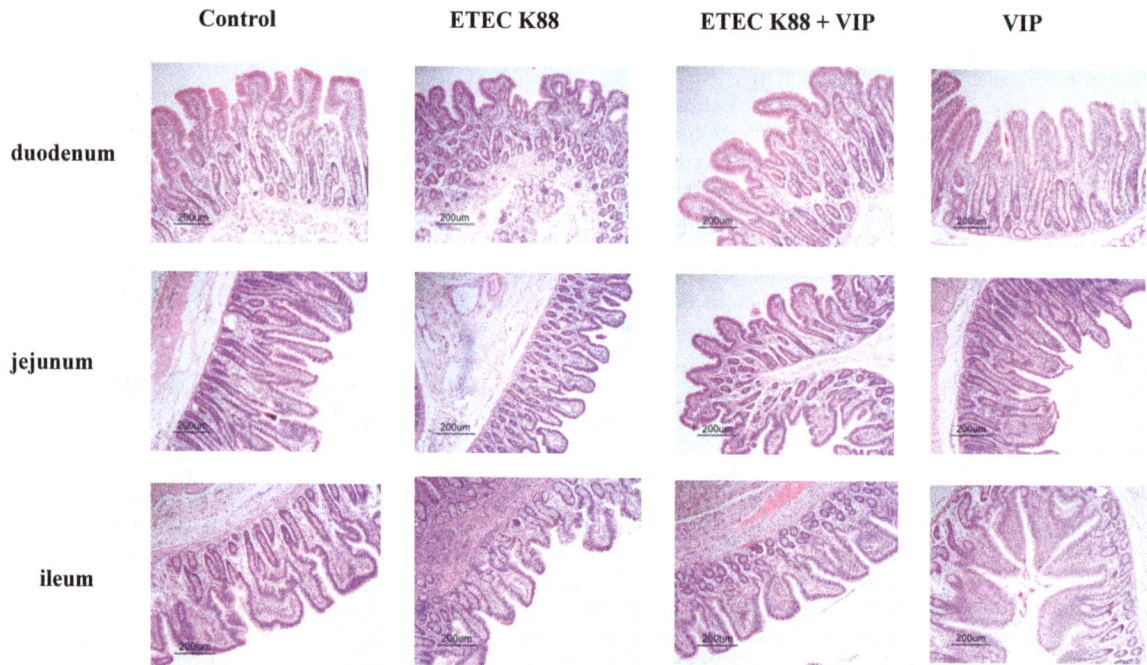

Figure 1. Influence of VIP on morphology of intestine in piglets infected by ETEC K88 (H&E).

were obtained in all of the samples. All sequences were classified from phylum to genus according to the program Mothur using the default setting. 14 different phyla and 50 different genuses were identified from these samples. The eight libraries showed very dissimilar 16S rRNA profiles even in phylum level distributions (Figure 4). The most abundant OTUs associated with the colon digesta from the VIP treatment alone group were *Xylanibacter* (15.56%) and *Lachnospiraceae* (15.28%). The OUT composition and abundance was relatively similar between the colon and caecum content in the same group, two ETEC K88 infection groups, and the control and VIP treatment alone group (data not shown). The bacterial species in the colon and caecum digesta libraries were further investigated for the presence of a core gut microbiota. Figure 5 and Table 3 showed that the colon and

Table 2. Effect of VIP on morphology of the intestines in weaned piglets infected by ETEC K88.

Items	Groups			
	Control	ETEC K88	ETEC K88+VIP	VIP
Duodenum				
Villous height (VH), μm	327.80±11.78	232.10±25.83##	414.10±23.16***	355.50±12.22
Crypt depth (CD), μm	270.20±11.73	173.20±16.95###	305.90±13.24***	271.50±16.67
Total mucosal thickness, μm	640.70±7.25	455.20±9.91###	691.10±27.96***	631.80±17.04
VH:CD	1.23±0.08	1.37±0.15	1.37±0.10	1.33±0.06
Jejunum				
Villous height (VH), μm	281.10±12.13	215.30±10.99##	314.30±18.48***	307.60±12.96
Crypt depth (CD), μm	172.70±4.72	145.80±7.16	203.30±3.31***	181.31±15.30
Total mucosal thickness, μm	596.70±16.49	396.9±11.72###	572.60±10.12***	607.70±18.90
VH:CD	1.64±0.09	1.51±0.14	1.54±0.08	1.70±0.05
Ileum				
Villous height (VH), μm	276.10±12.56	214.6±18.15#	288.10±15.32**	285.10±12.94
Crypt depth (CD), μm	159.40±5.48	140.40±8.29	169.40±6.57	168.20±11.34
Total mucosal thickness, μm	424.80±5.56	400.00±16.01	450.00±17.29*	476.80±9.81#
VH:CD	1.75±0.11	1.52±0.06	1.71±0.10	1.75±0.14

Note: #P<0.05, ##P<0.01, ###P<0.001 compared to Control; *P<0.05, **P<0.01, ***P<0.001 compared to ETEC K88. Values are expressed as mean ± SEM (n = 6, each group).

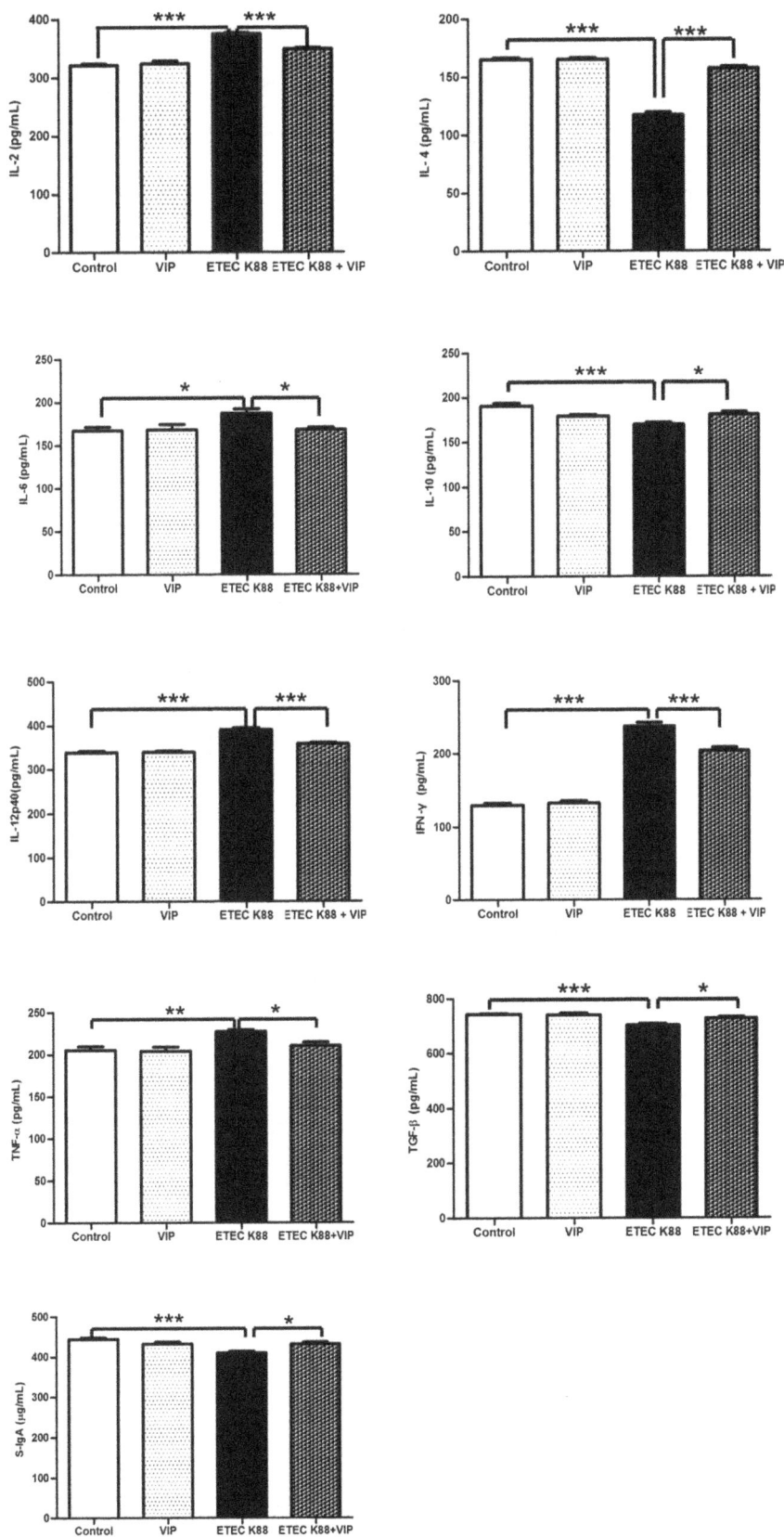

Figure 2. Effect of VIP on expression of immune-related molecules in serum from piglets infected with ETEC K88. Each results is the mean (n = 6) ± S.E.M. of cytokines levels determined in triplication. *P<0.05, **P<0.01, ***P<0.001.

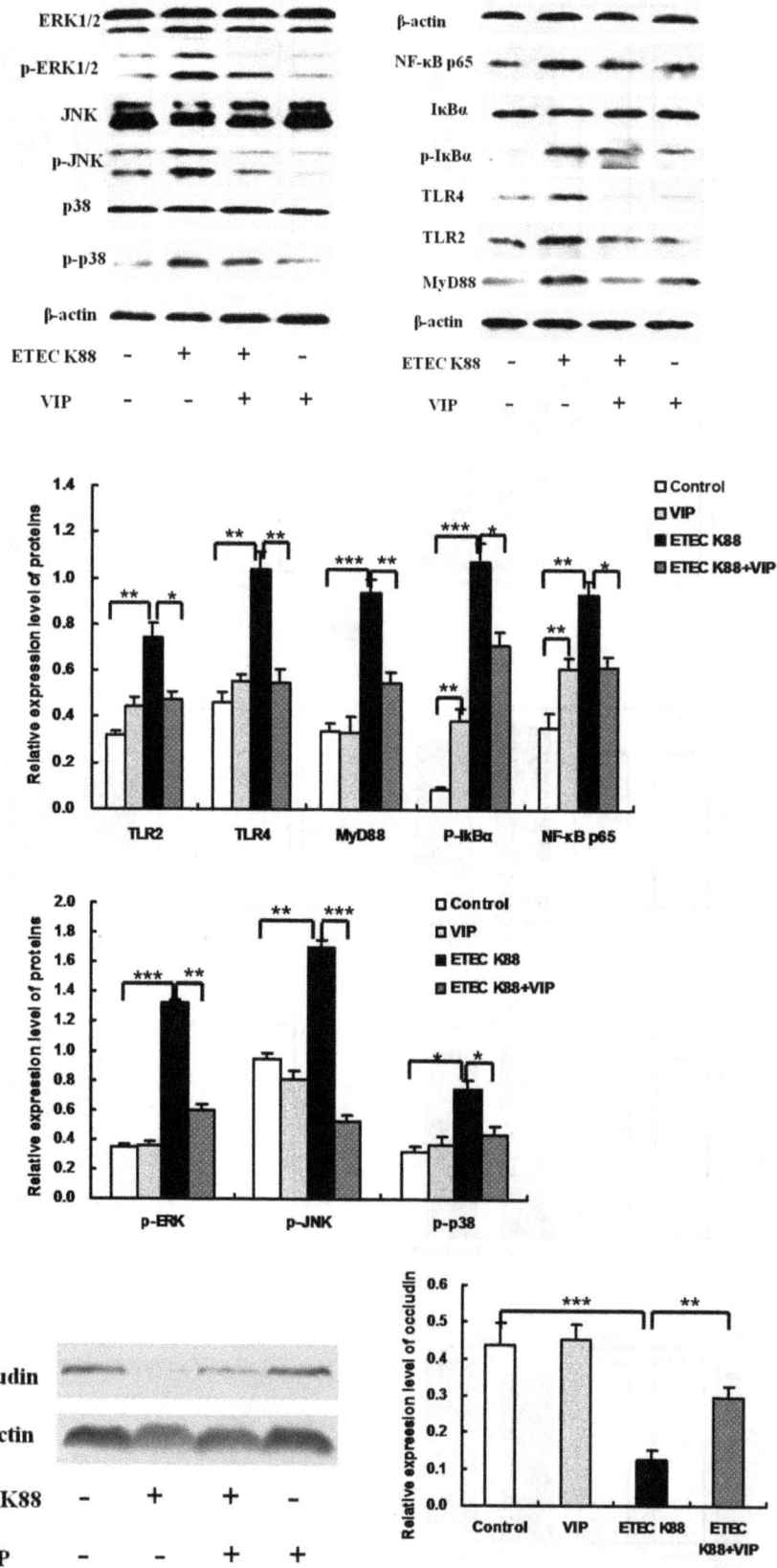

Figure 3. Effect of VIP on degradation and phosphorylation of IκBα, ERK1/2 (p44/p42) MAPK, p38 MAPK, and JNK/SAPK, and expression of TLRs, NF-κB p65, MyD88 and occludin in the ileum. Cytosolic occludin, IκB-α, p-IκB-α, p44/p42 (ERK1/2), p-p44/p42, p38, p-p38, JNK/SAPK, p-JNK/SAPK, p65, TLR4, TLR2, MyD88, nuclear NF-κB p65 proteins and actin were detected by western blot analysis. Each results is the mean (n = 6)±S.E.M. *P<0.05, **P<0.01, ***P<0.001.

caecum content libraries from each experimental group have 135 and 125 OTUs in common, respectively. *Bacteroidetes* and Firmicutes included 112 (colon content, 82.96% in proportion) and 101 (caecum content, 80.80% in proportion) of the shared OTUs, and 30013 (colon content) and 28852 (caecum content) shared reads. Within these two phyla, *Bacteroidia*, *Bacilli*, *Clostridia* and *Erysipelotrichi* represented the most abundant classes common to the eight libraries. For *Actinobacteria*, *Proteobacteria*, *Tenericutes* and *Spirochaetes*, OTUs common was very little, and they tended to be low in abundance. Hierarchically clustered heatmap analysis based on the bacterial community profiles at family level disclosed that the samples from the same group grouped together firstly except for VIP treatment alone group, and they then clustered with samples from VIP treatment alone, ETEC K88 plus VIP and control groups in order (Figure 6). In addition, the significant differences analysis between groups showed that the bacterial composition in the ETEC K88 infected groups was significantly different from the control groups, and administration with VIP in the weaned piglets challenged with ETEC K88 significantly changed the bacterial composition and community compared with the ETEC K88 infection group. The different bacterial at the genus level between each groups were shown in Table 4 and 5.

Discussion

Diarrhea in neonatal and early-weaned piglets due to ETEC is an important problem in the pig farming industry. The VIP is a well-characterized endogenous anti-inflammatory neuropeptide with therapeutic potential for a variety of immune disorders. The experiment was aimed to investigate whether exogenous VIP would protect against ETEC infection of piglets fed a diet without supplemental antibiotics. The current results indicated that the growth performance was impaired, and incidence of diarrhea was increased in piglets challenged by enterotoxigenic ETEC K88, which was in consistent with previous observation [17,18,21]. ETEC K88 is a major cause of diarrhea and death in neonatal and weaned pigs [22]. ETEC K88 not only colonize in the small intestine, but also release enterotoxins to stimulate the epithelial cells to secrete fluid into the lumen of the gut to cause diarrhea [23]. However, treatment with VIP significantly improved the ETEC K88 challenge-caused signs as indicated by attenuated growth depression and decreased diarrhea incidence in piglets.

The intestine of weaned piglet is very susceptible to pathogenic microorganisms, and severe changes occur in the intestinal epithelium after this insult. Furthermore, reductions in VH have been associated with poor growth performance and increased incidences of scouring in pigs challenged with ETEC [24]. A feature of ETEC infection is effacing of the intestinal mucosa, which often leads to shorter villous and deeper crypts [2]. The morphometric evaluation showed that a reduction in mucosal thickness in the ETEC K88 group. This reduction was mainly attributable to the loss in VH, with a relative sparing of the CD. However, longer VH in ETEC K88 infected-piglets receiving VIP than in ETEC K88 infected-piglets alone was observed in the study. Longer VH are often used as an indicator of an increased absorptive capacity of the small intestinal and a healthy gut [25]. The experiment demonstrated that VIP effectively alleviated the magnitude of the mucosal damage. However, no significant differences were observed among treatments in VCR. Moreover, enteric pathogen and endotoxin translocations are known to increase paracellular permeability through tight junction (TJs) alterations [26]. Numerous studies using animals and cell cultures indicate that occludin plays crucial roles in the TJs structure and

permeability in the intestinal epithelia [27–29]. In the study, administration with VIP alleviated ETEC K88 induced reduction of occludin expression in the ileum. Previous research also indicates that VIP has an important role in the nerve-mediated maintenance of intestinal barrier function by acting on ZO-1 [30]. Clarke et al. reported that invasive bacteria could lead to changes in TJ protein expression via TLRs-mediated pathways [31]. VIP protects the colonic epithelial barrier by minimizing bacterial-induced redistribution of tight junction proteins in part through actions on myosin light chain kinase (MLCK) and myosin light chain phosphorylation (p-MLC) [32].

Studies have shown that the function of the intestinal barrier may be regulated by a network of multiple cytokines, including ILs, IFNs and TNF-α [33]. An imbalance of pro-inflammatory cytokines and anti-inflammatory cytokines is another important mechanism of intestinal mucosal injury. The primary function of S-IgA is referred to as immune exclusion, a process that limits the access of numerous microorganisms and mucosal antigens to these thin and vulnerable mucosal barriers [34]. In the current study, the serum levels of S-IgA, IL-4, IL-10 and TGF-β from the ETEC K88 infected-pigs receiving VIP were higher than those from the ETEC K88 infected-pigs alone. It has been shown that VIP increase production of anti-inflammatory cytokines such as IL-10, TGF-β and IL-1Ra [12,35]. TNF-α, IL-6 and IFN-γ play important roles in various inflammatory reactions and are highly correlated with the severity of inflammation. IFN-γ is the main Th1-type cytokine produced by T effector lymphocytes. Under pathophysiological conditions, pro-inflammatory cytokines, antigens, and pathogens contribute to barrier impairment [36,37]. Moreover, weaning is associated with upregulation of IL-1, Il-6, and TNF-α in the intestine, and this early inflammatory response may contribute to both anatomical and functional intestinal disorders in piglets [38]. However, treatment with VIP significantly decreased the levels of TNF-α, IL-6 and INF-γ, suggesting that VIP may improve the permeability of the intestinal mucosa and protect the intestinal. The results are consistent with the report that VIP/PACAP protect mice from the lethal effect of high endotoxemia through the inhibition of TNF-α and IL-6 [39]. Modulatory effect of VIP on immune abnormalities mitigated the damage and inflammation of the intestinal immune response, which may also be one of the mechanisms VIP reducing rates of diarrhea in infected-piglets. Postnatal development of porcine IMIS was accompanied by a substantial increase in the secretion of neuropeptides/enzyme tested and that these molecules may participate in the functional maturation of immunoregulatory/ bactericidal mechanisms of the local (intestinal) immune defense in young pigs [40]. Recent study indicated that inhaled VIP exerts immunoregulatory effects in sarcoidosis [41]. VIP and urocortin protect from the lethal effect of *E.coli* and cecal ligation and puncture (CLP)-induced sepsis and this protection is paralleled by a decrease in the systemic levels of high mobility group box 1 (HMGB1) [42]. The therapeutic effect of VIP was initially attributed to the down-regulation of a wide panel of inflammatory mediators and to the inhibition of autoreactive T_H1 cells [43,44]. VIP is now recognized as playing a major role in the regulation of Th1/Th2 balance [45]. Mounting evidence indicates that VIP via multiple mechanisms to counter inflammatory factors. VIP is also produced by lymphoid cells and exerts a wide variety of immunological functions, including control of homeostasis of the immune system by ligand-receptor signaling to immunocompetent cells, regulation of the production of anti- or pro-inflammatory mediators, changing of expression of co-stimulatory molecules leading to switching of Th1 to Th2 response, and stimulation of B cell differentiation and production of IgA antibodies [46,47]. Anti-

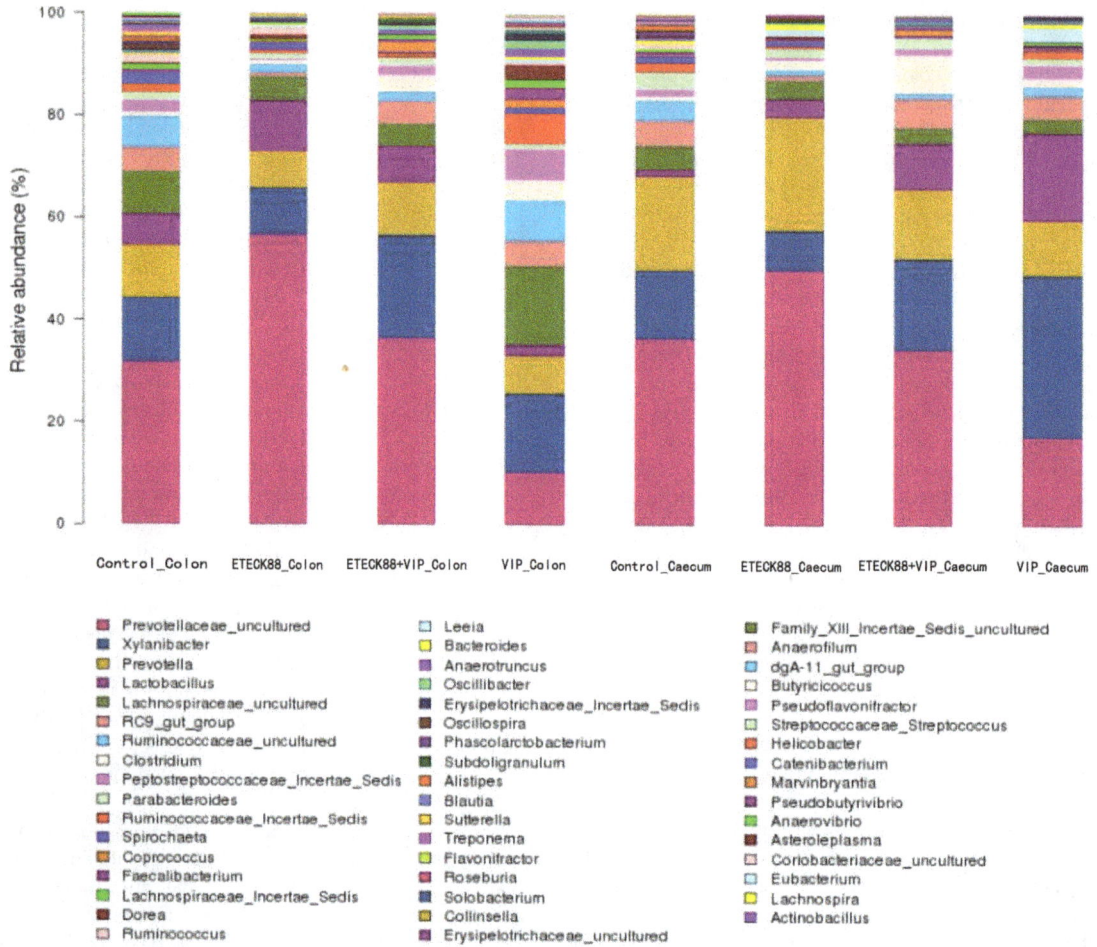

Figure 4. Bacterial composition of the different communities. Relative read abundance of different bacterial genus within the different communities. Sequences that could not be classified into any known group were assigned as "unclassified bacteria". The ETEC K88-challenged pigs and unchallenged pigs with same breed and age, and similar weight were not from the same litter and were assigned to the four treatments in a randomized complete block design. All pigs were housed in stainless steel pens (three piglets per pen) in the same unit.

A.

B.

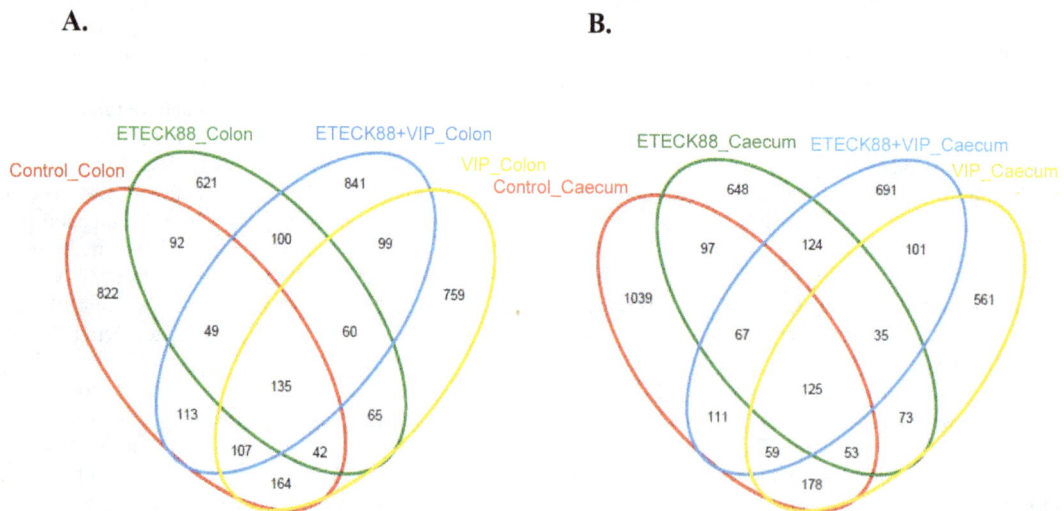

Figure 5. Shared OUT analysis of the different libraries. Venne diagram showing the unique and shared OTUs (3% distance level) in the different libraries (A) for the colon libraries from different treatments, and (B) for the caecum libraries from different treatments.

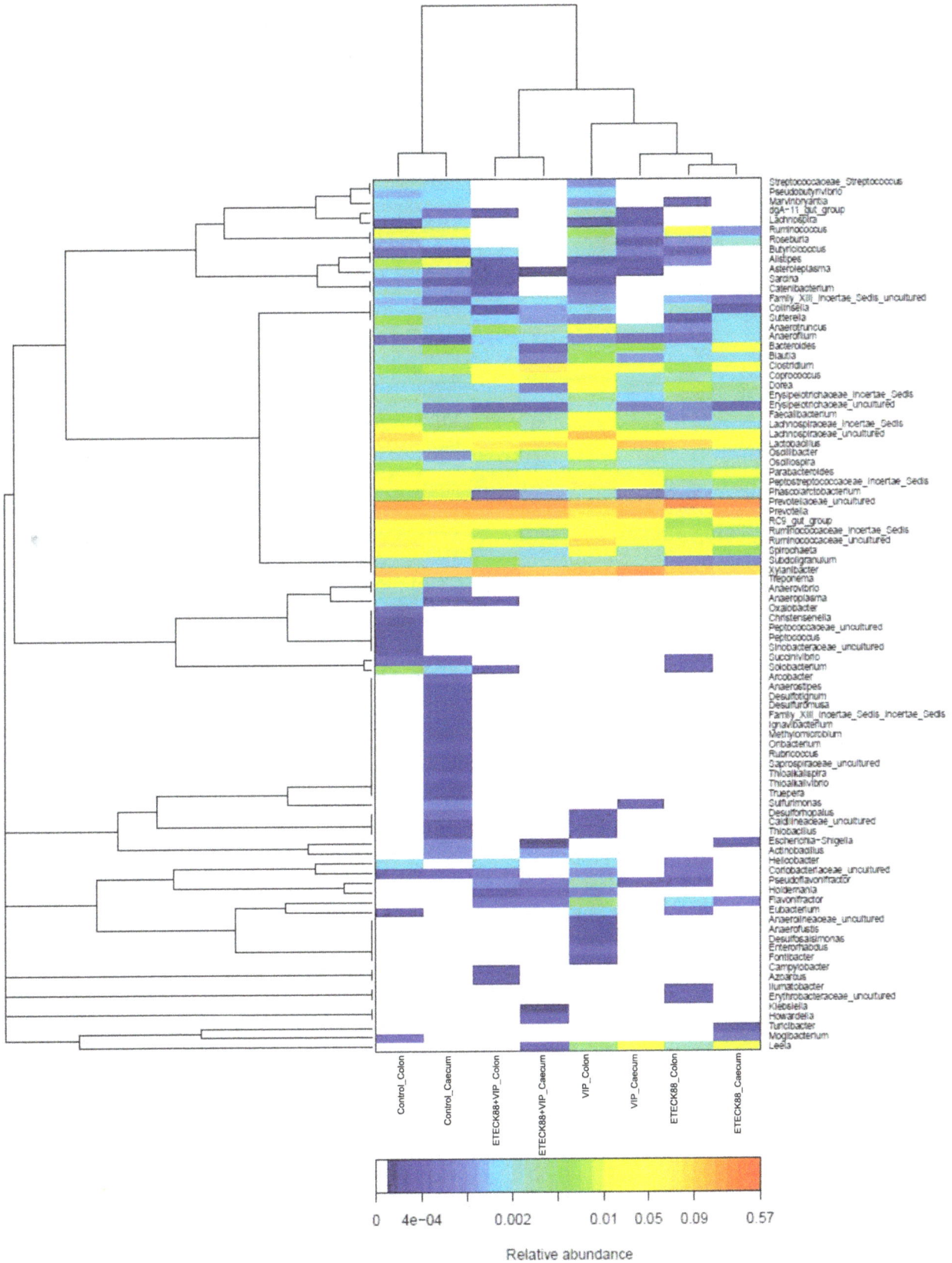

Figure 6. Bacterial distribution among the eight samples. Double hierarchical dendrogram showing the bacterial distribution among the samples. The bacterial phylogenetic tree was calculated using the neighbor-joining method and the relationship among samples was determined by Bray distance and the complete clustering method. The heatmap plot depicts the relative percentage of each bacterial family are depicted by color intensity with the legend indicated at the bottom of the figure. Clusters based on the distance of the eight samples along the X-axis and the bacterial families along the Y-axis are indicated in the upper and left of the figure, respectively.

Table 3. Shared phyla among the colon content and caecum content libraries*.

Phylum	Shared OTUs	Shared reads (colon content)				Shared OTUs	Shared reads (caecum content)			
		Control	ETEC K88	ETEC K88+VIP	VIP		Control	ETEC K88	ETEC K88+VIP	VIP
Actinobacteria	1	7	15	4	14	1	19	1	5	3
Bacteroidetes	68	3762	5408	5789	3093	62	6773	5981	5871	4610
Firmicutes	44	3437	1605	2257	4662	39	3297	1342	2161	2114
Proteobacteria	3	43	24	18	45	3	55	76	14	134
Spirochaetes	4	139	76	14	56	3	90	38	8	17
Tenericutes	2	413	318	12	246	2	215	207	21	71
unclassified	13	4	8	10	8	15	10	4	7	2
Total shared sequences	135	7801	7446	8094	8116	125	10449	7645	8080	6949
Total reads		7844	7485	8138	8165		10515	7696	8106	6975
Shared reads/Total reads (%)		99.45	99.48	99.46	99.4		99.37	99.34	99.68	99.63

*The phyla in bold letters represent core gut microbiota.

inflammatory effect of VIP is ascribed to its ability to abrogate phagocytosis and chemotaxis of macrophages [48] and to inhibit T cell proliferation and migration [49].

Intestinal microorganisms participate in various physiological functions, by which they influence their hosts. Enteric pathogens may cause several damages to intestinal cells, including interference in the epithelial cell signaling that controls both the transcellular and paracellular secretion pathways; concequently, protection against pathogenic and conditionally pathogenic microorganisms in the form of colonization resistance is most important [50]. In the current study, the microbial community of piglets in each treatment has been determined in detail. The obtained results indicated that ETEC K88 challenge diminished colon and caecum contents bacterial diversity and abundance. Administration with VIP increased these measurements, which may be associated with its capability of stimulating diverse microbial communities to colonize the GIT. An increase in microbial diversity has been associated with increased ecosystem stability and resistance to pathogen invasion [51]. The effect of VIP on intestinal bacterial community may be significant for its role in improving growth performance, reducing diarrhea ratio, and exerting immunoregulation function. Many researches demonstrate that the gut microflora plays an important role in the maintenance of animal health, improving immunity, participating in the absorption and metabolism of nutrients. Although the involved mechanisms remain unclear, similar to other neuropeptides [52], VIP shares some properties with antimicrobial peptides, such as small size, cationic charge, and amphipathic design. In addition, VIP is abundantly present in physical barriers of the body, physiological fluids, and immunoprivileged sites [53]. VIP is released under microbial-induced inflammation [54,55]. *Bacteroidetes* and *Firmicutes* were prevalent members of the intestinal bacterial communities in each treatment. These results were consistent with a previous report. The gut microbiota of pigs mainly consists of the *Bacteroidetes* and *Firmicutes* divisions [56], just as mice and humans. In the study, ETEC K88 challenge increased abundance of *Bacteroidetes* in colon content, increased the relative proportion of *Prevotellaceae_uncultured* in colon and caecum content compared with the control group. The proportion of *Bacteroidetes* had a negative correlation with the body weight [57]. Interesting, although administration of VIP alone did not change the intestinal morphology and the mucosal immune function, it could reshape the community structure in colon and caecum content. The possible mechanism of VIP affecting the gut microbial community structure may be associated with antimicrobial activity against certain groups of microorganisms and its secretory effects on intestinal epithelia. VIP displayed antimicrobial activity against *Escherichia coli* ATCC25922 and *Pseudomonas aeruginosa* ATCC 27853 in vitro [15]. Two VIP derivatives kill various non-pathogenic and pathogenic Gram-positive and Gram-negative bacteria through a mechanism that depends on the interaction with certain components of the microbial surface, the formation of pores, and the disruption of the surface membrane [16]. VIP binds to crypt cell receptors and triggers secretion of NaCl and water [58,59]. VIP strongly potentiated carbachol-induced mucin secretin [60]. Mourad and Nassar (2000) showed that VIP plays a role in heat labile enterotoxin (LT) and heat stable enterotoxin type A (STa) induced intestinal secretion and may be the final putative neurotransmitter in the pathophysiology of these toxins [61]. The potential advantages of the secretory effect for the host can be the flushing of the intestinal lumen and the clearing of pathogenic microbes. In pigs, the microbial ecosystem undergoes massive fluctuations in the time after weaning, and pigs are prone to enteric dysbiosis until a stable autochthonous microbiota has

Table 4. Differentially Abundant Features of Colon Contents*.

Control vs. ETEC K88	ETEC K88 vs. ETEC K88+VIP	Control vs. VIP
Alistipes	*Anaerotruncus*	*Alistipes*
Anaerotruncus	*Butyricicoccus*	Anaeroplasma
Anaerovibrio	*Clostridium*	*Anaerotruncus*
Catenibacterium	Collinsella	Anaerovibrio
Coprococcus	*Coprococcus*	*Blautia*
Dorea	Dorea	*Butyricicoccus*
Faecalibacterium	Erysipelotrichaceae_Incertae_Sedis	*Catenibacterium*
Flavonifractor	*Faecalibacterium*	Clostridium
Lachnospiraceae_Incertae_Sedis	*Flavonifractor*	Coprococcus
Lachnospiraceae_uncultured	Helicobacter	Dorea
Lactobacillus	*Lachnospiraceae_Incertae_Sedis*	Eubacterium
Leeia	*Lactobacillus*	Faecalibacterium
No_Rank	Leeia	Flavonifractor
Oscillospira	*No_Rank*	Lachnospiraceae_Incertae_Sedis
Peptostreptococcaceae_Incertae_Sedis	Oscillibacter	Lachnospiraceae_uncultured
Phascolarctobacterium	Parabacteroides	Lactobacillus
Prevotellaceae_uncultured	*Peptostreptococcaceae_Incertae_Sedis*	Leeia
Prevotella	Prevotellaceae_uncultured	No_Rank
RC9_gut_group	Prevotella	Oscillibacter
Ruminococcaceae_Incertae_Sedis	RC9_gut_group	Peptostreptococcaceae_Incertae_Sedis
Ruminococcaceae_uncultured	Ruminococcus	Prevotellaceae_uncultured
Solobacterium	Spirochaeta	Prevotella
Streptococcaceae_Streptococcus	*Subdoligranulum*	Pseudoflavonifractor
Sutterella	Xylanibacter	RC9_gut_group
Treponema		*Roseburia*
dgA-11_gut_group		*Ruminococcaceae_Incertae_Sedis*
		Ruminococcaceae_uncultured
		Ruminococcus
		Solobacterium
		Spirochaeta
		Streptococcaceae_Streptococcus
		Sutterella
		Treponema
		Xylanibacter

*Bacterial community comparison between the groups in the level of genus; The genus listed in the table are significant between the groups. Among of them, shared genus of bacteria between groups is shown in italics bold.

been developed [62]. The impact of bacteria on intestinal barrier function is clearly illustrated by the action of specific pathogenic enteric bacteria that have evolved remarkable means to penetrate and circumvent this important host defense mechanism [63]. Some bacteria such as *Lactobacillus plantarum* appear to modulate the epithelial barrier through the action of secreted protein (LGG p40) whereas other such as *Clostridium* likely influence the barrier through production of metabolites (SCFA). In view of the richness and diversity of the microbiota, it would be important to identify microorganisms with barrier protective function. Understanding the intricate relationship between epithelial barrier, microbe, and VIP would undeniably contribute key knowledge that could be harness for therapeutic purpose.

TLRs are one of the most important pattern recognition receptors (PRR) in innate immunity [64] and play a critical role in pathogen recognition and host defense [65,66]. However, inappropriate TLR signaling can contribute to loss of tolerance and result in tissue injury, the best example of such injury is the intestinal damage ediated by the inflammatory response triggered by the interaction between lipopolysaccharide (LPS) and TLR4. LPS present in the outer membranes of some Gram-negative pathogens such as ETEC triggers the production of proinflammatory mediators that may contribute to intestinal inflammation and damage during the infection [67]. The modulation of TLR expression is one of the most recent functions in immunity attribute to VIP [68–70]. The current results showed that ETEC K88 infection increased the expression of TLR2, TLR4 and MyD88, and induced the phosphorylation of IKBα), p-ERK, p-JNK and p38. The best known signaling pathway activated by TLRs is associated with the MyD88 adapter. Key points in this

Table 5. Differentially Abundant Features of Caecum Contents*.

Control vs. ETEC K88	ETEC K88 vs. ETEC K88+VIP	Control vs. VIP
Alistipes	*Anaerotruncus*	*Alistipes*
Anaerofilum	*Bacteroides*	*Blautia*
Bacteroides	*Clostridium*	*Clostridium*
Clostridium	*Coprococcus*	*Collinsella*
Dorea	*Dorea*	*Lachnospiraceae_uncultured*
Erysipelotrichaceae_Incertae_Sedis	*Family_XIII_Incertae_Sedis_uncultured*	*Lactobacillus*
Lachnospiraceae_Incertae_Sedis	*Lachnospiraceae_Incertae_Sedis*	*Leeia*
Lachnospira	*Lactobacillus*	*Marvinbryantia*
Lactobacillus	*Leeia*	*No_Rank*
Leeia	*No_Rank*	*Oscillibacter*
Marvinbryantia	*Oscillibacter*	*Parabacteroides*
No_Rank	*Peptostreptococcaceae_Incertae_Sedis*	*Peptostreptococcaceae_Incertae_Sedis*
Oscillospira	*Prevotellaceae_uncultured*	*Phascolarctobacterium*
Parabacteroides	*Prevotella*	*Prevotellaceae_uncultured*
Peptostreptococcaceae_Incertae_Sedis	*RC9_gut_group*	*Prevotella*
Phascolarctobacterium	*Roseburia*	*Ruminococcaceae_uncultured*
Prevotellaceae_uncultured	*Spirochaeta*	*Ruminococcus*
Prevotella	*Subdoligranulum*	*Solobacterium*
Pseudobutyrivibrio	*Xylanibacter*	*Spirochaeta*
RC9_gut_group		*Streptococcaceae_Streptococcus*
Roseburia		*Subdoligranulum*
Ruminococcaceae_Incertae_Sedis		*Sutterella*
Ruminococcaceae_uncultured		*Treponema*
Ruminococcus		*Xylanibacter*
Solobacterium		
Streptococcaceae_Streptococcus		
Treponema		
Xylanibacter		

*Bacterial community comparison between the groups in the level of genus; The genus listed in the table are significant between the groups. Among of them, shared genus of bacteria between groups is shown in italics bold.

pathway are TRAF6 activation by ubiquitination, IKK phosphorylation and activation of NF-κB and MAPK. Actually, many genes induced by TLR activation are controlled by both NF-κB and activator protein1 (AP-1). However, VIP treatment decreased the expression of TLR2, TLR4 and MyD88, and inhibited NF-κB and MAPK activation. Moreover, the activation of TLRs/NF-κB and TLRs/MAPK signaling was consistent with changes in the serum levels of IL-2, Il-6, IL-12p40, IFN-γ, and TNF-α. NF-κB is an essential transcription factor that regulates transcription of genes involved in the early inflammatory responses such as cytokines, chemokines and adhesion molecules and plays a central role in the pathobiology of inflammation [71]. Once activated, MAPK can phosphorylate transcription factors or transcriptional co-regulators or phosphorylate downstream kinases that induce expression of inflammatory mediators by extracellular stimuli [72]. The expression of proinflammatory genes such as TNF-α, IL-6 and IL-12 are induced via activation of NF-κB and MAPKs [73]. TGF-β is an anti-inflammatory cytokine produced in response to LPS stimulation that can attenuate the TLR-induced inflammatory response. Moreover, TGF-β is reported to produce ubiquitination and degradation of MyD88 protein, leading to a downregulation of MyD88-dependent activation of NF-κB and

TNF-α production [74]. The present results suggested that modulatory effect of VIP on intestinal mucosal immunity may be by inhibition of TLR2/4-MyD88/NF-κB, and the inhibition of TLR2/4-MyD88/MAPK pathway. The negative effects of VIP signaling on NF-κB activation have been well described in the mouse. In *vivo* VIP treatment in the collagen-induced arthritis model prevents NF-κB nuclear translocation through the inhibition of IκB-α phosphorylation and degradation [75]. VIP downregulates the activity of several transduction pathways and their associated transcription factors essential for the transcriptional activation of most inflammatory cytokines, chemokines and costimulatory factors, including NF-κB, MAPK, interferon regulatory factor 1 (IRF1) and AP1 [76,77]. As a small and hydrophilic molecule, VIP possesses excellent permeability properties that permit rapid access to the site of inflammation. Its high-affinity binding to specific receptors makes VIP very potent in exerting its immunomodulating and anti-inflammatory activities [78]. Although the exact mechanism of VIP-induced interference in TLRs expression and function in weaned piglets infected by ETEC K88 remains to be elucidated, emerging evidence suggests that the use of this neuroimmunopeptide represents one of the most promising future strategies for combating infections.

Conclusion

The current study contributes to an understanding of the mechanisms through which VIP may benefit piglets during ETEC challenge. In general, these results confirmed that exogenous neuropeptide VIP improved the intestinal mucosal immunity and microbial community of weaning piglet after an oral challenge with ETEC (K88). The TLR2/4-MyD88 mediated NF-κB and MAPK signaling pathway may be critical to the mechanism underlying the modulatory effect of VIP on intestinal mucosal immune function and bacterial community. Although further studies are needed to evaluate the mechanisms involved, our observation supports the hypothesis that VIP down-mediated multiple proinflammatory pathways, including TLR-mediated pathways. Hence, such potentials of these molecular elements of porcine IMIS should be also monitored when an exogenous immunomodulation is applied to enhance defense of intestinal mucosal surface of weaned pigs against enteric pathogens. The research provides new insight into its use in the animal husbandry.

Acknowledgments

We are grateful to Professor Yizhen Wang of Zhejiang University for kindly donating us the ETEC K88 strain, and Mingliang Jin, Feifei Han, Zeqing Lu for their technical help.

Author Contributions

Conceived and designed the experiments: CLX. Performed the experiments: YMW RS XJQ. Analyzed the data: RS. Contributed reagents/materials/analysis tools: XYS WNN. Contributed to the writing of the manuscript: CLX.

References

1. Stokes CR, Bailey M, Haverson K, Harris C, Jones P, et al. (2004) Postnatal development of intestinal immune system in piglets: implications for the process of weaning. Anim Res 53: 325–334.
2. Fairbrother JM, Nadeau E, Gyles CL (2005) *Escherichia coli* in postweaning diarrhea in pigs: an update on bacterial types, pathogenesis, and prevention strategies. Anim Health Res Rev 6: 17–39.
3. Konstantinov SR, Favier CF, Zhu WY, Williams BA, Klub J, et al. (2004) Microbial diversity studies of the porcine gastrointestinal ecosystem during weaning transition. Anim Res 53: 317–24.
4. Bailey M, Haverson K, Inman C, Harris C, Jones P, et al. (2005) The development of the mucosal immune system pre- and post-weaning: balancing regulatory and effector function. Proc Nutr Soc 64: 451–457.
5. Round JL, Mazmanian SK (2009) The gut microbiota shapes intestinal immune responses during health and disease. Nat Rev Immunol 9: 313–323.
6. Keita AV, Soderholm JD (2010) The intestinal barrier and its regulation by neuroimmune factors. Neurogastroenerol Motil 22: 718–733.
7. Gomariz RP, Gutierrez-Canas I, Arranz A, Carrion M, Juarranz Y, et al. (2010) Peptides targeting toll-like receptor signaling pathway for novel immune therapeutics. Current Pharmaceutical Design 16: 1063–1080.
8. Pozo D, Gonzalez-Rey E, Chorny A, Anderson P, Varela N, et al. (2007) Tuning immune tolerance with vasoactive intestinal peptide: a new therapeutic approach for immune disorders. Peptides 28: 1833–1846.
9. Sherwood NM, Krueckl SL, McRory JE (2000) The origin and function of the pituitary adenylate cyclase-activating polypeptide (PACAP)/glucagon superfamily. Endocr Rev 21: 619–670.
10. Kojima M, Ito T, Oono T, Hisano T, Igarashi H, et al. (2005) VIP attenuation of the severity of experimental pancreatitis is due to VPAC1 receptor-mediated inhibition of cytokine production. Pancreas 30: 62–70.
11. Delgado M, Gomariz RP, Martinez C, Abad C, Leceta J (2000) Antiinflammatory properties of the type 1 and type 2 vasoactive intestinal peptide receptors: role in lethal endotoxic shock. Eur J Immunol 30: 3236–46.
12. Delgado M, Abad C, Martinez C, Leceta J, Gomariz RP (2001) Vasoactive intestinal peptide prevents experimental arthritis by downregulating both autoimmune and inflammatory components of the disease. Nat Med 7: 563–568.
13. Abad C, Martinez C, Juarranz MG, Arranz A, Leceta J, et al. (2003) Therapeutic effects of vasoactive intestinal peptide in the trinitrobenzene sulfonic acid mice model of Crohn's disease. Gastroenterology 124: 961–971.
14. Bik W, Wolinska-Witort E, Chmielowska M, Baranowska-Bik A, Rusiecka-Kuczalek E, et al. (2004) Vasoactive intestinal peptide can modulate immune and endocrine responses during lipopolysaccharide-induced acute inflammation. Neuroimmunomodulation 11: 358–364.
15. El-Karim IA, Linden GJ, Orr DF, Lundy FT (2008) Antimicrobial activity of neuropeptides against a range of micro-organisms from skin, oral, respiratory and gastrointestinal tract sites. J Neuroimmunol 200: 11–16.
16. Campos-Salinas J, Cavazzuti A, O'Valle F, Forte-Lago I, Caro M, et al. (2014) Therapeutic efficacy of stable analogues of vasoactive intestinal peptide against pathogens. J Biol Chem 289: 14583–14599.
17. Liu P, Piao XS, Thacker PA, Zeng ZK, Li PF, et al. (2010) Chito-oligosaccharide reduces diarrhea incidence and attenuates the immune response of weaned pigs challenged with *Escherichia coli* K88. J Anim Sci. 88: 3871–3879.
18. Kiarie E, Bhandari S, Scott M, Krause DO, Nyachoti CM (2011) Growth performance and gastrointestinal microbial ecology responses of piglets receiving saccharomyces cerevisiae fermentation products after an oral challenge with *Escherichia coli* (K88). J Anim Sci. 89: 1062–1078.
19. Arranz A, Juarranz Y, Leceta J, Gomariz RP, Martinez C (2008) VIP balances innate and adaptive immune responses induced by specific stimulation of TLR2 and TLR4. Peptide. 29: 948–956.
20. Schmidt PT, Eriksen L, Loftager M, Rasmussen TN, Holst JJ (1999) Fast acting nervous regulation of immunoglobulin A secretion from isolated perfused porcine ileum. Gut 45: 679–685.
21. Nyachoti CM, Kiarie E, Bhandari SK, Zhang G, Krause DO (2012) Weaned pig responses to *Escherichia coli* K88 oral challenge when receiving a lysozyme supplement. J Anim Sci. 90: 252–260.
22. Francis DH, Grange PA, Zeman DH, Baker DR, Sun RG, et al. (1998) Expression of mucin-type glycoprotein K88 receptor strongly correlates with piglet susceptibility to K88 enterotoxigenic *Escherichia coli*, but adhesion of this bacterium to brush border does not. Infect. Immun. 66: 4050–4055.
23. Gaastra W, de Graaf FK (1982) Host-specific fimbrial adhensins of noninvasive enterotoxigenic *Escherichia coli* strains. Microbiol Rev 46: 129–161.
24. Owusu-Asiedu A, Nyachoti CM, Marquardt RR (2003) Response of early-weaned pigs to an enterotoxigenic *Escherichia coli* (K88) challenge when fed diets containing spray-dried porcine plasma or pea protein isolate plus egg yolk antibody, zinc oxide, fumaric acid, or antibiotic. J Anim Sci 81: 1790–1798.
25. Nyachoti CM, Omogbenigun FO, Rademacher M, Blank G (2006) Performance responses and indicators of gastrointestinal health in early-weaned pigs fed low-protein amino acid-supplemented diets. J Anim Sci 84: 125–134.
26. Groschwitz KR, Hogan SP (2009) Intestinal barrier function: molecular regulation and disease pathogenesis. J Allergy Clin Immunol 124: 3–20.
27. Kim JC, Hansen CF, Mullan BP, Pluske JR (2012) Nutrition and pathology of weaner pigs: Nutrional strategies to support barrier function in the gastrointestinal tract. Anim Feed Sci Technol 173: 3–16.
28. Al-Sadi R, Khatib K, Guo S, Ye D, Youssef M, et al. (2011) Occludin regulates macromolecule flux across the intestinal epithelial tight junction barrier. Am J Physiol Gastrointest Liver Physiol 300: G1054–G1064.
29. Wong V, Gumbiner BM (1997) A synthetic peptide corresponding to the extracellular domain of occluding perturbs the tight junction permeability barrier. J Cell Biol 136: 399–409.
30. Neunlist M, Toumi F, Oreshkova T, Denis M, Leborgne J, et al. (2003) Human ENS regulates the intestinal epithelial barrier permeability and a tight junction-associated protein ZO-1 via a VIPerigic pathway. Am J Physiol Gastrointest Liver Physiol 285: G1028–G1036.
31. Clarke TB, Francella N, Huegel A, Weiser JN (2011) Invasive bacterial pathogens exploit TLR-mediated downregulation of tight junction components to facilitate translocation across the epithelium. Cell Host Microbe, 9: 404–414.
32. Conlin VS, Wu X, Nguyen C, Dai C, Vallance BA, et al. (2009) Vasoactive intestinal peptide ameliorates intestinal barrier disruption associated with *Citrobacter rodentium*-induced colitis. Am J Physiol Gastrointest Liver Physiol 297: G735–G750.
33. Xavier RJ, Podolsky DK (2007) Unravelling the pathogenesis of inflammatory bowel disease. Nature 448: 427–434.
34. Corthesy B (2013) Multi-faceted functions of secretory IgA at mucosal surfaces. Front. Immunol. 4: 1–11.
35. Delgado M, Munoz-Elias EJ, Gomariz RP, Ganea D (1999) Vasoactive intestinal peptide and pituitary adenylate cyclase-activating polypeptide enhance IL-10 production by murine macrophages: in vitro and in vivo studies. J Immunol 162: 1707–1716.
36. Nusrat A, Turner JR, Madara JL (2000) Molecular physiology and pathophysiology of tight junctions. IV. Regulation of tight junctions by extracellular stimuli: nutrients, cytokines, and immune cells. Am J Physiol Gastrointest Liver Physiol 279: G851–G857.
37. Capaldo CT, Nusrat A (2009) Cytokine regulation of tight junctions. Biochim Biophys Acta 1788: 864–871.
38. Pie S, Lalles JP, Blazy F, Laffitte J, Seve B, et al. (2004) Weaning is associated with an upregulation of expression of inflammatory cytokines in the intestine of piglets. J Nutrition 134: 641–647.
39. Delgado M, Martinez C, Pozo D, Calvo JR, Leceta J, et al. (1999) Vasoactive intestinal peptide (VIP) and pituitary adenylate cyclase-activation polypeptide

(PACAP) protect mice from lethal endotoxemia through the inhibition of TNF-α and IL-6. J Immunol 162: 1200–1205.

40. Kovsca Janjatovic A, Valpotic H, Kezic D, Lackovic G, Gregorovic G, et al. (2012) Secretion of immunomodulating neuropeptides (VIP, SP) and nitric oxide synthase in porcine small intestine during postnatal development. Eur J Histochem 56: e30.

41. Prasse A, Zissel G, Lutzen N, Schupp J, Schmiedlin R, et al. (2010) Inhaled vasoactive intestinal peptide exerts immunoregulatory effects in sarcoidosis. Am J Respir Crit Care Med 182: 540–548.

42. Chorny A, Delgado M (2008) Neuropeptides rescue mice from lethal sepsis by down-regulating secretion of the late-acting inflammatory mediator high mobility group box 1. Am J Pathol 172: 1297–1302.

43. Delgado M, Pozo D, Ganea D (2004) The significance of vasoactive intestinal peptide in immunomodulation. Pharmacol Rev 56: 249–290.

44. Gonzale-Rey E, Chorny A, Delgado M (2007) Regulation of immune tolerance by anti-inflammatory neuropeptides. Nat Rev Immunol 7: 52–63.

45. Delgado M, Ganea D (2001) Gutting edge: is vasoactive intestinal peptide a type 2 cytokine? J Immunol 166: 2907–2912.

46. Kimata H, Fujimoto M (1994) Vasoactive intestinal peptide specifically induces human IgA1 and IgA2 production. Eur J Immunol 24: 2262–2265.

47. Delgado M, Abad C, Martinez C, Juarranz MG, Arranz A, et al. (2002) Vasoactive intestinal peptide in the immune system: potential therapeutic role in inflammatory and autoimmune diseases. J Mol Med 80: 16–24.

48. De la Fuente M, Delgado M, Gomariz RP (1996) VIP modulation of immune cell function. Adv Neuroimmunol 6: 75–91.

49. Delgado M, De la Fuente M, Martinez C, Gomariz RP (1995) Pituitary adenylate cyclaseactivating polypeptides (PACAP27 and PACAP38) inhibit the mobility of murine thymocytes and splenic lymphocytes: comparison with VIP and implication of cAMP. J Neuroimmunol 62: 137–146.

50. Roselli M, Finamore A, Britti MS, Bosi P, Oswald I, et al (2005) Alternatives to in-feed antibiotics in pigs: Evaluation of probiotics, zinc or organic acids as protective agents for the intestinal mucosa. A comparison of in vitro and in vivo results. Anim Res 54: 203–218.

51. Konstantinov SR, Favier CF, Zhu WY, Williams BA, Klüβ J, et al. (2004) Microbial diversity studies of the porcine gastrointestinal ecosystem during weaning transition. Anim Res 53: 317–324.

52. Augustyniak D, Nowak, Lundy FT (2012) Direct and indirect antimicrobial activities of neuropeptides and their therapeutic potential. Curr. Protein Pept Sci. 13: 723–738.

53. Vaudry D, Gonzalez BJ, Basille M, Yon L, Fournier A, et al. (2000) Pituitary adenylate cyclase-activating polypeptide and its receptors: from structure to functions. Pharmacol Rev. 52: 269–324.

54. Delgado M, Anderson P, Garcia-Salcedo JA, Caro M, Gonzalez-Rey E (2009) Neuropeptides kill African trypanosomes by targeting intracellular compartments and inducing autophagic-like cell death. Cell Death Differ. 16: 406–416.

55. Brogden KA, Guthmiller JM, Salzet M, Zasloff M (2005) The nervous system and innate immunity: the neuropeptide connection. Nat Immunol 6: 558–564.

56. Leser TD, Amernuvor JZ, Jensen TK, Lindecrona RH, Boye M, et al. (2004) Culture-independent analysis of gut bacteria: the pig gastrointestinal tract microbiota revisited. Appl Environ Microbiol 68, 673–690.

57. Guo X, Xia X, Tang R, Zhou J, Zhao H, et al. (2008) Development of a real-time PCR method for Firmicutes and Bacteroidetes in faeces and its application to quantify intestinal population of obese and lean pigs. Lett Appl Microbiol 47: 367–373.

58. Goyal RK, Hirano I (1996) The enteric nervous system. N Engl J Med 334: 1106–1115.

59. Mccabe RD, Dharmsathaphorn K (1988) Mechanism of VIP-stimulated chloride secretion by intestinal epithelial cells. Annals of the New York Academy of Sciences 527: 326–345.

60. Laburthe M, Auqeron C, Rouyer-Fessard C, Roumaqnac I, Maoret JJ, et al. (1989) Functional VIP receptors in the human mucus-secreting colonic epithelial cell line CL.16E. Am J Physiol 256: G443–G450.

61. Mourad FH, Nassar CF (2000) Effect of vasoactive intestinal polypeptide (VIP) antagonism on rat jejuna fluid and electrolyte secretion induced by cholera and Escherichia coli enterotoxins. Gut 47: 382–386.

62. Lallès JP, Bosi P, Janczyk P, Koopmans SJ, Torrallardona D (2009) Impact of bioactive substances on the gastrointestinal tract and performance of weaned piglets: a review. Animal 3: 1625–1643.

63. Guzman JR, Conlin VS, Jobin C (2013) Diet, microbiome, and the intestinal epithelium: an essential triumvirate? BioMed Res Intern. 2013: 1–12.

64. Westendorf AM, Fleissner D, Hansen W, Buer J (2010) T cells, dendritic cells and epithelial cells in intestinal homeostasis. Int J Med Microbiol 300: 11–18.

65. Alvarez S, Villena J, Tohno M, Salva S, Kitazawa H (2009) Modulation of innate immunity by lactic acid bacteria: impact on host response to infections. Curr Res Immunol 3: 87–126.

66. Kitazawa H, Tohno M, Shimosato T, Saito T (2008) Development of molecular immunoassay system for probiotics via toll-like receptors based on food immunology. Anim Sci 79: 11–21.

67. Long KZ, Rosado JL, Santos JI, Haas M, AI Mamun A, et al. (2010) Associations between mucosal innate and adaptive immune responses and resolution of diarrheal pathogen infections. Infect Immun 78: 1221–1228.

68. Gomariz RP, Arranz A, Juarranz Y, Gutierrez-Canas I, Garcia-Gomez M, et al. (2007) Regulation of TLR expression, a new perspective for the role of VIP in immunity. Peptides 28: 1825–1832.

69. Arranz A, Juarranz Y, Leceta J, Gomariz RP, Martinez C (2008) VIP balances innate and adaptive immune responses induced by specific stimulation of TLR2 and TLR4. Peptides 29: 948–956.

70. Gonzalez-Rey E, Chorny A, Delgado M (2007) Regulation of immune tolerance by anti-inflammatory neuropeptides. Nat Rev 7: 52–63.

71. Dokladny K, Lobb R, Wharton W, Ma TY, Moseley PL (2010) LPS-induced cytokine levels are repressed by elevated expression of HSP70 in rats: possible role of NF-kappa B. Cell Stress Chaperones 15: 153–163.

72. Hwang MH, Damte D, Lee JS, Gebru E, Chang ZQ, et al. (2011) Mycoplasma hyopneumoniae induces pro-inflammatory cytokine and nitric oxide production through NF-κB and MAPK pathways in RAW264.7 cells. Vet Res Commun 35: 21–34.

73. Gonzalez-Rey E, Chorny A, Delgado M (2007) Regulation of immune tolerance by anti-inflammatory neuropeptides. Nat Rev 7: 52–63.

74. Naiki Y, Michelsen KS, Zhang W, Chen S, Doherty TM, et al. (2005) Transforming growth factor-β differentially inhibits MyD88-dependent, but not TRAM-and TRIF-dependent, lipopolysaccharide-induced TLR4 signaling. J Biol Chem 280: 5491–5495.

75. Juarranz Y, Abad C, Martinez C, Arranz A, Gutierrez-Carias I, et al. (2005) Protective effect of vasoactive intestinal peptide on bone destruction in the collagen-induced arthritis model of rheumatoid arthritis. Arthritis Res Ther 7: R1034–1045.

76. Delgado M, Ganea D (2000) Vasoactive intestinal peptide and pituitary adenylate cyclase-activating polypeptide inhibit the MEKK/MEK4/JNK signaling pathway in LPS-activated macrophages. J Neuroimmunol 110: 97–105.

77. Delgado M, Ganea D (2003) Vasoactive intestinal peptide inhibits IL-8 production in human monocytes by downregulating nuclear factor kappaB-dependent transcriptional activity. Biochem Biophys Res Commun 302: 275–283.

78. Laburthe M, Couvineau A (2002) Molecular pharmacology and structure of VPAC receptors for VIP and PACAP. Regulaory Peptides. 108: 165–173.

6

Effects of Chitosan on Intestinal Inflammation in Weaned Pigs Challenged by Enterotoxigenic *Escherichia coli*

Dingfu Xiao[1], Yongfei Wang[2], Gang Liu[3], Jianhua He[1], Wei Qiu[4], Xionggui Hu[5], Zemeng Feng[2], Maoliang Ran[1], Charles M. Nyachoti[6], Sung Woo Kim[7], Zhiru Tang[8]*, Yulong Yin[3]*

1 College of Animal Science and Technology, Hunan Agricultural University, Changsha, China, 2 Research and Development Center, Twins Group Co., Ltd, Nanchang, Jiangxi, China, 3 Hunan Engineering and Research Center of Animal and Poultry Science and Key Laboratory for Agro-ecological Processes in Subtropical Region, Institute of Subtropical Agriculture, the Chinese Academy of Sciences, Hunan, China, 4 Hunan New Wellful Co., LTD, Changsha, Hunan, China, 5 Hunan Institute of Animal and Veterinary Science, Changsha, China, 6 Department of Animal Science, Faculty of Agricultural and Food Sciences, University of Manitoba, Winnipeg, Manitoba, Canada, 7 Department of Animal Science, North Carolina State University, Raleigh, North Carolina, United States of America, 8 College of Animal Science and Technology, Southwest University, Chongqing, China

Abstract

The aim of this study was to investigate whether supplementation with chitosan (COS) could reduce diarrhea and to explore how COS alleviates intestinal inflammation in weaned pigs. Thirty pigs (Duroc×Landrace×Yorkshire, initial BW of 5.65±0.27) weaned at age 21 d were challenged with enterotoxigenic Escherichia coli during a preliminary trial period, and then divided into three treatment groups. Pigs in individual pens were fed a corn-soybean meal diet, that contained either 0 (control), 50 mg/kg chlortetracycline, or 300 mg/kg COS for 21 days. The post-weaning diarrhea frequency, calprotectin levels and TLR4 protein expression were decreased ($P<0.05$) in both the COS and chlortetracycline groups compared with control. Simultaneously, supplemental COS and chlortetracycline had no effect on the mRNA expression of TNF-α in the jejunal mucosa, or on the concentrations of IL-1β, IL-6 and TNF-α in serum. However, COS supplementation improved ($P<0.05$) the mRNA expression of IL-1β and IL-6 in the jejunal mucosa. The results indicate that supplementation with COS at 300 mg/kg was effective for alleviating intestinal inflammation and enhancing the cell-mediated immune response. As feed additives, chitosan and chlortetracycline may influence different mechanisms for alleviating inflammation in piglets.

Editor: Dipshikha Chakravortty, Indian Institute of Science, India

Funding: This study was supported by National Natural Science Foundation of China (31330075, 31301985), Scientific Research Fund of Hunan Provincial Education Department Project of China (12B058), the National Program on Key Basic Research Project of China (2013CB127303), Natural Science Foundation Project of CQ CSTC (cstc2012jjA80001) and Chinese Academy of Sciences (ISACX-LYQY-QN-1205) and Chinese Academy of Sciences visiting professorship for senior international scientists (Grant no. 2013T2S0014, 2013T2S0015, 2013T2S0012, 2013T1S0010 and 2011T2S15). The funders had no role in study design, data collection and analysis, decision to publish, or preparation of the manuscript.

Competing Interests: The authors have declared that no competing interests exist.

* Email: yinyulong@isa.ac.cn (YY); tangzhiru2326@sina.com (ZT)

Introduction

Weaning removes young pigs from the passive immune protection they receive from the milk of the sow and increases their susceptibility to enterotoxigenic *E. coli* infection [1]. Early-weaned pigs often exhibit an underdeveloped immune system, digestive disorders and post-weaning diarrhea [2]. Enterotoxigenic *E. coli* not only colonize the small intestine, but can also release enterotoxins to stimulate epithelial cells to secrete fluid into the lumen of the gut to cause diarrhea [3]. Therefore, antibiotics are often added to the diet of weanling piglets to prevent infectious disease and improve growth. However, it has been suggested that the continuous use of antibiotics may contribute to a reservoir of drug-resistant bacteria which may be capable of transferring their resistance to pathogenic bacteria in both animals and humans [4]. In addition, consumers are becoming increasingly concerned about the presence of drug residues in livestock products. As a result, many countries have either banned or are in the process of banning the use of antibiotics in pig diets as a routine method for promoting growth.

The pro-inflammatory cytokines IL-1β, IL-6 and TNF-α play a central role in the cell-mediated immune response, and also participate in the maintenance of tissue integrity [5]. The level of fecal calprotectin is a sensitive and non-invasive marker of active inflammation in the gastrointestinal system [6]. Fecal calprotectin may be increased under various conditions, such as inflammatory bowel disease. TLR4, a key receptor for commensal recognition in gut innate immunity, is over-expressed in inflamed colonocytes and is the subject of therapy (target inhibition) in inflammatory bowel disease [7].

Several reports have described the effects of COS on growth [8], immunity [1], and oxidative stress [9], as well as the antimicrobial [10], hypolipidemic [11], and particularly the anti-inflammatory activities of COS both *in vitro* [12,13] and *in vivo* [14,15]. The anti-inflammatory effect of COS *in vitro* has been shown to positively correlate with its molecular weight (MW) and degree of deacetylation (DD) [16]. Chitosan has been shown to have specific immunomodulatory effects: i.e., it can polarize the cytokine balance toward Th1 cytokines, decrease the production of the inflammatory cytokines IL-6 (interleukin-6) and TNF-α, down-regulate CD44 and TLR4 receptor expression, and inhibit

T cell proliferation [17]. However, it is still unclear whether dietary supplementation with COS can alleviate inflammatory bowel diseases and how COS affects intestinal inflammation. Our previous studies showed that supplemental COS in weaned piglets decreased the feed conversion ratio and improved the intestinal morphology, intestinal connectivity, and intestinal mucosal immunity [18]. We established an *Escherichia coli* model of post-weaning diarrhea in early-weaned piglets, and used this new model to investigate the effects of COS on intestinal inflammation by daily monitoring of diarrhea and analyzed the effects of COS on inflammatory responses by determining TLR4 and calprotectin protein expression, as well as the concentration and mRNA expression of IL-1β, IL-6 and TNF-α.

Materials and Methods

Animals and experimental design

Animals and experimental design were same with the previous reported paper [18]. Thirty 21-day-old piglets (Duroc×Landrace×Yorkshire, initial BW of 5.65±0.27) were challenged with enterotoxigenic *Escherichia coli* during a preliminary trial period. The piglets were then randomly assigned into three groups with 10 piglets in each group. The piglets in the control group (A group) were fed the basal diet without any supplement, those in the chlortetracycline group (B group) were fed the basal diet plus 50 mg/kg chlortetracycline, and those in the COS group (C group) were fed the basal diet plus 300 mg/kg COS. The basal diets were formulated based on NRC requirements (National Research Council, 1998), and their compositions and nutritional levels are listed in Table 1. Each group of piglets was fed their respective diet for 21 days. COS (molecular weight <5,000 Da and degree of deacetylation >90%) was provided by Dalian Chemical and Physical Institute (Chinese Academy of Sciences, city, China) and has a 6-sugar unit of N-acetyl glucosamine with β-(1–4)-linkages. Chlortetracycline was provided by Jinhe Biotechnology Co., Ltd. (city, China).

Piglets were randomly allocated into pens with one pig per pen in a temperature-controlled room, as described by Tang et al. Feed was provided to the piglets three times per day at 8:00, 12:00 and 18:00, and any uneaten food was weighed in the morning of the next day. Feed and water were provided *ad libitum*. The piglets were checked daily for signs of disease and mortality. The animals were weighed individually, and feed intake and feed efficiency were determined for each pen on a weekly basis to monitor the growth of animals fed the different diets. At the end of the 21-day period of feeding with the experimental diets, six piglets per treatment were sacrificed for sampling. The animal protocol was approved by the Animal Care Committee of the Institute of Subtropical Agriculture, the Chinese Academy of Sciences.

Sampling and sample processing procedures

Six piglets from each treatment group were sacrificed after feed deprivation for 12 h by the injection of 4% sodium pentobarbital solution (40 mg/kg BW) for the collection of tissue samples on day 21 post-weaning. Blood samples were taken from the heart, and were centrifuged at 3000 rpm for 10 minutes, then, the serums were collected and stored at −80°C. The small intestine (SI) was removed and its length was determined; the jejunum was considered to be located at about 50% of the length of the SI. About 3 g of jejunal mucosa was collected immediately, frozen in liquid nitrogen, and stored at −80°C until the extraction of total RNA. Four cm-long segments were excised from the jejunum and fixed in 4% formaldehyde for subsequent morphological and immunohistochemical analysis.

Table 1. Composition and nutrient levels of the basal diet (DM basis) %.

Items	Content
Ingredients	
Corn	58.42
Soybean meal	25.00
Fish meal	5.00
Whey powder	4.00
Cream powder	5.00
Limestone	0.30
CaHPO$_4$	1.10
Moldproofant	0.10
Antioxidant	0.02
Vitamin premix[1]	0.04
Choline chloride	0.08
Mineral premix[2]	0.30
NaCl	0.30
Flavor	0.06
L-Lys HCl	0.23
Met	0.05
Total	100.00
Calculation composition	
DE (MJ/kg)	14.3
CP (%)	19.00
Ca (%)	0.58
AP (%)	0.42
Lys (%)	1.20
Met (%)	0.40
Thr (%)	0.85

[1]Provided additional vitamins per kilogram diet: VA 11 000 IU, VD$_3$ 1 100 IU, VE 16 IU, VK 1 mg, pantothenate 6 mg, retinoic acid 2 mg, folic acid 0.8 mg, nicotinic acid 10 mg, thiamine 0.6 mg, VB$_1$ 0.6 mg, biotin 0.08 mg, VB$_{12}$ 0.03 mg.
[2]Provided with additional trace elements per kilogram diet: Zn 165 mg, Fe 165 mg, Mn 33 mg, Cu 16.5 mg, I 297 μg, Se 297 μg.

Diarrhea index

The piglets' stool was observed when they were fed, and those that had thin, soft feces were considered to have diarrhea. Diarrhea index (%) was calculated as 100× number of piglets that had diarrhea/total number of piglets.

Enzyme-linked immunosorbent assay (ELISA)

Cytokines including IL-1β, IL-6 and TNF-α in serum were measured by an ELISA kit (R & D Systems, Wiesbaden-Nordenstadt, Germany) according to the manufacturer's instructions.

Immunohistochemistry and relative quantitative real-time PCR

Calprotectin and TLR4 protein expression in the jejunal mucosa were detected by immunohistochemistry. The mRNA expression of IL-1β, IL-6 and TNF-α in the jejunal mucosa were detected by relative quantitative real-time PCR and the results were presented as fold changes using the $2^{-\Delta\Delta CT}$ method

Table 2. Sequences (5'–3') of the primers used for the detection of mRNA specific for IL-1β, IL-6, TNF-α and GAPDH.

Gene	Accession number	Primer sequences (5' to 3')	Product size (bp)
GAPDH	AF017079	F: GAAGGTCGGAGTGAACGGAT	149
		R: CATGGGTAGAATCATACTGGAACA	
IL-1β	NM_214055.1	F: GAAAGATAACACGCCCACCC	165
		R: TCTGCTTGAGAGGTGCTGATGT	
IL-6	NM_214399.1	F: TCCAGAAAGAGTATGAGAGCA	177
		R: TCTTCATCCACTCGTTCTGT	
TNF-α	NM_214022.1	F: CCACGCTCTTCTGCCTACTGC	168
		R: GCTGTCCCTCGGCTTTGAC	

Notes: F = forward primer; R = reverse primer.

(Table 2). Those methods were reported in the previous paper [18].

Statistical Analysis

The data was analyzed by analysis of variance (ANOVA) using the general linear model (GLM) procedure of the statistical analysis system (SAS) programs (9.1). Duncan's multiple range test was applied for comparing the differences among treatments. The difference was considered to be significant at $P<0.05$, and be very significant at $P<0.01$.

Results

Diarrhea

As presented in Fig. 1, the diarrhea frequency slowly decreased as the experiment progressed, and four piglets had diarrhea at the end of the feeding trial in the control group. In the chlortetracycline group, five piglets had diarrhea on the fifth day, and from day 17 to the end, two piglets had diarrhea; In the COS group, from day 14 to the end, none of the piglets had diarrhea. The results showed that 300 mg/kg COS had a similar effect ($P>0.05$) on reducing diarrhea as 50 mg/kg chlortetracycline.

Inflammatory cytokines

The concentrations of IL-1β, IL-6 and TNF-α in serum were not affected by any of the treatments (Table 3).

Jejunal mucosal calprotectin and TLR4 protein expression

The color signals of jejunal mucosal calprotectin and TLR4 protein expression in the COS group were lighter than those in both the control and chlortetracycline groups (Figure 2). The integral optical density of calprotectin and TLR4 protein expression in the COS group was lower ($P<0.05$) than those in both the control and chlortetracycline groups, and there was no difference between the chlortetracycline group and the control group (Table 4).

Jejunal mucosal IL-1β, IL-6 and TNF-α mRNA expression

There was no difference in the relative expression level of jejunal mucosal TNF-α mRNA among the three groups (Figure 3). The relative expression level of jejunal mucosal IL-6 mRNA in the COS group was higher ($P<0.05$) than that in the control group. There was no difference between the chlortetracycline group and the COS group (Figure 3). The relative expression level of jejunal mucosal IL-1β mRNA in the COS group was higher ($P<0.05$)

than that in the chlortetracycline group. There was no difference between the chlortetracycline group and the COS group (Figure 3).

Discussion

The present study established an excellent piglet diarrhea model for intestinal disorder and demonstrated a clear difference between the effects of COS or chlortetracycline on intestinal inflammation. Chito-oligosaccharide reduced the incidence of diarrhea, but the growth performance of E. coli-challenged pigs supplemented with 160 mg of chito-oligosaccharide was not better than that of unsupplemented pigs challenged with E. coli K88. Dietary supplementation with COS at 100 and 200 mg/kg enhanced growth performance by increasing apparent digestibility, decreasing the incidence of diarrhea, and improving the small intestine morphology [19].

In essence, the danger model proposes that endogenous host-derived molecules from damaged cells and tissues activate the immune system to cause a systemic inflammatory response. Activation of the corresponding receptors in turn results in the production of pro-inflammatory and tissue-injurious mediators [20]. Toll-like receptors (TLRs) are an important class of pattern recognition receptors (PRRs) in innate immunity, and play a critical role in pathogen recognition and host defense [21]. TLR4

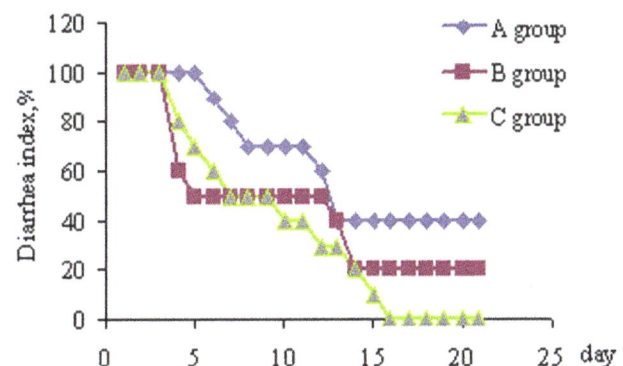

Figure 1. Changes in diarrhea index in piglets. Piglets challenged by enterotoxigenic Escherichia coli were fed either a control diet (A group, n = 10), or control diet plus chlortetracycline (B group, n = 10) or control diet plus chitosan (C group, n = 10) for 21 days. Diarrhea index (%) was calculated as 100× number of piglets that had diarrhea/total number of piglets.

Table 3. Serum IL-1β, IL-6 and TNF-α levels in weaned piglets.

Items	Treatments[1]			SEM	P-value
	A group	B group	C group		
IL-1β (ng/L)	58.36	65.14	61.65	1.783	0.3000
IL-6 (ng/L)	57.20	63.35	67.30	1.808	0.133
TNF-α (ng/L)	54.84	60.01	61.34	1.709	0.441
Number of observations	6	6	6		

[1]A group means the control group, B group means the chlortetracycline group, C group means the COS group.

activation and cytokine production by intestinal epithelial cells (IECs) can induce the recruitment and activation of inflammatory cells, and prolonged or dysregulated pro-inflammatory cytokine production may lead to tissue damage and epithelial barrier dysfunction [22]. TLR4 plays a major role in controlling inflammation through the inhibition of mitogen-activated protein kinase (p38 and c-Jun N-terminal kinase) and NF-κB signaling pathways [23]. TLR4 activation has been shown to be involved in the pathogenesis of acute tissue injury and the induction of a systemic inflammatory state [24]. An important biological consequence of TLR signalling is the production of chemoat-tractants, which leads to the recruitment of inflammatory cells to the site of exposure [25]. Therefore, this piglet diarrhea model was useful for studying TLR4-mediated inflammatory responses in the intestine. Our earlier work showed that COS supplementation decreased the expression of *TLR4* mRNA, and our current work extends these findings by demonstrating that COS supplementa-tion decreased TLR4 protein expression, which indicates that

COS supplementation can efficiently activate an inflammatory immune response, thus reducing intestinal infection.

Calprotectin is a cytosolic protein in the S-100 protein group; its levels increase under conditions such as inflammation, infection, and malignancy. It has immunomodulatory, antimicrobial and antiproliferative action and is predominantly found in neutrophils, monocytes and macrophages, as well as (to a lesser extent) in T and B lymphocytes [26]. Fecal calprotectin is a promising marker of neutrophilic intestinal inflammation [27], and correlates well with the severity of inflammation, as judged by both endoscopic and histological scoring systems [28]. It has been consistently shown to be elevated in patients with known irritable bowel disease (IBD), and has an excellent negative predictive value in ruling out IBD in under-diagnosed symptomatic patients. The degree of inflammation has been shown to be strongly associated with calprotectin-positive cells in the stomach [29]. *E. coli* elicited a significant increase in the calprotectin level, which was confirmed by immunofluorescence and immunohistochemistry, and the

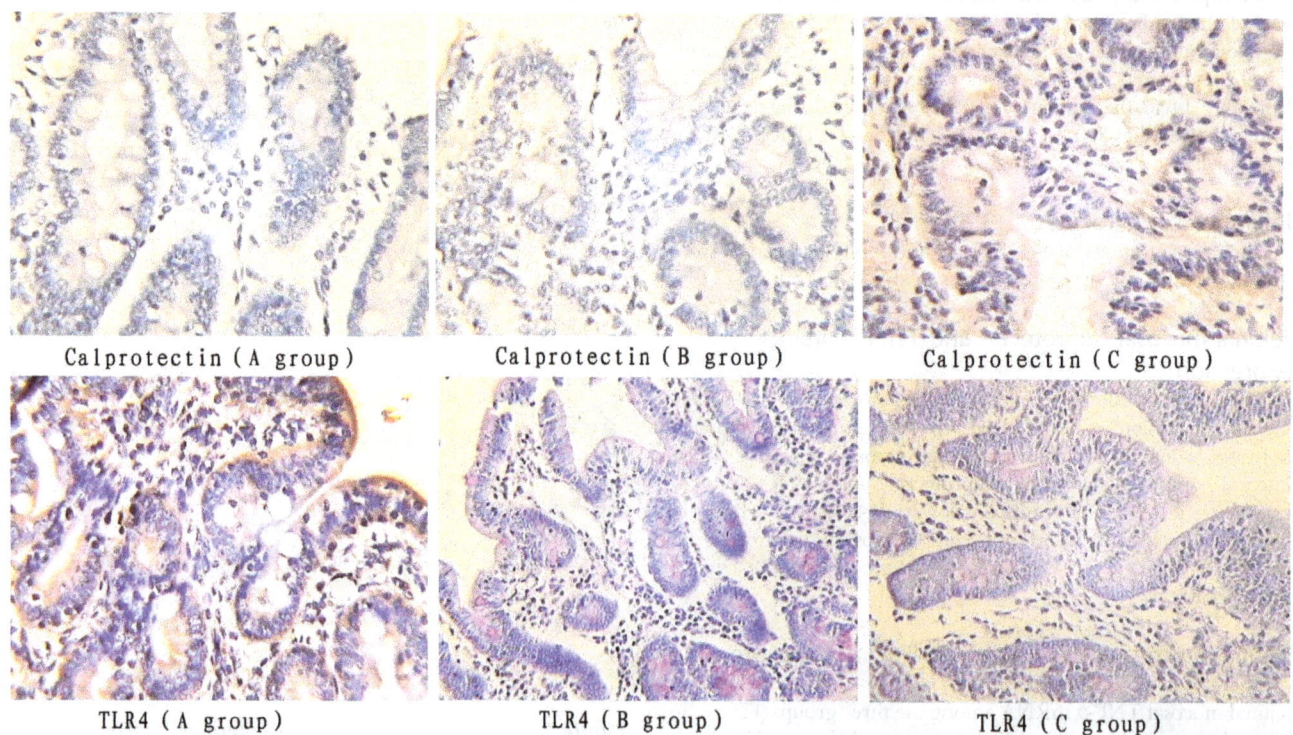

Figure 2. Calprotectin and TLR4 protein expression in jejunal mucosa (immunohistochemical staining, ×400). Piglets challenged by enterotoxigenic *Escherichia* coli were fed either a control diet (A group, n = 6), or control diet plus chlortetracycline (B group, n = 6) or control diet plus chitosan (C group, n = 6) for 21 days and 6 pigs per treatment were killed to excise the jejunum.

Table 4. Integral optical density of Calprotectin and TLR4 protein expression in jejunal mucosa.

Items	Treatments[1]			SEM	P-value
	A group	B group	C group		
Integral optical density of Calprotectin protein expression	389.68[a]	327.54[b]	338.65[b]	17.49	0.0285
Integral optical density of TLR4 protein expression	250.51[a]	202.30[b]	212.94[b]	12.52	0.0397
Number of observations	6	6	6		

[a, b]Means with different superscripts in the same row differ ($P<0.05$).
[1]A group means the control group, B group means the chlortetracycline group, C group means the COS group.

calprotectin level is an important indicator of inflammatory bowel disease [5]. Calprotectin is an abundant neutrophil protein that is released during inflammation. Since calprotectin correlates well with the degree of inflammation, the results of the current study demonstrated that supplementation with COS and chlortetracycline efficiently decreased calprotectin protein expression, and therefore inhibited inflammation and decreased diarrhea in piglets.

Proinflammatory cytokines emanating from the immune system can have profound effects on the neuroendocrine system, either by gaining direct access to the central nervous system or by triggering the synthesis of cytokines by cells in the central nervous system [30]. Inflammatory activation (IL-1β or TNF-α) of astrocytes results in the transient production of key inflammatory mediators including IL-6, cell surface adhesion molecules, and various leukocyte chemoattractants [31]. Lower levels of IL-6 help to regulate the recruitment and activity of inflammatory cells and

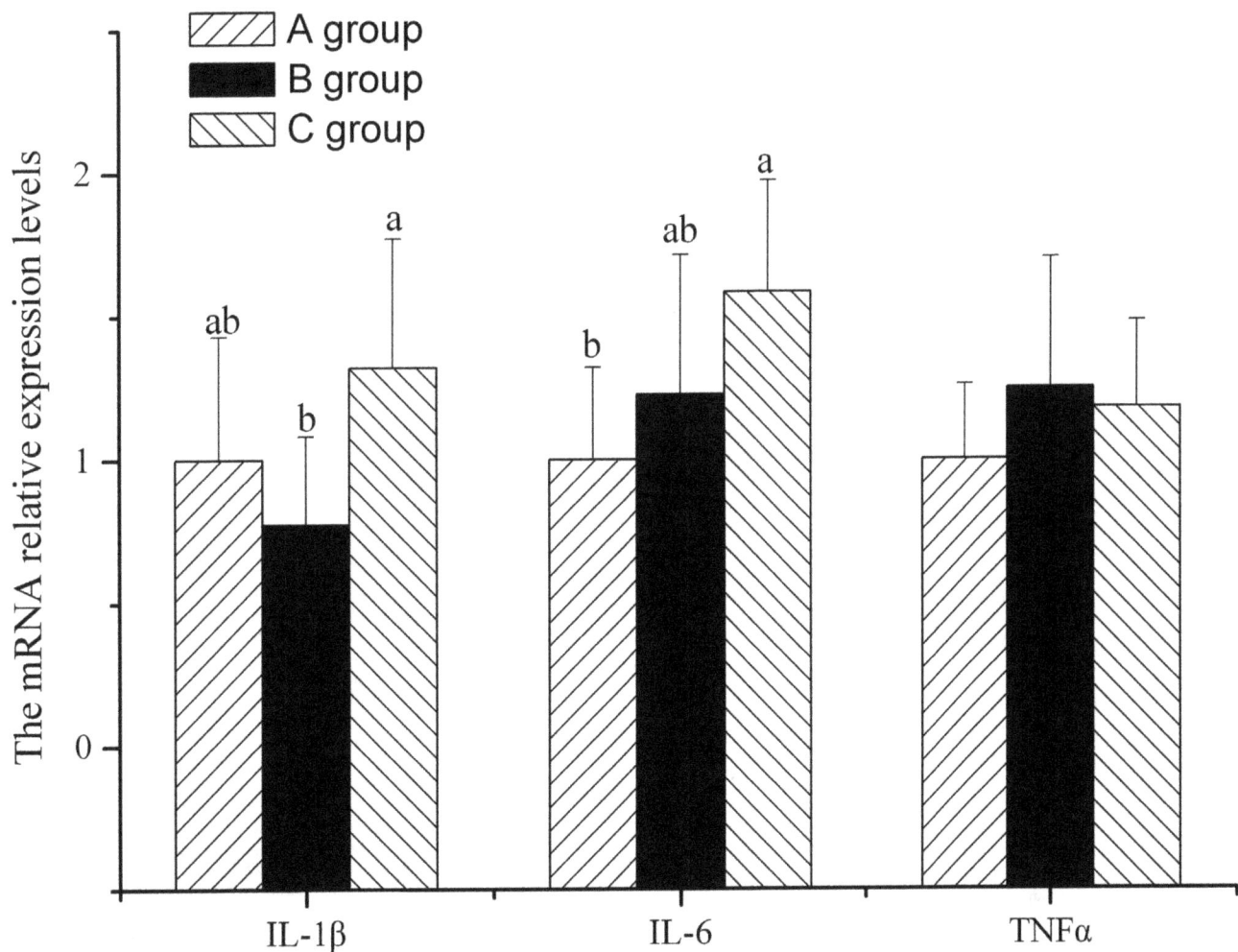

Figure 3. The relative expression of IL-1β, IL-6 and TNF-α mRNA in jejunal mucosa. Piglets challenged by enterotoxigenic *Escherichia* coli were fed either a control diet (A group, n = 6), or control diet plus chlortetracycline (B group, n = 6) or control diet plus chitosan (C group, n = 6) for 21 days and 6 pigs per treatment were killed to excise the jejunum.

limit inflammatory damage. As an innate immune receptor, TLR4 activates NF-κB through recruitment of the adaptor proteins myeloid differentiation primary response gene 88 (MyD88) and Toll/interleukin 1 receptor domain-containing adaptor protein inducing IFN-β (TRIF), which leads to the subsequent induction of NF-κB signalling genes, such as TNF-α, IL-1 and IL-6 [32]. The complex network of cytokines regulates the immune response in the host to prevent susceptibility to disease and enhance resistance to infections. Logically, up-regulation of the protein expression of TLR4 should indicate that the TLR4 signaling pathway is inhibited, and its downstream cytokines including IL-1β, IL-6 and TNF-α should decrease. However, IL-1β and IL-6 mRNA expression improved in that study. Moreover, that study supported our present study in that COS supplementation promoted IL-1β and IL-6 expression, while COS did not affect either TNF-α mRNA expression in the jejunal mucosa, or the levels of IL-1β, IL-6 and TNF-α in serum. We can speculate on possible reasons for these results: In response to peripheral challenge with enterotoxigenic *E. coli*, comprehensive inflammation may have been elicited in weaned piglets; a variety of cells in the immune system may have secreted high concentrations of proinflammatory cytokines. COS supplementation enhances the cell-mediated immune response by modulating the production of cytokines, but some time is needed before TLR4 can activate its downstream signaling pathway. Therefore, IL-1β and IL-6 mRNA expression in intestinal mucosa were still quite high when the piglets were slaughtered. This result is consistent with a previous report that supplementation with COS and chlortetracycline have similar effects in reducing intestinal inflammation, but different effects on intestinal mucosal barrier function [18].

In summary, we can propose a mechanism by which COS can inhibit diarrhea: after chitosan adheres to the intestinal mucosa, its amine is recognized by the immune system. Immune response pathways are activated, and the gut-associated lymphoid immune system is stimulated to produce lymphokines and inflammatory mediators, secrete cytokines IL-1, IL-6, etc., reduce calprotectin and TLR4 protein expression, and enhance the cell-mediated immune response. Therefore, COS helps to prevent inflammatory intestinal disorders, including weaning-associated intestinal inflammation. Furthermore, our previous paper reported that diets supplemented with COS or chlortetracycline could improve intestinal mucosal morphology and occludin protein expression [18]. Thus, the digestion and absorption of nutrients in the intestine are improved in piglets. These may be contributing factors for chitosan to decrease diarrhea.

In conclusion, we have demonstrated that supplementation with COS and chlortetracycline can decrease the occurrence of diarrhea and alleviate intestinal inflammation by up-regulating TLR4 and calprotectin protein expression in weaned piglets challenged with enterotoxigenic *Escherichia* coli. In addition, COS can enhance the cell-mediated immune response by modulating the production of inflammatory cytokines.

Author Contributions

Conceived and designed the experiments: ZT YY JH CMN SWK. Performed the experiments: DX ZF MR. Analyzed the data: XH WY. Contributed reagents/materials/analysis tools: ZT YY GL WQ YW. Wrote the paper: DX YW.

References

1. Yin YL, Tang ZR, Sun ZH, Liu ZQ, Li TJ, et al. (2008) Effect of Galacto-mannan-oligosaccharides or chitosan supplementation on cytoimmunity and humoral immunity in early-weaned piglets. Asian-Aust J Anim Sci 21: 723–731.

2. Fairbrother JM, Nadeau E, Gyles CL (2005) Escherichia coli in postweaning diarrhea in pigs: an update on bacterial types, pathogenesis, and prevention strategies. Anim Health Res Rev 6: 17–39.

3. Liu P, Piao XS, Thacker PA, Zeng ZK, Li PF, et al. (2010) Chito-oligosaccharide reduces diarrhea incidence and attenuates the immune response of weaned pigs challenged with Escherichia coli K88. J Anim Sci 88: 3871–3879.

4. van der Fels-Klerx HJ, Puister-Jansen LF, van Asselt ED, Burgers SL (2011) Farm factors associated with the use of antibiotics in pig production. J Anim Sci 89: 1922–1929.

5. Splichal I, Fagerhol MK, Trebichavsky I, Splichalova A, Schulze J (2005) The effect of intestinal colonization of germ-free pigs with Escherichia coli on calprotectin levels in plasma, intestinal and bronchoalveolar lavages. Immunobiology 209: 681–687.

6. von Roon AC, Karamountzos L, Purkayastha S, Reese GE, Darzi AW, et al. (2007) Diagnostic precision of fecal calprotectin for inflammatory bowel disease and colorectal malignancy. Am J Gastroenterol 102: 803–813.

7. Heimesaat MM, Fischer A, Jahn HK, Niebergall J, Freudenberg M, et al. (2007) Exacerbation of murine ileitis by Toll-like receptor 4 mediated sensing of lipopolysaccharide from commensal Escherichia coli. Gut 56: 941–948.

8. Tang ZR, Yin YL, Nyachoti CM, Huang RL, Li TJ, et al. (2005) Effect of dietary supplementation of chitosan and galacto-mannan-oligosaccharide on serum parameters and the insulin-like growth factor-I mRNA expression in early-weaned piglets. Domest Anim Endocrinol 28: 430–441.

9. Anandan R, Ganesan B, Obulesu T, Mathew S, Kumar RS, et al. (2012) Dietary chitosan supplementation attenuates isoprenaline-induced oxidative stress in rat myocardium. Int J Biol Macromol 51: 783–787.

10. Rabea EI, Badawy ME, Stevens CV, Smagghe G, Steurbaut W (2003) Chitosan as antimicrobial agent: applications and mode of action. Biomacromolecules 4: 1457–1465.

11. Kobayashi S, Terashima Y, Itoh H (2002) Effects of dietary chitosan on fat deposition and lipase activity in digesta in broiler chickens. Br Poult Sci 43: 270–273.

12. Yoon HJ, Moon ME, Park HS, Im SY, Kim YH (2007) Chitosan oligosaccharide (COS) inhibits LPS-induced inflammatory effects in RAW 264.7 macrophage cells. Biochem Biophys Res Commun 358: 954–959.

13. Pangestuti R, Bak SS, Kim SK (2011) Attenuation of pro-inflammatory mediators in LPS-stimulated BV2 microglia by chitooligosaccharides via the MAPK signaling pathway. Int J Biol Macromol 49: 599–606.

14. Fernandes JC, Spindola H, de Sousa V, Santos-Silva A, Pintado ME, et al. (2010) Anti-inflammatory activity of chitooligosaccharides in vivo. Mar Drugs 8: 1763–1768.

15. Qiao Y, Bai XF, Du YG (2011) Chitosan oligosaccharides protect mice from LPS challenge by attenuation of inflammation and oxidative stress. Int Immunopharmacol 11: 121–127.

16. Lee SH, Senevirathne M, Ahn CB, Kim SK, Je JY (2009) Factors affecting anti-inflammatory effect of chitooligosaccharides in lipopolysaccharides-induced RAW264.7 macrophage cells. Bioorg Med Chem Lett 19: 6655–6658.

17. Chen CL, Wang YM, Liu CF, Wang JY (2008) The effect of water-soluble chitosan on macrophage activation and the attenuation of mite allergen-induced airway inflammation. Biomaterials 29: 2173–2182.

18. Xiao D, Tang Z, Yin Y, Zhang B, Hu X, et al. (2013) Effects of dietary administering chitosan on growth performance, jejunal morphology, jejunal mucosal sIgA, occluding, claudin-1 and TLR4 expression in weaned piglets challenged by enterotoxigenic Escherichia coli. Int Immunopharmacol 17: 670–676.

19. Liu P, Piao XS, Kim SW, Wang L, Shen YB, et al. (2008) Effects of chito-oligosaccharide supplementation on the growth performance, nutrient digestibility, intestinal morphology, and fecal shedding of Escherichia coli and Lactobacillus in weaning pigs. J Anim Sci 86: 2609–2618.

20. Reino DC, Palange D, Feketeova E, Bonitz RP, Xu da Z, et al. (2012) Activation of toll-like receptor 4 is necessary for trauma hemorrhagic shock-induced gut injury and polymorphonuclear neutrophil priming. Shock 38: 107–114.

21. Shimazu T, Villena J, Tohno M, Fujie H, Hosoya S, et al. (2012) Immunobiotic Lactobacillus jensenii elicits anti-inflammatory activity in porcine intestinal epithelial cells by modulating negative regulators of the Toll-like receptor signaling pathway. Infect Immun 80: 276–288.

22. Hormannsperger G, Haller D (2010) Molecular crosstalk of probiotic bacteria with the intestinal immune system: clinical relevance in the context of inflammatory bowel disease. Int J Med Microbiol 300: 63–73.

23. Byun EB, Sung NY, Byun EH, Song DS, Kim JK, et al. (2013) The procyanidin trimer C1 inhibits LPS-induced MAPK and NF-kappaB signaling through TLR4 in macrophages. Int Immunopharmacol 15: 450–456.

24. Mollen KP, Anand RJ, Tsung A, Prince JM, Levy RM, et al. (2006) Emerging paradigm: toll-like receptor 4-sentinel for the detection of tissue damage. Shock 26: 430–437.

25. Sahlander K, Larsson K, Palmberg L (2012) Daily exposure to dust alters innate immunity. PLoS One 7: e31646.

26. Beser OF, Sancak S, Erkan T, Kutlu T, Cokugras H, et al. (2014) Can Fecal Calprotectin Level Be Used as a Markers of Inflammation in the Diagnosis and Follow-Up of Cow's Milk Protein Allergy? Allergy Asthma Immunol Res 6: 33–38.

27. Costa F, Mumolo MG, Bellini M, Romano MR, Ceccarelli L, et al. (2003) Role of faecal calprotectin as non-invasive marker of intestinal inflammation. Dig Liver Dis 35: 642–647.

28. Konikoff MR, Denson LA (2006) Role of fecal calprotectin as a biomarker of intestinal inflammation in inflammatory bowel disease. Inflamm Bowel Dis 12: 524–534.

29. Choi HK, Lee YH, Park JP, Min K, Park H (2013) Inflammatory responses in the muscle coat of stomach and small bowel in the postoperative ileus model of guinea pig. Yonsei Med J 54: 1336–1341.

30. Liu Y, Chen F, Li Q, Odle J, Lin X, et al. (2013) Fish oil alleviates activation of the hypothalamic-pituitary-adrenal axis associated with inhibition of TLR4 and NOD signaling pathways in weaned piglets after a lipopolysaccharide challenge. J Nutr 143: 1799–1807.

31. van Kralingen C, Kho DT, Costa J, Angel CE, Graham ES (2013) Exposure to Inflammatory Cytokines IL-1beta and TNFalpha Induces Compromise and Death of Astrocytes; Implications for Chronic Neuroinflammation. PLoS One 8: e84269.

32. Dou W, Zhang J, Sun A, Zhang E, Ding L, et al. (2013) Protective effect of naringenin against experimental colitis via suppression of Toll-like receptor 4/ NF-kappaB signalling. Br J Nutr 110: 599–608.

7

Efficacy and Safety of Gemcitabine-Fluorouracil Combination Therapy in the Management of Advanced Pancreatic Cancer

Qin Li[1], Han Yan[1], Wenting Liu[1,2,3], Hongchao Zhen[1,2,3], Yifan Yang[1,2,3], Bangwei Cao[1,2,3]*

1 Department of Oncology, Beijing Friendship Hospital, Capital Medical University, Beijing, China, 2 Beijing Key Laboratory for Precancerous Lesion of Digestive Diseases, Beijing Friendship Hospital, Capital Medical University, Beijing, China, 3 Beijing Digestive Diseases Center, Beijing Friendship Hospital, Capital Medical University, Beijing, China

Abstract

Background: Gemcitabine (GEM) is the standard first-line chemotherapy that provides limited clinical benefits for patients with locally advanced/metastatic pancreatic adenocarcinoma (LA/MPC). However, the fluorouracil derivatives (CAP and S-1) show promising efficacy in these patients. This study compared the efficacy and safety of GEM with GEM plus fluorouracil drugs in the treatment of LA/MPC.

Methods: Pubmed, EMBASE and Cochrane Library databases were searched for relevant randomized controlled trials published on or before January 2014. The Cochrane Collaboration's tool was used to assess the risk of bias in randomized trials. The primary end point was overall survival (OS); the secondary end points were one-year survival rate, objective response rate (ORR) and toxicity rates (TRs).

Results: A total of 8 randomized controlled trials involving 2,126 patients were included in the systematic evaluation. The results showed that OS was significantly improved (HR 0.83, $P<0.01$; HR 0.87, $P = 0.03$; HR 0.80, $P = 0.01$; respectively) and ORR was significantly increased (OR 0.51, $P<0.01$; OR 0.66, $P = 0.03$; OR 0.35, $P<0.01$; respectively) in the GEM+5-FU/CAP/S-1, GEM+CAP and GEM+S-1 groups compared to the GEM alone group. In addition, the one-year survival rate was significantly increased (OR 0.78 $P = 0.01$; OR 0.47, $P = 0.04$; respectively) in the GEM+5-FU/CAP/S-1 and GEM+S-1 groups compared to the GEM alone group. The frequency of grade 3/4 TRs were higher in GEM+5-FU/CAP/S-1 group, the significant increase of grade 3/4 neutropenia, thrombocytopenia and diarrhea were observed.

Conclusions: GEM combined with fluorouracil drugs significantly improved OS and increased one-year survival rate and ORR compared to GEM alone in LA/MPC patients. GEM combined with fluorouracil drugs may be considered as an acceptable alternative treatment for LA/MPC patients.

Editor: Jonathan R. Brody, Thomas Jefferson University, United States of America

Funding: This work was supported by grants from Beijing Municipal Health System High-level Health Person Foundation Project (No. 2011-3-007 to Bangwei Cao), National Nature Science Foundation of China (No. 81272615; No. 81301912) and Capital Medical University Sciences-clinical Research Cooperation Foundation (No. 12JL33). The funders had no role in study design, data collection and analysis, decision to publish, or preparation of the manuscript.

Competing Interests: The authors have declared that no competing interests exist.

* Email: oncologychina@163.com

Introduction

Pancreatic cancer is the eighth leading cause of cancer-related mortality worldwide. More than 80% of patients with pancreatic cancer have late-stage disease when diagnosed. Patients with locally advanced/metastatic pancreatic adenocarcinoma (LA/MPC) have missed the opportunity to be managed surgically [1]. Gemcitabine (GEM) is the standard first-line chemotherapy for patients with LA/MPC, offering a statistically longer survival compared to 5-fluorouracil (5-FU) [2,3]. However, the prognosis of patients with LA/MPC remains poor. In order to achieve a better survival benefit for LA/MPC patients, GEM combined with cytotoxic drugs or molecular-targeted agents has been intensely investigated.

Many studies on GEM-based combination scheme have failed to demonstrate an improvement in overall survival (OS) [2,4,5]. Only a minority of combination therapies such as GEM plus erlotinib or GEM plus nab-paclitaxel showed a significant improvement of OS compared to GEM alone in LA/MPC patients [6,7]. Three meta-analyses showed that GEM combination chemotherapy conferred a significant benefit in terms of OS or a modest improvement of one-year survival rate compared to GEM mono-therapy in LA/MPC patients. However, these combination therapies were associated with increased toxicity [8–10]. This combination therapy offers some viable options for the management of LA/MPC patients with good performance status.

The aforementioned meta-analyses included GEM combined with biologics or cytotoxic agents, however, our study focused on GEM combined with fluorouracil drugs compared to GEM alone. Fluorouracil drugs including 5-FU, Capecitabine (CAP) and S-1 have proven to be effective in LA/MPC treatment. Two randomized controlled trials (RCTs) reported that the median survival times (MST) were 4.2 months and 5.1 months respectively and one-year survival rates were 26% and 23% respectively for LA/MPC patients receiving protracted venous 5-FU infusion [11,12]. Similar survival rates were obtained using protracted venous infusion of 5-FU and GEM, and this supported further exploration of the role of fluorouracil in LA/MPC patients. CAP is an oral fluorouracil pro-drug that has selective activity against tumor cells and it exerts sustained antitumor effects when transformed into 5-FU. Cartwright et al. reported that treatment with CAP resulted in a clinically significant benefit, with a MST of 6 months in LA/MPC patients [13]. This result together with its generally tolerable safety profile and the added advantage of oral administration provide the basis for further evaluating CAP in combination with GEM in this patient population. S-1 is a newly developed oral 5-FU derivative, which contains tegafur, gimeracil and oteracil potassium. Gimeracil enhances S-1 anti-tumor effect by preventing its degradation and oteracil potassium reduces digestive tract reactions by protecting the gastrointestinal mucosa. The efficacy of S-1 has already been demonstrated on a variety of solid tumors [14,15]. A phase II trial of S-1 alone in MPC showed a response rate of 37.5% and a MST up to 9.2 months, which far exceeded the efficacy of GEM [16].

Because fluorouracil drugs have shown promising activity in LA/MPC patients, many RCTs have been designed to evaluate whether GEM combined with fluorouracil drugs is superior to GEM alone, but the conclusions are not consistent. Therefore, we undertook a systematic assessment of relevant RCTs in this study.

Materials and Methods

Literature search strategy

This meta-analysis was performed according to the Preferred Reporting Items for Systematic Reviews and Meta-analysis (PRISMA) criteria [17]. PubMed, EMBASE and the Central Registry of Controlled Trials of the Cochrane Library were searched for original articles written in English and published before January 31, 2014. Abstracts presented at the annual meeting of the American Society of Clinical Oncology and the European Cancer Conference were also searched. Prospective studies were allowed in this assessment to minimize the risk of selection or information bias. The initial search used the MeSH terms "Pancreatic neoplasm OR Pancreas neoplasm OR Pancreas Cancers OR Pancreatic Cancer OR Pancreatic Carcinoma" AND "Gemcitabine OR Gemzar" AND "Fluorouracil OR 5-Fluorouracil OR 5-FU; Capecitabine OR Xeloda; S-1 OR S1".

RCT selection and exclusion criteria

The inclusion criteria were as follows: (1) the trials were required to be prospective, properly randomized and well-designed, which we defined as matched for age, gender, tumor stage and performance status (PS) or Karnofsky performance status (KPS); (2) the subjects of the trials were patients with LA/MPC, and histologic or cytologic confirmation of pancreatic adenocarcinoma was required; (3) the patients received GEM monotherapy in the control arm, while patients received GEM combined with 5-FU/CAP/S-1 therapy in the experimental arm;

(4) the primary end point was OS, secondary end points were one-year survival rate, objective response rate (ORR) and toxicity rates (TRs); (5) the original article had explicit survival information included as follow-up censored or explicit survival curves, and the follow-up rate was greater than 95%; and (6) whenever trials with overlapping patient populations were encountered, only the trial with the longest follow-up was included.

The exclusion criteria were: (1) trials that included patients with major comorbidities or second tumors were excluded; and (2) if a trial included adjuvant chemotherapy within six months or concomitant interventions such as radiotherapy that differed systematically between the investigated arms, it was excluded.

Data collection and extraction

All identified abstracts were assessed independently by two investigators (Qin Li and Yi-fan Yang). If one investigator considered that an abstract was eligible, the full text of the article was retrieved and reviewed in detail by both investigators. Any discrepancy was resolved by an arbiter (Han Yan) or by contacting the authors of the original study. Different variables including authors' names, journal, year of publication, original country, sample size per arm, performance status, regimens, line of treatment, median age of patients, gender ratio, tumor stage and pre-specified outcomes of efficacy and safety were extracted and evaluated.

Assessment of methodological quality

Following the Cochrane Handbook for Systematic Reviews of Interventions [18], the methodological quality of the included studies was independently assessed by two authors. Any disagreements were resolved by discussion. The corresponding author was the arbiter when no consensus could be achieved. We evaluated the risk of bias in the studies using the Review Manager software (RevMan Version 5.1; The Nordic Cochrane Center, The Cochrane Collaboration, Copenhagen, Denmark), which included the following key domains: random sequence generation (selection bias), allocation concealment (selection bias), blinding of participants and personnel (performance bias), blinding of outcome assessment (detection bias), incomplete outcome data (attrition bias), selective reporting (reporting bias) and other bias. The publication bias was assessed using funnel plots.

Within a trial, low risk of bias for all key domains indicated a low risk of bias, low or unclear risk of bias for all key domains indicated an unclear risk of bias, and high risk of bias for one or more key domains indicated a high risk of bias. Across trials, most information from trials at low risk of bias indicated a low risk of bias, most information from trials at low or unclear risk indicated an unclear risk of bias, and that the proportion of information from trials at high risk of bias was sufficient to affect the interpretation of results indicated a high risk of bias.

Statistical analysis

The systematic assessment was performed using Review Manager Version 5.1.7 (http://ims.cochrane.org/revman). Heterogeneity between the trials was assessed to determine which model should be used. The Cochrane's Q-test was performed and I^2 statistics were obtained, with a predefined significance threshold of 0.05. A P value of more than 0.05 suggested that the studies were homogeneous, and the pooled estimation of hazard ratio (HR) and odds ratio (OR) for each study were calculated using the fixed effects model (FEM). A P value of less than 0.05 for the Q-test suggested that the studies were heterogeneous, and the random effects model (REM) was applied. HR and OR were the principal measurements of effect and were presented with 95%

confidence interval (CI); a *P* value of less than 0.05 was considered statistically significant. All reported *P* values were from two-sided versions of the respective tests. If a trial provided only a Kaplan-Meier curve, the HR and 95% CI were estimated utilizing the Engauge Digitizer V4.1 screenshot tool and a formula proposed by Parmar [19,20]. The potential presence of publication bias was evaluated visually by inspecting funnel plots and statistically using the Egger's test.

Results

Selection of the trials

The inclusion and exclusion of RCTs for this systematic assessment are shown in a flow chart (Figure 1). In accordance with our search strategy, 137 abstracts were screened. Primary screening led to the exclusion of 126 abstracts for the following reasons: 105 abstracts were unrelated studies and 21 abstracts were only single-arm studies about GEM combined with 5-FU or CAP or S-1. The remaining 11 articles were retrieved for more detailed evaluation. Of these, 3 articles were excluded due to incomplete data, repetitive study or small sample size. In the end, 8 RCTs were eligible for inclusion in this meta-analysis. The PRISMA checklist is shown in Checklist S1.

The risk of bias in the included studies

Four RCTs were assessed to have an unclear risk of selection bias due to insufficient detail on random sequence generation or allocation concealment. Three RCTs were assessed to have a high risk of performance and detection bias due to open label in trial design. Six RCTs were assessed to have an unclear risk of other bias due to insufficient details, such as lacking an adequate description of patients' the uptake of the therapeutic drug monitoring recommendations by physicians (Figure 2).

Main characteristics of RCTs included in the systematic assessment

The main characteristics of all eligible RCTs are listed in Table 1. Of the eight trials, four were randomized phase II trials and four were randomized phase III trials. A total of 2,126 patients were included in this assessment, of which 1,059 patients received GEM+5-FU/CAP/S-1 therapy and 1,067 patients received GEM alone therapy. In subgroup analysis, 416 patients received GEM+5-FU versus GEM alone therapy, 935 patients received GEM+CAP versus GEM alone therapy, and 775 patients received GEM+S-1 versus GEM alone therapy. The data on OS, ORR and TRs were extracted from eight trials and the data on one-year survival rates were extracted from seven trials.

Efficacy analysis

Four RCTs, including one GEM+CAP versus GEM trial and three GEM+S-1 versus GEM trials, provided complete data on OS [HR (95% CI)]. Four RCTs, including two GEM+5-FU versus GEM trials and two GEM+CAP versus GEM trials, provided only the OS and Kaplan-Meier curves. The Engauge Digitizer V4.1 screenshot tool and the formula proposed by Parmar et al were used to estimate the HR (95% CI).

There was no significant difference in the heterogeneity for OS between the GEM combination group and the GEM alone group (*P*>0.05), and therefore FEM was selected for this systemic assessment. The analysis indicated a significant improvement in OS when the GEM+5-FU/CAP/S-1, GEM+CAP, GEM+S-1, GEM+5-FU groups were compared to the GEM alone group (HR 0.83, 95% CI: 0.76–0.91, *P*<0.01; HR 0.87, 95% CI: 0.76–0.99, *P*=0.03; HR 0.80, 95% CI: 0.67–0.95, *P*=0.01; HR 0.81, 95% CI: 0.68–0.96, *P*=0.02; respectively) (Figure 3).

There was no significant difference in the heterogeneity for one-year survival rates between the GEM+5-FU/CAP/S-1, GEM+CAP groups and the GEM alone group (*P*>0.05), and therefore

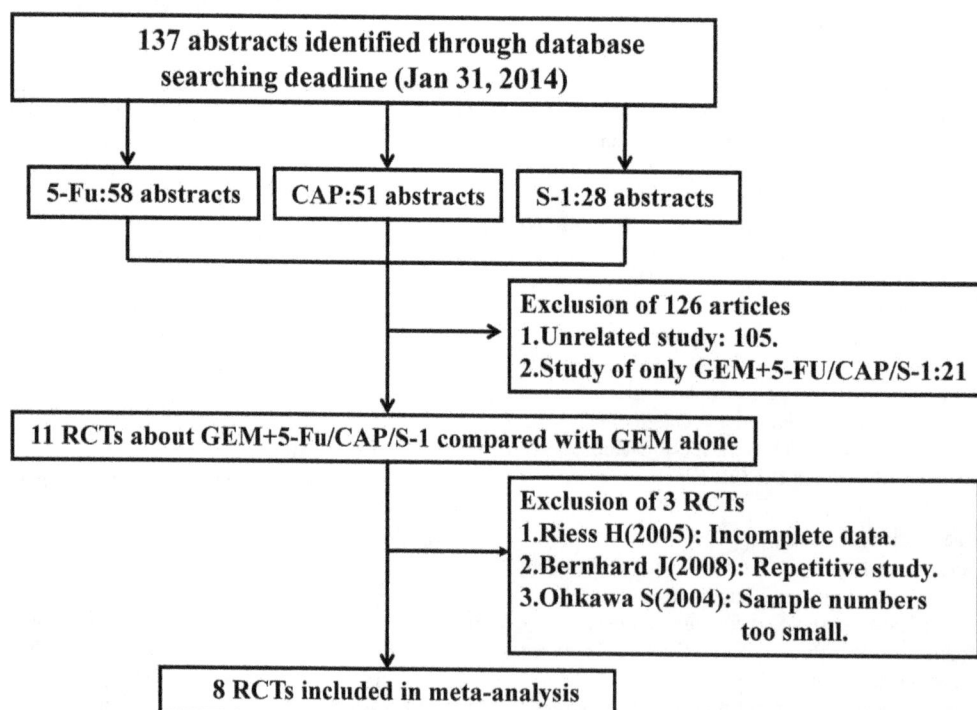

Figure 1. PRISMA flow diagram showing the exclusion and inclusion of trials in the meta-analysis.

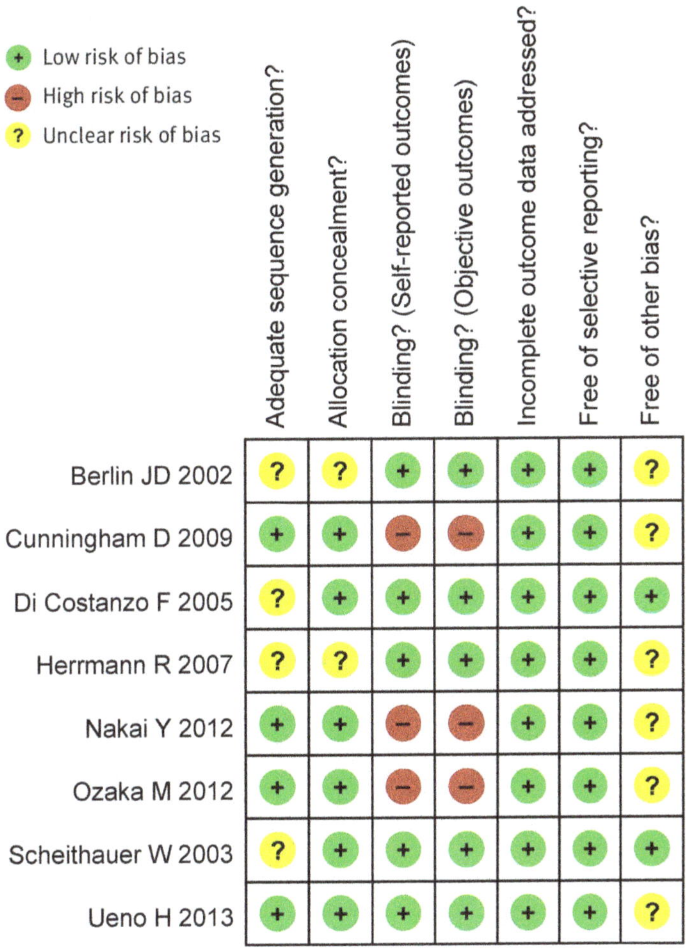

Figure 2. The risk of bias for the included studies.

FEM was selected. However, there was a significant difference in the heterogeneity for one-year survival rates between the GEM+S-1 group and the GEM alone group ($P<0.05$), so REM was applied. The analysis indicated a significant increase in one-year survival rate when the GEM+5-FU/CAP/S-1 and GEM+S-1 groups were compared to the GEM alone group (OR 0.78, 95% CI: 0.64–0.95, $P=0.01$; OR 0.47, 95% CI: 0.23–0.96, $P=0.04$; respectively) (Figure 4). However, there was no significant difference in one-year survival rate when the GEM+CAP group was compared to the GEM alone group (OR 0.95, 95% CI: 0.71–1.27, $P=0.72$) (Figure 4).

There was no significant difference in the heterogeneity for ORR between the GEM combination groups and the GEM alone group ($P>0.05$), and therefore FEM was applied. The analysis demonstrated a significant increase in ORR when the GEM+5-FU/CAP/S-1, GEM+CAP and GEM+S-1 groups were compared to the GEM alone group (OR 0.51, 95% CI: 0.39–0.65, $P<0.01$; OR 0.66, 95% CI: 0.45–0.96, $P=0.03$; OR 0.35, 95% CI: 0.23–0.52, $P<0.01$; respectively) (Figure 5).

Efficacy analysis of phase III trials

The efficacy of four phase III trials, including one GEM+5-FU versus GEM trial, two GEM+CAP versus GEM trials and one GEM+S-1 versus GEM trial, was analyzed. The analysis showed a significant improvement in OS (HR 0.86, 95% CI: 0.78–0.94, $P<0.01$) and a significant increase in ORR (OR 1.91, 95% CI: 1.43–

2.54, $P<0.01$) when the GEM+5-FU/CAP/S-1 group was compared to the GEM alone group (Figure 6).

Grade 3–4 toxicity analysis

Grade 3–4 hematologic adverse events, gastrointestinal reactions and other toxicities were extracted from the eight RCTs. There was no significant difference in the heterogeneity for TRs ($P>0.05$), and therefore FEM was used. The analysis showed a significant increase in grade 3–4 neutropenia (OR 1.90, 95% CI: 1.54–2.34, $P<0.01$), grade 3–4 thrombocytopenia (OR 1.62, 95% CI: 1.20–2.18, $P<0.01$) and grade 3–4 diarrhea (OR 2.04, 95% CI: 1.28–3.26, $P<0.01$), but significant increase in grade 3–4 anemia, nausea and vomiting were not observed when the GEM+5-FU/CAP/S-1 group was compared to the GEM alone group (Table 2, Figure 7). The dropout rates due to toxicity were 0–7.1% in the GEM alone group and 0.6–8.9% in the GEM+5-FU/CAP/S-1 group. However, there were no significant differences in the dropout rates between the two groups.

Discussion

GEM is a therapy cornerstone for patients with LA/MPC. However, LA/MPC patients receiving GEM therapy have a MST of only 5.65 months [3]. In order to improve the survival benefit for LA/MPC patients, many RCTs evaluated the efficacy of GEM combined with 5-FU/CAP/S-1. In this study, we compared the

Table 1. Characteristics of the eligible trials included in the systematic assessment.

Trial	Phase	Arms	Case (n)	Male (%)	Median age (y)	LA (%)/MPC (%)	Regimens
Berlin JD	III	GEM+5-FU	160	51.8	65.8	11/89	GEM 1000 mg/m², then 5-FU 600 mg/m² d1,8,15, q4w, IV.
2002 [21]	Multicenter	GEM alone	162	53.7	64.3	10/90	GEM 1000 mg/m² d1,8,15, q4w, IV.
Scheithauer W	II	GEM+CAP	41	66.0	64.0	0/100	GEM 2200 mg/m² d1, q2w, IV; CAP 2500 mg/m² d1-7, q2w, PO.
2003 [22]	Multicenter	GEM alone	42	55.0	66.0	0/100	GEM 2200 mg/m² d1, q2w, IV.
Di Costanzo F	II	GEM+5-FU	45	63.0	62.0	33/67	GEM 1000 mg/m²/w, 5-FU 200 mg/m²/d×6weeks followed by 1-week rest; then d1,8,15, q4w. IV.
2005 [23]	Multicenter	GEM alone	49	48.0	64.0	27/73	GEM 1000 mg/m²/w×7 weeks followed by 2-weeks rest, then d1,8,15, q4w, IV.
Herrmann R	III	GEM+CAP	160	54.0	Unknown	20/80	GEM 1000 mg/m² d1,8, q3w, IV; CAP 650 mg/m² twice daily d1-14, q3w, PO.
2007 [24]	Multicenter	GEM alone	159	53.0	Unknown	21/79	GEM 1000 mg/m²/w×7 weeks followed by 1-week rest, then d1,8,15, q4w, IV.
Cunningham D	III	GEM+CAP	267	60.0	62.0	30/70	GEM 1000 mg/m² d1,8,15, q4w, IV; CAP 830 mg/m² twice daily d1-21, q4w, PO.
2009 [25]	Multicenter	GEM alone	266	58.0	62.0	29/71	GEM 1000 mg/m²/w×7 weeks followed by 1-week rest, then d1,8,15, q4w, IV.
Nakai Y	II	GEM+S-1	53	79.2	63.0	28/72	GEM 1000 mg/m² d1,15, q4w, IV; S-1 40 mg/m² twice daily d1-14, q4w, PO.
2012 [26]	Multicenter	GEM alone	53	62.3	67.0	24/76	GEM 1000 mg/m² d1,8,15, q4w, IV.
Ozaka M	II	GEM+S-1	58	60.3	Unknown	25/75	GEM 1000 mg/m² d1,8, q3w, IV; S-1 40 mg/m² twice daily d1-14, q3w, PO.
2012 [27]	Multicenter	GEM alone	59	59.3	Unknown	31/69	GEM 1000 mg/m² d1,8,15, q4w, IV.
Ueno H	III	GEM+S-1	275	57.5	Unknown	25/75	GEM 1000 mg/m² d1,8, IV; S-1 60/80/100 mg/m² d1-14, q3w, PO.
2013 [28]	Multicenter	GEM alone	277	61.4	Unknown	24/76	GEM 1000 mg/m² d1,8,15, q4w, IV.

GEM, gemcitabine; 5-FU, 5-fluorouracil; CAP, capecitabine; LA/MPC, locally advanced/metastatic pancreatic adenocarcinoma; OS, overall survival.

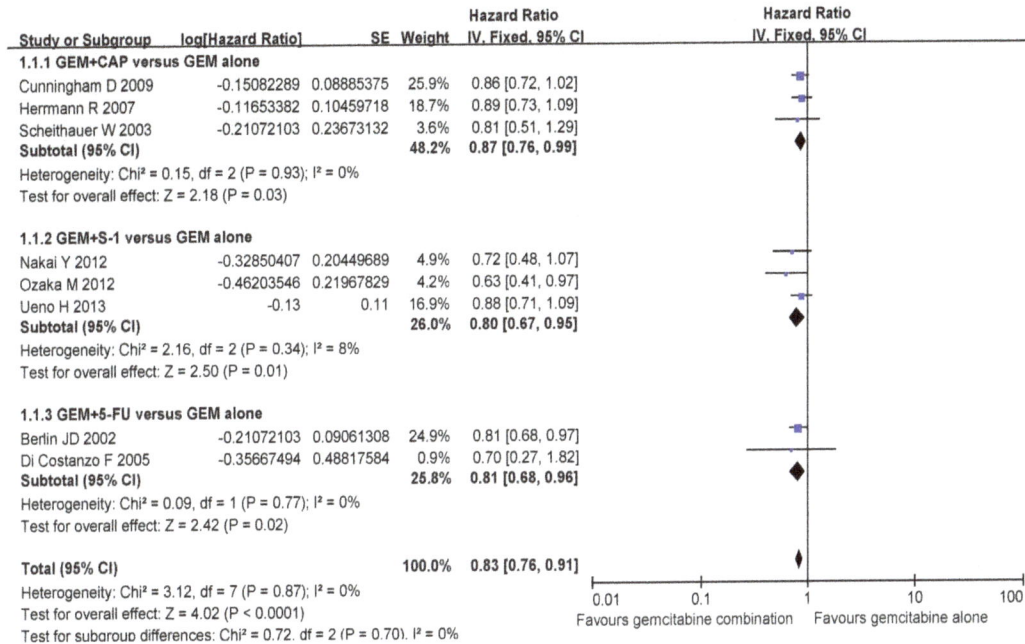

Figure 3. Comparison of overall survival between GEM combination therapy and GEM alone therapy.

efficacy and safety profile of GEM combined with 5-FU/CAP/S-1 versus GEM alone in LA/MPC patients.

Berlin's phase III study reported that the median OS was 6.7 months for GEM combined with 5-FU and 5.4 months for GEM alone ($P = 0.09$) [21]. Di Costanzo's phase II study reported that treatment with GEM combined with 5-FU obtained a median OS of 31 weeks and 30 weeks in GEM alone. But our subgroup meta-analysis obtained a meaningful conclusion that GEM combined

with 5-FU significantly improved the OS and ORR compared with GEM alone [23,29]. This conclusion supports that the addition of 5-FU to GEM maybe replace GEM in the management of LA/MPC patients.

CAP, an oral tumor-selective fluoropyrimidine, has been verified as efficacious as continuous-infusion 5-FU [30]. Both single-arm studies about GEM combined with CAP reported that the median OS were 8.7 and 10.0 months respectively in LA/

GEM+5-FU/CAP/S-1 versus GEM alone

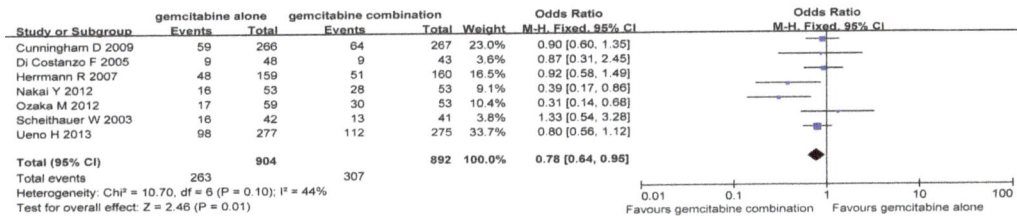

GEM+CAP versus GEM alone

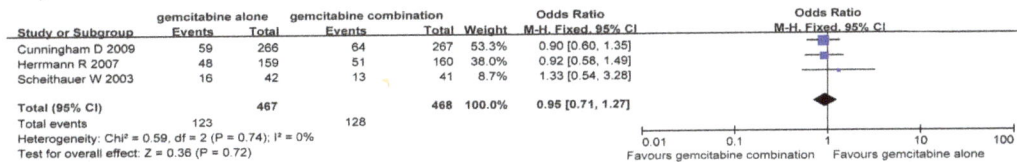

GEM+S-1 versus GEM alone

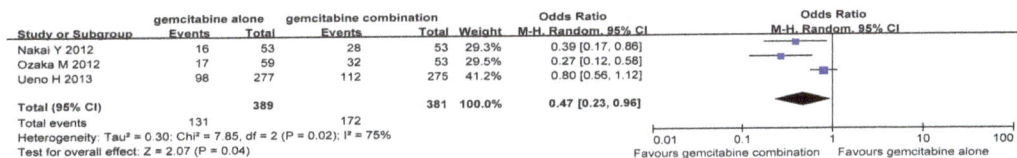

Figure 4. Comparison of one-year survival rate between GEM combination therapy and GEM alone therapy.

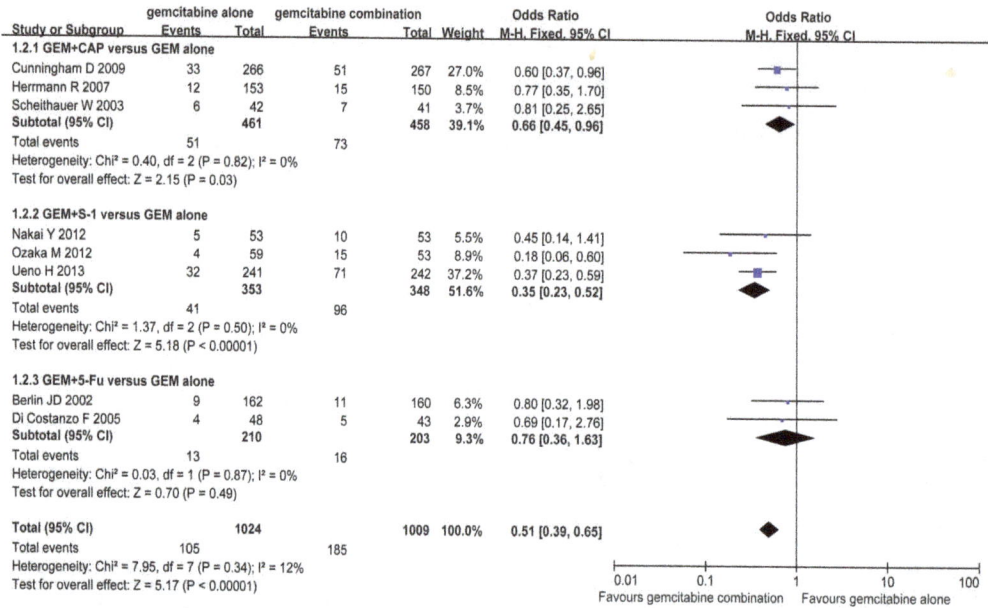

Figure 5. Comparison of objective response rate between GEM combination therapy and GEM alone therapy.

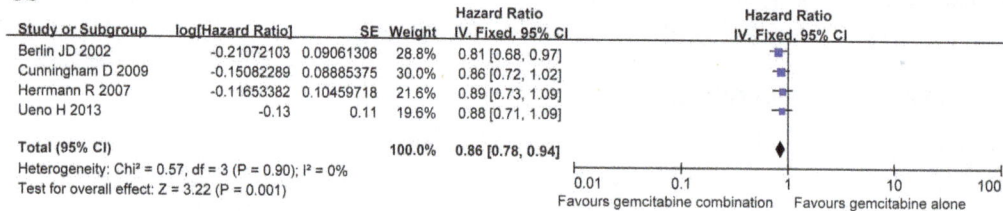

MPC patients [31,32]. Phase II and III comparison studies confirmed that the combination therapy of GEM and CAP resulted in an improved OS compared to GEM monotherapy (9.5 vs 8.2 months, 8.4 vs 7.2 months, 7.1 vs 6.2 months, respectively) in LA/MPC patients [22,24,25]. Moreover, Herrmann's analysis in patients with good KPS (90 to 100) showed a significant prolongation of median OS in the GEM-CAP arm compared to the GEM arm (10.1 vs 7.4 months, $P = 0.014$) [24]. In our subgroup meta-analysis, there was a significant improvement in OS (HR 0.87, $P = 0.03$) and a significant increase in ORR (OR 0.66, $P = 0.03$), but there was no significant difference in one-year survival rates between the two groups. This indicates that GEM

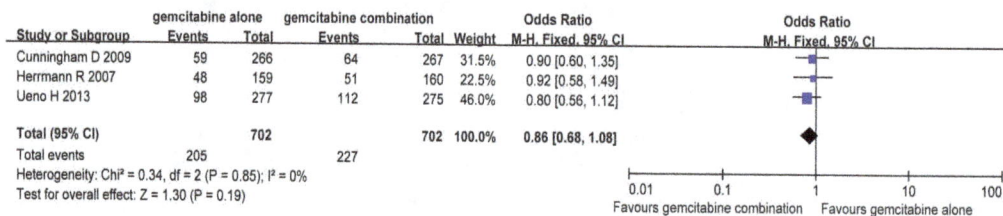

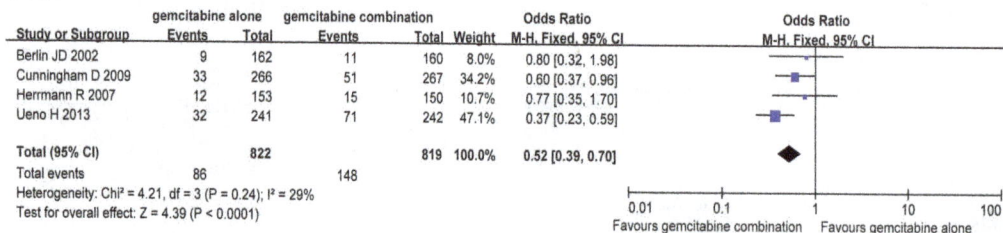

Figure 6. Efficacy sub-analysis of the phase III trials.

Table 2. Comparison of Grade 3–4 toxicity rates between GEM combination therapy and GEM alone therapy.

Grade 3–4 TRs	No of Grade 3–4 TRs/Total patients (%)		OR	95%CI	Significance test	
	GEM combination	GEM alone			Z	P
Neutropenia	350/979 (35.8)	238/984 (24.2)	1.90	1.54–2.34	6.03	<0.01
Thrombocytopenia	122/1021 (11.9)	80/1035 (7.7)	1.62	1.20–2.18	3.19	<0.01
Anemia	98/1020 (9.6)	91/1003 (9.1)	1.11	0.82–1.50	0.66	0.51
Diarrhea	53/979 (5.4)	26/984 (2.6)	2.04	1.28–3.26	2.99	<0.01
Nausea	57/986 (5.8)	42/994 (4.2)	1.37	0.91–2.06	1.53	0.13
Vomiting	46/882 (5.2)	39/883 (4.4)	1.18	0.76–1.83	0.76	0.45

GEM, gemcitabine; TRs, toxicity rates; OR, odds ratio; CI, confidence interval.

combined with CAP maybe considered as an alternative to GEM alone, and further stratification studies are required.

S-1 is an oral 5-FU derivative with high efficiency and low toxicity. A single-arm phase II study reported that the MST was 12.5 months and one-year survival rate was 54% in LA/MPC patients receiving GEM combined with S-1 therapy [16]. Phase II and III comparison studies reported that GEM combined with S-1 did not significantly improve OS compared to GEM alone (13.5 vs 8.8 months, $P = 0.102$; 10.1 vs 8.8 months, $P = 0.15$; respectively) [26,28]. However, in Ozaka's phase II study, the OS of patients in the GEM combined with S-1 group was significantly longer than that in the GEM alone group (13.7 vs 8.0 months, $P = 0.035$) [27]. However, two of the three studies mentioned above are open-label studies, which may result in potential bias to the conclusion. Our subgroup meta-analysis revealed that there was a significant improvement in OS and a significant increase in both one-year survival rate and ORR when the GEM combined with S-1 group

was compared to the GEM group. Given these promising and surprising results, the combination of GEM and S-1 may become a valuable and acceptable alternative treatment for LA/MPC patients.

GEM combined with fluorouracil drugs brings significant clinical benefits to LA/MPC patients. Whether combination therapy leads to more side effects is also a concern for the clinican. Although this systematic assessment demonstrated a significant increase of grade 3–4 neutropenia, thrombocytopenia and diarrhea in the GEM combination group, these TRs were generally tolerable and reversible. 3 RCT (2 GEM+CAP versus GEM trials; 1 GEM+S-1 versus GEM trial) reported that the addition of CAP/S-1 to GEM did not compromise patients' quality of life or quality-adjusted life-years [22,25,28].

GEM-based combination therapy improved the survival benefit in LA/MPC patients. Non-GEM-based combination schemes, for example the combination of oxaliplatin, irinotecan, fluorouracil

A. Grade 3–4 neutropenia

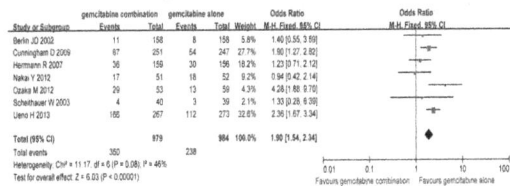

B. Grade 3–4 thrombocytopenia

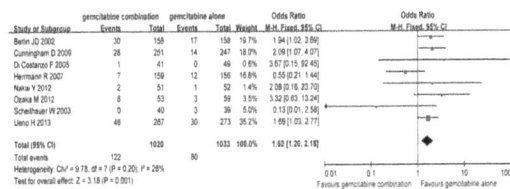

C. Grade 3–4 anemia

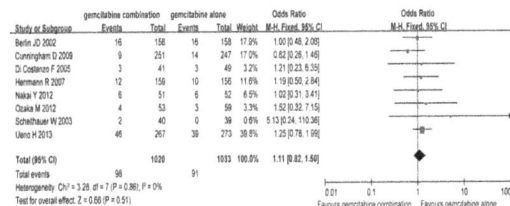

D. Grade 3–4 diarrhea

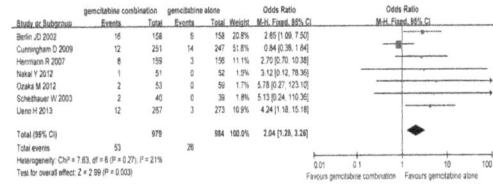

E. Grade 3–4 nausea

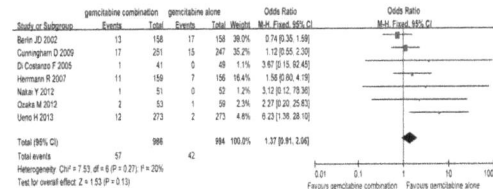

F. Grade 3–4 vomiting

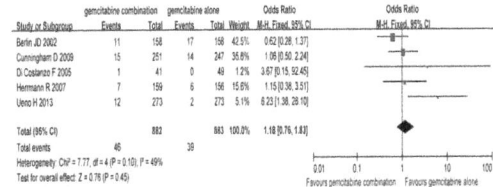

Figure 7. Comparison of Grade 3–4 toxicity rates between GEM combination therapy and GEM alone therapy.

and leucovorin (FOLFIRINOX), also significantly improved OS and PFS compared to GEM alone [33]. There have been some positive results confirmed by phase III trials, and our study does not suggest that GEM combined with fluorouracil drugs surpasses other treatment schemes in certain patients [7,33]. Rigorous phase III clinical trials are needed to further explore the potential benefits of GEM combined with fluorouracil drugs in LA/MPC patients.

This study revealed a significant improvement in OS and a significant increase in ORR when GEM combined with 5-FU/CAP/S-1 or 5-FU or CAP or S-1 were compared to GEM alone in LA/MPC patients. There was a significant increase in the one-year survival rate when GEM combined with 5-FU/CAP/S-1 or

S-1 was compared to GEM alone. Grade 3–4 neutropenia, thrombocytopenia and diarrhea were significantly increased in GEM combined with 5-FU/CAP/S-1 group. The combination of GEM and fluorouracil drugs may be considered as a valuable and acceptable alternative treatment for medically fit patients with LA/MPC.

Author Contributions

Conceived and designed the experiments: BC. Performed the experiments: QL. Analyzed the data: HY QL. Contributed reagents/materials/analysis tools: WL HZ YY. Wrote the paper: QL.

References

1. Goulart BH, Clark JW, Lauwers GY, Ryan DP, Grenon N, et al. (2009) Long term survivors with metastatic pancreatic adenocarcinoma treated with gemcitabine: a retrospective analysis. J Hematol Oncol 2: 13.
2. Bria E, Milella M, Gelibter A, Cuppone F, Pino MS, et al. (2007) Gemcitabine-based combinations for inoperable pancreatic cancer: have we made real progress? A meta-analysis of 20 phase 3 trials. Cancer 110: 525–533.
3. Burris HR, Moore MJ, Andersen J, Green MR, Rothenberg ML, et al. (1997) Improvements in survival and clinical benefit with gemcitabine as first-line therapy for patients with advanced pancreas cancer: a randomized trial. J Clin Oncol 15: 2403–2413.
4. Choi JH, Oh SY, Kwon HC, Kim JH, Lee JH, et al. (2008) Gemcitabine versus gemcitabine combined with cisplatin treatment locally advanced or metastatic pancreatic cancer: a retrospective analysis. Cancer Res Treat 40: 22–26.
5. Xie DR, Yang Q, Chen DL, Jiang ZM, Bi ZF, et al. (2010) Gemcitabine-based cytotoxic doublets chemotherapy for advanced pancreatic cancer: updated subgroup meta-analyses of overall survival. Jpn J Clin Oncol 40: 432–441.
6. Moore MJ, Goldstein D, Hamm J, Figer A, Hecht JR, et al. (2007) Erlotinib plus gemcitabine compared with gemcitabine alone in patients with advanced pancreatic cancer: a phase III trial of the National Cancer Institute of Canada Clinical Trials Group. J Clin Oncol 25: 1960–1966.
7. Von Hoff DD, Ervin T, Arena FP, Chiorean EG, Infante J, et al. (2013) Increased survival in pancreatic cancer with nab-paclitaxel plus gemcitabine. N Engl J Med 369: 1691–1703.
8. Ciliberto D, Botta C, Correale P, Rossi M, Caraglia M, et al. (2013) Role of gemcitabine-based combination therapy in the management of advanced pancreatic cancer: a meta-analysis of randomised trials. Eur J Cancer 49: 593–603.
9. Hu J, Zhao G, Wang HX, Tang L, Xu YC, et al. (2011) A meta-analysis of gemcitabine containing chemotherapy for locally advanced and metastatic pancreatic adenocarcinoma. J Hematol Oncol 4: 11.
10. Sun C, Ansari D, Andersson R, Wu DQ (2012) Does gemcitabine-based combination therapy improve the prognosis of unresectable pancreatic cancer? World J Gastroenterol 18: 4944–4958.
11. Maisey N, Chau I, Cunningham D, Norman A, Seymour M, et al. (2002) Multicenter randomized phase III trial comparing protracted venous infusion (PVI) fluorouracil (5-FU) with PVI 5-FU plus mitomycin in inoperable pancreatic cancer. J Clin Oncol 20: 3130–3136.
12. Chau I, Cunningham D, Russell C, Norman AR, Kurzawinski T, et al. (2006) Gastrazole (JB95008), a novel CCK2/gastrin receptor antagonist, in the treatment of advanced pancreatic cancer: results from two randomised controlled trials. Br J Cancer 94: 1107–1115.
13. Cartwright TH, Cohn A, Varkey JA, Chen YM, Szatrowski TP, et al. (2002) Phase II study of oral capecitabine in patients with advanced or metastatic pancreatic cancer. J Clin Oncol 20: 160–164.
14. Saif MW, Syrigos KN, Katirtzoglou NA (2009) S-1: a promising new oral fluoropyrimidine derivative. Expert Opin Investig Drugs 18: 335–348.
15. Shirasaka T (2009) Development history and concept of an oral anticancer agent S-1 (TS-1): its clinical usefulness and future vistas. Jpn J Clin Oncol 39: 2–15.
16. Nakamura K, Yamaguchi T, Ishihara T, Sudo K, Kato H, et al. (2006) Phase II trial of oral S-1 combined with gemcitabine in metastatic pancreatic cancer. Br J Cancer 94: 1575–1579.
17. Moher D, Liberati A, Tetzlaff J, Altman DG (2009) Preferred reporting items for systematic reviews and meta-analyses: the PRISMA statement. BMJ 339: b2535.
18. Higgins JP, Altman DG, Gotzsche PC, Juni P, Moher D, et al. (2011) The Cochrane Collaboration's tool for assessing risk of bias in randomised trials. BMJ 343: d5928.

19. Parmar MK, Torri V, Stewart L (1998) Extracting summary statistics to perform meta-analyses of the published literature for survival endpoints. Stat Med 17: 2815–2834.
20. Tierney JF, Stewart LA, Ghersi D, Burdett S, Sydes MR (2007) Practical methods for incorporating summary time-to-event data into meta-analysis. Trials 8: 16.
21. Berlin JD, Catalano P, Thomas JP, Kugler JW, Haller DG, et al. (2002) Phase III study of gemcitabine in combination with fluorouracil versus gemcitabine alone in patients with advanced pancreatic carcinoma: Eastern Cooperative Oncology Group Trial E2297. J Clin Oncol 20: 3270–3275.
22. Scheithauer W, Schull B, Ulrich-Pur H, Schmid K, Raderer M, et al. (2003) Biweekly high-dose gemcitabine alone or in combination with capecitabine in patients with metastatic pancreatic adenocarcinoma: a randomized phase II trial. Ann Oncol 14: 97–104.
23. Di Costanzo F, Carlini P, Doni L, Massidda B, Mattioli R, et al. (2005) Gemcitabine with or without continuous infusion 5-FU in advanced pancreatic cancer: a randomised phase II trial of the Italian oncology group for clinical research (GOIRC). Br J Cancer 93: 185–189.
24. Herrmann R, Bodoky G, Ruhstaller T, Glimelius B, Bajetta E, et al. (2007) Gemcitabine plus capecitabine compared with gemcitabine alone in advanced pancreatic cancer: a randomized, multicenter, phase III trial of the Swiss Group for Clinical Cancer Research and the Central European Cooperative Oncology Group. J Clin Oncol 25: 2212–2217.
25. Cunningham D, Chau I, Stocken DD, Valle JW, Smith D, et al. (2009) Phase III randomized comparison of gemcitabine versus gemcitabine plus capecitabine in patients with advanced pancreatic cancer. J Clin Oncol 27: 5513–5518.
26. Nakai Y, Isayama H, Sasaki T, Sasahira N, Tsujino T, et al. (2012) A multicentre randomised phase II trial of gemcitabine alone vs gemcitabine and S-1 combination therapy in advanced pancreatic cancer: GEMSAP study. Br J Cancer 106: 1934–1939.
27. Ozaka M, Matsumura Y, Ishii H, Omuro Y, Itoi T, et al. (2012) Randomized phase II study of gemcitabine and S-1 combination versus gemcitabine alone in the treatment of unresectable advanced pancreatic cancer (Japan Clinical Cancer Research Organization PC-01 study). Cancer Chemother Pharmacol 69: 1197–1204.
28. Ueno H, Ioka T, Ikeda M, Ohkawa S, Yanagimoto H, et al. (2013) Randomized phase III study of gemcitabine plus S-1, S-1 alone, or gemcitabine alone in patients with locally advanced and metastatic pancreatic cancer in Japan and Taiwan: GEST study. J Clin Oncol 31: 1640–1648.
29. Xie DR, Liang HL, Wang Y, Guo SS, Yang Q (2006) Meta-analysis on inoperable pancreatic cancer: a comparison between gemcitabine-based combination therapy and gemcitabine alone. World J Gastroenterol 12: 6973–6981.
30. Ling W, Fan J, Ma Y, Ma Y, Wang H (2011) Capecitabine-based chemotherapy for metastatic colorectal cancer. J Cancer Res Clin Oncol 137: 927–938.
31. Hubner RA, Worsnop F, Cunningham D, Chau I (2013) Gemcitabine plus capecitabine in unselected patients with advanced pancreatic cancer. Pancreas 42: 511–515.
32. Choi JG, Seo JH, Oh SC, Choi CW, Kim JS (2012) A Phase II Trial of Gemcitabine plus Capecitabine for Patients with Advanced Pancreatic Cancer. Cancer Res Treat 44: 127–132.
33. Gourgou-Bourgade S, Bascoul-Mollevi C, Desseigne F, Ychou M, Bouche O, et al. (2013) Impact of FOLFIRINOX compared with gemcitabine on quality of life in patients with metastatic pancreatic cancer: results from the PRODIGE 4/ACCORD 11 randomized trial. J Clin Oncol 31: 23–29.

8

Porcine Epidemic Diarrhea Virus RNA Present in Commercial Spray-Dried Porcine Plasma is not Infectious to Naïve Pigs

Tanja Opriessnig[1,2]*, Chao-Ting Xiao[2], Priscilla F. Gerber[1], Jianqiang Zhang[2], Patrick G. Halbur[2]

1 The Roslin Institute and The Royal (Dick) School of Veterinary Studies, University of Edinburgh, Roslin, Midlothian, United Kingdom, 2 Department of Veterinary Diagnostic and Production Animal Medicine, College of Veterinary Medicine, Iowa State University, Ames, Iowa, United States of America

Abstract

Porcine epidemic diarrhea virus emerged in North America in April 2013 and has since been identified in 30 U.S. States, Canada and Mexico. The rapid spread of PEDV has raised concerns about the role of feed and particularly pork-by-product components such as spray-dried porcine plasma (SDPP) in PEDV transmission. The aim of this study was to determine the infectivity of PEDV RNA present in commercial SDPP. Specifically, 40 3-week-old PEDV naïve pigs were randomly assigned to one of five treatment groups. At day post inoculation (dpi) 0, NEG-CONTROL pigs were sham-inoculated, PEDV-CONTROL pigs received cell culture propagated PEDV, and SDPP-CONTROL pigs were switched to a diet with 5% SDPP containing 5.1 ± 0.1 $\log_{10}$ PEDV RNA copies/g. To evaluate a potential positive effect of anti-PEDV antibodies in SDPP on PEDV challenge, four days prior to PEDV challenge the pigs in the SDPP-PEDV group were switched to and remained on a 5% SDPP diet through dpi 28. Another group, EGG-PEDV, was orally administered a commercial egg-derived liquid PEDV globulin product from dpi -4 through 6. All PEDV-CONTROL pigs began shedding PEDV in feces by dpi 3 and seroconverted between dpi 7 and 14, whereas pigs in NEG-CONTROL and SDPP-CONTROL groups remained PEDV RNA negative and did not seroconvert to PEDV for the study duration. This indicates no evidence of infectivity of the PEDV RNA in the SDPP lot utilized. Furthermore, under the study conditions SDPP or egg-derived liquid PEDV globulin addition did not significantly alter PEDV-shedding or overall disease course after experimental challenge.

Editor: Karol Sestak, Tulane University, United States of America

Funding: Funding for this study was provided in part by APC, Inc., Ankeny, Iowa, United States of America and EPFX/EGCO Protein, Provanco Feeds, Le Center, Minnesota, United States of America. The funders had no role in study design, data collection and analysis, decision to publish, or preparation of the manuscript.

* Email: Tanja.Opriessnig@roslin.ed.ac.uk

Introduction

Porcine epidemic diarrhea virus emerged in North America in April 2013 [1]. Since the initial discovery, PEDV has spread rapidly through the pig population and is present in 30 U.S. States, Canada and Mexico as of May 2014. PEDV, an *Alphacoronavirus*, is a member of the *Coronaviridae* family which is a group of single-stranded, positive-sense RNA viruses [2]. PEDV isolates can be divided into genogroups 1 and 2 [3].

Spray-dried porcine plasma (SDPP) is a common feed additive to nursery pig diets to promote growth and improve overall pig health [4]. The raw plasma utilized is commonly collected in slaughter house plants from healthy pigs, transported to spray drying facilities and immediately processed. While it is possible that the plasma contains trace amounts of viral DNA or RNA [5], experimental feed trials using a much higher than normal percentage of SDPP over prolonged periods of time have indicated no infectivity of common viruses such as porcine circovirus type 2 (PCV2) [5,6]. Moreover, SDPP also contains high levels of

neutralizing antibodies [7] which ultimately contribute to the biosafety of the final SDPP.

With the rapid spread of PEDV in North America, concerns over SDPP as a possible source of PEDV introduction into herds were raised and led to the recommendation to discontinue use in some countries such as the UK [8]. While PEDV as an RNA virus is unlikely to survive the commercial spray-drying process, controlled experimental studies are needed to further prove or disprove these transmission speculations as SDPP is an important component of nursery diets in many production systems.

Effective vaccines for PEDV are still urgently needed and the current lack of vaccines or other tools for prevention and control of PEDV in North America has forced producers to utilize alternative strategies such as avian derived immunoglobulins to attempt to mitigate the effects of PEDV. However, little information is available on the efficacy of these products to protect pigs against PEDV in the U.S. or elsewhere. Past studies also demonstrated that the use of SDPP improved average daily weight gain and decreased severity of enteric disease in piglets challenged with pathogenic *Escherichia coli* [9,10]; therefore, a reduction of the negative effects associated with PEDV due to SDPP appeared reasonable. The objectives of this study were (1) to determine the infectivity of commercial SDPP confirmed positive for PEDV RNA and (2) to evaluate a potential protective effect of commercial SDPP and an egg-derived liquid PEDV globulin product.

Materials and Methods

Ethic statement

The experimental protocol was approved by the Iowa State University Institutional Animal Care and Use Committee (Approval No. 2-14-7742-S; approved on the 5th of March 2014).

Animals and housing

Forty, 2-week-old, colostrum-fed, crossbred piglets from a commercial herd free of PEDV and porcine reproductive and respiratory syndrome (PRRSV) were arbitrarily selected, transported to the Iowa State University Livestock Infectious Disease Isolation Facility, and housed in four separate biosecurity level 2 rooms. Three of the rooms contained a 3.8×1.5 m pen on a solid concrete floor, a self-feeder, and one nipple drinker. Two similar pens were placed at opposite ends of a larger 4th room with 3.5 m separation between the two pens. Personnel handling the pigs were required to shower and change clothes, boots, gloves before entering each room. Prior to start of the experiment, all pigs were fed an age appropriate starter diet free of animal protein (produced on the 13th of February 2014; Heartland Coop, Prairie City, Iowa, USA).

Spray-dried porcine plasma (SDPP) production

The SDPP used for this study was from lot No. A4051110 (APC Inc., Ankeny, Iowa, USA) and was produced on the 20th of February 2014. The inlet temperature in the spray drier was $204 \pm 5^{\circ}C$ and the outlet temperature was $79 \pm 1.9^{\circ}C$. The moisture of the product during the run was $7.35 \pm 0.7\%$. This product was within normal production conditions and can be considered typical of commercial SDPP protein. Three different SDPP samples were collected; from the beginning, the middle, and at the end of the batch production cycle. The SDPP plasma lot used in this trial contained 5.1 ± 0.1 $\log_{10}$ PEDV RNA copies/g and had IgG antibodies against PEDV at the ELISA optical density (OD) value of 0.45 ± 0.0 at a dilution of 1:10 in phosphate-buffered saline (PBS).

Feed formulation

The selected commercial SDPP was incorporated into a non-pelleted, complete feed, at a final inclusion of 5%. Based on average intake of 215 g/d for a 28 day old pig fed for 28 d, average plasma consumption was 10.5 g/d, for a total consumption of 301 g of SDPP per pig. In addition, a diet without SDPP was also produced to provide equivalent dietary energy and lysine compared to the diet containing SDPP.

The SDPP diet contained 3.3 ± 0.3 $\log_{10}$ PEDV RNA copies/g whereas the negative control diet was PEDV RT-PCR negative. After arrival at the research facility the bagged feed was stored in separate anterooms for each group at ambient room temperature (approximately 18°C). The interval from SDPP production to initiation of feeding the pigs in this trial at -4 dpi (20th March 2014) for the SDPP-PEDV group or 0 dpi for the SDPP-CONTROL group (24th March 2014) was between 28 and 32 days which can be considered typical in the U.S. and accounts for the time from production, transport to the feed mill, distribution to the farm, and administration to the pigs. Feed samples were obtained on a weekly basis from each anteroom and confirmed to (1) be PEDV negative (negative control feed) or (2) to contain 3.2 ± 0.5 $\log_{10}$ PEDV genomic equivalent copies/g (SDPP positive feed ratio) without apparent reduction over time.

Experimental design

After a one-week acclimation period, the pigs were randomly divided into five groups (Table 1) with eight pigs in each group including: Treatment 1 NEG-CONTROL (no SDPP in the feed; pigs not inoculated with PEDV), Treatment 2 PEDV-CONTROL (no SDPP in the feed; pigs inoculated with PEDV), Treatment 3 SDPP-CONTROL (5% commercial SDPP in the feed from dpi 0 to 28; pigs not inoculated with PEDV), Treatment 4 SDPP-PEDV (5% commercial SDPP in the feed from dpi -4 to 28; pigs inoculated with PEDV), and Treatment 5 EGG-PEDV (no SDPP in the feed; 5 ml per day orally from dpi -4 to 6 of EPFX/EGCO Protein's Farrow X1, Provanco Feeds, Le Center, Minnesota, USA; pigs inoculated with PEDV). The negative control diet used for treatments 1, 2 and 5 did not contain any blood-derived protein. All diets were formulated to meet the nutritional requirements of the pig [11] and were provided in self-feeders to assure ad libitum consumption. Treatment 2, 4 and 5 pigs were inoculated orally with 10 ml of a cell-culture propagated PEDV inoculum by slowly dripping the inoculum into the oral cavity of the pig. Blood samples were collected in serum separator tubes (Fisher Scientific, Pittsburgh, Pennsylvania, USA) at arrival, on the day of inoculation, and at dpi 3, 7, 14, 21 and 28, centrifuged at $2000 \times g$ for 10 min at 4°C, and tested for the presence of anti-PEDV-IgG antibodies and PEDV RNA. Similarly, fecal swabs were collected at arrival and dpi 0, 3, 5, 7, 14, 21 and 28 and tested for the presence of PEDV RNA. Specifically, the swabs were collected using polyester swabs (Fisher Scientific, Inc.) and stored in 5 ml plastic tubes (Fisher Scientific, Inc.) containing 1 ml of sterile saline solution (Fisher Scientific, Inc.). All pigs were weighed at -4 dpi and at dpi 28.

Treatments

SDPP-free, PEDV-negative control feed. Pigs in the NEG-CONTROL, PEDV-CONTROL, and the EGG-PEDV groups were feed a diet free of SDPP and PEDV RNA from dpi 0 through 28.

SDPP (5%), PEDV-positive control feed. Pigs in the SDPP-PEDV group were fed the 5% SDPP diet from dpi -4 through 28 and pigs in the SDPP-CONTROL group received the SDPP diet from dpi 0 until 28.

Anti-PEDV globulin. A liquid egg protein formulation (EPFX/EGCO Protein's Farrow X1, Provanco Feeds, Le Center, Minnesota, USA; Lot# LS 60030614-1) was obtained from a commercial source and was administered daily in a 5 ml volume orally from dpi -4 to dpi 6. According to company specifications, the product was tested for anti-coronavirus antibodies and had an OD value of 1.0 based on incubating the liquid egg protein formulation diluted 1:10 in PBS on ELISA plates coated with various coronavirus antigens. In that test, samples with OD values greater than 0.2 were considered positive.

PEDV inoculation

PEDV-CONTROL, SDPP-PEDV and EGG-PEDV pigs were experimentally infected with 10 ml of the 5th passage of the PEDV isolate 13-19338E [12] at a tissue culture infective dose (TCID$_{50}$) of 5×10^2 per ml via the oral route on dpi 0.

Table 1. Experimental design.

Group Designation	No. of pigs	Diet or treatment	Inoculation	Necropsy	
			dpi 0	dpi 3	dpi 28
NEG-CONTROL	8	No SDPP or other treatment	PBS	3	5
SDPP-CONTROL	8	5% SDPP[1] (dpi 0 to dpi 28)	PBS	3	5
PEDV-CONTROL	8	No SDPP or other treatment	PEDV	3	5
SDPP-PEDV	8	5% SDPP (dpi -4 to dpi 28)	PEDV	3	5
EGG-PEDV	8	Ab[2] treatment (dpi -4 to dpi 6)	PEDV	3	5

Abbreviations: dpi, day post inoculation; SDPP, spray-dried porcine plasma; PBS, phosphate-buffered saline; PEDV, porcine epidemic diarrhea virus.
[1]Spray-dried porcine plasma from APC, Inc., Ankeny, Iowa, USA.
[2]EPFX/EGCO Protein's Farrow X1, Provanco Feeds, Le Center, Minnesota, USA.

Serology

Sera from blood samples collected at arrival and at dpi -4, 0, 7, 14, 21 and 28 were tested for the presence of anti-PEDV IgG antibodies by an *in-house* spike gene 1 (S1)-based indirect ELISA and by indirect immunofluorescence assay (IFA). Briefly for the S1-ELISA, an immunogenic fragment spanning amino acids 1 through 718 of the S1 domain of the PEDV IA1 strain [3] expressed in an eukaryotic expression vector was used as antigen. Microtiter plates were coated with the S1 polypeptide diluted in carbonate coating buffer and incubated overnight at 4°C. Plates were then blocked with 1% bovine serum albumin for 2 h at 22°C and incubated with samples diluted 1:100 in PBS containing 10% goat serum for 30 min at 37°C. After a washing step, a 1:20,000 diluted peroxidase-conjugated goat anti-swine IgG (Jackson ImmunoResearch) was added and incubated at 37°C for 30 min. The peroxidase reaction was visualized by using tetramethylbenzidine-hydrogen peroxide solution as the substrate for 10 min at room temperature and stopped by adding 50 µl of 2.5 M sulfuric acid to each well. For the S1-ELISA, samples with an OD value greater than 0.3 were considered positive, samples with OD values between 0.2 and 0.3 were considered as indeterminate, and samples with OD values below 0.2 were considered negative. Samples were tested in 2-fold dilutions with the IFA ranging from 1:40 to 1:320. Positive signals at a sample dilution of 1:40 or higher were considered positive.

RNA extraction

Total nucleic acids were extracted from serum samples, fecal swab suspensions and inoculation materials (raw plasma samples and reconstituted spray-dried porcine plasma powders) using the MagMax Pathogen RNA/DNA Kit (Applied Biosystems, Life Technologies, Carlsbad, California, USA) and an automated DNA/RNA extraction system (Thermo Scientific Kingfisher Flex, Thermo Fisher Scientific, Pittsburgh, Pennsylvania, USA) according to the instructions of the manufacturer.

Quantitative real-time RT-PCR for PEDV

For development of the quantitative PEDV real-time RT-PCR assay 31 genomic sequences of PEDV were downloaded from GenBank and aligned with the Lasergene package (DNAStar Inc., Madison, Wisconsin, USA). A pair of PEDV detection primers (PEDVDF: 5′-GTGGCTCTCAAACTGTTTTACGTTG-3′; PEDVDR: 5′-GACACCACAATCTGAAGCACAACAC-3′) and a TaqMan probe (PEDVprob: 5′-6-FAM-ACGGCGTCC-TATGCTTTGTACTAAGTGTG-BHQ-3′) were designed within the conservative ORF1b gene by Primer Express software

(version 3.0; Applied Biosystems, Foster City, California, USA) to cover a region of 149 nucleotides. The probe was labeled with 6-Carboxyfluorescein (FAM) at the 5′ end and Black Hole Quencher (BHQ) at the 3′ end.

The real-time RT-PCR was carried out in 96-well plates, with each reaction consisting of a total volume of 25 µl, containing 12.5 µl TaqMan One-Step RT-PCR Master Mix Reagent (Applied Biosystems), 6 µl RNA, 0.625 µl 40× MultiScribe and RNase Inhibitor, 1 µl each of the two primers (10 µM), 0.5 µl probe (10 µM) and 3.375 µl RNase-free water. Amplification reactions were performed using an Applied Biosystems 7500 Fast Real-Time PCR System (Applied Biosystems) under universal conditions: 30 min at 50°C, 10 min at 95°C, followed by 40 cycles of 15 s at 95°C and 1 min at 60°C. A sample was considered negative if no cycle threshold (Ct) was detected during the 40 amplification cycles. PEDV genomic loads per fecal swab were calculated by multiplying the individual results from the quantitative real-time RT-PCR by 166.7 (50 µl RNA preparation eluted from 50 µl fecal swab suspension ×20 (1 ml saline per 50 µl elution buffer) per 6 µl PCR input).

To obtain standards, the PCR products with primers PEDVDF/DR were purified and cloned into pGEM-T Easy Vector System (Promega). The recombinant plasmids were transformed into TOP10 *Escherichia coli* competent cells (Invitrogen) and propagated following the instructions of the cloning kit manual. The plasmids were extracted using a QIAprep Spin Minipreps Kit (Qiagen) according to the manufacturer's instructions, quantified using a spectrophotometer (NanoPhotometer; Implen) and sequenced. The confirmed plasmids were used as standards in the real-time RT-PCR assay to determine assay sensitivity and to quantify viral loads in the fecal swabs. The standard curve and the sensitivity of the real-time RT-PCR were carried out and determined as described previously [13]. The real-time RT-PCR assay was used on 10-fold serial dilutions of the PEDV plasmid, with a detection limit of 5 genome equivalents which occurred around a Ct of 36. The determined slope, R2 and intercept value of the standard curve were −3.455, 0.99 and 38.3. The specificity of the probe was confirmed by BLAST analysis and by testing samples positive for other RNA viruses available in the laboratory, including PRRSV, transmissible gastroenteritis virus, porcine respiratory coronavirus, porcine deltacoronavirus, porcine astrovirus and swine hepatitis E virus. No cross-amplification was observed, indicating that this real-time RT-PCR assay allowed specific, efficient and sensitive detection of PEDV. All RNA extracts were tested for the presence of PEDV RNA by the quantitative real-time RT-PCR assay.

Sequencing

To confirm that the PEDV from the experimentally infected pigs was the same as the virus in the inocula, the S1 gene and nucleocapsid gene were amplified and sequenced utilizing the following primers: PEDVS1F (5-TTCTAATCATTTGGT-CAACGTAAAC-3), PEDVS1R (5-TACTCATACTAAAGT-TGGTGGGAATAC-3), PEDVNF (5- GTGCTTCATTTAGT-CTAAACAGAAAC-3) and PEDVNR (5-GACATTACCACT-GGCTTACCGT-3). The PCR products were purified using the QIAquick PCR Purification Kit (Qiagen) according to the manufacturers' directions and sequenced at the Iowa State University DNA facility. The sequences were aligned with published data using BLAST at the National Center for Biotechnology Information (NCBI) (http://www.ncbi.nlm.nih.gov/) and compiled using Lasergene software and the Clustal W alignment algorithm (DNAStar, Madison, Wisconsin, USA).

Necropsy

All pigs were humanely euthanized by pentobarbital overdose (Fatal-plus, Vortech Pharmaceuticals, LTD, Dearborn, Michigan, USA) and three pigs per group were necropsied at dpi 3 and the remaining five pigs were necropsied at dpi 28. Severity of macroscopic lesions in the small and large intestines and consistency of the colon content (normal, fluid, liquid) were estimated by a pathologist blinded to the treatment status. Six sections of small intestines, three sections of large intestines, and one section of lung were collected at necropsy and fixed in 10% neutral-buffered formalin and routinely processed for histological examination. In addition, intestinal content was collected from the cecum of each animal and stored in individual 50 ml plastic centrifuge tubes (Fisher Scientific, Inc.). Sections of small and large intestines were also collected fresh and stored at -80°C.

Histopathology

Microscopic lesions were evaluated by a veterinary pathologist blinded to treatment status. Sections of small and large intestines were evaluated for the presence of inflammation, villus atrophy, and necrosis and scored from 0 (none) to 3 (severe). Lung sessions were evaluated for presence of interstitial pneumonia and bronchiolitis.

PEDV immunohistochemistry (IHC)

PEDV-specific antigen was detected by immunohistochemistry (IHC) on selected formalin-fixed and paraffin-embedded sections of intestinal sections using monoclonal antibody specific for PEDV (BioNote, Hwaseong-si, Gyeonggi-do, Korea) as described [1,14]. The amount of PEDV antigen was scored by a pathologist blinded to treatment status. Scores ranged from 0 (no signal) to 3 (abundant, diffuse staining).

Statistical analysis

For data analysis, JMP software version 10.0.2 (SAS Institute, Cary, North Carolina, USA) was used. Summary statistics were calculated for all the groups to assess the overall quality of the data set including normality. Statistical analysis of the data was performed by one-way analysis of variance (ANOVA) for continuous data ($\log_{10}$ transformed RT-PCR data, ELISA data, and average daily weight gain). A p-value of less than 0.05 was set as the statistically significant level. Pairwise test using Tukey's adjustment was subsequently performed to determine which differences among groups were statistically significant. Non-repeated nominal data (histopathology scores and IHC scores) were assessed using a non-parametric Kruskal-Wallis one-way ANOVA, and if there was a significant difference, pairwise Wilcoxon tests were used to evaluate differences among groups. Differences in prevalence were determined by using chi-square tests.

Results

Clinical presentation

The average daily weight gain is summarized in Table 2. There were no significant differences among groups. Clinical signs were characterized by development of mild diarrhea defined by semi-solid to fluid feces around dpi 2 in PEDV-infected groups. By dpi 4, PEDV-infected pigs were lethargic and had moderate amounts of liquid greyish diarrhea. Between dpi 6 to 9 the degree of clinical signs appeared less severe in SDPP-PEDV pigs compared to EGG-PEDV and PEDV-CONTROL. Clinical signs between dpi 10 to 11 and feces composition returned to normal standards. There were no remarkable clinical signs in any of the NEG-CONTROL pigs or SDPP-CONTROL pigs.

Anti-PEDV antibody levels

Classification of individual pigs as antibody positive or negative was identical for the S1-ELISA and the IFA. Antibodies against PEDV were initially detected by dpi 7 in the PEDV-CONTROL pigs (2/8) (Fig. 1). By dpi 14, 100% (5/5) of PEDV-CONTROL pigs, 80% (4/5) of the SDPP-PEDV pigs and 60% (3/5) of the EGG-PEDV pigs had seroconverted to PEDV. At dpi 21 and 28, all PEDV-infected pigs were seropositive. Using the S1-ELISA, EGG-PEDV pigs had lower anti-PEDV OD values compared to PEDV-CONTROL and SDPP-PEDV pigs at dpi 14, 21 and 28; however, the difference was not significant (Fig. 1A). PEDV-antibodies were not detected in any of the NEG-CONTROL pigs or the SDPP-CONTROL pigs throughout the study.

PEDV shedding in feces

PEDV RNA was not detected in any of the NEG-CONTROL or SDPP-CONTROL pigs throughout the study (Table 3). PEDV RNA was detected in fecal swabs of all PEDV-infected groups at dpi 3, 5 and 7. By dpi 14, fewer pigs were shedding PEDV RNA in the SDPP-PEDV (1/5) and EGG-PEDV (4/5) groups. At dpi 28, the only PEDV inoculated group that did not contain PEDV RNA in feces was the EGG-PEDV group. Prevalence and mean group amount of PEDV RNA in feces are summarized in Table 3 and Fig. 2. Further sequencing of PCR positive samples confirmed 100% identity of the PEDV compared to the strain used for inoculation.

PEDV viremia

PEDV RNA was detected in low amounts in individual PEDV-infected pigs at dpi 3 and 7 but not at dpi 14, 21, or 28. Specifically, 2/8 PEDV-CONTROL pigs, 1/8 SDPP-PEDV pigs and 4/8 EGG-PEDV pigs were positive for PEDV RNA on dpi 3, and 1/5 positive controls, 2/5 SDPP-PEDV pigs and 1/5 EGG-PEDV pigs were RT-PCR positive on dpi 7. The PEDV load in positive serum samples ranged from 2.2 to 3.2 $\log_{10}$ genomic equivalent copies per ml. PEDV RNA was not detected in any of the serum samples obtained from the NEG-CONTROL pigs or the SDPP-CONTROL pigs.

Macroscopic lesions

By dpi 3, gross lesions were limited to thin-walled small intestines containing fluid grey-green intestinal content in PEDV-infected pigs (Table 4). By dpi 28, no remarkable macroscopic lesions were observed and the intestinal content appeared normal.

Table 2. Average daily gain in grams (±SEM) as determined on all pigs that were kept until 28 days post inoculation.

Group designation	No. of pigs	Average daily gain from dpi -4 to 28
NEG-CONTROL	5	381.3±41.9
SDPP-CONTROL	5	446.6±39.9
PEDV-CONTROL	**5**	**358±53.0**
SDPP-PEDV	**5**	**360±19.0**
EGG-PEDV	**5**	**348.6±45.8**

Bold areas indicate the pigs experimentally inoculated with PEDV

Microscopic lesions and PEDV antigen in tissues

By dpi 3, the majority of the PEDV-infected pigs had segmental, mild to severe villous atrophy and fusion in the small intestines associated with abundant PEDV antigen in the enterocytes along the tip and sides of the villi (Fig. 3). PEDV antigen staining was also observed in isolated cells in the lamina propria and Peyer's patches. Staining was not observed in the crypts of the small intestines or in any cells of the colon. Individual pigs had very mild multifocal necrosuppurative colitis associated with attaching and effacing *E. coli* (Table 4). The prevalence of PEDV antigen as determined by IHC stains in the PEDV-infected pigs is summarized in Table 4. PEDV antigen was not detected in any of the NEG-CONTROL pigs or SDPP-CONTROL pigs (Fig. 3).

By dpi 28, no microscopic lesions were observed in intestinal sections and PEDV antigen was not detected in any of the groups.

Discussion

The emergence of PEDV in North America in April 2013 and the apparent inability to prevent the virus from spreading rapidly through the swine population has raised important questions on transmission between farms and countries. Concerns over the role of SDPP in PEDV transmission were raised, when geographically unrelated pig operations without known contact points, but with a common commercial feed source almost simultaneously became infected with PEDV [15,16]. SDPP is derived from slaughter age pigs without clinical signs of disease. Recently it has been determined that under extreme experimental conditions, PCV2, a small, non-enveloped DNA virus that is very resistant to temperature changes, can survive the spray-drying process and retain infectivity [17]; however, the PCV2 in commercial product has been repeatedly demonstrated to not be infective [5,6,18]. Under similar conditions, RNA viruses like porcine reproductive and respiratory syndrome virus (PRRSV) were inactivated successfully [19]. The main objective of this study was to determine the infectivity of commercial SDPP positive for PEDV RNA in a conventional pig model.

In this study, PEDV-negative pigs were divided into five groups and four rooms and fed either a diet containing 5% SDPP confirmed positive for PEDV RNA or a control diet. One group was experimentally infected with PEDV by the oral route and served as positive control. Under the study conditions, none of the SDPP-CONTROL pigs developed clinical signs consistent with PEDV-infection, they did not shed PEDV RNA in feces and they did not seroconvert to PEDV indicating that the PEDV in the SDPP was not infectious. In contrast, the PEDV-CONTROL pigs had diarrhea from dpi 2 through dpi 10, shed PEDV RNA in feces from dpi 3 through 28, and seroconverted to PEDV.

Porcine plasma is obtained from blood collected in abattoirs. Presence of a virus in plasma is typically associated with an ongoing viremia. Previously, PEDV viremia has been reported in gnotobiotic pigs experimentally infected with PEDV genogroup 2 [20]. Similarly, in the present study PEDV RNA was detected in serum at the peak of disease, but viremia was short and of low magnitude (low numbers of PEDV genomic copies in real-time RT-PCR positive pigs at single time points). Therefore it appears unlikely that PEDV viremia and utilization of blood from viremic pigs is a main source of PEDV contamination of SDPP. Another potential source of PEDV RNA in raw blood may be attributed to contamination from swine carcasses during the blood withdrawal process. Sources of secondary contamination of the SDPP or swine feed throughout the distribution chain should be further investigated to reduce or prevent feed-associated transmission of PEDV.

Due to the lack of effective intervention tools against PEDV in North America, alternative methods are being investigated. Chicken egg antibodies have been used for prophylaxis and therapy of infectious disease in pigs for some time and have been suggested as a viable alternative to commonly used antimicrobial therapy [21]. Oral administration of IgY has been demonstrated to be cost effective and convenient [22]. Studies with *Escherichia coli* K88 [23] or F18 [24] indicated performance improvements and inhibition of bacterial shedding in treated pigs compared to untreated controls. Chicken egg yolk globulin against PEDV was found to reduce mortality in piglets after experimental PEDV challenge (2–3 ml were administered orally three times for one day) and also significantly improved survival rates of piglets during a field study in Korea [25]. In order to mimic what is done in the U.S. field, the liquid egg protein formulation (Farrow X1) obtained from hens immunized against PEDV and transmissible gastroenteritis virus (TGEV) was administered orally for 10 consecutive days to the EGG-PEDV group starting at 4 days prior to PEDV challenge. Due to presence of anti-chicken IgY antibody rather than pig IgG, Farrow X1 was not tested with the *in house* IgG ELISA, as results would not have been comparable due to using a different conjugate. However, based on company specifications, anti-coronavirus antibodies in high levels were present in the product. There was no significant clinical improvement and except for dpi 14 there was no significant reduction in PEDV shedding in treated (EGG-PEDV) versus untreated pigs (PEDV-CONTROL) although there was a numerical difference in the early phase of infection (dpi 3 and dpi 5). Reasons for this may include pathogen type, challenge route and dose, and timing/dosing of the EGG-PEDV treatment under the study conditions. Of note, PEDV shedding in this study was evaluated by RT-PCR which cannot distinguish between virus fragments or live virus. It is therefore unknown if the treatment would have affected transmission rates to naïve pigs and the overall environmental virus load.

Another potential way to neutralize infectious viruses present in the intestinal lumen is by feeding SDPP containing high levels of immunoglobulins [26–28]. It has also been determined that the

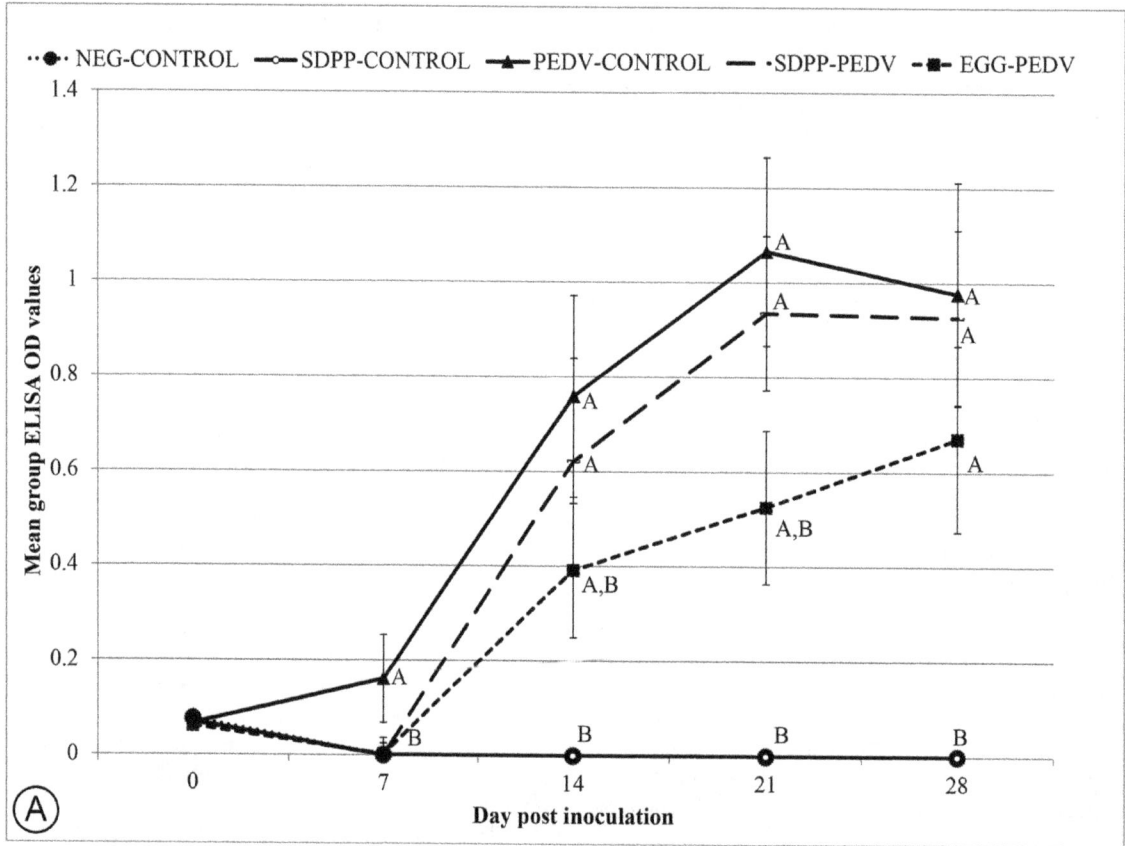

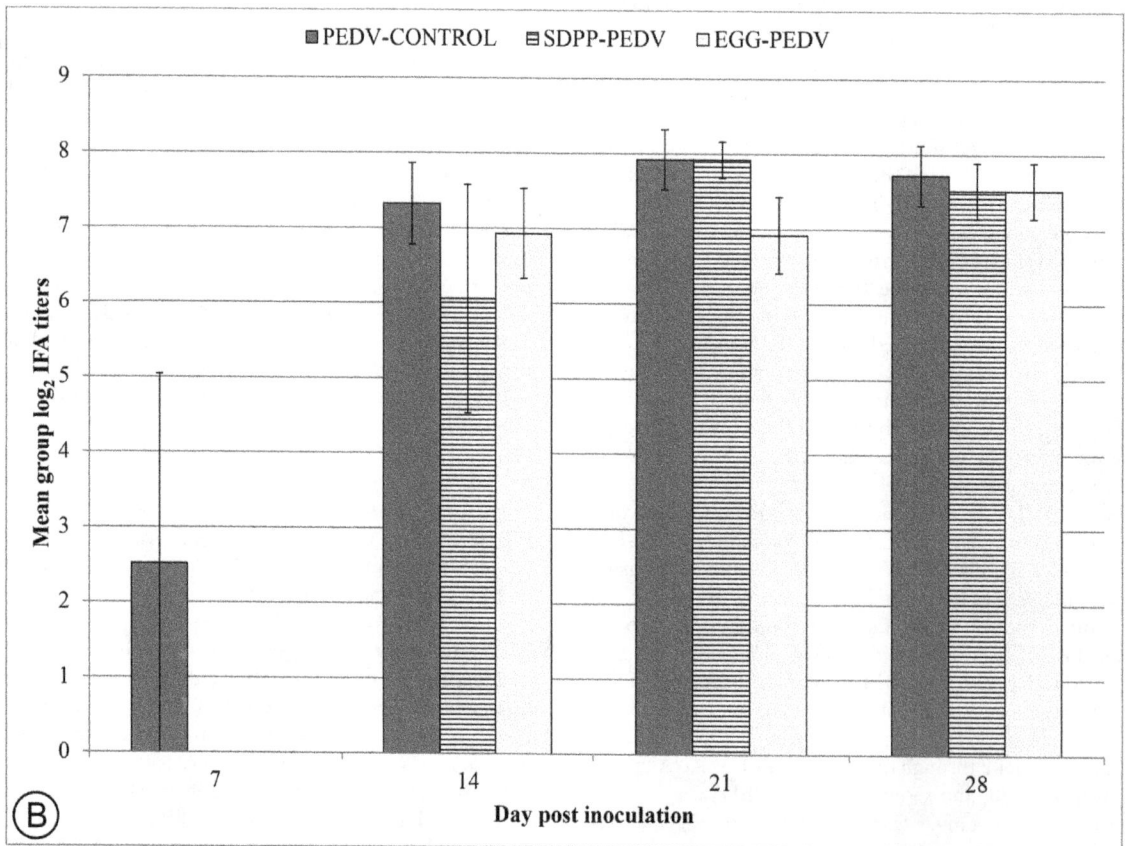

Figure 1. Group mean antibody response in serum over time. (A) Group mean S1 ELISA OD values ±SEM. An OD value greater than 0.3 was considered positive, samples with OD values between 0.2 and 0.3 were considered suspect, and samples with OD values less than 0.2 were considered negative. **(B)** Group mean IFA titers (±SEM). Samples were tested in 2-fold dilutions with the IFA ranging from 1:40 to 1:320. Positive signals at a sample dilution of 1:40 or higher were considered positive. The data were analyzed by one-way ANOVA method followed by Tukey's pairwise test using the JMP software version 10.0.2 (SAS Institute, Cary, North Carolina, USA). Different superscripts (^{A,B}) indicate significant different group means on selected days (p<0.05).

dietary inclusion of SDPP enhanced the intestinal barrier function and reduced inflammation and subsequent presence of diarrhea in weaned pigs [26]. Some of the benefits were attributed to promotion of the intestinal development, increased antioxidant capacity and decreased production of inflammatory factors in the intestinal mucosa [29]. Interestingly, during acute PEDV infection at 3 dpi, adherent *E. coli* was not observed in any of the SDPP-PEDV pigs but was present in 2/3 EGG-PEDV pigs and in 2/3 PEDV-CONTROL pigs (Table 4). In addition, at dpi 14 there was significantly reduced PEDV shedding in the SDPP-PEDV group versus the EGG-PEDV group.

In this study, the SDPP-PEDV pigs were given the SDPP diet for 32 consecutive days starting at dpi -4 until dpi 28. This is longer than SDPP is typically fed in the field; however, it was done in this experiment to mimic the SDPP-CONTROL group which

received the SDPP diet from challenge to dpi 28. Similar to the results for the EGG-PEDV group, the kinetics of PEDV infection was essentially no different in the SDPP-PEDV group compared to PEDV-CONTROL pigs except that the SDPP group appeared more active during the acute PEDV disease stage with less pronounced diarrhea as determined by several independent observers. It has been determined that apparent and standardized ileal digestibility of egg derived amino acids is lower when compared to SDPP [30] and a higher amino acid digestion could have contributed to the milder clinical signs in the present study. However, larger studies to evaluate this further are needed.

Under the conditions of this study, which were designed to mimic field conditions, a commercial PEDV positive SDPP product was not capable of transmitting PEDV to pigs. However, in contrast to anecdotal reports from the field, SDPP or anti-

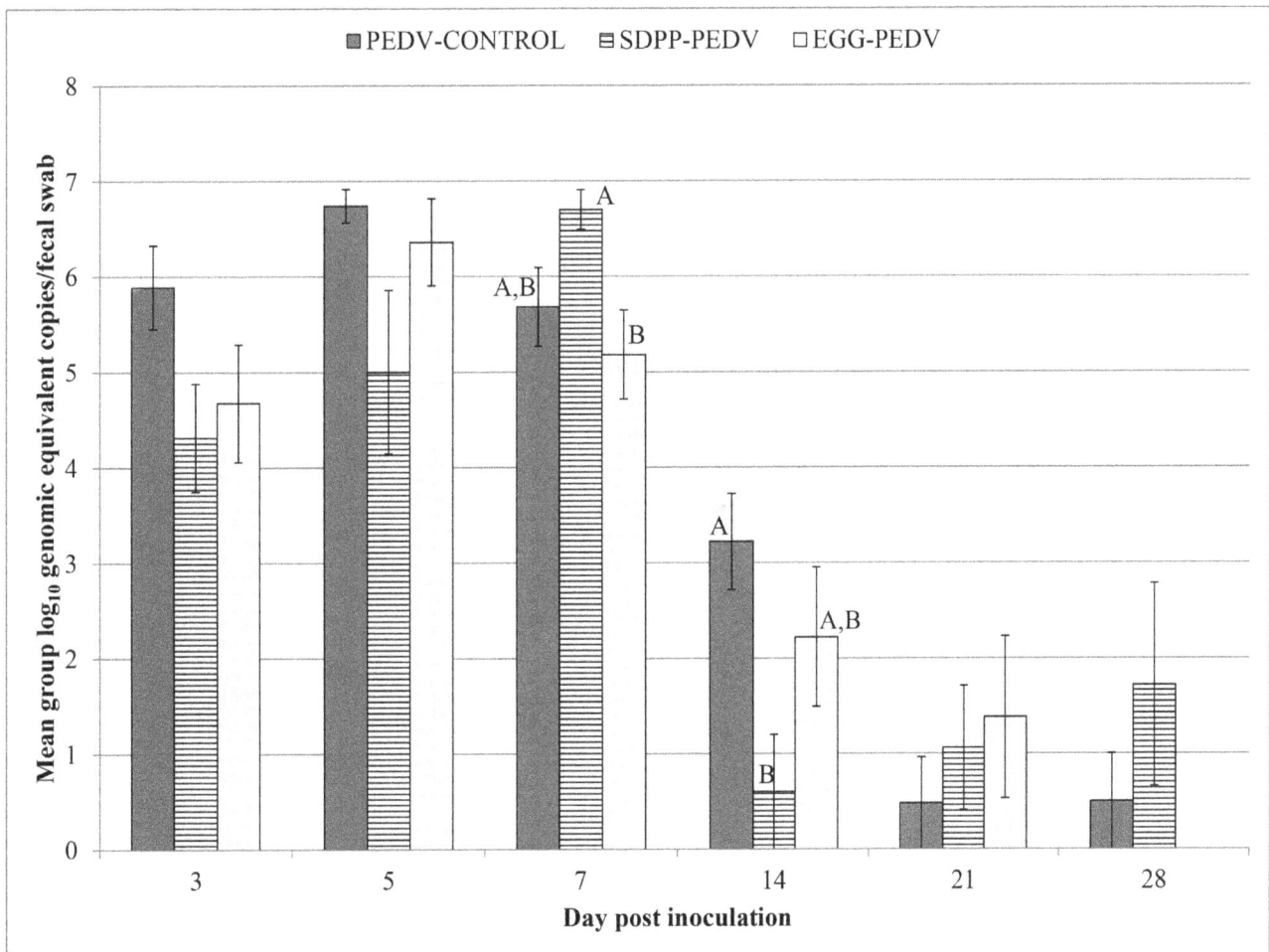

Figure 2. Group mean PEDV RNA levels in fecal samples over time. Group mean $\log_{10}$ PEDV RNA levels (±SEM) were determined in fecal samples from PEDV-infected pigs (PEDV-CONTROL, SDPP-PEDV, EGG-PEDV) collected from day post inoculation (dpi) 3 through 28. The data were analyzed by one-way ANOVA method followed by Tukey's pairwise test using the JMP software version 10.0.2 (SAS Institute, Cary, North Carolina, USA). Different superscripts (^{A,B}) indicate significant different group means on selected days (p<0.05).

Table 3. Prevalence of PEDV RNA in fecal swabs at different days post PEDV inoculation.

Group	0	3	5	7	14	21	28
NEG-CONTROL	0/8	0/8	0/5	0/5	0/5	0/5	0/5
SDPP-CONTROL	0/8	0/8	0/5	0/5	0/5	0/5	0/5
PEDV-CONTROL	0/8	8/8	5/5	5/5	5/5	1/5	1/5
SDPP-PEDV	0/8	8/8	5/5	5/5	1/5	2/5	2/5
EGG-PEDV	0/8	8/8	5/5	5/5	4/5	2/5	0/5

Bold areas indicate the pigs experimentally inoculated with PEDV.

Table 4. Macroscopic appearance of the intestinal content, prevalence of PEDV antigen as determined by IHC and microscopic lesions in pigs euthanized at 3 days post inoculation.

Group designation	No. of pigs	Appearance of the intestinal content			PEDV IHC	Microscopic lesions		
		Normal	Semi-solid	Fluid		Villus Atrophy	Colitis	Presence of adherent E. coli
NEG-CONTROL	3	1	2	0	0/3 (0)[1]	0/3	0/3	0/3
SDPP-CONTROL	3	3	0	0	0/3 (0)	0/3	0/3	0/3
PEDV-CONTROL	3	0	0	3	3/3 (3)	3/3 (3)	1/3 (1)	2/3
SDPP-PEDV	3	2	0	1	2/3 (1.5)	2/3 (1.7)	0/3	0/3
EGG-PEDV	3	0	1	2	1/3 (0.3)	2/3 (1.3)	2/3 (0.7)	2/3

Bold areas indicate the pigs experimentally inoculated with PEDV.
[1]Number of pigs affected/total number of pigs (group mean score).

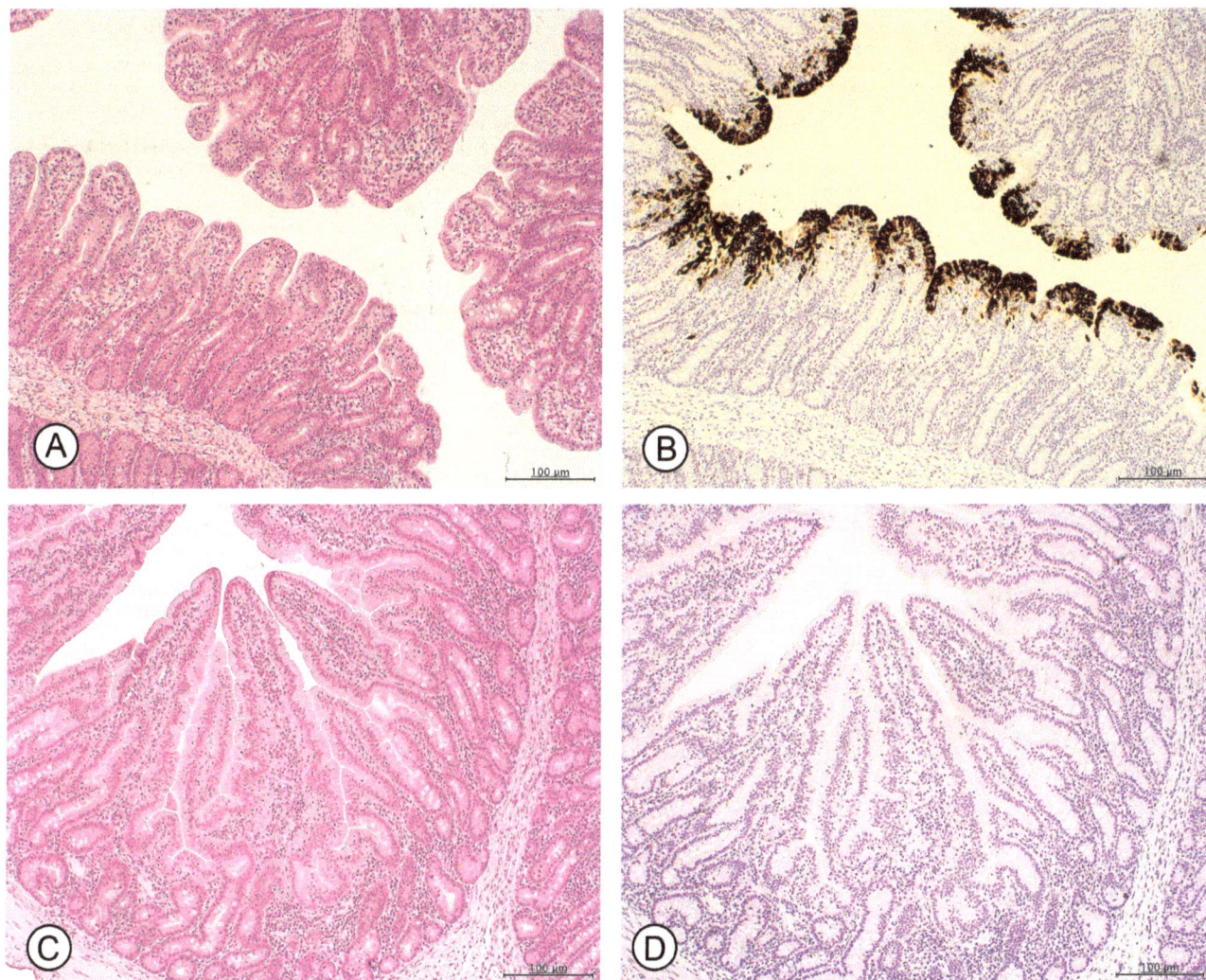

Figure 3. Microscopic lesions in the small intestines at 3 days post PEDV inoculation. (A) PEDV-CONTROL. HE. There is severe diffuse atrophy and fusion of villi of the small intestine. **(B)** PEDV-CONTROL. PEDV IHC. The majority of the enterocytes contain abundant PEDV antigen as indicated by brown staining of enterocytes. **(C)** SDPP-CONTROL. HE. The intestinal mucosa is normal and the villi are of normal length. **(D)** SDPP-CONTROL. PEDV IHC. PEDV antigen is not present.

PEDV globulin addition did not significantly alter PEDV disease course or PEDV shedding after experimental challenge. However, fecal PEDV shedding in treated pigs (EGG-PEDV and SDPP-PEDV) was about 1 log lower compared to the POSITIVE-CONTROL pigs in the early stage of infection which could contribute to lower environmental PEDV loads and lower transmission rates to uninfected contact pigs.

Author Contributions

Conceived and designed the experiments: TO PGH. Performed the experiments: TO PFG JZ CTX PGH. Analyzed the data: TO. Contributed reagents/materials/analysis tools: JZ. Contributed to the writing of the manuscript: TO PFG JZ CTX PGH.

References

1. Stevenson GW, Hoang H, Schwartz KJ, Burrough ER, Sun D, et al. (2013) Emergence of Porcine epidemic diarrhea virus in the United States: clinical signs, lesions, and viral genomic sequences. J Vet Diagn Invest 25: 649–654.
2. de Groot RJ, Baker SC, Baric R, Enjuanes L, Gorbalenya AE, et al. (2011) Coronaviridae. In: King AMQ, Adams MJ, Carstens EB, Leftkowitz EJ, editors. Virus taxonomy: ninth report of the International Committee on Taxonomy of Viruses.London: Elsevier Academic. pp. 806–828.
3. Huang YW, Dickerman AW, Pineyro P, Li L, Fang L, et al. (2013) Origin, evolution, and genotyping of emergent porcine epidemic diarrhea virus strains in the United States. MBio 4: e00737–13.
4. Ferreira AS, Barbosa FF, Tokach MD, Santos M. (2009) Spray dried plasma for pigs weaned at different ages. Recent Pat Food Nutr Agric 1: 231–235.
5. Shen HG, Schalk S, Halbur PG, Campbell JM, Russell LE, et al. (2011) Commercially produced spray-dried porcine plasma contains increased concentrations of porcine circovirus type 2 DNA but does not transmit porcine circovirus type 2 when fed to naive pigs. J Anim Sci 89: 1930–1938.
6. Pujols J, Lorca-Oro C, Diaz I, Russell LE, Campbell JM, et al. (2011) Commercial spray-dried porcine plasma does not transmit porcine circovirus type 2 in weaned pigs challenged with porcine reproductive and respiratory syndrome virus. Vet J 190: e16–e20.
7. Polo J, Opriessnig T, O'Neill KC, Rodriguez C, Russell LE, et al. (2013) Neutralizing antibodies against porcine circovirus type 2 in liquid pooled plasma contribute to the biosafety of commercially manufactured spray-dried porcine plasma. J Anim Sci 91: 2192–2198.
8. Anonymous (2014) Pig producers warned to be wary when using spray-dried porcine plasma. Vet Rec 174: 291.
9. Van Dijk AJ, Enthoven PM, Van den Hoven SG, Van Laarhoven MM, Niewold TA, et al. (2002) The effect of dietary spray-dried porcine plasma on clinical

response in weaned piglets challenged with a pathogenic *Escherichia coli*. Vet Microbiol 84: 207–218.

10. Niewold TA, Van Dijk AJ, Geenen PL, Roodink H, Margry R, et al. (2007) Dietary specific antibodies in spray-dried immune plasma prevent enterotoxigenic *Escherichia coli* F4 (ETEC) post weaning diarrhoea in piglets. Vet Microbiol 124: 362–369.

11. NRC (1998) Nutrient requirements of swine, 10th ed. Natl Acad Press, Washington, D.C.

12. Chen Q, Li G, Stasko J, Thomas JT, Stensland WR, et al. (2014) Isolation and characterization of porcine epidemic diarrhea viruses associated with the 2013 disease outbreak among swine in the United States. J Clin Microbiol 52: 234–243.

13. Xiao CT, Gimenez-Lirola L, Huang YW, Meng XJ, Halbur PG, et al. (2012) The prevalence of Torque teno sus virus (TTSuV) is common and increases with the age of growing pigs in the United States. J Virol Methods 183: 40–44.

14. Kim O, Chae C, Kweon CH (1999) Monoclonal antibody-based immunohistochemical detection of porcine epidemic diarrhea virus antigen in formalin-fixed, paraffin-embedded intestinal tissues. J Vet Diagn Invest 11: 458–462.

15. Lundeen T, Muirhead S (20 Feb 2014) Ontario feed company provides details on PEDV-related recall. Available: http://feedstuffs.com/story-ontario-feed-company-provides-details-pedv-related-recall-45-109035. Accessed 2014 May 1.

16. Canadian Food Inspection Agency (3 Mar 2014) Porcine Epidemic Diarrhea (PED) situation in Canada. Available: http://www.inspection.gc.ca/animals/terrestrial-animals/diseases/other-diseases/ped/eng/1392762503272/1392762576176. Accessed 2014 May 1.

17. Patterson AR, Madson DM, Opriessnig T (2010) Efficacy of experimentally-produced spray-dried plasma on infectivity of porcine circovirus type 2 (PCV2). J Anim Sci 88: 4078–4085.

18. Pujols J, López-Soria S, Segalés J, Fort M, Sibila M, et al. (2008) Lack of transmission of porcine circovirus type 2 to weanling pigs by feeding them spray-dried porcine plasma. Vet Rec 163: 536–538.

19. Polo J, Quigley JD, Russell LE, Campbell JM, Pujols J, et al. (2005) Efficacy of spray-drying to reduce infectivity of pseudorabies and porcine reproductive and respiratory syndrome (PRRS) viruses and seroconversion in pigs fed diets containing spray-dried animal plasma. J Anim Sci 83: 1933–1938.

20. Jung K, Wang Q, Scheuer KA, Lu Z, Zhang Y, et al. (2014) Pathology of US porcine epidemic diarrhea virus strain PC21A in gnotobiotic pigs. Emerg Infect Dis 20: 662–665.

21. Wiedemann V, Linckh E, Kuhlmann R, Schmidt P, Losch U (1991) Chicken egg antibodies for prophylaxis and therapy of infectious intestinal diseases. V. *In vivo* studies on protective effects against *Escherichia coli* diarrhea in pigs. Zentralbl Veterinarmed B 38: 283–291.

22. Xu Y, Li X, Jin L, Zhen Y, Lu Y, et al. (2011) Application of chicken egg yolk immunoglobulins in the control of terrestrial and aquatic animal diseases: a review. Biotechnol Adv 29: 860–868.

23. Owusu-Asiedu A, Nyachoti CM, Baidoo SK, Marquardt RR, Yang X (2003) Response of early-weaned pigs to an enterotoxigenic *Escherichia coli* (K88) challenge when fed diets containing spray-dried porcine plasma or pea protein isolate plus egg yolk antibody. J Anim Sci 81: 1781–1789.

24. Imberechts H, Deprez P, Van DE, Pohl P (1997) Chicken egg yolk antibodies against F18ab fimbriae of *Escherichia coli* inhibit shedding of F18 positive *E. coli* by experimentally infected pigs. Vet Microbiol 54: 329–341.

25. Kweon CH, Kwon BJ, Woo SR, Kim JM, Woo GH, et al. (2000) Immunoprophylactic effect of chicken egg yolk immunoglobulin (Ig Y) against porcine epidemic diarrhea virus (PEDV) in piglets. J Vet Med Sci 62: 961–964.

26. Peace RM, Campbell J, Polo J, Crenshaw J, Russell L, et al. (2011) Spray-dried porcine plasma influences intestinal barrier function, inflammation, and diarrhea in weaned pigs. J Nutr 141: 1312–1317.

27. Campbell J, Jacobi S, Liu Y, Robertson KH, Drayton J, et al. (2012) Evaluation of immunoglobulin G absorption from colostrum supplements gavaged to newborn piglets. J Anim Sci 90 Suppl 4: 299–301.

28. Polo J, Campbell JM, Crenshaw J, Rodriguez C, Pujol N, et al. (2012) Half-life of porcine antibodies absorbed from a colostrum supplement containing porcine immunoglobulins. J Anim Sci 90 Suppl 4: 308–310.

29. Gao YY, Jiang ZY, Lin YC, Zheng CT, Zhou GL, et al. (2011) Effects of spray-dried animal plasma on serous and intestinal redox status and cytokines of neonatal piglets. J Anim Sci 89: 150–157.

30. Heo JM, Kiarie E, Kahindi RK, Maiti P, Woyengo TA, et al. (2012) Standardized ileal amino acid digestibility in egg from hyperimmunized hens fed to weaned pigs. J Anim Sci 90 Suppl 4: 239–241.

9

Application of a Combination of a Knowledge-Based Algorithm and 2-Stage Screening to Hypothesis-Free Genomic Data on Irinotecan-Treated Patients for Identification of a Candidate Single Nucleotide Polymorphism Related to an Adverse Effect

Hiro Takahashi[1,2,3]*, Kimie Sai[4], Yoshiro Saito[4], Nahoko Kaniwa[4], Yasuhiro Matsumura[5], Tetsuya Hamaguchi[6], Yasuhiro Shimada[6], Atsushi Ohtsu[7], Takayuki Yoshino[7], Toshihiko Doi[7], Haruhiro Okuda[4], Risa Ichinohe[3,8], Anna Takahashi[2], Ayano Doi[3,8], Yoko Odaka[3], Misuzu Okuyama[3], Nagahiro Saijo[9¤a], Jun-ichi Sawada[10¤b], Hiromi Sakamoto[3], Teruhiko Yoshida[3]

1 Graduate School of Horticulture, Chiba University, Matsudo, Chiba, Japan, 2 Plant Biology Research Center, Chubu University, Kasugai, Aichi, Japan, 3 Division of Genetics, National Cancer Center Research Institute, Tokyo, Japan, 4 Division of Medicinal Safety Science, National Institute of Health Sciences, Tokyo, Japan, 5 Division of Developmental Therapeutics, Research Center for Innovative Oncology, National Cancer Center Hospital East, Kashiwa, Chiba, Japan, 6 Gastrointestinal Medical Oncology Division, National Cancer Center Hospital, Tokyo, Japan, 7 Department of Gastrointestinal Oncology, National Cancer Center Hospital East, Kashiwa, Chiba, Japan, 8 Faculty of Horticulture, Chiba University, Matsudo, Chiba, Japan, 9 National Cancer Center Hospital East, Kashiwa, Chiba, Japan, 10 Division of Functional Biochemistry and Genomics, National Institute of Health Sciences, Tokyo, Japan

Abstract

Interindividual variation in a drug response among patients is known to cause serious problems in medicine. Genomic information has been proposed as the basis for "personalized" health care. The genome-wide association study (GWAS) is a powerful technique for examining single nucleotide polymorphisms (SNPs) and their relationship with drug response variation; however, when using only GWAS, it often happens that no useful SNPs are identified due to multiple testing problems. Therefore, in a previous study, we proposed a combined method consisting of a knowledge-based algorithm, 2 stages of screening, and a permutation test for identifying SNPs. In the present study, we applied this method to a pharmacogenomics study where 109,365 SNPs were genotyped using Illumina Human-1 BeadChip in 168 cancer patients treated with irinotecan chemotherapy. We identified the SNP rs9351963 in potassium voltage-gated channel subfamily KQT member 5 (KCNQ5) as a candidate factor related to incidence of irinotecan-induced diarrhea. The p value for rs9351963 was 3.31×10^{-5} in Fisher's exact test and 0.0289 in the permutation test (when multiple testing problems were corrected). Additionally, rs9351963 was clearly superior to the clinical parameters and the model involving rs9351963 showed sensitivity of 77.8% and specificity of 57.6% in the evaluation by means of logistic regression. Recent studies showed that KCNQ4 and KCNQ5 genes encode members of the M channel expressed in gastrointestinal smooth muscle and suggested that these genes are associated with irritable bowel syndrome and similar peristalsis diseases. These results suggest that rs9351963 in KCNQ5 is a possible predictive factor of incidence of diarrhea in cancer patients treated with irinotecan chemotherapy and for selecting chemotherapy regimens, such as irinotecan alone or a combination of irinotecan with a KCNQ5 opener. Nonetheless, clinical importance of rs9351963 should be further elucidated.

Editor: Olga Y. Gorlova, Geisel School of Medicine at Dartmouth College, United States of America

Funding: This work was supported in part by the Ministry of Education, Culture, Sports, Science, and Technology of Japan (MEXT): Grants-in-Aid for Scientific Research for Young Scientists (B) (nos. 21710211 and 24710222 to H.T.) and Grant-in-Aid for Scientific Research on Innovative Areas (no. 26114703 to H.T.). This work was also supported by the Advanced Research for Medical Products Mining Program of the National Institute of Biomedical Innovation (NIBIO ID10-41), the Futaba Electronics Memorial Foundation, the Research Foundation for the Electrotechnology of Chubu, and the Nakajima Foundation. The funders had no role in study design, data collection and analysis, decision to publish, or preparation of the manuscript.

Competing Interests: The authors have declared that no competing interests exist.

* Email: hiro.takahashi@chiba-u.jp

¤a Current address: Japanese Society of Medical Oncology, Tokyo, Japan
¤b Current address: Pharmaceutical and Medical Devices Agency, Tokyo, Japan

Introduction

Genomic information has been proposed to be utilized as the basis for "personalized" health care. Interindividual variation in a drug response among patients has been well documented to cause serious problems in pharmacotherapy. This variation may be due to multiple factors such as disease phenotypes, genetic and clinical parameters (or environmental factors), and variability in the drug target or allergic response; all of these factors may affect both main and side effects [1,2]. Although some biomarkers [3–9] have been proposed, it is still difficult to determine which group of patients will respond positively, which patients are nonresponders, and which may experience adverse reactions in cases where patients are administered the same medication dose. For effectiveness of personalized medicine in cancer chemotherapy, it is critically important to observe interindividual differences in a drug response and the role of genetic polymorphisms relevant to the drug metabolic pathways and drug response biology in pharmacogenomics [10].

Irinotecan (CPT-11), an anticancer prodrug, is widely used for the treatment of a broad range of carcinomas, such as colorectal, lung, ovarian, and cervical cancers. Unexpected severe diarrhea and neutropenia are prominent adverse effects of irinotecan treatment. The active metabolite SN-38 (7-ethyl-10-hydroxycamptothecin), a topoisomerase I inhibitor, is generated via hydrolysis of the parent compound by carboxylesterases [11], and is subsequently glucuronidated by uridine diphosphate glucuronosyltransferases (UGTs), such as UGT1A1, UGT1A7, or UGT1A9, to form an inactive metabolite, SN-38 glucuronide (SN-38G) [12–14]. Irinotecan is also inactivated by CYP3A4 to produce 7-ethyl-10- [4-N-(5-aminopentanoic acid)-1-piperidino] carbonyloxycamptothecin (APC; a major CYP3A4 product) and 7-ethyl-10-(4-amino-1-piperidino) carbonyloxycamptothecin (NPC; a minor product) [15,16]. Irinotecan and its metabolites are excreted into the bile and urine via the action of ATP-binding cassette (ABC) transporters, such as P-glycoprotein (P-gp/ABCB1), multiple resistance-associated protein 2 (MRP2/ABCC2), and breast cancer resistance protein (BCRP/ABCG2) [17]. Transport of SN-38 from the plasma into the liver is mediated by the organic anion transporting polypeptide C (OATP-C/SLCO1B1) [18]. Most of the previous pharmacogenetic studies of irinotecan have been focused on UGT1A1 polymorphisms and have shown clinical relevance of UGT1A1*28, a repeat polymorphism in the TATA box [-54_-39A(TA)$_6$TAA>A(TA)$_7$TAA or -40_-39ins TA], to severe adverse effects [3,19,20]. Based on these findings, in 2005, the Food and Drug Administration (FDA) of the United States approved an amendment for the formulation called Camptosar (irinotecan-HCl) (NDA 20-571/S-024/S-027/S-028) and for clinical use of a genetic diagnostic kit for the *28 allele. In parallel with this advance in the USA, clinical relevance to severe neutropenia of UGT1A1*6 [211G>A(G71R)], another low-activity allele detected specifically in East Asians, as well as *28, was demonstrated in several studies on Asian patients [5,21–23]. Accordingly, in June 2008, the Ministry of Health, Labor, and Welfare of Japan approved changes to irinotecan formulations (Campto and Topotecin) by adding a warning about the risk of severe adverse effects in patients either homozygous or compound-heterozygous for UGT1A1*28 and *6 (*28/*28, *6/*6, *28/*6) and also approved clinical use of a diagnostic kit for UGT1A1*28 and *6. Severe adverse effects, however, are reported in patients without the genetic variations *6/*6, *28/*28, and *28/*6; therefore, several clinical studies have suggested that polymorphisms of the drug transporter genes, such as ABCB1, ABCC2, ABCG2, and SLCO1B1, might affect irinotecan pharmacokinetics

(PK)/pharmacodynamics (PD) in Caucasian and Asian patients [22,24–35], as shown in Fig. 1. Nonetheless, the almost all reported results deal with PK in patients and neutropenia induced by irinotecan as an adverse reaction not but with diarrhea. Therefore, other factors responsible for other irinotecan adverse effects, such as diarrhea should be identified.

Diarrhea induced by irinotecan is classified into early- and delayed-onset diarrhea, occurring within 24 hr or ≤24 hr after irinotecan administration, respectively [36]. Irinotecan induces early-onset diarrhea as one of adverse cholinergic effects (acetylcholinelike effects) by inhibiting acetylcholinesterase (AChE) and binding to muscarinic acetylcholine receptors (mAChR) [37,38]. These inhibitory actions are induced by irinotecan, which has an amino group at the C-10 position [37]. Other than that, irinotecan induces delayed-onset diarrhea via rapid deconjugation of SN38G and adsorption of released free SN-38 by β-glucuronidase of intestinal flora [39–41], as shown in Fig. 1. In the present study, we focused on polymorphisms of genes with transporter activity to identify predictive factors of diarrhea induced by irinotecan because there are many genes related to transporter activity in both pathways.

A genome-wide association study (GWAS), also known as a whole-genome association study (WGA study, or WGAS), is an examination of many common genetic variants in different individuals to determine whether a particular variant is associated with a trait. GWAS using hypothesis-free genomic data is a powerful technique for identifying interindividual variation among patients. On the other hand, multiple testing problems are a limitation of this approach. To address this issue, we recently proposed a combined method consisting of a knowledge-based algorithm, 2 stages of screening, and a permutation test for identifying single nucleotide polymorphisms (SNPs) [7]. In general, the objective of a statistical or bioinformatic analysis is the enrichment of important information in a large dataset [42–47]. The use of a knowledge-based algorithm is not a novel concept, but is both practical and useful [48–66]. In the previous study, we found that rs2293347 in the gene of human epidermal growth factor receptor (EGFR) is a candidate SNP related to the chemotherapeutic response; we achieved this result by applying our combined method to gastric cancer patients who were treated with fluoropyrimidine [7]. However, our combined method was applied to only 1 dataset. Therefore, the usability of our combined method as a novel approach was still unclear.

We used the combined method in an actual genome-wide pharmacogenomics study of antitumor drugs, particularly irinotecan. We found that rs9351963 in the gene of potassium voltage-gated channel subfamily KQT member 5 (KCNQ5) is a candidate SNP related to the adverse response. Rs9351963 may be a potential predictive factor of incidence of diarrhea in cancer patients treated with the cancer prodrug irinotecan.

Materials and Methods

Ethics statement

The study was conducted according to the principles expressed in the Declaration of Helsinki, and the ethics committees of the National Cancer Center and National Institute of Health Sciences, Japan, approved the study protocol. All patients provided written informed consent to participate.

Preparation of hypothesis-free genomic data for cancer patients treated with irinotecan

This study was performed within the framework of the Millennium Genome Project in Japan, and 4 antitumor drugs

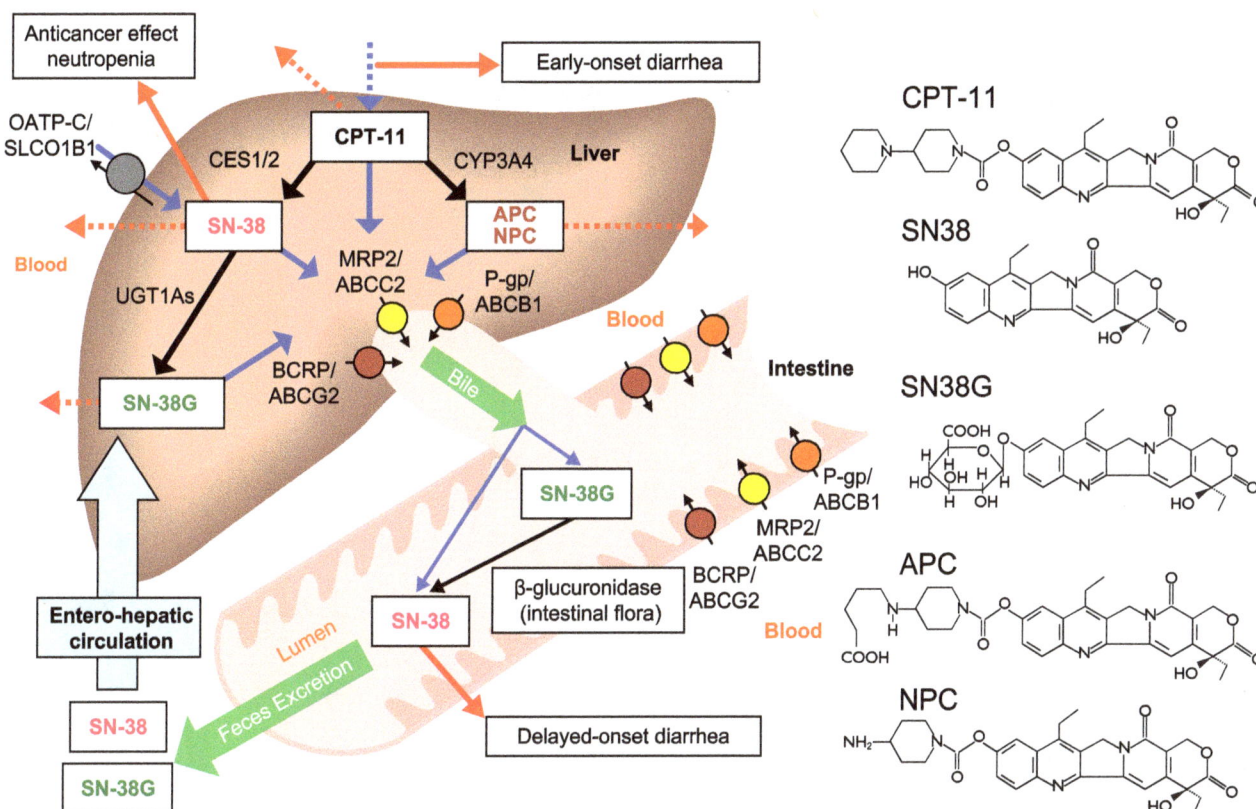

Figure 1. Drug metabolic pathways and the drug response of irinotecan.

were chosen as project targets: gemcitabine, paclitaxel, fluoropyrimidine, and irinotecan. These drugs (alone or in some combination) were administered to approximately 1,000 cancer patients at the National Cancer Center, Japan. Additionally, approximately 1,000 DNA samples were extracted from peripheral blood mononuclear cells and 109,365 SNPs were genotyped using the Illumina Human-1 BeadChip. In this study, we focused on pharmacogenomic properties of irinotecan. Participants included 177 Japanese irinotecan-naïve cancer patients (56 cancer patients treated with irinotecan monotherapy and 121 cancer patients treated with irinotecan combination therapy) at the National Cancer Center Hospital and National Cancer Center Hospital East. A summary of the characteristics of the 176 patients is listed in Table S1. We excluded 1 patient who refused grading of adverse reactions. Furthermore, we excluded 8 patients who did not have genotyping data. Therefore, we analyzed the remaining 168 patients (53 cancer patients treated with irinotecan monotherapy and 115 cancer patients treated with irinotecan combination therapy) in the present study. We defined the 53 patients treated with irinotecan monotherapy as the first dataset and the 168 patients treated with irinotecan chemotherapy (consisting of irinotecan monotherapy and combination therapy) as the second dataset for 2 stages of screening.

Monitoring and adverse effects

A complete medical history and data on physical examination were recorded before the irinotecan therapy. Complete blood cell counts with differentials and platelet counts, as well as blood biochemical variables, were measured once a week during the first 2 months of irinotecan treatment. Adverse events were graded according to the National Cancer Institute - Common Toxicity Criteria (NCI-CTC Version 2.0). Only the highest grade of adverse events was recorded during the first 2 months of irinotecan treatment for each patient and adverse event.

Patient characteristics and clinical parameters

A summary of the patients' characteristics in the two datasets for diarrhea is shown in Table 1. The association of genetic or clinical parameters with incidence of grade ≥ 2 diarrhea was examined on the basis of Spearman's rank correlation coefficient. "UGT1A1*6 or *28" is an effective genetic predictive factor of irinotecan-induced neutropenia and pharmacokinetics in cancer patients [5]. This factor was constructed from 2 polymorphisms: UGT1A1*6 and *28.

Fisher's exact test

This statistical test is usually used to determine nonrandom associations between 2 categorical variables [67]. Fisher's exact test is similar to the chi-squared test. If a sample size is large, then the chi-squared test is suitable. Nevertheless, significance values from the chi-squared test are only approximated. Fisher's exact test is used in to analyze contingency tables when the sample sizes are small [67]. We used Fisher's exact test in the present study. The odds ratio (OR) is defined as $a \times d / (b \times c)$, where a is the number of patients that had adverse events with a minor allele, b is the number of patients that did not have adverse events with a minor allele, c is the number of patients that had adverse events with a major allele, and d is the number of patients that did not have adverse events with a major allele. The null hypothesis for Fisher's exact test is OR = 1.

Table 1. Irinotecan-treated cancer patients with SNP information, genetic factor, and clinical parameters for incidence of diarrhea.

Parameters		Diarrhea							
		Irinotecan monotherapy				Irinotecan chemotherapy (including monotherapy)			
		Number of patients		Spearman's rank correlation		Number of patients		Spearman's rank correlation	
		Grade <2	Grade ≥2	ρ	p value	Grade <2	Grade ≥2	ρ	p value
UGT1A1*6 or *28	0	15	5	0.056	6.89E-01	64	17	0.009	9.06E-01
	1	21	7			57	16		
	2	3	2			11	3		
Gender	Male	26	11	-0.114	4.15E-01	101	28	-0.012	8.75E-01
	Female	13	3			31	8		
Age		39	14	0.013	9.29E-01	132	36	0.080	3.02E-01
Area		39	14	0.010	9.45E-01	132	36	-0.054	4.88E-01
PS	<2	38	13	0.106	4.50E-01	130	35	0.039	6.15E-01
	≥2	1	1			2	1		
Smoking	0	37	14	-0.119	3.97E-01	111	30	0.008	9.13E-01
	1	2	0			21	6		
Alcohol	0	33	10	0.149	2.88E-01	90	26	-0.036	6.44E-01
	1	6	4			42	10		
Alb	0	18	10	-0.223	1.08E-01	71	24	-0.108	1.62E-01
	1	21	4			60	12		
	2	0	0			1	0		
Hg	0	14	4	0.061	6.65E-01	58	14	0.040	6.05E-01
	1	22	9			67	20		
	2	3	0			6	1		
	3	0	1			0	1		
	4	0	0			1	0		
GOT	0	33	12	-0.014	9.23E-01	108	32	-0.080	3.05E-01
	1	6	2			22	4		
	2	0	0			2	0		
ALP	0	28	8	0.117	4.05E-01	89	23	0.026	7.38E-01
	1	9	6			38	12		
	2	0	0			2	1		
	3	2	0			3	0		
Cr	0	31	13	-0.157	2.62E-01	124	35	-0.060	4.41E-01
	1	8	1			8	1		
C_{max}/dose		39	14	0.049	7.31E-01	132	36	0.019	8.10E-01
AUC ratio		39	14	-0.078	5.81E-01	132	36	-0.109	1.60E-01

Table 1. Cont.

Parameters		Diarrhea							
		Irinotecan monotherapy				Irinotecan chemotherapy (including monotherapy)			
		Number of patients		Spearman's rank correlation		Number of patients		Spearman's rank correlation	
		Grade <2	Grade ≥2	ρ	p value	Grade <2	Grade ≥2	ρ	p value
Concomitant drug - 5-FU	0	39	14	NA	NA	106	28	0.026	7.40E-01
	1	0	0			26	8		
Concomitant drug - CDDP	0	39	14	NA	NA	76	24	−0.076	3.28E-01
	1	0	0			56	12		
Concomitant drug - MMC	0	39	14	NA	NA	121	36	−0.138	7.40E-02 †
	1	0	0			11	0		
Concomitant drug - VP16	0	39	14	NA	NA	129	35	0.014	8.61E-01
	1	0	0			3	1		
Concomitant drug - Amrubicin	0	39	14	NA	NA	132	34	0.210	6.25E-03 *
	1	0	0			0	2		

"UGT1A1*6 or *28" is a genetic factor constructed from 2 polymorphisms (UGT1A1*6 and *28); "2" indicates *6/*6, *28/*28 or *6/*28, "1" indicates *6 or *28, and "0" indicates "other than 2 and 1." Area: body surface area (m²), PS: performance status, Cr: grade of creatinine, Hg: grade of hemoglobin, Alb: grade of albumin, ALP: grade of alkaline phosphatase, and GOT: grade of glutamic oxaloacetic transaminase. Each laboratory test value (Alb, Hg, GOT, ALP, and Cr) was recorded before the irinotecan therapy. For each type of clinical tests the grade and aberrant values were defined according to the National Cancer Institute - Common Toxicity Criteria (NCI-CTC, Version 2.0). C_{max}/dose: SN38 C_{max}/dose [$10^{-3} \times m^2/L$]. AUC: area under the concentration-time curve. AUC ratio: Ratio of AUC_{SN38}/AUC_{CPT-11}. 5-FU: 5-fluorouracil, CDDP: cisplatin, MMC: mitomycin C, VP16: etoposide. * and † indicate $p<0.05$ and $0.05 \leq p < 0.10$, respectively. For each concomitant drug, 0 means "not administered," 1 indicates administered.

The permutation test

The permutation test theory evolved from the works of Fisher and Pitman in the 1930s [68]. In this study, p values of multiple-comparison analyses were adjusted by applying the permutation test to 2 stages of screening. The case–control (or phenotype) labels were randomly shuffled for the 2 screening stages, and p values were calculated using Fisher's exact test. The lowest p value was selected for the randomized data. This procedure was repeated 100,000 times. Exact p values for the permutation test were calculated based on the distribution of the lowest p values.

Multiple testing correction

The Bonferroni correction is a method used to address the problem of multiple comparisons (also known as the multiple testing problem). It is considered the simplest and most conservative method for control of the family-wise error rate (FWER). In addition, false discovery rate (FDR) controlling procedures, such as the Benjamini-Hochberg (BH) method [69], are more powerful (i.e., less conservative) than the FWER procedures, such as the Bonferroni correction, at the cost of increasing the likelihood of false positives within the rejected hypothesis. In the present study, the BH method was used to calculate the q value. The q value is defined as an FDR analog of the p value.

The Akaike information criterion (AIC)

The AIC is a measure of the relative goodness of fit of a statistical model [70]. A smaller AIC indicates a better fit when comparing fitted objects. The AIC is defined according to the formula $-2 \times$ (log likelihood) + ($2 \times n_{par}$), where n_{par} represents the number of parameters in the fitted model, and the log-likelihood value [71] is obtained from the logistic regression model.

The receiver operating characteristic (ROC)

ROC analysis is a graphical plot that illustrates the performance of a binary classifier system as its discrimination threshold is varied. It is built by plotting sensitivity (the number of true positive results divided by the number of true positive samples) against (1 minus specificity) at various threshold settings. (Specificity is the number of true negative results divided by the number of true negative samples.) The area under the curve (AUC) of a ROC curve is an indicator of expected performance of the test. A higher AUC is more desirable, with a value of 1.00 denoting perfect performance (sensitivity and specificity are both 100%), while a value of 0.50 indicates random performance.

Gene set based on gene ontology GO terms

GO has been developed to provide scientists with a controlled terminology system for labeling gene functions in a precise, reliable, computer-readable manner. Data for annotated genes and associated GO terms were obtained from the GO website (http://www.geneontology.org). We compiled a GO term list to select polymorphisms in genes with transporter activity (GO:0005215) and related activities, as shown in Table S2. The numbers of GO terms obtained was 943. GO data were obtained on July 1, 2010.

Results

Association analysis of adverse affects and clinical parameters (or a genetic factor)

The association between clinical parameters (or a genetic factor) and incidence of grade ≥ 2 diarrhea was examined on the basis of

Spearman's rank correlation coefficient, as shown in Table 1. This table shows that no parameter was associated with the adverse response to chemotherapy (incidence of grade ≥ 2 diarrhea) in the first dataset (patients treated with irinotecan monotherapy). Nonetheless, Amrubicin ($p = 0.00625$) was significantly associated with the response in the second dataset (patients treated with any irinotecan chemotherapy: a combination or monotherapy). Mitomycin C (MMC; $p = 0.0740$) was weakly associated with the response. These clinical factors should be evaluated when constructing diagnostic models involving multiple factors.

Extraction of candidate SNPs using the combined method consisting of the knowledge-based algorithm, 2 stages of screening, and the permutation test

In this study, we applied the combined method to hypothesis-free genomic data on cancer patients treated with irinotecan chemotherapy as shown in Fig. 2. Figure 2A shows an outline of the knowledge-based algorithm for identifying SNPs (KB-SNP). In the previous study, we extracted rs numbers (SNP IDs) related to cancer using a combination of National Center for Biotechnology Information (NCBI) dbSNP and NCBI PubMed [7]. In the present study, we extracted rs numbers from genes linked to specific GO terms instead of the combination of NCBI dbSNP and PubMed. In this analysis, we defined specific GO terms as the terms related to transporter activity.

A total of 6,506 SNPs related to transporter activity were extracted from 109,365 SNPs using KB-SNP (Fig. 2B). Furthermore, we excluded SNPs with a p value <0.2 in the Hardy-Weinberg equilibrium (HWE) or the minor allele frequency (MAF) <0.05. Then the extracted 5,242 SNPs were used in the association study.

We analyzed 53 patients treated with irinotecan monotherapy as the first dataset for first-stage screening in the association study (Fig. 2C). Each p value was calculated using Fisher's exact test for the allele model. A total of 24 SNPs with $p<0.005$ were extracted. In the second stage of screening, 168 patients treated with irinotecan chemotherapy (including 53 patients treated with irinotecan monotherapy) were analyzed to validate these 24 SNPs. Adjustment of a calculated p value for the second stage of screening was conducted using the permutation test for these 2 stages of screening (Fig. 2D). Only rs9351963 in *KCNQ5* showed a statistically significant p value (0.0289), which was determined using the permutation test. The rs9351963 is a common variant (MAF = 0.328). Furthermore, we conducted Fisher's exact test and used the Benjamini-Hochberg method [69] to calculate p and q values for the second dataset only. Seven SNPs had a q value <1, as shown in Table 2. Six SNPs (rs11022922, rs3918305, rs3813627, rs768172, rs3813628, and rs10815019) had $q = 0.802$ as shown in Table 2. This result indicates that 5 out of 6 SNPs were false positive; however, we assessed performance of only rs9351963 in the process of model construction.

Comparison of models based on rs9351963 in *KCNQ5*

We analyzed not only an allele model but also dominant and recessive models of rs9351963 in *KCNQ5* in relation to the first dataset (irinotecan monotherapy), the second dataset (any irinotecan chemotherapy), and the dataset of irinotecan combination chemotherapy (excluding irinotecan monotherapy), as shown in Figure 3. Figure 3A shows that the p value of the allele model was the lowest ($p = 8.86 \times 10^{-5}$, OR = 6.3), and the p value ($p = 1.29 \times 10^{-4}$, OR = 24) of the dominant model was lower than the p value ($p = 0.0358$, OR = 7.0) of the recessive model in the first dataset. In addition, Figure 3B shows that the p value of the

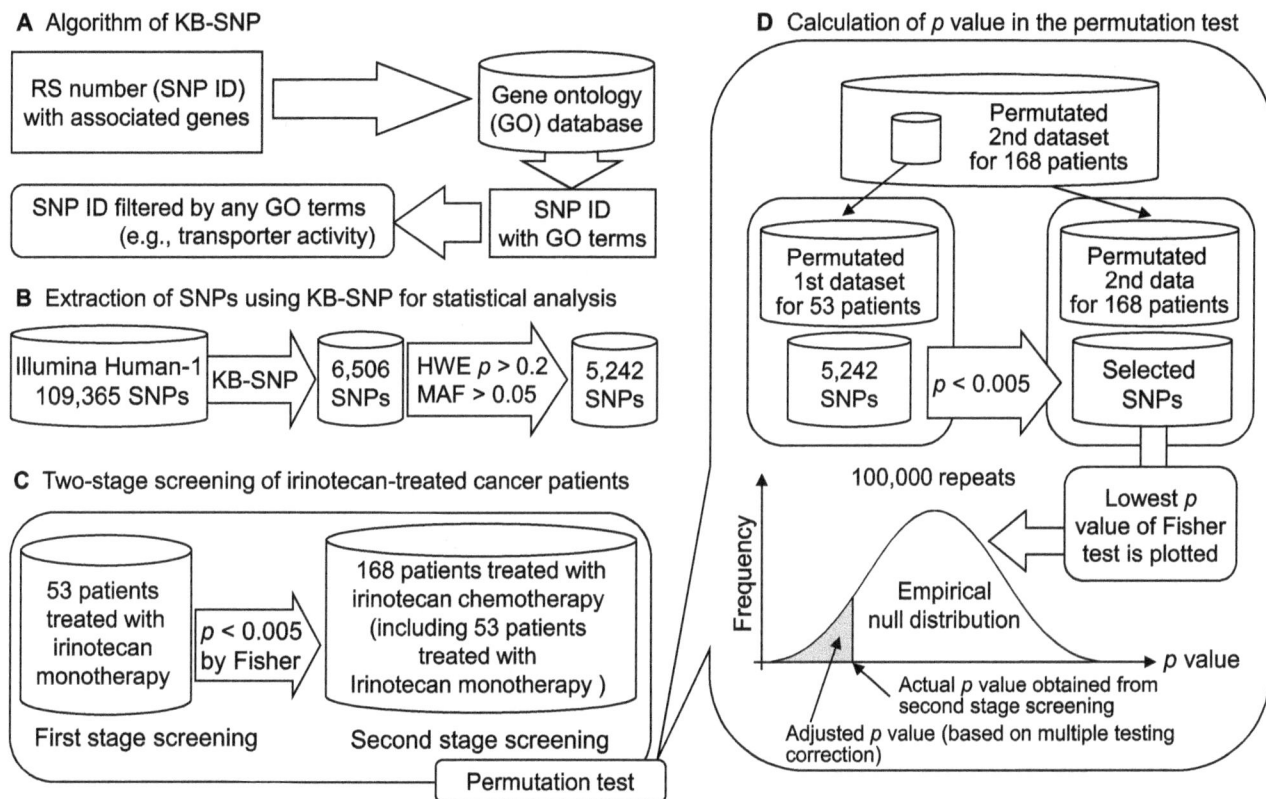

Figure 2. An outline of chemotherapeutic response analysis in irinotecan-treated cancer patients using a combined method consisting of a knowledge-based algorithm for identifying SNPs (KB-SNP), 2 stages of screening, and the permutation test. (A) The KB-SNP algorithm. (B) Extraction of SNPs using KB-SNP for statistical analysis. (C) Two-stage screening of irinotecan-treated cancer patients. (D) Calculation of the p value in the permutation test based on the 2 stages of screening. The second dataset (includes first dataset) was permutated. The permutated first dataset was extracted from the permutated second dataset. By using Fisher's exact test, SNPs with $p<0.005$ for the first dataset were selected from among 5,242 SNPs. Among the selected SNPs, those with the lowest p value in Fisher's exact test for the second dataset were selected. This procedure was repeated 100,000 times and empirical null distribution was constructed. Using the distribution, the actual p value obtained from the second stage of screening was converted to the adjusted p value (based on correction of multiple testing problems). At these screening steps, allele models were used for each SNP.

allele model was the lowest ($p = 3.31 \times 10^{-5}$, OR = 3.1), and the p value ($p = 1.28 \times 10^{-4}$, OR = 6.7) of the recessive model was lower than the p value ($p = 4.44 \times 10^{-3}$, OR = 3.3) of the dominant model in the second dataset. Therefore, we evaluated the 3 models using the dataset of irinotecan combination chemotherapy (excluding irinotecan monotherapy; Fig. 3C). Figure 3C shows that the p value ($p = 1.44 \times 10^{-3}$, OR = 6.9) of the recessive model meant strong statistical significance and the OR was almost equal to OR (= 7.0) in the first dataset, as shown in Figure 3A. Although ORs of the recessive models seemed to have high homogeneity among all 3 datasets, there was no statistical evidence. Therefore, the proportional odds model was used to construct multiple logistic regression models.

Selection of the model of rs9351963 in *KCNQ5* and construction of multiple regression models

We compared the AICs and AUCs using the second dataset in the 8 models: NULL (without parameter), "*UGT1A1*6* or *28*" (an integrated predictive factor based on polymorphisms related to neutropenia), and rs9351963 (genotype of rs9351963 in *KCNQ5*), Amrubicin, MMC, rs9351963+Amrubicin, rs9351963+MMC, and rs9351963+Amrubicin+MMC (Fig. 4A). Figure 4A shows that performance of all models except *UGT1A1 *6* or *28* is better than the performance of the NULL model. Although the

Amrubicin+MMC (combination of Amrubicin and MMC) model was better than Amrubicin alone or MMC, the rs9351963 models were clearly better than the Amrubicin+MMC model, as shown in Figures 4A and 4B. Performance of rs9351963+Amrubicin and rs9351963+MMC models was better than performance of the rs9351963 model. Furthermore, performance of the rs9351963+Amrubicin+MMC model was better than that of rs9351963+Amrubicin and rs9351963+MMC models. Therefore, we selected the rs9351963+Amrubicin+MMC model as the best one on the basis of AIC. AUC, sensitivity, and specificity of this model were 0.744, 77.8%, and 57.6% in in the ROC curve, respectively, as shown in Figures 4A and 4B.

Discussion

In the present study, we used 2 stages of screening: the method that is based on the concept of joint analysis. Joint analysis is more efficient than replication-based analysis [72]. The first dataset is a part of the second dataset in joint analysis (the latter includes the former). In contrast, the 2 datasets must be independent in a replication-based analysis (which we did not use here). Our 2 stages of screening derived from the joint analysis were used to increase statistical detection power. KB-SNP was performed prior to 2 stages of screening. KB-SNP reduced the number of

Table 2. Extracted 7 SNPs with $q<1$ for the second dataset.

RS number	Allele	MAF	SNP function		Chr	Position[a]	Associated gene symbol	For second dataset		Two stages of screening	
			Type	Location				p_F	q_{BH}		p_{per}
rs9351963	A/C	0.328	cSNP	intron	6	73749861	KCNQ5	3.31E-05	0.173	*	0.0289
rs11022922	C/T	0.376	cSNP	intron	14	63472498	KCNH5	3.21E-04	0.802		1.0000
rs3918305	A/G	0.402	cSNP	intron	12	109331162	SVOP	6.21E-04	0.802		1.0000
rs3813627	G/T	0.435	cSNP	NearGene-5	1	161195148	TOMM40L	7.62E-04	0.802		1.0000
rs768172	A/T	0.441	cSNP	intron	7	95805703	SLC25A13	7.87E-04	0.802		1.0000
rs3813628	A/C	0.436	cSNP	5'UTR	1	161196166	TOMM40L	1.02E-03	0.802		1.0000
rs10815019	A/G	0.222	cSNP	intron	9	4547288	SLC1A1	1.20E-03	0.802		1.0000

RS number: reference SNP identification number in dbSNP, MAF: minor allele frequency, Chr: chromosome number, i.e., a position in human genome GRCh37.p10 build 104, p_F indicates a p value calculated using Fisher's exact test, q_{BH} indicates adjusted p_F value by the Benjamini-Hochberg method, p_{per} indicates p values adjusted using a permutation test for multiple testing problems, * indicates $p_{per} < 0.05$. NearGene-5 indicates that the SNP is within 2 kb upstream of a gene.

candidate SNPs to 6,506 from 109,365. Approximately 80,000 SNPs can be extracted without knowledge-based reduction of the SNP number. Thus, statistically significant SNPs cannot be extracted from the present data. We could find the statistically significant rs9351963 in *KCNQ5* by applying the combined method to hypothesis-free genomic data.

The KCNQ/K(v)7 potassium channel family consists of 5 members of neural muscarine channel (M channel; from KCNQ1 to KCNQ5) which have a distinct expression pattern and a functional role. Although KCNQ1 is prevalently expressed in the cardiac muscle, KCNQ2, KCNQ3, KCNQ4, and KCNQ5 are expressed in neural tissue [73–75]. On the other hand, a recent study revealed that KCNQ4 and KCNQ5 are the most abundantly expressed KCNQ channels in smooth muscle throughout the gastrointestinal tract [76]. Furthermore, Jepps et al. opined that drugs that selectively block KCNQ4/KCNQ5 might be promising as therapeutics for the treatment of motility disorders such as constipation associated with irritable bowel syndrome [76]. In other words, drugs that selectively open KCNQ4/KCNQ5 might be effective against diarrhea. The KCNQ family gene products assemble as homomeric or heteromeric tetramers to form functional channels that mediate the M-current [77], a current that is suppressed by mAChR activation [78,79]. Irinotecan induces adverse cholinergic effects (acetylcholinelike actions) by inhibiting AChE and binding to mAChR [37,38,80]. Therefore, polymorphisms of *KCNQ5* genes possibly effect incidence of diarrhea as interindividual variation in the drug response among cancer patients treated with irinotecan chemotherapy.

In the present study, only the highest grade of adverse events is recorded during the first 2 months of irinotecan treatment for each patient and each adverse effect. Therefore, incidence of grade ≥ 2 diarrhea possibly includes cases caused partially by enterohepatic circulation of APC and NPC, but genotype of rs9351963 in *KCNQ5* correlates with the start date of treatment with antidiarrheal agents (Spearman's rank correlation coefficient $\rho = -0.198$, $p = 0.00995$). In other words, genotype of rs9351963 may correlates with the diagnosis (or presentiment) of irinotecan induced early-onset diarrhea (diagnosis is made by trained chemotherapists).

The rs9351963 A>C polymorphism is located in an intron, which does not change the amino acid sequence of the protein and may not influence the biological function of the protein itself. Nonetheless, some intronic polymorphisms are effective markers: For example, rs2237892 in intron 15 of *KCNQ1* is associated with susceptibility to type 2 diabetes mellitus in Japanese individuals [81], and the CA simple sequence repeat in intron 1 (CA-SSR1) of the gene of epidermal growth factor receptor (*EGFR*) is associated with the clinical outcome in gefitinib-treated Japanese patients with non-small cell lung cancer [82]. Furthermore, variations related to intronic or synonymous SNPs possibly affect mRNA stability, translational kinetics, and splicing, resulting in alterations at the protein level, e.g., changes of structure or function [83–89]. Although rs9351963 does not have a known function, this SNP is a possible predictive factor of adverse effects of irinotecan-based chemotherapy and is possibly linked to some functional polymorphisms in *KCNQ5*. Their clinical importance needs to be further elucidated.

In the present study, we extracted rs9351963, which showed a p value (0.0289) obtained using a combination of 2 stages of screening and a permutation test from SNPs selected by KB-SNP. In the second dataset, the p value of Fisher's exact test was 3.31×10^{-5}, and the q value was 0.173 calculated by correction of Benjamini-Hochberg method, as shown in Table 2. This value is

A Irinotecan monotherapy

Allele model

rs9351963	Diarrhea	
	Grade < 2	Grade ≥ 2
A	63	11
C	15	17

OR (95%CI): 6.3 (2.3-19)
$p = 8.86 \times 10^{-5}$

Dominant model

rs9351963	Diarrhea	
	Grade < 2	Grade ≥ 2
AA	26	1
AC+CC	13	13

OR (95%CI): 24 (3.1-1139)
$p = 1.29 \times 10^{-4}$

Recessive model

rs9351963	Diarrhea	
	Grade < 2	Grade ≥ 2
AA+AC	37	10
CC	2	4

OR (95%CI): 7.0 (0.87-89)
$p = 0.0358$

B Any irinotecan chemotherapy (including irinotecan monotherapy)

Allele model

rs9351963	Diarrhea	
	Grade < 2	Grade ≥ 2
A	192	33
C	72	39

OR (95%CI): 3.1 (1.8-5.6)
$p = 3.31 \times 10^{-5}$

Dominant model

rs9351963	Diarrhea	
	Grade < 2	Grade ≥ 2
AA	69	9
AC+CC	63	27

OR (95%CI): 3.3 (1.4-8.5)
$p = 4.44 \times 10^{-3}$

Recessive model

rs9351963	Diarrhea	
	Grade < 2	Grade ≥ 2
AA+AC	123	24
CC	9	12

OR (95%CI): 6.7 (2.3-20)
$p = 1.28 \times 10^{-4}$

C Irinotecan combination chemotherapy (excluding irinotecan monotherapy)

Allele model

rs9351963	Diarrhea	
	Grade < 2	Grade ≥ 2
A	129	22
C	57	22

OR (95%CI): 2.3 (1.1-4.7)
$p = 0.0211$

Dominant model

rs9351963	Diarrhea	
	Grade < 2	Grade ≥ 2
AA	43	8
AC+CC	50	14

OR (95%CI): 1.5 (0.53-4.5)
$p = 0.478$

Recessive model

rs9351963	Diarrhea	
	Grade < 2	Grade ≥ 2
AA+AC	86	14
CC	7	8

OR (95%CI): 6.9 (1.9-26)
$p = 1.44 \times 10^{-3}$

Figure 3. Contingency tables for rs9351963 in *KCNQ5* for each model using each dataset. (A) irinotecan monotherapy (first dataset), (B) any irinotecan chemotherapy (including irinotecan monotherapy; second dataset), and (C) irinotecan combination chemotherapy (excluding irinotecan monotherapy). OR: odds ratio. The *p* values were calculated using Fisher's exact test. CI: confidence interval.

statistically insignificant. Therefore, during the 2 stages of screening, it is statistically sufficient to extract rs9351963.

The calculation of probability of occurrence in Bernoulli trials is suitable to for estimation of validity of the repetition number in the permutation process. In this trial, occurrence probability is defined as $_nC_k \times (p_B)^k \times (1 - p_B)^{(n-k)}$, where k is the occurrence number, n is the repetition number, and p_B represents probability. If the repetition number is 100,000 for rs9351963 ($p = 0.02891$ [2891/100000]) and the significance level of the test (α) is 0.05, the occurrence probability is $_{100000}C_{2891} \times (0.05)^{2891} \times (1-0.05)^{(100000-2891)} = 4.89 \times 10^{-241}$. In statistics, the 99% (or 95%) confidence interval should be considered. The significance level of $\alpha = 0.05$ does not exist in the 99% confidence interval of the p value for rs9351963, because the occurrence probability 4.89×10^{-241} is clearly lower than 0.01. Similarly, if the repetition number is 10,000, the occurrence probability is 3.41×10^{-26}. This way, the occurrence probability is sufficiently low for 10,000 permutations. Nevertheless, we conducted 100,000 permutations to estimate p values more accurately for the permutation test.

Using our combined method involving KB-SNP, we identified rs9351963 as a potential predictive factor of diarrhea in cancer patients treated with irinotecan chemotherapy; however, the comprehensiveness of KB-SNP was limited. Therefore, statistical information regarding the adverse effects of cancer patients treated with irinotecan chemotherapy is shown in Table S3 for incidence of diarrhea ($p<0.05$) and in Table S4 for incidence of neutropenia ($p<0.05$). The relevant data are also provided on the website

Genome Medicine Database of Japan (GeMDBJ) [90] (https://gemdbj.nibio.go.jp/). These data will be useful for replication studies or meta-analyses in the future.

In conclusion, in the present study, we applied the combined method to hypothesis-free genomic data on cancer patients treated with irinotecan chemotherapy. By means of this method, rs9351963 in *KCNQ5* was extracted as a candidate SNP related to the incidence of diarrhea. For example, the association of rs9351963 with irinotecan-related diarrhea (OR of 3.14) showed a p value of 3.31×10^{-5} in Fisher's exact test (allele model). Even if this p value were adjusted by means of the permutation test for the effects of multiple testing problems, the adjusted p value would still indicate statistical significance (adjusted p value of 0.0289<0.05). Additionally, we evaluated the performance of rs9351963 using multiple regression models. rs9351963 was clearly superior to clinical parameters (or environmental factors) and showed a sensitivity of 77.8% and specificity of 57.6% in the multiple regression model, including rs9351963. Recent studies showed that the *KCNQ4* and *KCNQ5* genes encode components of the M channel expressed in gastrointestinal smooth muscles and suggested that these genes are associated with irritable bowel syndrome and similar peristalsis diseases. These results suggest that rs9351963 may be a predictive factor of diarrhea in cancer patients treated with irinotecan chemotherapy. This SNP may also be useful for selection of chemotherapy regimens, such as irinotecan monotherapy or a combination of irinotecan chemo-

A

Parameter	AIC	AUC	Sens.	Spec.
NULL	177	0.500	50.0	50.0
UGT1A1*6 or *28	179	0.506	52.8	48.5
rs9351963	162	0.690	75.0	52.3
MMC	173	0.542	100.0	8.3
Amrubicin	172	0.528	5.6	100.0
MMC+Amrubicin	169	0.567	100.0	8.3
rs9351963 + Amrubicin	156	0.718	38.9	93.2
rs9351963 + MMC	159	0.718	75.0	57.6
rs9351963 + Amrubicin + MMC	153	0.744	77.8	57.6

B

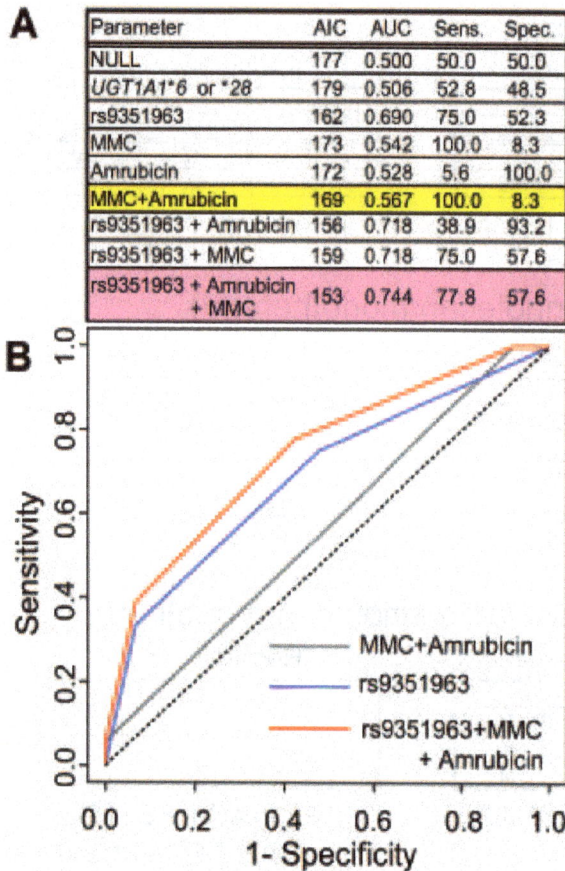

Figure 4. Comparison of AIC, AUC, and ROC curves for logistic regression models. (A) Parameters of each model. (B) The ROC curve of a model consisting of rs9351963+MMC+ Amrubicin. ROC: receiver operating characteristic, AUC: area under the ROC curve, NULL indicates the model without parameters. Each genetic factor conforms to the proportional odds model, AIC: Akaike's information criterion, AUC: area under the ROC curve, Sens.: Sensitivity (%), Spec.: Specificity (%).

therapy with KCNQ5 opener. Furthermore, the result of the present analysis supports usability of our combined method.

Supporting Information

Table S1   Irinotecan-treated cancer patients, genetic factor, and clinical parameters for incidence of diarrhea

References

1. Evans WE, McLeod HL (2003) Pharmacogenomics–drug disposition, drug targets, and side effects. N Engl J Med 348: 538–549.
2. Ingelman-Sundberg M (2008) Pharmacogenomic biomarkers for prediction of severe adverse drug reactions. N Engl J Med 358: 637–639.
3. Ando Y, Saka H, Ando M, Sawa T, Muro K, et al. (2000) Polymorphisms of UDP-glucuronosyltransferase gene and irinotecan toxicity: a pharmacogenetic analysis. Cancer Res 60: 6921–6926.
4. Ma F, Sun T, Shi Y, Yu D, Tan W, et al. (2009) Polymorphisms of EGFR predict clinical outcome in advanced non-small-cell lung cancer patients treated with Gefitinib. Lung Cancer 66: 114–119.
5. Minami H, Sai K, Saeki M, Saito Y, Ozawa S, et al. (2007) Irinotecan pharmacokinetics/pharmacodynamics and UGT1A genetic polymorphisms in Japanese: roles of UGT1A1*6 and *28. Pharmacogenet Genomics 17: 497–504.
6. Sato Y, Laird NM, Nagashima K, Kato R, Hamano T, et al. (2009) A new statistical screening approach for finding pharmacokinetics-related genes in genome-wide studies. Pharmacogenomics J 9: 137–146.
7. Takahashi H, Kaniwa N, Saito Y, Sai K, Hamaguchi T, et al. (2013) Identification of a candidate single-nucleotide polymorphism related to

and neutropenia. "UGT1A1*6 or *28" is a genetic factor constructed from 2 polymorphisms (UGT1A1*6 and *28); "2" indicates *6/*6, *28/*28 or *6/*28, "1" indicates *6 or *28, and "0" indicates "other than 2 and 1." Area: body surface area (m^2), PS: performance status, Cr: grade of creatinine, Hg: grade of hemoglobin, Alb: grade of albumin, ALP: grade of alkaline phosphatase, and GOT: grade of glutamic oxaloacetic transaminase. Each laboratory test value (Alb, Hg, GOT, ALP, and Cr) was recorded before the irinotecan therapy. For each type of clinical tests the grade and aberrant values were defined according to the National Cancer Institute - Common Toxicity Criteria (NCI-CTC, Version 2.0). C_{max}/dose: SN38 C_{max}/dose $[10^{-3} \times m^2/L]$. AUC: area under the concentration-time curve. AUC ratio: Ratio of AUC_{SN38}/AUC_{CPT-11}. 5-FU: 5-fluorouracil, CDDP: cisplatin, MMC: mitomycin C, VP16: etoposide. * and † indicate $p < 0.05$ and $0.05 \leq p < 0.10$, respectively. For each concomitant drug, 0 means "not administered," 1 indicates administered.

Table S2   GO term list for transporter activity and the related functions.

Table S3   Statistical information on the chemotherapeutic response (incidence of grade ≥ 2 diarrhea) of irinotecan-treated cancer patients ($p < 0.05$). RS number: reference SNP identification number in dbSNP; p values were calculated using Fisher's exact test and q values were calculated using the Benjamini-Hochberg (BH) method from p values.

Table S4   Statistical information on the chemotherapeutic response (incidence of grade ≥ 3 neutropenia) of irinotecan-treated cancer patients ($p < 0.05$). RS number: reference SNP identification number in dbSNP; p values were calculated using Fisher's exact test and q values were calculated using the Benjamini-Hochberg (BH) method from p values.

Acknowledgments

We thank Ms. Sumiko Ohnami for help with SNP genotyping.

Author Contributions

Conceived and designed the experiments: HT Y. Saito NS JS HS T. Yoshida. Performed the experiments: HT KS NK HO YO MO. Analyzed the data: HT RI AT AD. Contributed reagents/materials/analysis tools: HT YM TH Y. Shimada AO T. Yoshino TD. Contributed to the writing of the manuscript: HT.

chemotherapeutic response through a combination of knowledge-based algorithm and hypothesis-free genomic data. J Biosci Bioeng 116: 768–773.
8. van Kuilenburg AB, Muller EW, Haasjes J, Meinsma R, Zoetekouw L, et al. (2001) Lethal outcome of a patient with a complete dihydropyrimidine dehydrogenase (DPD) deficiency after administration of 5-fluorouracil: frequency of the common IVS14+1G>A mutation causing DPD deficiency. Clin Cancer Res 7: 1149–1153.
9. Raida M, Schwabe W, Hausler P, Van Kuilenburg AB, Van Gennip AH, et al. (2001) Prevalence of a common point mutation in the dihydropyrimidine dehydrogenase (DPD) gene within the 5'-splice donor site of intron 14 in patients with severe 5-fluorouracil (5-FU)- related toxicity compared with controls. Clin Cancer Res 7: 2832–2839.
10. Efferth T, Volm M (2005) Pharmacogenetics for individualized cancer chemotherapy. Pharmacol Ther 107: 155–176.
11. Slatter JG, Su P, Sams JP, Schaaf LJ, Wienkers LC (1997) Bioactivation of the anticancer agent CPT-11 to SN-38 by human hepatic microsomal carboxylesterases and the in vitro assessment of potential drug interactions. Drug Metab Dispos 25: 1157–1164.

12. Iyer L, King CD, Whitington PF, Green MD, Roy SK, et al. (1998) Genetic predisposition to the metabolism of irinotecan (CPT-11). Role of uridine diphosphate glucuronosyltransferase isoform 1A1 in the glucuronidation of its active metabolite (SN-38) in human liver microsomes. J Clin Invest 101: 847–854.

13. Ciotti M, Basu N, Brangi M, Owens IS (1999) Glucuronidation of 7-ethyl-10-hydroxycamptothecin (SN-38) by the human UDP-glucuronosyltransferases encoded at the UGT1 locus. Biochem Biophys Res Commun 260: 199–202.

14. Gagne JF, Montminy V, Belanger P, Journault K, Gaucher G, et al. (2002) Common human UGT1A polymorphisms and the altered metabolism of irinotecan active metabolite 7-ethyl-10-hydroxycamptothecin (SN-38). Mol Pharmacol 62: 608–617.

15. Haaz MC, Rivory L, Riche C, Vernillet L, Robert J (1998) Metabolism of irinotecan (CPT-11) by human hepatic microsomes: participation of cytochrome P-450 3A and drug interactions. Cancer Res 58: 468–472.

16. Sai K, Saito Y, Fukushima-Uesaka H, Kurose K, Kaniwa N, et al. (2008) Impact of CYP3A4 haplotypes on irinotecan pharmacokinetics in Japanese cancer patients. Cancer Chemother Pharmacol 62: 529–537.

17. Sparreboom A, Danesi R, Ando Y, Chan J, Figg WD (2003) Pharmacogenomics of ABC transporters and its role in cancer chemotherapy. Drug Resist Updat 6: 71–84.

18. Nozawa T, Minami H, Sugiura S, Tsuji A, Tamai I (2005) Role of organic anion transporter OATP1B1 (OATP-C) in hepatic uptake of irinotecan and its active metabolite, 7-ethyl-10-hydroxycamptothecin: in vitro evidence and effect of single nucleotide polymorphisms. Drug Metab Dispos 33: 434–439.

19. Iyer L, Das S, Janisch L, Wen M, Ramirez J, et al. (2002) UGT1A1*28 polymorphism as a determinant of irinotecan disposition and toxicity. Pharmacogenomics J 2: 43–47.

20. Innocenti F, Undevia SD, Iyer L, Chen PX, Das S, et al. (2004) Genetic variants in the UDP-glucuronosyltransferase 1A1 gene predict the risk of severe neutropenia of irinotecan. J Clin Oncol 22: 1382–1388.

21. Han JY, Lim HS, Shin ES, Yoo YK, Park YH, et al. (2006) Comprehensive analysis of UGT1A polymorphisms predictive for pharmacokinetics and treatment outcome in patients with non-small-cell lung cancer treated with irinotecan and cisplatin. J Clin Oncol 24: 2237–2244.

22. Jada SR, Lim R, Wong CI, Shu X, Lee SC, et al. (2007) Role of UGT1A1*6, UGT1A1*28 and ABCG2 c.421C>A polymorphisms in irinotecan-induced neutropenia in Asian cancer patients. Cancer Sci 98: 1461–1467.

23. Sai K, Saito Y, Sakamoto H, Shirao K, Kurose K, et al. (2008) Importance of UDP-glucuronosyltransferase 1A1*6 for irinotecan toxicities in Japanese cancer patients. Cancer Lett 261: 165–171.

24. Sai K, Saito Y, Maekawa K, Kim SR, Kaniwa N, et al. (2010) Additive effects of drug transporter genetic polymorphisms on irinotecan pharmacokinetics/pharmacodynamics in Japanese cancer patients. Cancer Chemother Pharmacol 66: 95–105.

25. Mathijssen RH, Marsh S, Karlsson MO, Xie R, Baker SD, et al. (2003) Irinotecan pathway genotype analysis to predict pharmacokinetics. Clin Cancer Res 9: 3246–3253.

26. Sai K, Kaniwa N, Itoda M, Saito Y, Hasegawa R, et al. (2003) Haplotype analysis of ABCB1/MDR1 blocks in a Japanese population reveals genotype-dependent renal clearance of irinotecan. Pharmacogenetics 13: 741–757.

27. Zhou Q, Sparreboom A, Tan EH, Cheung YB, Lee A, et al. (2005) Pharmacogenetic profiling across the irinotecan pathway in Asian patients with cancer. Br J Clin Pharmacol 59: 415–424.

28. de Jong FA, Marsh S, Mathijssen RH, King C, Verweij J, et al. (2004) ABCG2 pharmacogenetics: ethnic differences in allele frequency and assessment of influence on irinotecan disposition. Clin Cancer Res 10: 5889–5894.

29. de Jong FA, Scott-Horton TJ, Kroetz DL, McLeod HL, Friberg LE, et al. (2007) Irinotecan-induced diarrhea: functional significance of the polymorphic ABCC2 transporter protein. Clin Pharmacol Ther 81: 42–49.

30. Xiang X, Jada SR, Li HH, Fan L, Tham LS, et al. (2006) Pharmacogenetics of SLCO1B1 gene and the impact of *1b and *15 haplotypes on irinotecan disposition in Asian cancer patients. Pharmacogenet Genomics 16: 683–691.

31. Takane H, Miyata M, Burioka N, Kurai J, Fukuoka Y, et al. (2007) Severe toxicities after irinotecan-based chemotherapy in a patient with lung cancer: a homozygote for the SLCO1B1*15 allele. Ther Drug Monit 29: 666–668.

32. Han JY, Lim HS, Shin ES, Yoo YK, Park YH, et al. (2008) Influence of the organic anion-transporting polypeptide 1B1 (OATP1B1) polymorphisms on irinotecan-pharmacokinetics and clinical outcome of patients with advanced non-small cell lung cancer. Lung Cancer 59: 69–75.

33. Han JY, Lim HS, Park YH, Lee SY, Lee JS (2009) Integrated pharmacogenetic prediction of irinotecan pharmacokinetics and toxicity in patients with advanced non-small cell lung cancer. Lung Cancer 63: 115–120.

34. Michael M, Thompson M, Hicks RJ, Mitchell PL, Ellis A, et al. (2006) Relationship of hepatic functional imaging to irinotecan pharmacokinetics and genetic parameters of drug elimination. J Clin Oncol 24: 4228–4235.

35. Sai K, Itoda M, Saito Y, Kurose K, Katori N, et al. (2006) Genetic variations and haplotype structures of the ABCB1 gene in a Japanese population: an expanded haplotype block covering the distal promoter region, and associated ethnic differences. Ann Hum Genet 70: 605–622.

36. Yang X, Hu Z, Chan SY, Chan E, Goh BC, et al. (2005) Novel agents that potentially inhibit irinotecan-induced diarrhea. Curr Med Chem 12: 1343–1358.

37. Kawato Y, Sekiguchi M, Akahane K, Tsutomi Y, Hirota Y, et al. (1993) Inhibitory activity of camptothecin derivatives against acetylcholinesterase in dogs and their binding activity to acetylcholine receptors in rats. J Pharm Pharmacol 45: 444–448.

38. Hyatt JL, Tsurkan L, Morton CL, Yoon KJ, Harel M, et al. (2005) Inhibition of acetylcholinesterase by the anticancer prodrug CPT-11. Chem Biol Interact 157–158: 247–252.

39. Takakura A, Kurita A, Asahara T, Yokoba M, Yamamoto M, et al. (2012) Rapid deconjugation of SN-38 glucuronide and adsorption of released free SN-38 by intestinal microorganisms in rat. Oncol Lett 3: 520–524.

40. Yamamoto M, Kurita A, Asahara T, Takakura A, Katono K, et al. (2008) Metabolism of irinotecan and its active metabolite SN-38 by intestinal microflora in rats. Oncol Rep 20: 727–730.

41. Kuhn JG (1998) Pharmacology of irinotecan. Oncology (Williston Park) 12: 39–42.

42. Takahashi H, Honda H (2006) Modified signal-to-noise: a new simple and practical gene filtering approach based on the concept of projective adaptive resonance theory (PART) filtering method. Bioinformatics 22: 1662–1664.

43. Takahashi H, Kobayashi T, Honda H (2005) Construction of robust prognostic predictors by using projective adaptive resonance theory as a gene filtering method. Bioinformatics 21: 179–186.

44. Takahashi H, Iwakawa H, Nakao S, Ojio T, Morishita R, et al. (2008) Knowledge-based fuzzy adaptive resonance theory and its application to the analysis of gene expression in plants. J Biosci Bioeng 106: 587–593.

45. Takahashi H, Honda H (2006) Prediction of peptide binding to major histocompatibility complex class II molecules through use of boosted fuzzy classifier with SWEEP operator method. J Biosci Bioeng 101: 137–141.

46. Kawamura T, Takahashi H, Honda H (2008) Proposal of new gene filtering method, BagPART, for gene expression analysis with small sample. J Biosci Bioeng 105: 81–84.

47. Takahashi H, Takahashi A, Naito S, Onouchi H (2012) BAIUCAS: a novel BLAST-based algorithm for the identification of upstream open reading frames with conserved amino acid sequences and its application to the Arabidopsis thaliana genome. Bioinformatics 28: 2231–2241.

48. Chiba Y, Mineta K, Hirai MY, Suzuki Y, Kanaya S, et al. (2013) Changes in mRNA stability associated with cold stress in Arabidopsis cells. Plant Cell Physiol 54: 180–194.

49. Iwasaki M, Takahashi H, Iwakawa H, Nakagawa A, Ishikawa T, et al. (2013) Dual regulation of ETTIN (ARF3) gene expression by AS1-AS2, which maintains the DNA methylation level, is involved in stabilization of leaf adaxial-abaxial partitioning in Arabidopsis. Development 140: 1958–1969.

50. Kojima S, Iwasaki M, Takahashi H, Imai T, Matsumura Y, et al. (2011) ASYMMETRIC LEAVES2 and Elongator, a histone acetyltransferase complex, mediate the establishment of polarity in leaves of Arabidopsis thaliana. Plant Cell Physiol 52: 1259–1273.

51. Kotooka N, Komatsu A, Takahashi H, Nonaka M, Kawaguchi C, et al. (2013) Predictive value of high-molecular weight adiponectin in subjects with a higher risk of the development of metabolic syndrome: From a population based 5-year follow-up data. Int J Cardiol 167: 1068–1070.

52. Matsuo N, Mase H, Makino M, Takahashi H, Banno H (2009) Identification of ENHANCER OF SHOOT REGENERATION 1-upregulated genes during in vitro shoot regeneration. Plant Biotechnol 26: 385–393.

53. Nakagawa A, Takahashi H, Kojima S, Sato N, Ohga K, et al. (2012) Berberine enhances defects in the establishment of leaf polarity in asymmetric leaves1 and asymmetric leaves2 of Arabidopsis thaliana. Plant Mol Biol 79: 569–581.

54. Nakayama R, Nemoto T, Takahashi H, Ohta T, Kawai A, et al. (2007) Gene expression analysis of soft tissue sarcomas: characterization and reclassification of malignant fibrous histiocytoma. Mod Pathol 20: 749–759.

55. Sano M, Aoyagi K, Takahashi H, Kawamura T, Mabuchi T, et al. (2010) Forkhead box A1 transcriptional pathway in KRT7-expressing esophageal squamous cell carcinomas with extensive lymph node metastasis. Int J Oncol 36: 321–330.

56. Yajima I, Kumasaka MY, Naito Y, Yoshikawa T, Takahashi H, et al. (2012) Reduced GNG2 expression levels in mouse malignant melanomas and human melanoma cell lines. Am J Cancer Res 2: 322–329.

57. Yoshimura K, Mori T, Yokoyama K, Koike Y, Tanabe N, et al. (2011) Identification of alternative splicing events regulated by an Arabidopsis serine/arginine-like protein, atSR45a, in response to high-light stress using a tiling array. Plant Cell Physiol 52: 1786–1805.

58. Takahashi H, Iwakawa H, Ishibashi N, Kojima S, Matsumura Y, et al. (2013) Meta-analyses of microarrays of arabidopsis asymmetric leaves1 (as1), as2 and their modifying mutants reveal a critical role for the ETT pathway in stabilization of adaxial-abaxial patterning and cell division during leaf development. Plant Cell Physiol 54: 418–431.

59. Takahashi H, Murase Y, Kobayashi T, Honda H (2007) New cancer diagnosis modeling using boosting and projective adaptive resonance theory with improved reliable index. Biochem Eng J 33: 100–109.

60. Takahashi H, Nemoto T, Yoshida T, Honda H, Hasegawa T (2006) Cancer diagnosis marker extraction for soft tissue sarcomas based on gene expression profiling data by using projective adaptive resonance theory (PART) filtering method. BMC Bioinformatics 7: 399.

61. Takahashi H, Aoyagi K, Nakanishi Y, Sasaki H, Yoshida T, et al. (2006) Classification of intramural metastases and lymph node metastases of esophageal

cancer from gene expression based on boosting and projective adaptive resonance theory. J Biosci Bioeng 102: 46–52.

62. Takahashi H, Honda H (2006) Lymphoma prognostication from expression profiling using a combination method of boosting and projective adaptive resonance theory. J Chem Eng Jpn 39: 767–771.

63. Takahashi H, Honda H (2005) A new reliable cancer diagnosis method using boosted fuzzy classifier with a SWEEP operator method. J Chem Eng Jpn 38: 763–773.

64. Takahashi H, Masuda K, Ando T, Kobayashi T, Honda H (2004) Prognostic predictor with multiple fuzzy neural models using expression profiles from DNA microarray for metastases of breast cancer. J Biosci Bioeng 98: 193–199.

65. Takahashi H, Tomida S, Kobayashi T, Honda H (2003) Inference of common genetic network using fuzzy adaptive resonance theory associated matrix method. J Biosci Bioeng 96: 154–160.

66. Takahashi H, Nakayama R, Hayashi S, Nemoto T, Murase Y, et al. (2013) Macrophage migration inhibitory factor and stearoyl-CoA desaturase 1: potential prognostic markers for soft tissue sarcomas based on bioinformatics analyses. PLoS One 8: e78250.

67. Fisher RA (1922) On the interpretation of χ2 from contingency tables, and the calculation of P. J Roy Statistical Society 85: 87–94.

68. Pitman EJG (1938) Significance tests which may be applied to samples from any population. Part III. The analysis of variance test. Biometrika 29: 322–335.

69. Benjamini Y, Hochberg Y (1995) Controlling the false discovery rate: a practical and powerful approach to multiple testing. J R Statist Soc serB 57: 298–300.

70. Akaike H (1974) A new look at the statistical model identification. IEEE T Automat Contr 19: 716–723.

71. Sakamoto Y, Ishiguro M, Kitagawa G (1986) Akaike Information Criterion Statistics. Dordrecht: Reidel Publishing Company.

72. Skol AD, Scott LJ, Abecasis GR, Boehnke M (2006) Joint analysis is more efficient than replication-based analysis for two-stage genome-wide association studies. Nat Genet 38: 209–213.

73. Delmas P, Brown DA (2005) Pathways modulating neural KCNQ/M (Kv7) potassium channels. Nat Rev Neurosci 6: 850–862.

74. Miceli F, Soldovieri MV, Martire M, Taglialatela M (2008) Molecular pharmacology and therapeutic potential of neuronal Kv7-modulating drugs. Curr Opin Pharmacol 8: 65–74.

75. Brown DA, Passmore GM (2009) Neural KCNQ (Kv7) channels. Br J Pharmacol 156: 1185–1195.

76. Jepps TA, Greenwood IA, Moffatt JD, Sanders KM, Ohya S (2009) Molecular and functional characterization of Kv7 K+ channel in murine gastrointestinal smooth muscles. Am J Physiol Gastrointest Liver Physiol 297: G107–115.

77. Schwake M, Jentsch TJ, Friedrich T (2003) A carboxy-terminal domain determines the subunit specificity of KCNQ K+ channel assembly. EMBO Rep 4: 76–81.

78. Cavaliere S, Malik BR, Hodge JJ (2013) KCNQ channels regulate age-related memory impairment. PLoS One 8: e62445.

79. Perez C, Vega R, Soto E (2010) Phospholipase C-mediated inhibition of the M-potassium current by muscarinic-receptor activation in the vestibular primary-afferent neurons of the rat. Neurosci Lett 468: 238–242.

80. Blandizzi C, De Paolis B, Colucci R, Lazzeri G, Baschiera F, et al. (2001) Characterization of a novel mechanism accounting for the adverse cholinergic effects of the anticancer drug irinotecan. Br J Pharmacol 132: 73–84.

81. Yasuda K, Miyake K, Horikawa Y, Hara K, Osawa H, et al. (2008) Variants in KCNQ1 are associated with susceptibility to type 2 diabetes mellitus. Nat Genet 40: 1092–1097.

82. Ichihara S, Toyooka S, Fujiwara Y, Hotta K, Shigematsu H, et al. (2007) The impact of epidermal growth factor receptor gene status on gefitinib-treated Japanese patients with non-small-cell lung cancer. Int J Cancer 120: 1239–1247.

83. Seo S, Takayama K, Uno K, Ohi K, Hashimoto R, et al. (2013) Functional Analysis of Deep Intronic SNP rs13438494 in Intron 24 of PCLO Gene. PLoS One 8: e76960.

84. Sauna ZE, Kimchi-Sarfaty C, Ambudkar SV, Gottesman MM (2007) Silent polymorphisms speak: how they affect pharmacogenomics and the treatment of cancer. Cancer Res 67: 9609–9612.

85. Capon F, Allen MH, Ameen M, Burden AD, Tillman D, et al. (2004) A synonymous SNP of the corneodesmosin gene leads to increased mRNA stability and demonstrates association with psoriasis across diverse ethnic groups. Hum Mol Genet 13: 2361–2368.

86. Nackley AG, Shabalina SA, Tchivileva IE, Satterfield K, Korchynskyi O, et al. (2006) Human catechol-O-methyltransferase haplotypes modulate protein expression by altering mRNA secondary structure. Science 314: 1930–1933.

87. Nielsen KB, Sorensen S, Cartegni L, Corydon TJ, Doktor TK, et al. (2007) Seemingly neutral polymorphic variants may confer immunity to splicing-inactivating mutations: a synonymous SNP in exon 5 of MCAD protects from deleterious mutations in a flanking exonic splicing enhancer. Am J Hum Genet 80: 416–432.

88. Spasovski V, Tosic N, Nikcevic G, Stojiljkovic M, Zukic B, et al. (2013) The influence of novel transcriptional regulatory element in intron 14 on the expression of Janus kinase 2 gene in myeloproliferative neoplasms. J Appl Genet 54: 21–26.

89. Xue G, Aida Y, Onodera T, Sakudo A (2012) The 5′ flanking region and intron1 of the bovine prion protein gene (PRNP) are responsible for negative feedback regulation of the prion protein. PLoS One 7: e32870.

90. Yoshida T, Ono H, Kuchiba A, Saeki N, Sakamoto H (2010) Genome-wide germline analyses on cancer susceptibility and GeMDBJ database: Gastric cancer as an example. Cancer Sci 101: 1582–1589.

10

Methylglyoxal Induces Systemic Symptoms of Irritable Bowel Syndrome

Shuang Zhang[1], Taiwei Jiao[1], Yushuai Chen[2], Nan Gao[2], Lili Zhang[2], Min Jiang[1]*

1 Department of Gastroenterology, First Affiliated Hospital of China Medical University, Shenyang, China, **2** Department of Cadre Ward II, First Affiliated Hospital of China Medical University, Shenyang, China

Abstract

Patients with irritable bowel syndrome (IBS) show a wide range of symptoms including diarrhea, abdominal pain, changes in bowel habits, nausea, vomiting, headache, anxiety, depression and cognitive impairment. Methylglyoxal has been proved to be a potential toxic metabolite produced by intestinal bacteria. The present study was aimed at investigating the correlation between methylglyoxal and irritable bowel syndrome. Rats were treated with an enema infusion of methylglyoxal. Fecal water content, visceral sensitivity, behavioral tests and serum 5-hydroxytryptamine (5-HT) were assessed after methylglyoxal exposure. Our data showed that fecal water content was significantly higher than controls after methylglyoxal exposure except that of 30 mM group. Threshold volumes on balloon distension decreased in the treatment groups. All exposed rats showed obvious head scratching and grooming behavior and a decrease in sucrose preference. The serum 5-HT values were increased in 30, 60, 90 mM groups and decreased in 150 mM group. Our findings suggested that methylglyoxal could induce diarrhea, visceral hypersensitivity, headache as well as depression-like behaviors in rats, and might be the key role in triggering systemic symptoms of IBS.

Editor: John Green, University Hospital Llandough, United Kingdom

Funding: This work was supported by the Innovation Project of Shenyang Bureau of Science and Technology (F13-316-1-12) (http://www.systplan.gov.cn/Plan/planindex.aspx). The funders had no role in study design, data collection and analysis, decision to publish, or preparation of the manuscript.

Competing Interests: The authors have declared that no competing interests exist.

* Email: minjiangcmu@gmail.com

Introduction

Irritable bowel syndrome is one of the most frequently encountered disorders in outpatient gastroenterology practices, characterized by complex symptoms including abdominal pain and spasms, diarrhea, flatulence, altered bowel habits, headache, fatigue, loss of concentration, depression and heart palpitations, after excluding organic diseases [1]. Gastroenteric symptoms are associated with meals in almost two-thirds of patients suffering from IBS [2]. Elie Metchnikoff, who was awarded the 1908 Nobel Prize in Physiology or Medicine, proposed that bacteria in the colon could be the source of "toxicants" and toxic substances would lead to illness and aging [3]. A.K. Campbell and colleagues have made substantial progress in this theory. They indicated that carbohydrates not completely digested or absorbed in the small intestine reached the colon, where decomposed into hydrogen gas and other metabolites, methylglyoxal, methane, diacetyl, aldehydes and ketones [4].

Methylglyoxal has particular potential in all of the toxic metabolites [5]. Methylglyoxal is a natural substance in various organisms produced by the degradation of glycated proteins and monosaccharides [6], and detected in coffee, alcohol and foodstuffs. It is also a bacteria product from anaerobic glycolysis of carbohydrates in the large intestine. Previous studies have shown that methylglyoxal (0.1–10 mM) inhibits the growth of wild type *E. coli* cells via inducing rapid increase of cytosolic free Ca^{2+}, followed by altered expression of at least 90 genes [7]. Moreover, several recent investigations have suggested that methylglyoxal is involved in many diseases such as diabetes, cancer, and obesity [8–

10], and can also disrupt barrier function of brain microvascular endothelial cells [11]. These studies may provide a novel perspective on the pathogenesis of IBS. We therefore assumed that the toxic metabolites produced by gut bacteria might be the potential culprit for IBS. In the current study, we intended to investigate whether methylglyoxal had the potential to induce systemic symptoms in IBS via evaluations of abdominal reactions and behavioral tests as well as serum 5-HT level in rats, and to assess the evidence to clarify the association between methylglyoxal and IBS.

Materials and Methods

Ethics Statement

All procedures were approved by the Animal Care Committee of the Chinese Medical University and were in accordance with the principles outlined in the NIH Guide for the Care and Use of Laboratory Animals. All possible efforts were made to optimize the comfort and to minimize the use of the animals.

Animals

Adult female Wistar rats weighing 180–200 g, were purchased from the Experimental Animal Center, China Medical University. Animals were housed in groups of 8 rats in polyethylene cages (L×W×H: 48×35×20 cm) on aspen chip bedding, containing wood chips and paper towels as enrichment. All animals were acclimatized under standard housing conditions (12/12 h light-dark cycle starting at 7:00 AM, temperature at 23±2°C, relative

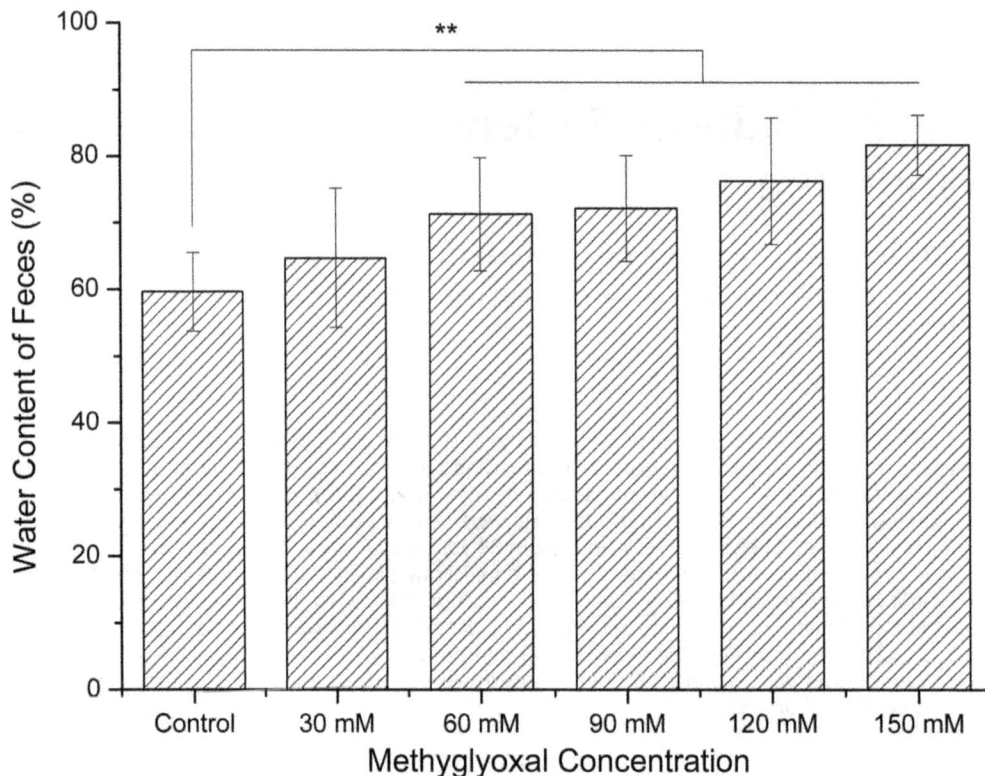

Figure 1. Effects of methylglyoxal on fecal water content. The fecal water content of 60 mM, 90 mM, 120 mM, 150 mM groups were significantly increased compared with controls. The 30 mM group showed no significant difference compared with controls. **$p<0.01$ versus controls.

humidity at 50–60%) for 1 week before the experiment, with access to standard pelleted rodent chow (Trophic Animal Feed High-tech Co., Ltd., China) and tap water ad libitum. The treatments and experimental testing were conducted during the light component of the cycle. Any rough pelages and signs of diarrhea were noted.

Treatments

The methylglyoxal stock solution (40%, Alfa Aesar, USA), which was freshly prepared before each experiment, was dissolved in saline and administrated as an enema (1 ml) at concentrations of 30 mM, 60 mM, 90 mM, 120 mM, and 150 mM. Rats were randomly divided into 6 groups (n = 8). The rats in the control group were treated with saline (1 ml).

Fecal Water Content

Each rat was transferred into an individual metabolic cage on day 9 (1350×400×1500 mm), under where a separate metabolism tray was placed to observe the appearance of feces. Fecal samples were collected and thoroughly oven-dried (80°C, 48 h) to calculate fecal water content according to the equation: water content = 100%×(wet weight − dry weight)/wet weight [12].

Rectal Distension

Visceral sensitivity was assessed by measuring the abdominal withdrawal reflex (AWR) using a semiquantitative score. The rats were lightly anesthetized with ether after fasting for 12 h. Distension balloons were inserted through the anus of the rats and positioned 2 cm from the anal verge. The rats were then housed in transparent cages (200 mm×80 mm×80 mm) individ-

ually after woke up, in which they were not allowed to swivel but only able to move forward-backward. The balloon was distended with water at 37°C after one-hour adaptation, and the threshold intensity was observed by AWR test as previously reported with some modification [13]. Visual observation of the animal response to ascending-limit distension was performed by blinded observers from minimum volume of 0.1 ml to maximum of 1.0 ml. The AWR score was assigned by blinded observers as follows: 0, no behavioral response to distension; 1, brief head movements followed by immobility; 2, contraction of abdominal muscle; 3, lifting of abdomen; 4, body arching and lifting of pelvic structure. The volumes on balloon distension were recorded when the rats reached an AWR score of 3 or more.

Behavioral Testing

Head scratching and grooming. On day 10, the severity of headache was assessed by measuring head scratching and head grooming. The procedures were performed as described [14,15]. The sum of movements were recorded, including head scratching, head grooming, washing the head and licking the fore paws. The behaviors were observed within 60 minutes after methylglyoxal administration.

Sucrose preference test (SPT). SPT was conducted to evaluate depression-like behavior [16,17]. All rats were first given weak (1%) sucrose solution in their home cage to reduce reaction to novel environment and to ensure stability of the experimental results. Training consisted of an initial 48 hours exposure to sucrose solution, followed by five 1-h tests in which sucrose was presented. On day 10, sucrose consumption was measured by weighing bottles before and after the test period. Sucrose

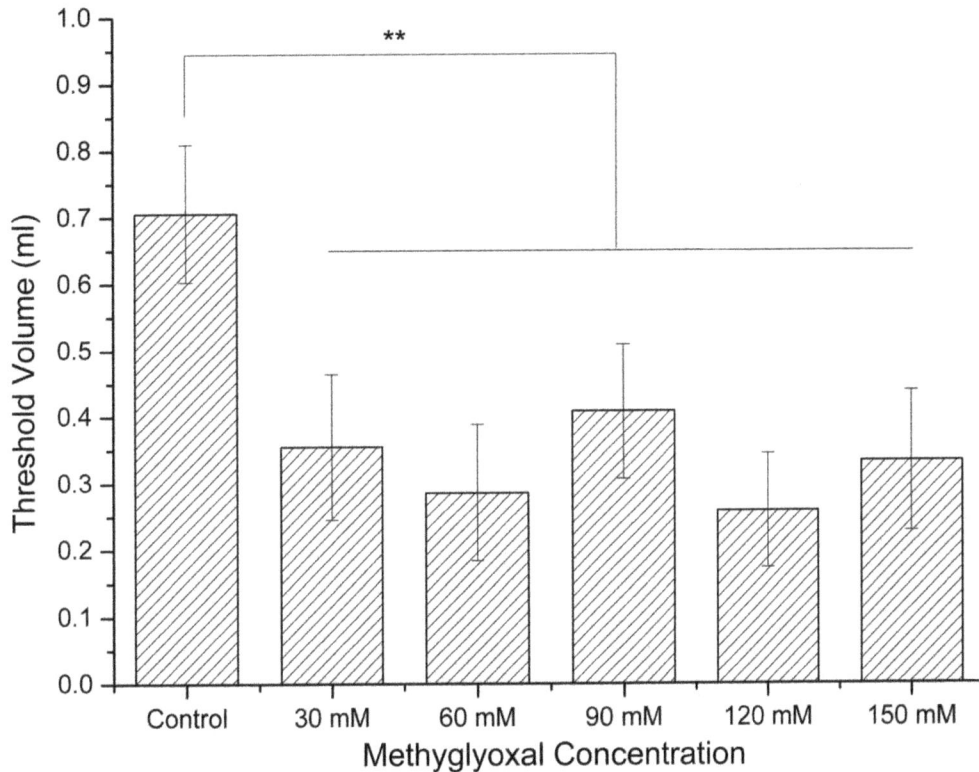

Figure 2. Effects of methylglyoxal on visceral sensitivity. The threshold volumes in all treatment groups were significant lower than controls. **$p < 0.01$ versus controls.

preference was calculated as: $100\% \times$(sucrose consumption)/(total fluid consumption).

Analysis of Serum 5-Hydroxytryptamine (5-HT)

Blood samples were collected from decapitated rats between 9:00AM and 11:00AM twenty-four hours after behavioral testing and separated in a refrigerated centrifuge at 4°C (3,000 rpm×15 min). Serum was stored at −80°C until used. The serum 5-HT was quantified using enzyme linked immunosorbent assay (ELISA) kits (Quantikine; R&D Systems, Minneapolis, MN, USA) according to the manufacturer's instructions.

Statistics

All data are presented as mean ± standard deviation. Parametric data were analyzed using the student's t test and ANOVA was used for multiple comparisons. Statistical analyses were performed using the SPSS 17.0 software. Results were considered to be statistically significant at $p < 0.05$.

Results

Defecation

Rat droppings of the control group were pellet shaped with a wet surface appearance and directly fell into metabolic tray without adhering to metabolic cage wall. However, feces adhered to the wall of metabolic cage in some rats of each treatment group. The time of rats first showing feces adhesion phenomenon in each group were day 4 (30 mM group), day 3 (60 mM group), day 3 (90 mM group), day 2 (120 mM group), day 2 (150 mM group), respectively. On day 10, the number of rats with feces adhesion in each treatment group was recorded, and the percentages of

occurrence were 37.5% (30 mM group), 62.5% (60 mM group), 87.5% (90 mM group), 100% (120 mM group), 100% (150 mM group), respectively. None was observed in the control group. There were no significant differences in the fecal water content between the 30 mM group and controls ($p > 0.05$) as shown in Figure 1. The fecal water contents of rats exposed to 60 mM, 90 mM, 120 mM and 150 mM methylglyoxal were significantly increased compared with controls ($p < 0.01$) (Fig. 1).

Visceral Sensitivity

The nociceptive threshold volume to elicit abdominal muscle contraction (AWR score is 3) was 0.70 ± 0.10 ml in the control group. The mean threshold volumes in rats were 0.35 ml (30 mM), 0.28 ml (60 mM), 0.40 ml (90 mM), 0.25 ml (120 mM) and 0.33 ml (150 mM) ($p < 0.01$) (Fig. 2).

Head Scratching and Grooming

All rats exposed to methylglyoxal performed more frequent head scratching and grooming activities than naive controls ($p < 0.01$). The amount of activities were 167 (60 mM), 139 (90 mM) and 125 (120 mM). The behaviors showed significant negative correlation to the concentrations of methylglyoxal except 30 mM group (Fig. 3).

Depression-Like Behaviors

The sucrose preference of the rats treated with 150 mM methylglyoxal (45%) was significantly decreased compared with controls (69%) as shown in Figure 4 ($p < 0.01$). However, the differences of the SPT between 30 mM, 60 mM, 90 mM, 120 mM groups and the control group were not significant ($p > 0.05$).

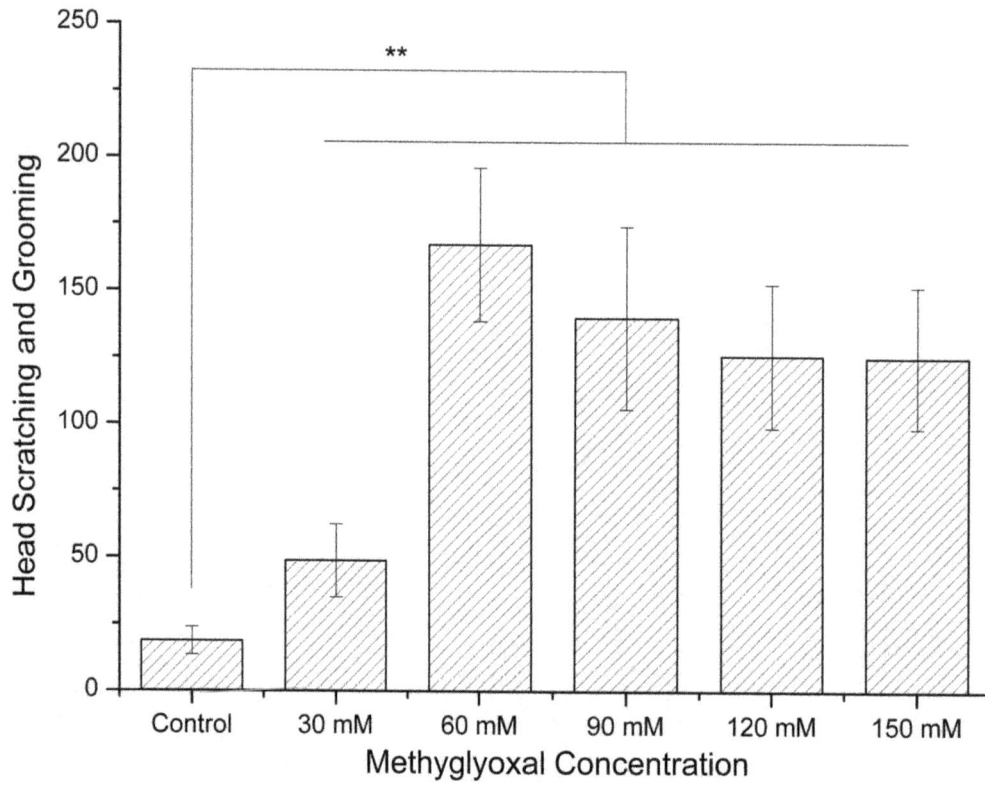

Figure 3. Effects of methylglyoxal on head scratching and grooming behaviors. The time of scratching behavior in all treatment groups markedly increased compared with controls. **$p<0.01$ versus controls.

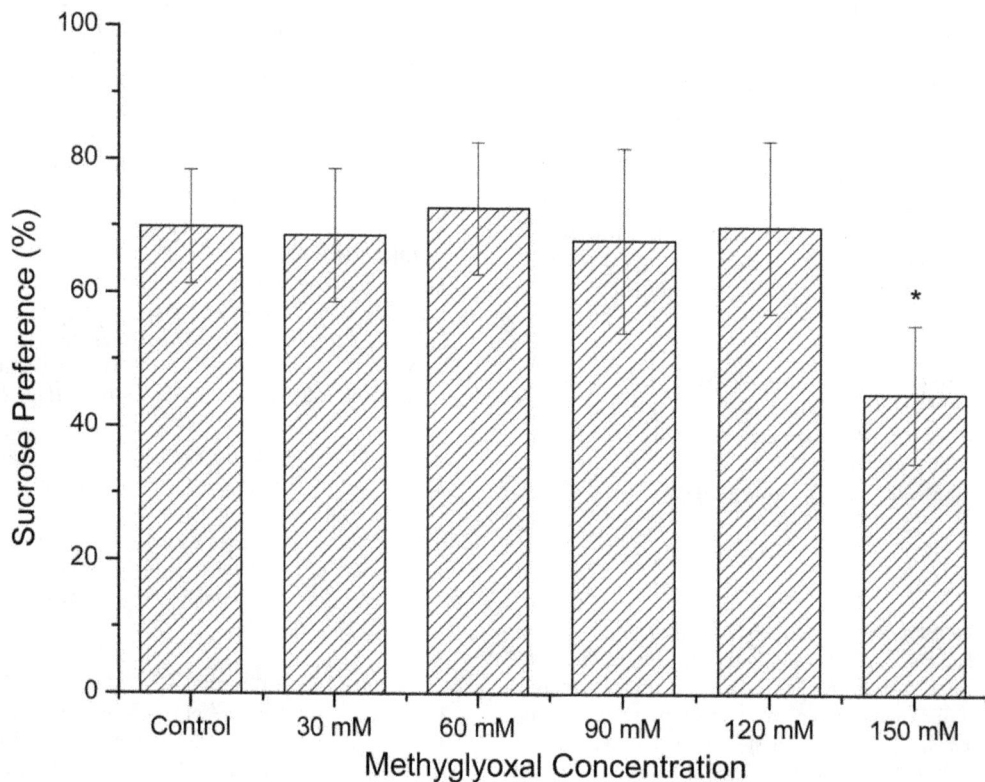

Figure 4. Effects of methylglyoxal on sucrose preference test. The SPT scores of the 150 mM group were decreased. *$p<0.05$ versus controls.

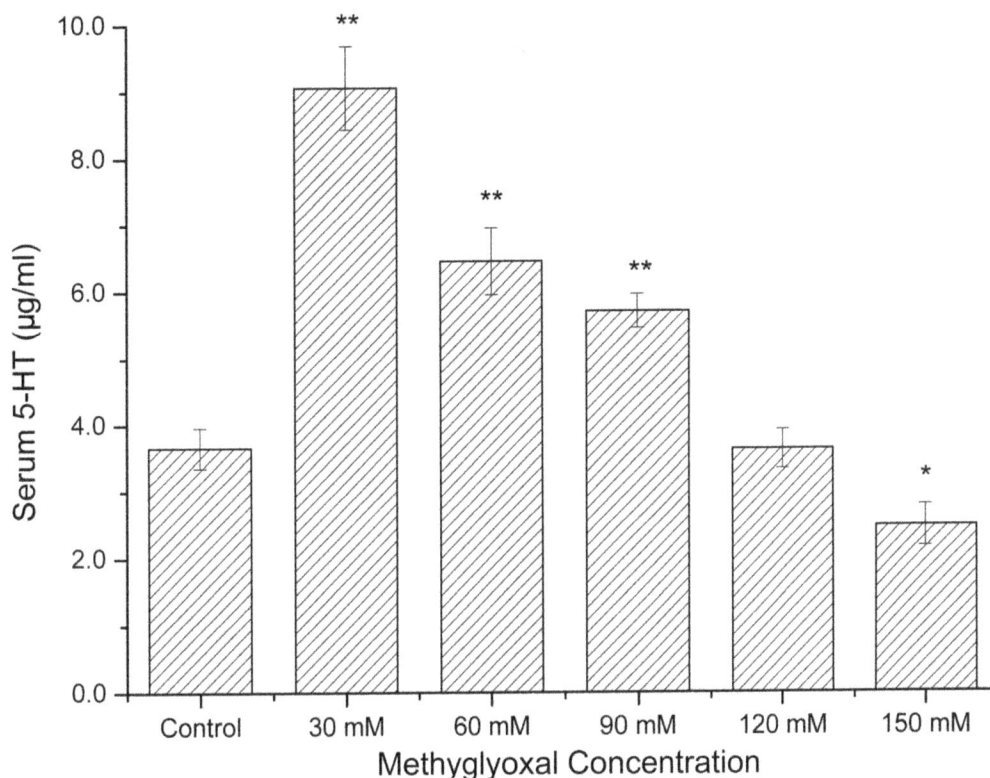

Figure 5. Effects of methylglyoxal on serum 5-HT level. The serum 5-HT levels of 30 mM, 60 mM and 90 mM groups were markedly higher than controls. The difference between 120 mM group and controls was not significantly. The level of 5-HT in 150 mM group rats was decreased than controls. **$p<0.01$ versus controls, *$p<0.05$ versus controls.

Serum 5-HT Levels

Rats exposed to 30 mM, 60 mM, 90 mM methylglyoxal presented significantly higher serum 5-HT levels than controls ($p<0.01$) with a dose-dependent decline. The serum level of 5-HT in 150 mM group was significantly decreased compared with the control group ($p<0.01$). There was no statistically significant difference between 120 mM group and controls ($p>0.05$) (Fig. 5).

Discussion

IBS is the most common functional gastrointestinal disorder with worldwide incidence of up to 10%–20%. The clinical profile of patients with IBS is characterized by bowel symptoms such as abdominal pain, change in bowel habit, passing gas, accompanied by a range of other symptoms including tiredness, nausea, depression [18]. IBS is conventionally regarded as the outcome of a complex interaction between psychological and physical factors, however, a bacterial metabolic toxin hypothesis is now proposed, which postulates that gastrointestinal and systemic symptoms of IBS may be induced by intestinal bacterial metabolic toxins, the anaerobic products of carbohydrates not digested and absorbed in the small intestine [5]. The biological effects of methylglyoxal have been revealed in earlier studies. Cytotoxicity of methylglyoxal was investigated in some researches indicating severe inhibition of DNA, RNA and protein syntheses. The division of bacteria, cells in tissue culture and fertilized sea urchin eggs was inhibited by a low concentration of methylglyoxal [19]. It was reported to have pharmacological potential of antiviral, antimalarial and antibacterial activities [20]. Campbell pointed out that methylglyoxal could affect the intestinal microflora via

calcium signaling, and also affect the signaling within the whole body. It offers a new perspective on the cause of intricate complex of symptoms of IBS.

The densities of microflora in the large intestine achieve concentrations of up to 10^{11} or 10^{12} cells/g, and the composition pattern of an individual flora usually remains constant [21]. There are various functions of the normal gut microflora: fermentation of undigested food and endogenous mucus, supplement of short-chain fatty acids (SCFAs), participating in iron absorption, trophic effect on the intestinal epithelium, protection against pathogens, and influence on the homoeostasis of the immune system [22]. It is understood that the population of bacteria in lower gastrointestinal tract is much more complex than upper gastrointestinal tract. In patients with IBS, undigested and low-digestible carbohydrates which cannot be absorbed by the small intestine reach the large intestine, where contains little oxygen and large numbers of bacteria. Methylglyoxal and other intestinal bacteria metabolites, such as hydrogen and methane, are produced via anaerobic fermentation, suggesting why patients with IBS suffer from excessive gas and bloating. Our data showed that the fecal water content of rats treated with methylglyoxal was significantly higher than controls except the 30 mM group, and positively correlated with enemas concentration. During the observation on defecation, we noticed that the rat droppings were softer and more moisture in each treatment group than controls with the naked eye. Rat feces in the 120 mM and 150 mM groups were mushy and aqueous, and could not roll in the metabolic tray but stick to the bottom of the cage after discharging. Although there was no increase in fecal water content of the 30 mM group compared with controls, feces adhesion to the cage was also observed. Meanwhile this

Diarrhea: A Clinical Guide

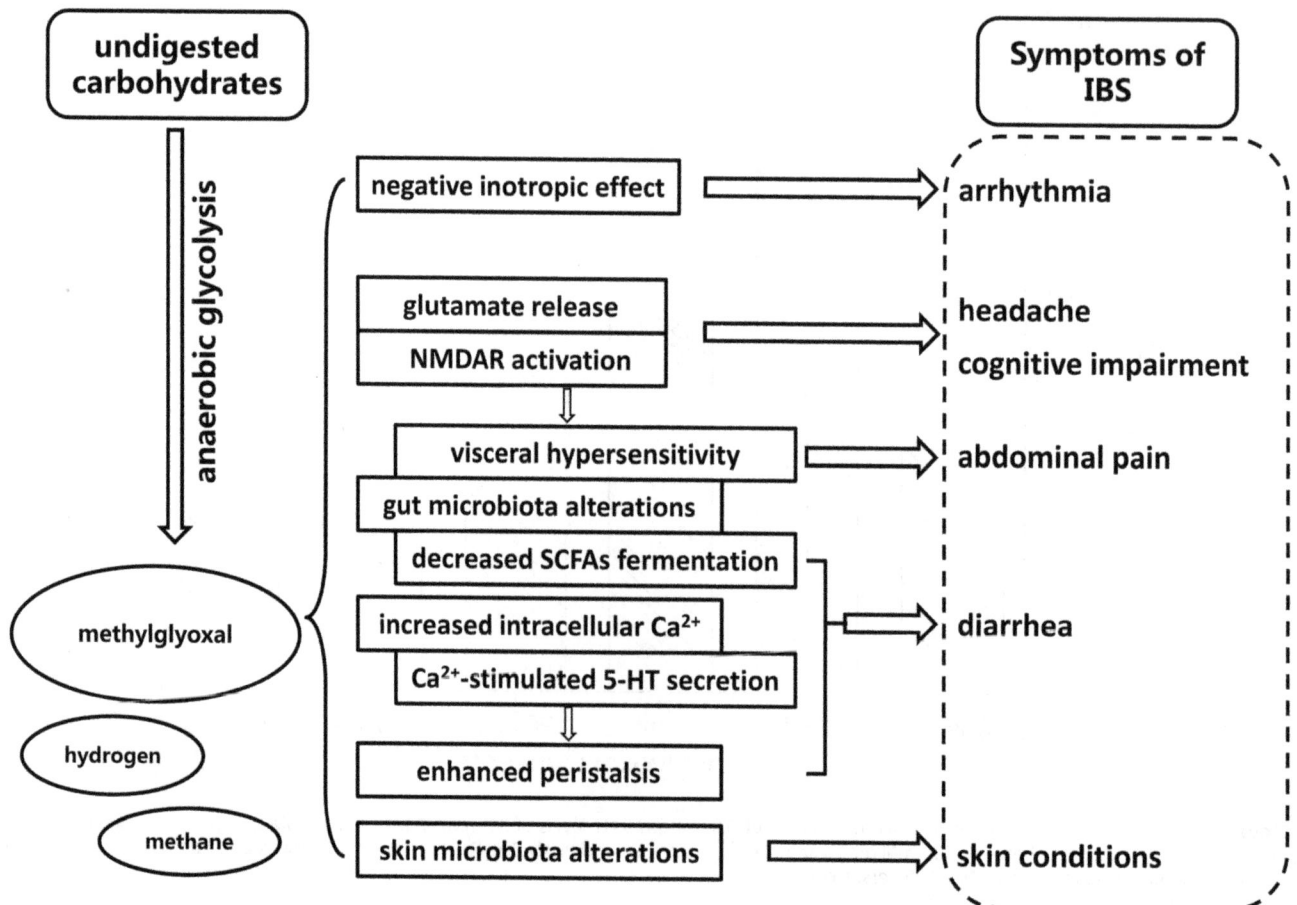

Figure 6. Diagram showing the mechanism that methylglyoxal induces various symptoms of IBS.

phenomenon had never been observed in the control rats, which suggested that methylglyoxal exposure had a positive effect on diarrhea in rats. It was shown that methylglyoxal (10 mM) induced contraction of guinea pig ileum in a standard organ bath preparation [5]. Stimulation of colonic transit determines insufficient time for intestine to absorb the water and leads to diarrhea. There is also a possibility that methylglyoxal induces diarrhea via alteration of intestinal microflora. Methylglyoxal is cytotoxic and growth of bacteria such as *E. coli* is inhibited by 0.2–1.2 mM methylglyoxal [23]. E. Mavric demonstrated that Manuka honey had notable antimicrobial activity which originates directly from the high level of methylglyoxal it contains [24]. The alteration of intestinal microbiota caused by methylglyoxal may depress the fermentation of SCFAs, and the decrease of SCFAs in the intestinal lumen will reduce water and sodium absorption in the colon and induce diarrhea eventually.

Serotonin (5-HT) is an essential monoamine neurotransmitter mainly located in the enterochromaffin (EC) cells lining the intestinal mucosa and the remainder is produced in central serotonergic neurons. Numerous studies have provided us with an in-depth understanding of the complex regulation of 5-HT on gastrointestinal functions. Abnormal regulation of 5-HT results in unusual motility and secretory activities of alimentary tract, diarrhea, visceral hypersensitivity, chronic constipation, and other gastrointestinal disorders. Previous studies have confirmed that methylglyoxal induces a rise in intracellular Ca^{2+} concentration by activating Ca^{2+} channels in membrane of eukaryotic cells [25–27]. Ca^{2+}-dependent secretion of 5-HT in EC cells is mediated by

activation of Ca^{2+} channels [28] and the release and secretion of 5-HT could be inhibited by calcium antagonist nifedipine [29]. Taken together, these findings suggest that methylglyoxal may stimulate 5-HT release by induction of Ca^{2+} influx in EC cells. Our results demonstrated that the serum levels of 5-HT were significantly increased in the 30, 60, 90 mM groups compared with controls ($p<0.01$), however, the difference between the 120 mM group and the control group was not significantly ($p>0.05$), while the serum level in the 150 mM group was lower than controls ($p<0.01$). It was consistent with the previous study, which showed that intracellular free calcium concentration was decreased with the increase of the concentration of methylglyoxal [30]. These data therefore reveal that methylglyoxal may modulate the serum 5-HT in a concentration-dependent manner. Serotonin is also known as a key agent that accelerates intestinal peristalsis in IBS via acting at specific serotonin-receptor subtypes. Nevertheless, the 5-HT level in rats treated with 30 mM methylglyoxal was significantly increased than all the other groups, and it implied that the 5-HT increase might not be the only trigger for diarrhea in rats. This situation could be interpreted as a combination of two factors, the toxic effects mediated by methylglyoxal including direct stimulation of intestinal motility and interfering with the ecological balance of the intestinal microflora, and the modulation of 5-HT. In the 30 mM group, stimulation of bowel movement due to increased 5-HT played a dominant role in the onset of diarrhea, while the toxic effects of methylglyoxal were secondary. In the 60 mM and 90 mM groups, the results suggested that the symptoms of the two groups were caused by both factors. The data of the 120 mM and 150 mM groups illustrated that diarrhea of the rats exposed to high concentrations of methylglyoxal was mainly maintained by the methylglyoxal toxicity.

Abdominal pain can be one of the most prominent symptoms of IBS and is attributed to visceral hypersensitivity. The data showed that the distension volumes to achieve an AWR score of 3 were remarkably lower in all rats exposed to methylglyoxal. A previous study revealed that visceral hypersensitivity involved the activation of spinal NMDA and non-NMDA receptors, meanwhile methylglyoxal could precisely induce the activation via a process which is discussed in the following passage. Another survey indicated that antibiotics could perturb intestinal microbiota, change the content of colon sensory neurotransmitter, and thus produce increased visceral sensitivity [31]. Investigation has shown that probiotics therapy prevents antibiotic-induced visceral hyperalgesia in mice [32]. Probiotics may locally control the nociceptive information transmitted to the intestinal nervous system by mediating the expression of receptors on epithelial cell such as opioid receptor and cannabinoid receptor type 2. Therefore, we infer that abdominal pain associated with IBS may result from methylglyoxal-induced visceral hypersensitivity and alterations of gut microflora.

A study of human neuroblastoma SH-SY5Y cells indicated that methylglyoxal was associated with the early plasma membrane depolarization and glutamate release and it could be prevented by N-methyl-d-aspartate (NMDA) receptors antagonists. The cell membrane was depolarized after a few minutes of exposure to methylglyoxal [33], followed by glutamate release, the relief of the Mg^{2+} block of NMDA receptors and Ca^{2+} influx, and afterwards it triggered a series of biochemical reactions in the neurons [34], and further changed the nature of the postsynaptic membrane and established the Long-term potentiation (LPT). Hippocampal LPT is involved in memory formation and consolidation. It may explain why patients with IBS exhibit symptoms of memory loss, poor concentration and other cognitive disorders. Glutamate is implicated in the development and maintenance of headache via interacting with its receptors [35]. The release of glutamate can activate the non-NMDA and NMDA receptors in spinal and supraspinal sites. The latter makes neurons more susceptible to nociceptive inputs and thus induces central sensitization, which is one of the putative mechanisms of headache [36,37]. Our results were consistent with the notion in that head scratching and grooming were significantly induced in all treatment groups.

Depression is a mood disorder with a variety of causes. The main characteristics is pervasive and lasting low mood and it is a common symptom in patients with IBS [38]. The prevalence of depression was up to 37.1% with the OR of 6.3 in a recent survey [39]. A clinical research involved one hundred eleven individuals found that the Beck's inventory depression scores were significantly high in female patients with isolated fructose malabsorption

and combined fructose/lactose malabsorption. The result was believed to be associated with increased fermentation of carbohydrates [40]. In support of this study, fructose elimination diet was found to improve symptoms of depression as well as gastrointestinal symptoms [41]. Likewise, probiotics could also alleviate the depression-like behaviors in adult mice [42]. The results in the present study showed that methylglyoxal might give rise to the occurrence of depression-like behaviors in rats. A newly proposed conceptual model of microbiota-gut-brain axis may explain the situation. Microbiota accesses the brain and influences behavior through bacterial products that gain access to the brain via the bloodstream, via the release of gut hormones such as 5-hydroxytryptamine (5-HT) from EC cells, via cytokine released from mucosal immune cells, or via afferent neural pathways [43]. Moreover, microbiota alters the expression of brain-derived neurotropic factor (BDNF), activity of Hypothalamic - pituitary-adrenal (HPA) axis, which has been confirmed to be closely related to depression-like behaviors [44,45]. In support of the proposition, a probiotic, *Bifidobacteria infantis*, may be beneficial in the treatment of depression [46].

Studies have hitherto revealed potential link between methylglyoxal and other diseases. Methylglyoxal was observed to induce a major negative inotropic effect on the isolated perfused guinea pig heart in vitro, followed by a small positive inotropic effect [5]. Moreover, skin conditions in patients with IBS may be closely related to the skin microflora. Gueniche et al. indicated that alteration of the enteric microbiota through ingested probiotics showed beneficial effects on maintaining skin homeostasis after ultraviolet exposure [47]. The outline of our hypothesis is summarized and illustrated in Fig 6. The limitations of the current study are that we focus exclusively on diarrhea-predominant IBS and only one bacterial metabolite. Whether metabolites besides methylglyoxal can induce symptoms in constipation-predominant IBS and other subtypes requires further investigation.

In conclusion, the present finding suggests that a wide range of systemic symptoms of IBS including diarrhea, abdominal pain, headache, depression, cognitive impairment, arrhythmia and skin problems may be induced by methylglyoxal, an intestinal bacterial toxic metabolite. The result offers a hopeful target in the search for a unitary view on the etiology of IBS.

Author Contributions

Conceived and designed the experiments: MJ SZ. Performed the experiments: SZ TJ YC NG. Analyzed the data: SZ LZ. Contributed reagents/materials/analysis tools: SZ LZ. Wrote the paper: SZ MJ.

References

1. Matthews SB, Campbell AK (2000) When sugar is not so sweet. Lancet 355: 1330.
2. Simren M, Mansson A, Langkilde AM, Svedlund J, Abrahamsson H, et al. (2001) Food-related gastrointestinal symptoms in the irritable bowel syndrome. Digestion 63: 108–115.
3. Metchnikoff E, Mitchell PC (1908) The prolongation of life: optimistic studies. New York & London,: G. P. Putnam's sons. l p.l., v -xx p., p.
4. Eadala P, Matthews SB, Waud JP, Green JT, Campbell AK (2011) Association of lactose sensitivity with inflammatory bowel disease—demonstrated by analysis of genetic polymorphism, breath gases and symptoms. Aliment Pharmacol Ther 34: 735–746.
5. Campbell AK, Matthews SB, Vassel N, Cox CD, Naseem R, et al. (2010) Bacterial metabolic 'toxins': a new mechanism for lactose and food intolerance, and irritable bowel syndrome. Toxicology 278: 268–276.
6. Degen J, Vogel M, Richter D, Hellwig M, Henle T (2013) Metabolic Transit of Dietary Methylglyoxal. J Agric Food Chem.
7. Naseem R, Wann KT, Holland IB, Campbell AK (2009) ATP regulates calcium efflux and growth in E. coli. J Mol Biol 391: 42–56.
8. Lee BH, Hsu WH, Hsu YW, Pan TM (2013) Dimerumic acid attenuates receptor for advanced glycation endproducts signal to inhibit inflammation and diabetes mediated by Nrf2 activation and promotes methylglyoxal metabolism into d-lactic acid. Free Radic Biol Med 60C: 7–16.
9. Antognelli C, Mezzasoma L, Fettucciari K, Talesa VN (2013) A novel mechanism of methylglyoxal cytotoxicity in prostate cancer cells. Int J Biochem Cell Biol 45: 836–844.
10. Matafome P, Sena C, Seica R (2012) Methylglyoxal, obesity, and diabetes. Endocrine.

11. Li W, Maloney RE, Circu ML, Alexander JS, Aw TY (2013) Acute carbonyl stress induces occludin glycation and brain microvascular endothelial barrier dysfunction: role for glutathione-dependent metabolism of methylglyoxal. Free Radic Biol Med 54: 51–61.

12. Lee do K, Jang S, Baek EH, Kim MJ, Lee KS, et al. (2009) Lactic acid bacteria affect serum cholesterol levels, harmful fecal enzyme activity, and fecal water content. Lipids Health Dis 8: 21.

13. Al-Chaer ED, Kawasaki M, Pasricha PJ (2000) A new model of chronic visceral hypersensitivity in adult rats induced by colon irritation during postnatal development. Gastroenterology 119: 1276–1285.

14. Kemper RH, Spoelstra MB, Meijler WJ, Ter Horst GJ (1998) Lipopolysaccha-ride-induced hyperalgesia of intracranial capsaicin sensitive afferents in conscious rats. Pain 78: 181–190.

15. Kemper RH, Meijler WJ, Ter Horst GJ (1997) Trigeminovascular stimulation in conscious rats. Neuroreport 8: 1123–1126.

16. D'Aquila PS, Brain P, Willner P (1994) Effects of chronic mild stress on performance in behavioural tests relevant to anxiety and depression. Physiol Behav 56: 861–867.

17. Ping F, Shang J, Zhou J, Zhang H, Zhang L (2012) 5-HT(1A) receptor and apoptosis contribute to interferon-alpha-induced "depressive-like" behavior in mice. Neurosci Lett 514: 173–178.

18. Malinen E, Krogius-Kurikka L, Lyra A, Nikkila J, Jaaskelainen A, et al. (2010) Association of symptoms with gastrointestinal microbiota in irritable bowel syndrome. World J Gastroenterol 16: 4532–4540.

19. Szent-Gyorgyi A, Egyud LG, McLaughlin JA (1967) Keto-aldehydes and cell division. Science 155: 539–541.

20. Talukdar D, Chaudhuri BS, Ray M, Ray S (2009) Critical evaluation of toxic versus beneficial effects of methylglyoxal. Biochemistry (Mosc) 74: 1059–1069.

21. Simon GL, Gorbach SL (1984) Intestinal flora in health and disease. Gastroenterology 86: 174–193.

22. Guarner F, Malagelada JR (2003) Gut flora in health and disease. Lancet 361: 512–519.

23. Egyud LG, Szent-Gyorgyi A (1966) Cell division, SH, ketoaldehydes, and cancer. Proc Natl Acad Sci U S A 55: 388–393.

24. Mavric E, Wittmann S, Barth G, Henle T (2008) Identification and quantification of methylglyoxal as the dominant antibacterial constituent of Manuka (Leptospermum scoparium) honeys from New Zealand. Mol Nutr Food Res 52: 483–489.

25. Jan CR, Chen CH, Wang SC, Kuo SY (2005) Effect of methylglyoxal on intracellular calcium levels and viability in renal tubular cells. Cell Signal 17: 847–855.

26. Mukohda M, Yamawaki H, Nomura H, Okada M, Hara Y (2009) Methylglyoxal inhibits smooth muscle contraction in isolated blood vessels. J Pharmacol Sci 109: 305–310.

27. Cook LJ, Davies J, Yates AP, Elliott AC, Lovell J, et al. (1998) Effects of methylglyoxal on rat pancreatic beta-cells. Biochem Pharmacol 55: 1361–1367.

28. Lomax RB, Gallego S, Novalbos J, Garcia AG, Warhurst G (1999) L-Type calcium channels in enterochromaffin cells from guinea pig and human duodenal crypts: an in situ study. Gastroenterology 117: 1363–1369.

29. Timar Peregrin A, Ahlman H, Jodal M, Lundgren O (1997) Effects of calcium channel blockade on intestinal fluid secretion: sites of action. Acta Physiol Scand 160: 379–386.

30. Campbell AK, Naseem R, Holland IB, Matthews SB, Wann KT (2007) Methylglyoxal and other carbonyl metabolites induce lanthanum-sensitive Ca2+ transients and inhibit growth in E. coli. Arch Biochem Biophys 468: 107–113.

31. Verdu EF, Bercik P, Verma-Gandhu M, Huang XX, Blennerhassett P, et al. (2006) Specific probiotic therapy attenuates antibiotic induced visceral hypersensitivity in mice. Gut 55: 182–190.

32. Eutamene H, Lamine F, Chabo C, Theodorou V, Rochat F, et al. (2007) Synergy between Lactobacillus paracasei and its bacterial products to counteract stress-induced gut permeability and sensitivity increase in rats. J Nutr 137: 1901–1907.

33. de Arriba SG, Krugel U, Regenthal R, Vissiennon Z, Verdaguer E, et al. (2006) Carbonyl stress and NMDA receptor activation contribute to methylglyoxal neurotoxicity. Free Radic Biol Med 40: 779–790.

34. Naarala J, Nykvist P, Tuomala M, Savolainen K (1993) Excitatory amino acid-induced slow biphasic responses of free intracellular calcium in human neuroblastoma cells. FEBS Lett 330: 222–226.

35. Urban MO, Gebhart GF (1999) Central mechanisms in pain. Med Clin North Am 83: 585–596.

36. Trist DG (2000) Excitatory amino acid agonists and antagonists: pharmacology and therapeutic applications. Pharm Acta Helv 74: 221–229.

37. Gallai V, Alberti A, Gallai B, Coppola F, Floridi A, et al. (2003) Glutamate and nitric oxide pathway in chronic daily headache: evidence from cerebrospinal fluid. Cephalalgia 23: 166–174.

38. Campbell AK, Matthews SB (2005) Darwin's illness revealed. Postgrad Med J 81: 248–251.

39. Kabra N, Nadkarni A (2013) Prevalence of depression and anxiety in irritable bowel syndrome: A clinic based study from India. Indian J Psychiatry 55: 77–80.

40. Ledochowski M, Widner B, Sperner-Unterweger B, Propst T, Vogel W, et al. (2000) Carbohydrate malabsorption syndromes and early signs of mental depression in females. Dig Dis Sci 45: 1255–1259.

41. Ledochowski M, Widner B, Bair H, Probst T, Fuchs D (2000) Fructose- and sorbitol-reduced diet improves mood and gastrointestinal disturbances in fructose malabsorbers. Scand J Gastroenterol 35: 1048–1052.

42. Bravo JA, Forsythe P, Chew MV, Escaravage E, Savignac HM, et al. (2011) Ingestion of Lactobacillus strain regulates emotional behavior and central GABA receptor expression in a mouse via the vagus nerve. Proc Natl Acad Sci U S A 108: 16050–16055.

43. Collins SM, Bercik P (2012) The interplay between the intestinal microbiota and the brain. Nat Rev Microbiol 10: 735–742.

44. Bercik P, Denou E, Collins J, Jackson W, Lu J, et al. (2011) The intestinal microbiota affect central levels of brain-derived neurotropic factor and behavior in mice. Gastroenterology 141: 599–609, 609 e591–593.

45. Ait-Belgnaoui A, Durand H, Cartier C, Chaumaz G, Eutamene H, et al. (2012) Prevention of gut leakiness by a probiotic treatment leads to attenuated HPA response to an acute psychological stress in rats. Psychoneuroendocrinology 37: 1885–1895.

46. Desbonnet L, Garrett L, Clarke G, Bienenstock J, Dinan TG (2008) The probiotic Bifidobacteria infantis: An assessment of potential antidepressant properties in the rat. J Psychiatr Res 43: 164–174.

47. Gueniche A, Benyacoub J, Buetler TM, Smola H, Blum S (2006) Supplemen-tation with oral probiotic bacteria maintains cutaneous immune homeostasis after UV exposure. Eur J Dermatol 16: 511–517.

11

A Novel Familial Mutation in the *PCSK1* Gene that Alters the Oxyanion Hole Residue of Proprotein Convertase 1/3 and Impairs its Enzymatic Activity

Michael Wilschanski[1]*, Montaser Abbasi[1], Elias Blanco[2,3], Iris Lindberg[2], Michael Yourshaw[3], David Zangen[4], Itai Berger[5], Eyal Shteyer[1], Orit Pappo[6], Benjamin Bar-Oz[7], Martin G. Martín[3], Orly Elpeleg[8]

1 Gastroenterology Unit, Division of Pediatrics, Hadassah Hebrew University Hospital, Jerusalem, Israel, 2 Department of Anatomy and Neurobiology, University of Maryland-Baltimore, Baltimore, Maryland, United States of America, 3 Department of Pediatrics, Division of Gastroenterology and Nutrition, Mattel Children's Hospital and the David Geffen School of Medicine, University of California Los Angeles, Los Angeles, California, United States of America, 4 Endocrinology Unit, Division of Pediatrics, Hadassah Hebrew University Hospital, Jerusalem, Israel, 5 Neurology Unit, Division of Pediatrics, Hadassah Hebrew University Hospital, Jerusalem, Israel, 6 Department of Pathology, Hadassah Hebrew University Hospital, Jerusalem, Israel, 7 Department of Neonatology, Hadassah Hebrew University Hospital, Jerusalem, Israel, 8 Monique and Jacques Roboh Department of Genetic Research, Hadassah Hebrew University Hospital, Jerusalem, Israel

Abstract

Four siblings presented with congenital diarrhea and various endocrinopathies. Exome sequencing and homozygosity mapping identified five regions, comprising 337 protein-coding genes that were shared by three affected siblings. Exome sequencing identified a novel homozygous N309K mutation in the proprotein convertase subtilisin/kexin type 1 (*PCSK1*) gene, encoding the neuroendocrine convertase 1 precursor (PC1/3) which was recently reported as a cause of Congenital Diarrhea Disorder (CDD). The *PCSK1* mutation affected the oxyanion hole transition state-stabilizing amino acid within the active site, which is critical for appropriate-proprotein maturation and enzyme activity. Unexpectedly, the N309K mutant protein exhibited normal, though slowed, prodomain removal and was secreted from both HEK293 and Neuro2A cells. However, the secreted enzyme showed no catalytic activity, and was not processed into the 66 kDa form. We conclude that the N309K enzyme is able to cleave its own propeptide but is catalytically inert against *in trans* substrates, and that this variant accounts for the enteric and systemic endocrinopathies seen in this large consanguineous kindred.

Editor: Stefan Strack, University of Iowa, United States of America

Funding: Funding provided by the National Institute of Diabetes and Digestive and Kidney Diseases (#DK083762), and California Institute of Regenerative Medicine (CIRM), RT2-01985 to MM and DA05084 to IL. The funders had no role in study design, data collection and analysis, decision to publish, or preparation of the manuscript.

Competing Interests: The authors have declared that no competing interests exist.

* Email: michaelwil@hadassah.org.il

Introduction

Congenital diarrheal disorders (CDDs) are a group of devastating and potentially fatal neonatal enteropathies that often require parenteral nutrition. Recently Canani *et al.* [1] proposed classifying these disorders into 4 groups: 1) defects in digestion, absorption, and transport of nutrients and electrolytes, such as glucose-galactose malabsorption or sucrase-isomaltase deficiency, caused by mutations in *SLC5A1* [2] and *SI* [3] respectively; 2) disorders of enterocyte differentiation and polarization, such as microvillus inclusion disease and tufting enteropathy, caused by mutations in *MYO5B* [4] and *EPCAM* [5] respectively; 3) dysregulation of the intestinal immune response, as in immune dysregulation, polyendocrinopathy, enteropathy, X-linked (IPEX) syndrome caused by mutations in *FOXP3* [6] and 4) defects of enteroendocrine cell differentiation, as may be caused, for example, by mutations in *NEUROG3* [7]. These patients frequently endure a complex and costly diagnostic odyssey that often fails to produce a definitive diagnosis. Once infection is ruled out, in most cases the disorder is found to be inherited in an autosomal recessive manner; mutations in any of a large number of genes may be responsible [8]. Identification of a causal mutation can lead to improved management of the disease but genome-wide screening for mutations has not yet entered standard practice [9].

Mild mutations in the *PCSK1* gene (proprotein convertase subtilisin/kexin type 1) are associated with obesity [10], and more severe, rare mutations have increasingly been recognized as a cause of malabsorptive diarrhea and other endocrinopathies in a disorder called proprotein convertase 1/3 (PC1/3) deficiency (OMIM: 600955) [11]. The enzyme encoded by *PCSK1*, the neuroendocrine convertase 1 precursor, cleaves itself into the active form, neuroendocrine convertase 1 (also called prohormone convertase 1, proprotein convertase 1, and PC1), which is responsible for processing multiple peptide hormones within the enteroendocrine cell. Other rare heterozygous mutations in *PCSK1* have been observed in the general population, which likely would be harmful in an individual with two damaged copies of the gene [12]. PC1/3 deficiency involves a significant risk of mortality and failure to thrive secondary to severe generalized malabsorptive diarrhea in early childhood. However, the requirement for parenteral nutritional support decreases after 18 months of age, while various major systemic endocrinopathies develop [9,11,13–15]. To date, 17 individuals in 15 families have been reported to have disease-causing mutations in *PCSK1*. Thus enteroendocrine cell dysfunction governs the early clinical phenotype, while malabsorption may actually lessen the severity of the obesity that develops at later ages. Growth hormone deficiency, adrenal insufficiency, central diabetes insipidus, and hypogonadism are commonly observed [11]. Here, we describe four siblings with PC1/3 deficiency resulting from a novel mutation in the *PCSK1* gene.

Material and Methods

Subjects

The study was approved by the ethical IRB of Hadassah Hebrew University Medical Center and the parents signed informed consent.

Genomic DNA Isolation

Genomic DNA was extracted from blood by standard procedures.

Linkage analysis

A search for common homozygous regions in the DNA samples of affected patients was performed, using Affymetrix GeneChip Human Mapping 250K Nsp Array, as previously described [16].

Whole exome analysis

Protein coding exon sequences were enriched in the DNA sample of patient II-5 (fig. 1) using the SureSelect Human All Exon 50 Mb Kit (Agilent Technologies, Santa Clara, CA, USA). 100 base, paired-end sequences were read by HiSeq2000 (Illumina, San Diego, CA, USA). Reads alignment and variant calling were performed with DNAnexus software (Palo Alto, CA) using the default parameters with the human genome assembly hg19 (GRCh37) as a reference.

Transient transfection of expression vectors

A wild-type human PC1/3 (NP_000430.3)-encoding plasmid, with a Flag-tag sequence inserted between the prodomain and the catalytic domain, was mutated at residue Asn309 to encode Lys (N309K AA$\underline{C}$ = >AA$\underline{G}$; Genscript, Piscataway NJ) and verified by sequencing in its entirety. No other mutations were present. The wild-type and mutant plasmids were transiently transfected into either HEK293 or Neuro2A cells using FuGene (Promega, Madison WI); two days later, the overnight conditioned Optimem (containing 100 μg/ml aprotinin) was assessed for protein expression by Western blotting and was tested for enzymatic activity using a fluorogenic substrate, pERTKR-AMC (Peptides International, Lexington, KY), as previously described [11–12].

Pulse-chase experiments. Neuro2A cells were transfected with either wild-type or mutant PC1/3 vectors and labeled with ^{35}S-methionine for 20 min, as described in Blanco et al. [17]. Cells were then chased for 2 h in medium containing cold methionine and lysed in boiling buffer for immunoprecipitation using N-terminal PC1/3 antisera (2B5) plus C-terminal PC1/3 antisera (3BF), and chase media were also immunoprecipitated. Immunoprecipitates were separated on 15% SDS-polyacrylamide gels, dried, and subjected to phosphoimaging.

Histology

Small bowel mucosal biopsies from subjects II-2 and II-5 were stained by standard hematoxylin and eosin.

Results

Clinical Phenotype

Following one early first trimester miscarriage, four children were born at normal birth weight to healthy parents, who were first cousins of Moslem Arab ethnicity. The first child (II-2) developed severe malabsorptive diarrhea during first week of life with steatorrhea but without evidence of a protein-losing enteropathy (Fig. 1). Various dietary manipulations were attempted including hydrosylate and amino acid based formulae which failed. She was started after the first month of life on parenteral nutrition (PN), which was continued until five years of age.

A residual metabolic acidosis, resulting most probably from the chronic diarrhea, was treated by bicarbonate until eight years of age. Repeated small intestinal biopsies showed non-specific enteropathy including mild villous atrophy, slight increase in number of intraepithelial lymphocytes, and chronic inflammation of lamina propria (Fig. 2). The usual serologies indicative of celiac disease were undetectable.

Initially her relatively low FT4 levels were attributed to sick euthyroid syndrome, but as they persisted into her second year of life in spite of an improving clinical condition she was diagnosed with mild central hypothyroidism (TSH levels of 2–3 mIU/ml despite low free T4 levels of 7–9 pmol/l) and received thyroid replacement therapy. Given her poor growth rate and decreased peak GH response in 2 stimulation tests (only 3.5 and 6.5 ng/ml) by 3–4 years of age she did also receive GH replacement therapy that resulted in adequate growth rate with a height of 156 cm at 12 years of age and breast and pubic hair development at Tanner stage 3–4.

Other remitting endocrinopathies included self-limited episodes of diabetes insipidus (DI) with polyuria, a low urine osmolarity (70–150 mOsm/l), and elevated serum osmolarity (>300 mOsm/l). These episodes ended spontaneously with a short course of intranasal desmopressin (ddAVP) treatment. Finally, a gradual weight gain was initially attributed to a better appetite. However, she became increasingly severely obese by six years of age (Body Mass Index (BMI) –21.6), (50th percentile 15.4) and continued to become more obese despite adequate GH and thyroid replacement, and intensive nutritional therapeutic guidance. Her neurologic development is normal and she has no convulsive disorder.

The two subsequent sisters (II-3, 4) were born after uneventful pregnancies and deliveries, but died at 9 days and 5 months of age respectively suffering from intractable seizures with left hemisphere rhythmic epileptiform activity by EEG. MR/MRS (at the age of 5 months) revealed periventricular white matter volume loss with ventricular dilatation. The second of these children had also recurrent episodes of diarrhea and hypothyroidism, and were treated with PN and thyroxine. Brain ultrasound scan in this infant was normal. The seizures were of multiple type (mainly clonic and myoclonic types) and unresponsive to all anti-epileptic drugs in various combinations. Both epileptic patients have neither permanent electrolyte nor metabolic imbalances associated with diarrhea. Epilepsy is an unexpected finding in patients with CDD especially in the absence of significant electrolyte or metabolic imbalances.

The youngest sibling (II-5) is now a one-year-old male who was born at normal birth weight following an uneventful pregnancy. He presented with neonatal diarrhea reminiscent of his two older

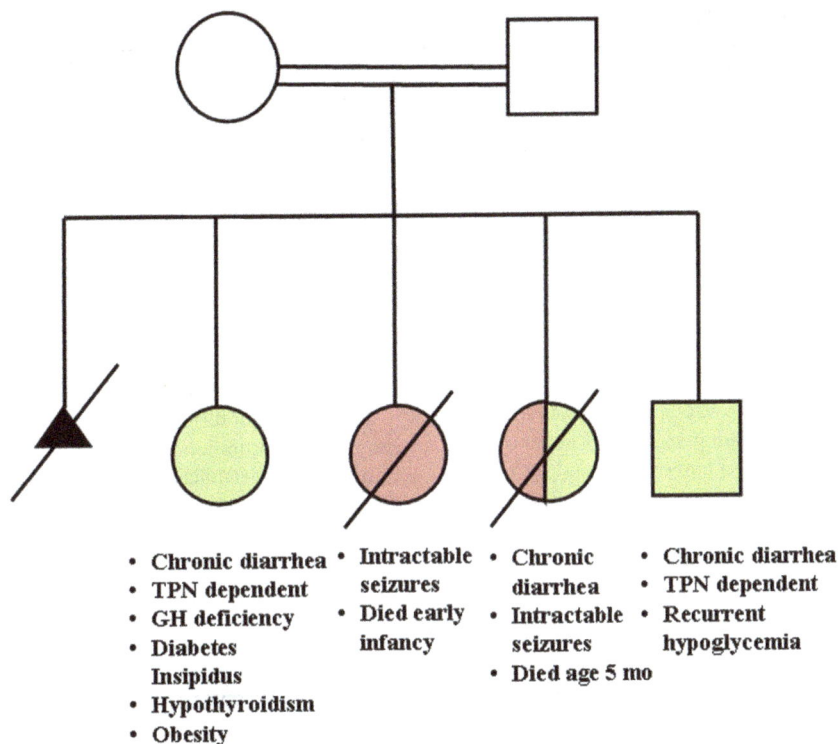

Figure 1. Family Pedigree. Pedigree showing intractable diarrhea (green) and seizures (red) and other clinical phenotypes. A slash through the symbol indicates that the subject is deceased, and a double line between the parents indicates a consanguineous union.

sisters and required home PN for one year. No endocrinopathies or convulsive disorders have been found thus far and his small bowel biopsy showed only non-specific changes.

Sequencing/Bioinformatics

The normal intestinal absorption of patient II-3, who suffered from severe epilepsy, suggested the presence of two non-linked disorders in the family, intractable diarrhea and drug-resistant epilepsy, both of which may have been transmitted in an autosomal-recessive manner, given the parental consanguinity. In order to identify the diarrhea-causing gene, we genotyped 250K SNPs in patients II-2 and II-4 who had intractable diarrhea and in patient II-3 who had normal bowel movement. This analysis

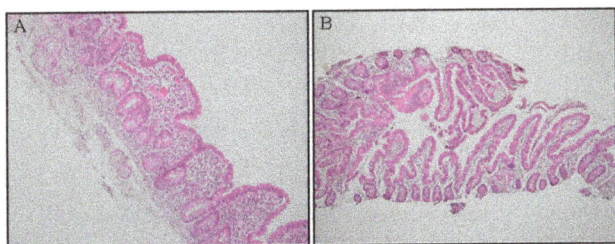

Figure 2. H&E staining of small bowel biopsies from patients II-2 and II-5. A) Mild villous atrophy associated with a slight increase in number of intraepithelial lymphocytes, and mild chronic inflammation of lamina propria (electron microscopy not shown-normal microvillous architecture); B) the villi appear normal without lymphocytic abnormalities in the intraepithelial and lamina propria compartments. Moreover, very few plasma cells were seen, and the epithelium was devoid of abnormal apoptosis, or abnormalities of microvilli.

resulted in the identification of five homozygous regions (Table 1) where the SNP genotype of patients II-2 and II-4 was identical and differed from that of patient II-3.

These regions encompassed 337 protein-coding genes and we therefore opted for whole exome sequencing of the DNA of patient II-5. The average coverage of the exons within the linked regions was 63X and 97.1% of the exons were covered >7X. Altogether we found 1089 missense or indel variants (only 46 of which were homozygous) that were not present in dbSNP version 129 or in the in-house dbSNP. Only four missense variants were located within the shared homozygosity blocks (Table 2).

One of these variants, the N309K mutation in the *PCSK1* gene, appeared to be the probable cause of the CDD and endocrinopathies, given that other mutations in *PCSK1* are known to cause similar symptoms, whereas the other three variants (HADHA, FBXL17 and GTF3C2) are not known to be involved in CDD. The N309K mutation in the *PCSK1* gene was predicted to be deleterious by multiple *in silico* methods: SIFT [18] , PolyPhen2 [19], LRT [20], MutationAssessor [21], MutationTaster [22], Condel [23], and CAROL [24]. The mutation was not reported in the 1092 genomes of the 1000 Genomes project [25] nor in the 6503 exomes in the NHLBI Exome Sequencing project [26] (Table 2) Moreover the probability of splicing changes due to the intronic variants in FBXL17 and GTF3C2 was predicted to be low. Interestingly, the rare, but predicted as deleterious HADHA variant is associated with long-chain 3-hydroxyl-CoA dehydrogenase (LCHAD) deficiency (OMIM: 609016), but malabsorptive diarrhea is not associated with this condition.

The enzyme encoded by *PCSK1*, prohormone convertase 1/3 (PC1/3), processes latent precursors to peptide hormones into their biologically active products within the enteroendocrine cell. The Asn residue at position 309 in the PC1/3 active site (the

Table 1. Homozygous regions linked to the enteric disease in the family.

chromosome	start	end	size (Mb)
2	18294643	30607011	12.31
3	178985197	190692992	11.71
5	89679361	109389770	19.71
10	87890424	95523820	7.63
13	19625269	24664802	5.04

peptidase S8 family domain) is conserved in all vertebrates (Fig 3). Sanger sequencing of other affected and unaffected family members confirmed that this mutation segregated in the family, with patients II-2, II-4 and II-5 being homozygous and the parents (I-1 and I-2) and patient II-3 heterozygous (Fig 4).

Functional Analysis and *In Vitro* Assessment

The position of this mutation corresponds to a residue critical to proprotein maturation and enzyme activity, the oxyanion hole transition state-stabilizing amino acid Asn309. To validate the functional significance of this rare variant, we expressed the wild type and the mutant PC1/3 protein in HEK293 and Neuro2A cells and tested its activity. Western blotting indicated that the N309K mutant protein exhibited apparently normal prodomain

Table 2. Homozygous variants within the diarrhea-linked regions of patient II-5.

Gene	HADHA	GTF3C2	PCSK1	FBXL17
CHROM	2	2	5	5
POS	26453084	27566454	95746646	107521954
ID	rs71441018	rs112001928	-	-
REF	C	A	G	G
ALT	G	G	C	A
Transcript	ENST00000380649	ENST00000359541	ENST00000311106	ENST00000542267
cDNA	c.652G>C	c.-24-9T>C	c.927C>G	c.1615-6C>T
Protein	p.Val218Leu	-	p.Asn309Lys	-
Exon	7/20	intron 1/18	8/14	intron 5/8
Amino acid	218/763	-/911	309/753	-/701
Consequence	missense_variant	intron_variant	missense_variant	splice_region_variant, intron_variant
Gene name	hydroxyacyl-CoA dehydrogenase/3-ketoacyl-CoA thiolase/enoyl-CoA hydratase (trifunctional protein), alpha subunit	general transcription factor IIIC, polypeptide 2, beta 110kDa	proprotein convertase subtilisin/kexin type 1	F-box and leucine-rich repeat protein 17
OMIM	LCHAD deficiency (609016; Trifunctional protein deficiency (609015)	-	Obesity and endocrinopathy due to impaired processing of prohormones (600955)	-
CAROL[24]	deleterious(1)	-	deleterious(1)	-
Condel[23]	deleterious(0.842)	-	deleterious(1)	-
LRT[20]	deleterious(1.03E-08)	-	deleterious(1.25E-10)	-
Mutation Assessor[21]	medium(2.76)	-	high(4)	-
Mutation Taster[22]	disease causing(1)	disease causing(0.98)	disease causing(1)	disease causing(0.85)
PolyPhen2[19]	probably_damaging(0.999)	-	probably_damaging(1)	-
SIFT[18]	deleterious(0.01)	-	deleterious(0)	-
African American AF(hom)*	0(0/2203)	0.003(0/2203)	0(2203)	-
European American AF(hom)*	0.000465(0/4300)	0.023(3/4297)	0(4300)	-

* Allele frequency (number of homozygous individuals) in the Exome Variant Server, NHLBI Exome Sequencing Project (ESP)[26].
REF – GRCh37 reference allele, ALT – variant allele, OMIM – Online Mendelian Inheritance in Man[36].

Organism	300##########309##########318
HUMAN	DCNDGQRGGNGSAWVFISG
RHESUS	DCNDGQRGGNGSAWVFISG
MOUSE	DCDDGQRGGNGSAWVFISG
DOG	DCNDGQRGGNGSAWVFISG
ELEPHANT	DCDDGQRGGNGSAWVFISG
OPOSSUM	DCNDGQRGGNGSAWVFISG
CHICKEN	DCNDGQRGGNGSAWVFISG
X_TROPICALIS	DCNDGQRGGNGSAWVFISG
ZEBRAFISH	DCNDGQRGGNGSAWVFISG

↑
N309K

Figure 3. Alignment of N309K missense variant to members of the PC1/3 gene family. The location of the missense mutation within a conserved region in the catalytic domain of the PC1/3 gene family.

removal and was efficiently secreted from both HEK293 and Neuro2A cells (Fig 5). However, the secreted enzyme showed no catalytic activity (panels A1–B1) and was not processed into the 66 kDa form independently of cell context (panels A2–B3), indicating no *in trans* activity.

In order to better assess prodomain removal, we performed radiolabeling experiments of *PCSK1*-transfected Neuro 2A cells. Fig 5, Panel C shows that the N309K mutant underwent only slight prodomain removal (prodomain = 94 kDa form; mature form = 87 kDa) within the 20 minute pulse period, but showed complete prodomain removal within the 2 h chase period in media samples. In agreement with the Western blots, the mature 87 kDa mature form of the N309K mutant was secreted. These results contrast with results obtained using the G593R *PCSK1* mutant, which is totally unable to remove its own propeptide and is retained in the endoplasmic reticulum [15]. In lysate samples from Neuro2A transfected cells, the G593R proprotein was unreactive against the M1 Flag antiserum (which is specific for N-terminal Flag sequences) but reacted with the M2 Flag antiserum which recognizes internal Flag sequences, while the N309K protein reacted with both antisera (panel D). These data corroborate the removal of the propeptide in N309K-transfected cells.

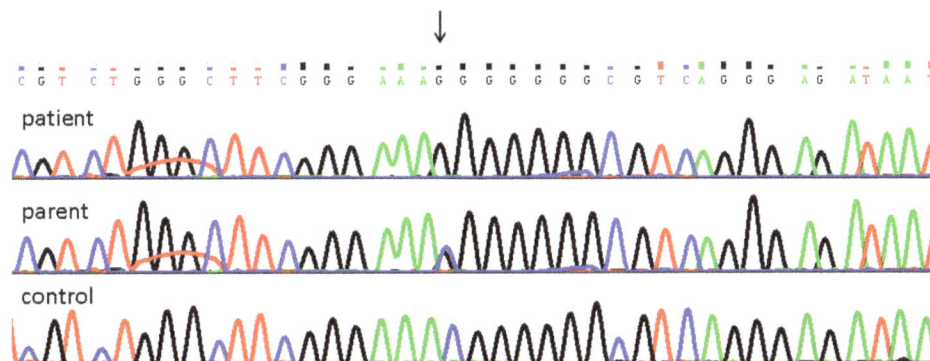

Discussion

The natural history of these children is consistent with the emerging clinical phenotype of proprotein convertase 1/3 deficiency, which typically involves CDD and an array of systemic endocrinopathies that develop in an age-dependent manner [11]. Neonates have severe generalized malabsorptive diarrhea and failure to thrive, and require prolonged total parenteral nutrition. As the disease progresses additional endocrine abnormalities develop, including diabetes insipidus, growth hormone deficiency, primary hypogonadism, adrenal insufficiency, and hypothyroidism. Moderate obesity, associated with severe polyphagia, generally appears despite early growth abnormalities. Patient II-2 required parenteral nutrition, and was diagnosed with diabetes insipidus, hypothyroidism and developed obesity in concordance with this disease phenotype [11].

In approximately 10–15% of infants who suffer from severe neonatal seizures the etiology is unknown, and it is assumed that these patients have genetic encephalopathies [27]. Several studies have elucidated the pathogenic role of genetic mutations involved in synaptogenesis, pruning, neuronal migration and differentiation, neurotransmitter synthesis and release, and structure and function of membrane receptors and transporters, but *PCSK1* variants have not been associated with a significant neurologic impairment [28–29].

PCSK1 point mutations associated with PC1/3 deficiency result in the absence or significant reduction of secreted PC1/3 enzymatic activity similar to that observed here [9,11–12]. However, the mutation presented herein, unlike previous reported cases, resulted in a secreted enzyme in which the propeptide was removed but no activity was present against synthetic substrates. The catalytic triad in eukaryotic subtilases consists of His-Ser-Asp; in addition, an Asn residue, which occupies a catalytic pocket site known as the oxyanion hole, is thought to stabilize the transition state of the product in both bacterial and eukaryotic subtilases [30]. Nearly all eukaryotic subtilases contain an Asn in this position; however, the prohormone convertase PC2 contains an Asp at this site. Substitution of the oxyanion hole Asn for Asp in the yeast subtilase kex2 resulted in a marked decrease in enzymatic activity [31]. However, substitution of the unusual Asp in PC2 with Asn did not result in measurable changes in enzyme activity [32], suggesting some flexibility in the oxyanion hole residue within prohormone convertases. By contrast, substitution of other catalytic residues in either PC1/3 or PC2 results in lack of prodomain removal, lack of secretion, and consequent loss of enzymatic activity [32–34].

↓

Figure 4. Sanger sequencing validation of the N309K variant. Sanger sequencing of the results for the proband, parent and unaffected control at nucleotide position 5: 95746646.

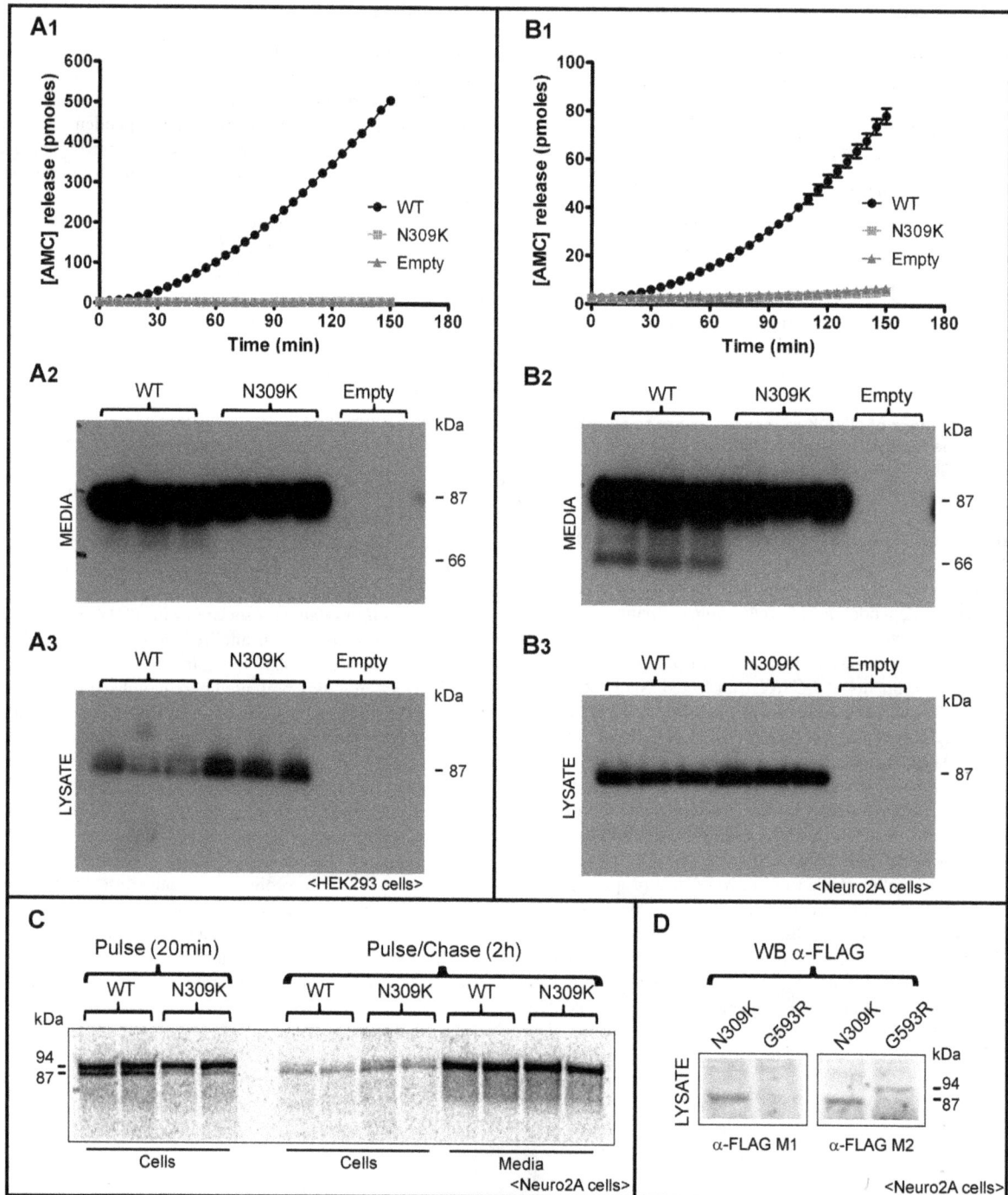

Figure 5. Lack of activity of N309K PC1/3 despite robust secretion. PC/3-encoding vectors were transfected into HEK (A panels, *left side*) or Neuro2A cells (B panels, *right side*) and the conditioned media subjected to either enzymatic assay (A1, B1) using the standard fluorogenic assay; or to Western blotting using PC1/3 antiserum (A2, B2). Cell extracts were also subjected to Western blotting (A3, B3). Panel C shows the maturation of ^{35}S-methionine-labeled wild-type and N309K precursor proteins during a 20-minute pulse followed by a 2 h chase in Neuro2A cells. WT, wild-type PC1/3. Panel D shows a Western blot of Neuro2A cell lysate, previously transfected with either N309K and G593R PC1/3 cDNAs and incubated with α-FLAG M1 or α-FLAG M2 antibodies to discriminate the 94 kDa PC1/3 prodomain ER-retained form.

The fact that the N309K mutant undergoes slowed prodomain removal implies that the identity of the oxyanion hole residue contributes to this intramolecular cleavage event. Interestingly, normal prodomain removal of a mouse PC1/3 N309D mutant was observed in *in vitro* translational experiments; in this work,

potential effects of this substitution on enzymatic activity using other substrates were not studied [35].

We conclude that replacing the oxyanion hole residue (N309) by Asp [35]. or Lys (this study) does not suppress prodomain removal, and PC1/3 continues to traffic through the secretory pathway. Nevertheless, the complete loss of activity of the resultant mature mutant enzyme supports a critical role for the oxyanion hole residue in intermolecular substrate catalysis. The total absence of the PC1/3 66 kDa form in the medium secreted from Neuro2A cells transfected with the N309K mutant corroborates the idea that this PC1/3 variant is unable to cleave its own C-terminal domain in the usual intermolecular interaction [36]. These unequivocal effects on enzyme activity would be expected to result in the loss of all PC1/3-mediated processing in patients with this oxyanion substitution.

References

1. Canani RB, Terrin G (2011) Recent progress in congenital diarrheal disorders. Curr Gastroenterol Rep 13: 257–264.
2. Turk E, Zabel B, Mundlos S, Dyer J, Wright EM (1991) Glucose/galactose malabsorption caused by a defect in the Na+/glucose cotransporter. Nature 350: 354–356.
3. Ouwendijk J, Moolenaar CE, Peters WJ, Hollenberg CP, Ginsel LA, et al. (1996) Congenital sucrase-isomaltase deficiency. Identification of a glutamine to proline substitution that leads to a transport block of sucrase-isomaltase in a pre-Golgi compartment. J Clin Invest 97: 633–641.
4. Muller T, Hess MW, Schiefermeier N, Pfaller K, Ebner HL, et al. (2008) MYO5B mutations cause microvillus inclusion disease and disrupt epithelial cell polarity. Nat Genet 40: 1163–1165.
5. Sivagnanam M, Mueller JL, Lee H, Chen Z, Nelson SF, et al. (2008) Identification of EpCAM as the gene for congenital tufting enteropathy. Gastroenterology 135: 429–437.
6. Bennett CL, Ochs HD (2001) IPEX is a unique X-linked syndrome characterized by immune dysfunction, polyendocrinopathy, enteropathy, and a variety of autoimmune phenomena. Curr Opin Pediatr 13: 533–538.
7. Wang J, Cortina G, Wu SV, Tran R, Cho JH, et al. (2006) Mutant neurogenin-3 in congenital malabsorptive diarrhea. N Engl J Med 355: 270–280.
8. Terrin G, Tomaiuolo R, Passariello A, Elce A, Amato F, et al. (2012) Congenital diarrheal disorders: an updated diagnostic approach. Int J Mol Sci 13: 4168–4185.
9. Yourshaw M, Solorzano-Vargas RS, Pickett LA, Lindberg I, Wang J, et al. (2013) Exome Sequencing Finds a Novel PCSK1 Mutation in a Child With Generalized Malabsorptive Diarrhea and Diabetes Insipidus. J Pediatr Gastroenterol Nutr 57: 759–767.
10. Benzinou M, Creemers JW, Choquet H, Lobbens S, Dina C, et al. (2008) Common nonsynonymous variants in PCSK1 confer risk of obesity. Nat Genet 40: 943–945.
11. Martin MG, Lindberg I, Solorzano-Vargas RS, Wang J, Avitzur Y, et al. (2013) Congenital proprotein convertase 1/3 deficiency causes malabsorptive diarrhea and other endocrinopathies in a pediatric cohort. Gastroenterology 145: 138–148.
12. Pickett LA, Yourshaw M, Albornoz V, Chen Z, Solorzano-Vargas RS, et al. (2013) Functional consequences of a novel variant of PCSK1. PLoS One 8: e55065.
13. Farooqi IS, Volders K, Stanhope R, Heuschkel R, White A, et al. (2007) Hyperphagia and early-onset obesity due to a novel homozygous missense mutation in prohormone convertase 1/3. J Clin Endocrinol Metab 92: 3369–3373.
14. Jackson RS, Creemers JW, Farooqi IS, Raffin-Sanson ML, Varro A, et al. (2003) Small-intestinal dysfunction accompanies the complex endocrinopathy of human proprotein convertase 1 deficiency. J Clin Invest 112: 1550–1560.
15. Jackson RS, Creemers JW, Ohagi S, Raffin-Sanson ML, Sanders L, et al. (1997) Obesity and impaired prohormone processing associated with mutations in the human prohormone convertase 1 gene. Nat Genet 16: 303–306.
16. Edvardson S, Shaag A, Kolesnikova O, Gomori JM, Tarassov I, et al. (2007) Deleterious mutation in the mitochondrial arginyl-transfer RNA synthetase gene is associated with pontocerebellar hypoplasia. Am J Hum Genet 81: 857–862.
17. Blanco EH, Peinado JR, Martin MG, Lindberg I (2014) Biochemical and cell biological properties of the human prohormone convertase 1/3 Ser357Gly mutation: a PC1/3 hypermorph. Endocrinology en20132151. [Epub ahead of print]
18. Kumar P, Henikoff S, Ng PC (2009) Predicting the effects of coding nonsynonymous variants on protein function using the SIFT algorithm. Nat Protoc 4: 1073–1081.
19. Adzhubei IA, Schmidt S, Peshkin L, Ramensky VE, Gerasimova A, et al. (2010) A method and server for predicting damaging missense mutations. Nat Methods 7: 248–249.
20. Chun S, Fay JC (2009) Identification of deleterious mutations within three human genomes. Genome Res 19: 1553–1561.
21. Reva B, Antipin Y, Sander C (2011) Predicting the functional impact of protein mutations: application to cancer genomics. Nucleic Acids Res 39: e118.
22. Schwarz JM, Rodelsperger C, Schuelke M, Seelow D (2010) MutationTaster evaluates disease-causing potential of sequence alterations. Nat Methods 7: 575–576.
23. Gonzalez-Perez A, Lopez-Bigas N (2011) Improving the assessment of the outcome of nonsynonymous SNVs with a consensus deleteriousness score, Condel. Am J Hum Genet 88: 440–449.
24. Lopes MC, Joyce C, Ritchie GR, John SL, Cunningham F, et al. (2012) A combined functional annotation score for non-synonymous variants. Hum Hered 73: 47–51.
25. Genomes Project Consortium, Abecasis GR, Auton A, Brooks LD, DePristo MA, et al. (2012) An integrated map of genetic variation from 1,092 human genomes. Nature 491: 56–65.
26. NHLBI Exome Sequencing Project. Exome Variant Server. Volume September 2011. Seattle WA: NHLBI Exome Sequencing Project (ESP), 2011.
27. Berger I, Dor T, Halvardson J, Edvardson S, Shaag A, et al. (2012) Intractable epilepsy of infancy due to homozygous mutation in the EFHC1 gene. Epilepsia 53: 1436–1440.
28. Zupanc ML (2009) Clinical evaluation and diagnosis of severe epilepsy syndromes of early childhood. J Child Neurol 24(8 Suppl): 6S–14S.
29. Mastrangelo M, Leuzzi V (2012) Genes of early-onset epileptic encephalopathies: from genotype to phenotype. Pediatr Neurol 46: 24–31.
30. Bryan P, Pantoliano MW, Quill SG, Hsiao HY, Poulos T (1986) Site-directed mutagenesis and the role of the oxyanion hole in subtilisin. Proc Natl Acad Sci U S A 83: 3743–3745.
31. Brenner C, Bevan A, Fuller RS (1993) One-step site-directed mutagenesis of the Kex2 protease oxyanion hole. Curr Biol 3: 498–506.
32. Zhou A, Paquet L, Mains RE (1995) Structural elements that direct specific processing of different mammalian subtilisin-like prohormone convertases. J Biol Chem 270: 21509–21516.
33. Goodman LJ, Gorman CM (1994) Autoproteolytic activation of the mouse prohormone convertase mPC1. Biochem Biophys Res Commun 201: 795–804.
34. Taylor NA, Shennan KI, Cutler DF, Docherty K (1997) Mutations within the propeptide, the primary cleavage site or the catalytic site, or deletion of C-terminal sequences, prevents secretion of proPC2 from transfected COS-7 cells. Biochem J 321: 367–373.
35. Scougall K, Taylor NA, Jermany JL, Docherty K, Shennan KI (1998) Differences in the autocatalytic cleavage of pro-PC2 and pro-PC3 can be attributed to sequences within the propeptide and Asp310 of pro-PC2. Biochem J 334: 531–537.
36. Online Mendelian Inheritance in Man OMIM®. Online Mendelian Inheritance in Man, OMIM®. Baltimore, MD: McKusick-Nathans Institute of Genetic Medicine, Johns Hopkins University.

Author Contributions

Conceived and designed the experiments: MW EB IL MY MM OE. Performed the experiments: MW MA EB IL MY DZ IB ES OP MM OE. Analyzed the data: MW EB IL MY OP MM BB OE. Contributed reagents/materials/analysis tools: EB IL MY OP MM BB OE. Wrote the paper: MW MA EB IL MY DZ IB ES OP MM OE.

12

Incidence of Rotavirus and Circulating Genotypes in Northeast Brazil during 7 Years of National Rotavirus Vaccination

Ricardo Q. Gurgel[1], Alberto De Juan Alvarez[2], Alda Rodrigues[1], Robergson R. Ribeiro[1], Sílvio S. Dolabella[1], Natanael L. Da Mota[1], Victor S. Santos[1], Miren Iturriza-Gomara[3], Nigel A. Cunliffe[3], Luis E. Cuevas[2]*

1 Federal University of Sergipe, Aracaju, Brazil, 2 Liverpool School of Tropical Medicine, Liverpool, United Kingdom, 3 Institute of Infection and Global Health, University of Liverpool, Liverpool, United Kingdom

Abstract

Background and Aims: Rotavirus causes severe diarrhoea and Brazil introduced the Rotarix G1P[8] vaccine in 2006. We aimed to describe changes in rotavirus incidence and diarrhoea epidemiology before and after vaccine introduction.

Methods: Design: (i) hospital-based survey of children with diarrhoea (2006–2012); (ii) diarrhea-mortality and hospitalization surveillance (1999–2012).

Setting: (i) Aracaju and (ii) state and national level.

Results: 1841 children were enrolled and 231 (12.5%) had rotavirus. Rotavirus was less frequent from January-June than from July-December (9.4% versus 20.9%, $p<0.01$), but the seasonal variation was less defined after 2009. Very few rotavirus cases (8–3.9%) were detected in 2011, with an increase in 2012 (13–18.5%). In 2006, unvaccinated children were more likely to have rotavirus, but thereafter unvaccinated and vaccinated children had equally low incidence. Older children and those with rotavirus were more likely to have severe diarrhea episodes. The most frequent genotype from 2006 to 2010 was G2P[4]; except in 2009, when most cases were G1P[8]. Very few G2P[4] were detected from 2011 and 50% cases in 2012 were G8P[4]. Diarrhoea-hospitalizations decreased nationally from 89,934 (2003) to 53,705 (2012; 40.3% reduction) and in the state from 1729 to 748 (56.7% reduction). Diarrhoea-deaths decreased nationally from 4368 in 1999 to 697 in 2012 (84% reduction, $p<0.001$) and in the state from 132 to 18 (86% reduction). These changes were much larger after vaccine introduction.

Conclusions: The vaccine was associated with substantial reductions in rotavirus incidence and diarrhoea-hospitalizations and deaths. The G2P[4] genotype predominance disappeared over time and may be replaced by other heterotypic genotypes.

Editor: Martyn Kirk, The Australian National University, Australia

Funding: Financial support for this study was received from CNPq/UFS-COPES/PIBIC- 2008-2012, calls Edital MCT/CNPq Universal 14/2009 (#478082/2006-9), Edital MCT/CNPq Universal 14/2011 (#475914/2011-2). The funders had no role in study design, data collection and analysis, decision to publish, or preparation of the manuscript.

Competing Interests: Prof Cunliffe received research grant support from GSK for the evaluation of rotavirus vaccination in Malawi and UK and has received honoraria from GSK for participation in rotavirus vaccine advisory board meetings. Dr. Iturriza Gomara reports grants from SPMSD and grants from GSK, outside the submitted work; all other authors have no conflicts of interest to declare.

* Email: lcuevas@liv.ac.uk

Introduction

The licensing of two rotavirus vaccines in 2006 and their large scale use in countries such as Brazil and the USA marked the beginning of a new era in paediatric diarrhoeal disease control [1,2]. Soon after their adoption, national immunisation programs reported significant reductions in diarrhoea-related hospitalisa-tions and ambulatory consultations. In 2012 following pivotal Phase III clinical trials, the World Health Organisation (WHO) recommended extension of their use to include countries with high diarrhoea burden in Africa and Asia [3]. Vaccine introduction in these continents is rapidly gaining momentum with support from international partners including the Global Alliance for Vaccines Initiative (GAVI).

Brazil was among the first countries to integrate a rotavirus vaccine into its national immunisation programme, the monovalent G1P[8] Rotarix vaccine (Glaxo Smith Kline Biologicals) in March 2006. Although Rotarix has good efficacy for most homotypic genotypes (91.8% for G1P[8]), efficacy against fully heterotypic genotype G2P[4] is only 41% [1]. Children were offered two oral doses free of charge and vaccine coverage reached 82% by 2008 and has since remained above this level (http://datasus.saude.gov.br/). The vaccine introduction coincided with a decline in severe rotavirus-diarrhoea episodes, all-cause diarrhoea-related hospitalisations and ambulatory consultations [4,5]. Although these reports were promising, Brazil reported a long-term decline in the incidence of childhood diarrhoea [6] and a longer period of observation was needed to elucidate the additional contribution of rotavirus vaccine to the control of childhood diarrhoea.

Early surveys following vaccine introduction described that nearly all rotavirus-diarrhoea episodes were associated with the heterotypic G2P[4] genotype [7,8]. Although this occurrence could have been due to a temporal coincidence, as this genotype was also circulating in several Latin American countries at that time including some without rotavirus vaccination [9], it could also be due to the immunological pressure exerted by the vaccine against other genotypes for which it has higher efficacy [10]. We now report long-term changes in the epidemiology of childhood diarrhoea, rotavirus incidence and genotypes in the first seven years after vaccine introduction.

Methods

Ethics statement

The study protocol was approved by the research ethics committees of the Liverpool School of Tropical Medicine, Sergipe's Federal University and the Brazilian National Commission for Ethics and Research (CONEP). Parents were requested provide written informed consent before enrolling their children in the study.

Study design

The study comprised (i) a hospital-based survey of the proportion, severity and genotypes of acute diarrhoea episodes due to rotavirus among children attending a reference hospital in Sergipe, Northeast Brazil and (ii) analysis of thirteen-year routinely generated regional and national surveillance data comprising seven years before and six years after rotavirus vaccine introduction.

Hospital-based survey

This was a prospective survey of children <12 years old presenting with diarrhea of <14 days duration to the pediatric emergency service of Sergipe Emergency Hospital (Hospital de Urgências de Sergipe - HUSE) from October 2006 to April 2012. HUSE is the largest reference hospital in Aracaju, the capital of Sergipe State in Northeast Brazil, containing 570,937 and 2,068,031 inhabitants, respectively [11]. Although HUSE provides 24-hour services, for logistical reasons only children attending between 8 am and 4 pm from Monday to Friday were included. We included a sample of these children to obtain a representative number of children for the month. We aimed to include a minimum of 300 specimens per year, assuming the prevalence of rotavirus would be 20% of cases per year and this sample size would allow establishing this proportion with +/−5% margin of error. After providing informed written consent, parents and children were interviewed to establish the clinical profile and

vaccination history. Parents were asked to collect a stool specimen in containers before leaving the services and the approximately 60% of parents able to provide specimens were included in the final dataset. Rotavirus vaccination status was verified against the child's vaccination card. In Brazil, most parents carry the child vaccination card because this is often requested when attending health services and it is therefore possible to confirm the vaccination status of most children. Children with two rotavirus vaccine doses recorded were considered vaccinated, while those without doses or only one dose were considered unvaccinated. Children without vaccination cards were classified as having an *unknown* vaccination status.

Stools specimens were stored at −70°C until tested using an enzyme linked immunosorbent assay (ELISA, Rotaclone; Meridian Diagnostics, Cincinnati, OH). Rotavirus genotypes were determined in ELISA-positive specimens using a hemi-nested reverse transcription-polymerase chain reaction using consensus and type-specific primers as described earlier [8].

Surveillance data

Rotavirus vaccine coverage data were obtained for 2007–2011 from the Expanded Program of Immunization databases at http://pni.datasus.gov.br/inf_estatistica_cobertura.asp and mortality data for 1999–2012 were obtained from the national surveillance system (Datasus) available at http://www2.datasus.gov.br/DATASUS/index.php?area=0205. Data were extracted for Aracaju, Sergipe and nationally using the International Diseases Classification (IDC) codes A08 and A09. Diarrhea-related hospitalization data were obtained from www.datasus.gov.br and the Hospital-based Information System (SUS-SIH/SUS) using the IDC codes J12–J18. Data were grouped by age (<1, 1 to 4, 5 to 10 and 10 to 14 years). Frequencies for 2012 were preliminary at the time of preparing the manuscript and thus may be revised once officially published in its final form in the website.

Descriptive statistics were used to ascertain changes in the distribution of diarrhea in vaccinated and unvaccinated children, clustering of genotypes over time and their association to disease severity. Differences in proportions were tested using Chi Squares. Diarrhea severity was described using a frequently used severity score [12]. Ninety five percent confidence intervals (95% CIs) and Student's T tests were used as appropriate.

Results

Characteristics of hospital participants

A total of 1841 children were enrolled at the HUSE survey from October 2006 to April 2012. Most children were young, with a median age of 12 months. Children in 2006–2009 were younger than children in 2010–2012 (p = 0.003– table 1) and more boys than girls were enrolled each year except in 2012. The median diarrhea duration before consultation was 3 days and the median number of stools before consultation varied from 4 to 5 episodes per day over the study period. The proportion of children vomiting was lower in 2006–2008 than in later years, increasing from 44.4% in 2007 to 73% in 2012 (p = <0.01). The diarrhea severity score was calculated for 1836 (99.7%) children and the mean severity score was 10.4, ranging from 9.2 in 2008 to 12.3 in 2012. In total 1108 (59%) children had mild/moderate (score <12) and 728 (38.9%) severe episodes (score ≥12). The proportion of children with scores ≥12 increased over the years from 27.6% in 2009 to 58.3% in 2012 (p<0.001). Diarrhea severity also increased with age, with 139/466 (29.8%) children <6 months, 160/438 (36.5%) 6−<12 months old, 178/405 (44%)

Table 1. Characteristics of the participants with acute diarrhea from 2006 to 2012.

	2006	2007	2008	2009	2010	2011	2012	Total
Number	73	324	416	387	363	206	72	1841
Male (%)	41 (56.2%)	185 (57.1%)	219 (52.6%)	217 (56.1%)	212 (58.4%)	110 (53.4%)	32 (44.4%)	1016 (55.2%)
Age, median [range], months	12 [1–144]	10 [1–144]	12 [0–138]	11 [0–131]	13 [1–132]	16 [1–144]	14 [1–131]	12 [0–144]
Age group, months (%) <6	22 (30.1%)	113 (34.9%)	126 (30.3%)	124 (32.0%)	87 (24.0%)	49 (23.8%)	18 (25.0%)	539 (29.3%)
6–<12	18 (24.7%)	70 (21.6%)	89 (21.4%)	87 (22.5%)	90 (24.8%)	36 (17.5%)	13 (18.1%)	403 (21.9%)
12–<24	13 (17.8%)	59 (18.2%)	76 (18.3%)	76 (19.6%)	93 (25.6%)	47 (22.8%)	24 (33.3%)	388 (21.1%)
≥24	20 (27.4%)	82 (25.3%)	125 (30.0%)	100 (25.8%)	93 (25.6%)	74 (35.9%)	17 (23.6%)	511 (27.8%)
Vaccination status								
Card available	73 (100%)	196 (60.5%)	204 (49.0%)	297 (76.7%)	259 (71.3%)	162 (78.6%)	60 (83.0%)	1451 (78.8%)
*Vaccinated	21 (28.8%)	103 (52.6%)	130 (63.7%)	184 (62.0%)	197 (76%)	117 (72.2%)	52 (86.7%)	804 (55.4%)
Not vaccinated	52 (71.2%)	93 (47.4%)	74 (36.3%)	113 (38.0%)	62 (24%)	45 (27.8%)	8 (13.3%)	647 (44.6%)
Diarrhoea								
**Median duration [range]	3 [1–13]	3 [1–15]	3 [0–60]	3 [1–17]	3 [0–30]	3 [1–15]	3 [1–15]	3 [1–15]
Frequency per day	5 [3–15]	5 [3–20]	4 [1–20]	4 [1–15]	4 [1–25]	5 [1–30]	5 [2–16]	4 [1–30]
Vomiting								
Present	41 (56.2%)	144 (44.4%)	230 (55.3%)	258 (66.7%)	244 (67.2%)	152 (73.8%)	53 (73.6%)	1122 (60.9%)
Median duration [range]**	1 [0–8]	0 [0–15]	1 [0–10]	1 [0–9]	1 [0–63]	1 [0–6]	1 [0–10]	1 [0–63]
Frequency per day	1 [0–15]	0 [0–15]	1 [0–20]	1 [0–15]	1 [0–20]	1 [0–30]	2 [0–18]	1 [0–30]
Severity score								
Mean	11.3	9.7	9.2	10.6	10.9	11.5	12.3	10.4
Score ≥12 (%)	33 (45.2%)	112 (34.6%)	115 (27.6%)	157 (40.6%)	158 (43.0%)	114 (54.9%)	43 (58.3%)	732 (39.6%)
Rotavirus ELISA positive (%)	18 (24.7%)	30 (9.3%)	77 (18.5%)	41 (10.6%)	43 (11.8%)	8 (3.9%)	14 (19.4%)	231 (12.5%)

*Only includes children with vaccination cards; **in days.

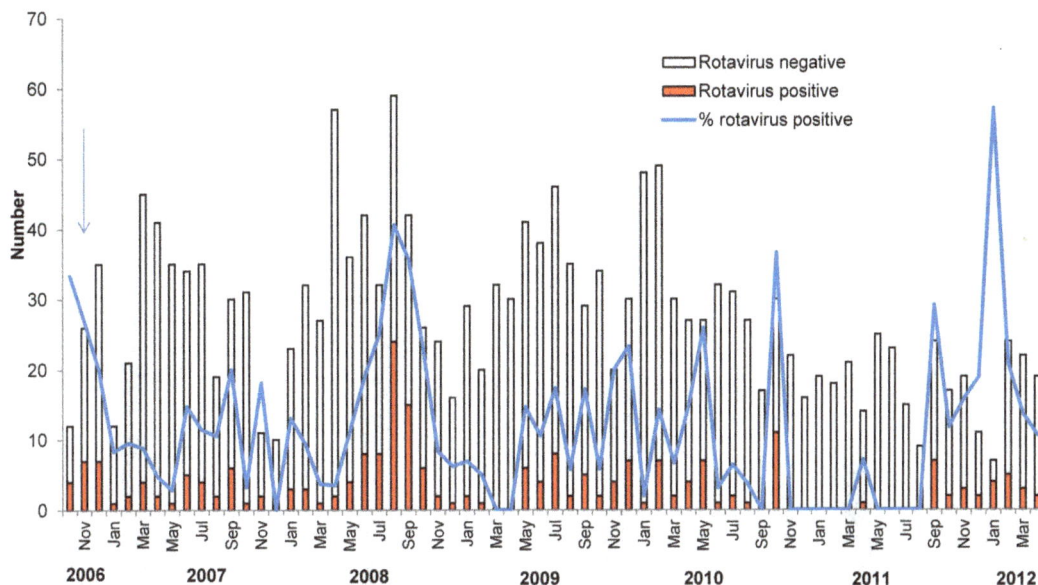

Figure 1. Number of children enrolled and proportion with rotavirus infection by month, November 2006 to April 2012. The arrow illustrates the date of vaccine introduction.

12−<24 months old and 255/531 (48%) children ≥24 months having severe episodes (p = <0.001).

Vaccination cards were available for 1451 (79%) children and rotavirus vaccines were recorded in 28.8% participants in 2006 and 86.7% in 2012, with an expected increase over time (p< 0.001).

Two-hundred and thirty one (12.5%) children were rotavirus-ELISA positive. The proportion of children with positive ELISAs varied by month and was lower during the months of January to June and higher from July to December (86/914 [9.4%] versus 145/695 [20.9%], respectively, p<0.01). This seasonal variation became less well defined since 2009 and very few rotavirus cases were detected in 2011 (Figure 1). The 2011 nadir however was then followed by an increase in the number of cases in 2012, when a much higher percentage of children had rotavirus.

The proportion of children with rotavirus by age and vaccination status is shown in figure 2. In 2006, unvaccinated children <24 months were more likely to have rotavirus than unvaccinated children ≥24 months old. Vaccinated children were also less likely to have rotavirus than unvaccinated children. This pattern changed after 2006, as a low percentage of both vaccinated and unvaccinated children had rotavirus. The change was observed in all age groups. The proportion of children with severe episodes increased with age in both children with and without rotavirus (p<0.001 for both) and children with rotavirus had more severe episodes than children without rotavirus, as shown in Figure 3. Generally, vaccinated children had less severe episodes than unvaccinated children, but this difference was only statistically significant in children <6 months.

Two-hundred twenty seven rotavirus-ELISA positive stools underwent G and P genotyping. Five G and three P types were identified over the six years, as shown in Table 2. The most prevalent G types were G2 (166, 73%), G1 (40, 17.6%) and G8 (13, 5.7%). Other G types identified included G3 (3, 1.5%), G12 (2, 0.9%) and four G non-typeable. The most frequent P types were P[4] (179, 78.9%), P[8] (35, 15.4%) and P[6] (8, 3.5%), and 10 were non-typeable. The most common G and P combinations were G2P[4] (160, 70.5%), G1P[8] (29, 12.7%), G8P[4] (12, 5.3%)

and G3P[8] (3, 1.3%). Less frequent combinations included G1P[4] and G1P[6], G2P[6], G8P[6] and G12P[4] and G12P[8]. Five stools had more than one genotype, including two G2P[4]P[8] and one each of G2G8P[1], G1G2P[4], with and G8G2P[4]. The frequency of the genotypes varied over time. G2P[4] was the only genotype identified from 2006 to 2009. Then in 2009, the majority of rotaviruses were G1P[8], with G2P[4] having a lower frequency. In 2010, G2P[4] was again the

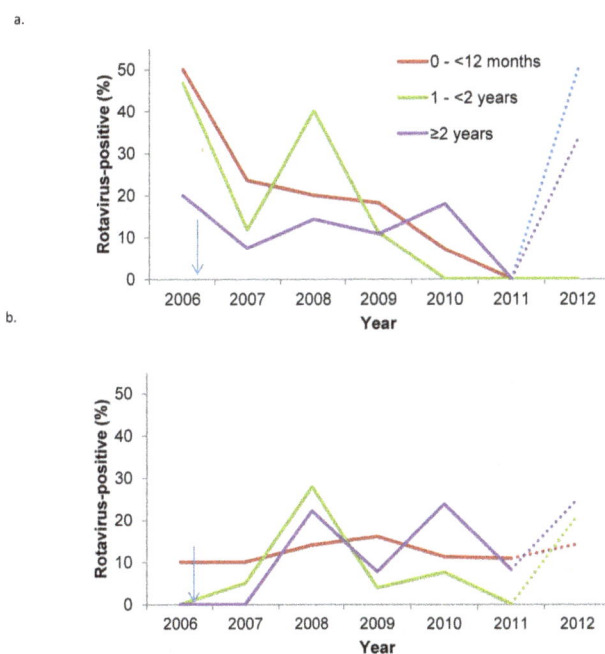

Figure 2. Proportion of (a) non-vaccinated and (b) vaccinated children attending the hospital with rotavirus, by age and year. Percentages for 2012 are incomplete (to March, represented by a dotted line). Arrows illustrate the vaccine introduction.

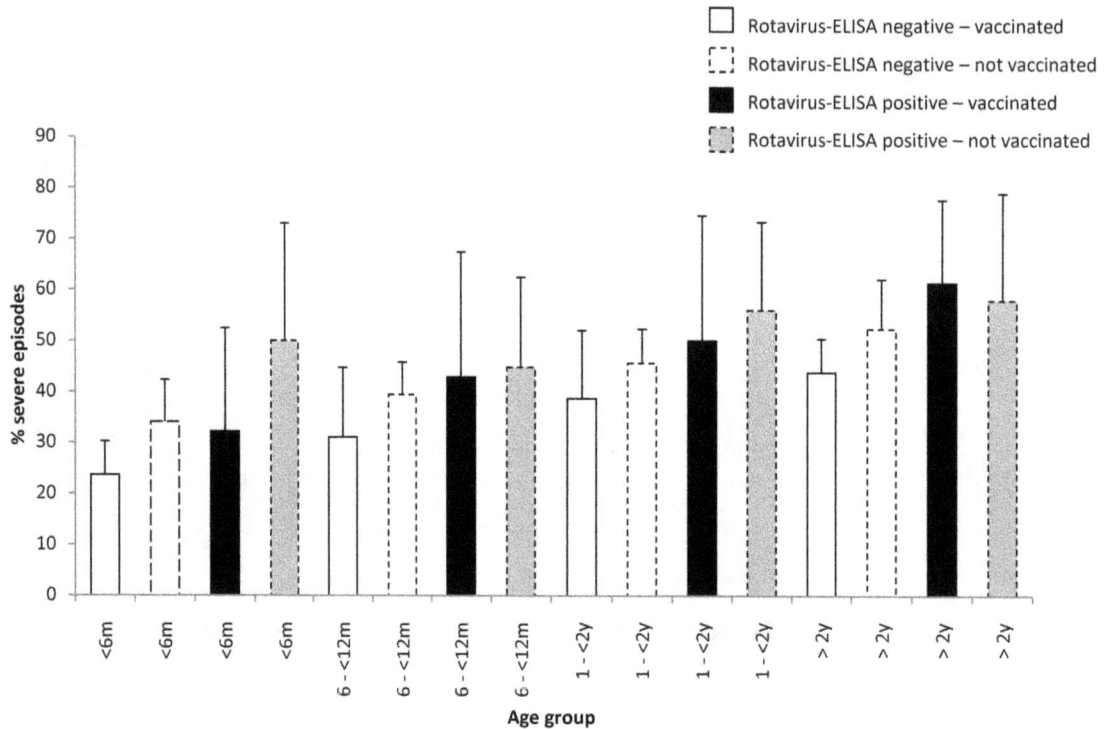

Figure 3. Proportion of vaccinated and non-vaccinated children attending the Emergency service with severe diarrhea, by age and presence of rotavirus.

predominant genotype and other genotypes had lower frequencies. A variety of genotypes were identified in 2011 but with low frequencies, while seven of 14 isolates in 2012 belonged to the uncommon G8P[4] genotype.

Surveillance data

All cause and diarrhoea-deaths occurring in children <5 years old in Brazil, Sergipe State and Aracaju from 1999 to 2012 are shown in Figure 4 (a) and (b). All-cause deaths decreased nationally from 81,391 deaths in 1999 to 45,101 in 2012 (45% reduction from the 1999 baseline). Sergipe State recorded 1,511 in 1999 and 639 in 2012 (58% reduction) and Aracaju had the largest percentage reduction with 450 deaths in 1999 and 167 in 2012 (63% reduction). The reduction trends for all-cause deaths were similar between 1999–2005 and 2006–2012 nationally and at state and city level.

Diarrhoea-specific deaths decreased more sharply than all-cause deaths, with a national reduction from 4368 deaths in 1999 and 697 in 2012 (84% reduction) (p<0.001). Sergipe State reported similar reductions, decreasing from 132 deaths in 1999 to 18 in 2012 (86% reduction). Aracaju city reported similar reductions, from 11 deaths in 1999 to two in 2012 (82% reduction). Percentage reductions in diarrhoea deaths were larger than for all-cause deaths (p<0.001 for national, state and city level). The decreasing trend for diarrhoea deaths were also different before and after 2006 at the national level, with a 45% reduction from 1999 to 2005 and an additional 71% reduction from 2006 to 2012 (p<0.001). Sergipe reported a 36.4% reduction between 1999 and 2005 and 78% reduction from 2006 to 2012 (p<0.001). Diarrhoea deaths therefore decreased more rapidly than all-cause deaths. The proportion of all-cause deaths due to diarrhoea changed nationally from 5.4% in 1999 to 1.5% in 2012. Similarly in Sergipe and Aracaju, diarrhoea deaths represented 8.7% and

6.9% of all deaths in 1999, but only 2.8% and 1.2% in 2012 (Figure 4c).

Diarrhoea-related hospitalisations in Brazil, Sergipe and Aracaju from 2003 to 2012 are shown in Figure 4d. Diarrhoea hospitalizations decreased nationally from 89,934 in 2003 to 53,705 in 2012 (40.3% reduction). The percentage decrease was also large in Sergipe and Aracaju, decreasing from 1729 to 748 (56.7% reduction) in Sergipe and from 483 to 296 (38.7% reduction) in Aracaju. The reduction in the number of diarrhoea-hospitalisations varied before and after vaccine introduction, with a 1.7% reduction in the national number of hospitalizations from 2003 to 2005 and a 39.2% reduction between 2006 and 2012. Similarly Sergipe State reported a 10% increase in diarrhoea hospitalizations between 2003 and 2005 but a 56.7% reduction between 2006 and 2012 (p<0.001).

Discussion

Diarrhoea is the second most important cause of child death globally, with most cases occurring in low and middle income countries and rotavirus is the pathogen most frequently associated with severe episodes [13], incurring substantial hospitalisation, medical consultations and parental costs [14]. The advent of rotavirus vaccines and their rapid adoption by national immunisation programmes heralded a new era of vaccine-based interventions for diarrhoea control [1,2] with enormous potential for health benefit. Brazil's adoption of a rotavirus vaccine created one of the largest rotavirus-vaccinated cohorts ever and monitoring changes in the burden of rotavirus and all cause-diarrhoea in the country could generate information for countries considering the adoption of the vaccines.

This study demonstrates that Brazil experienced major epidemiological changes in rotavirus-specific and all cause diarrhoea.

a.

b.

c.

d.

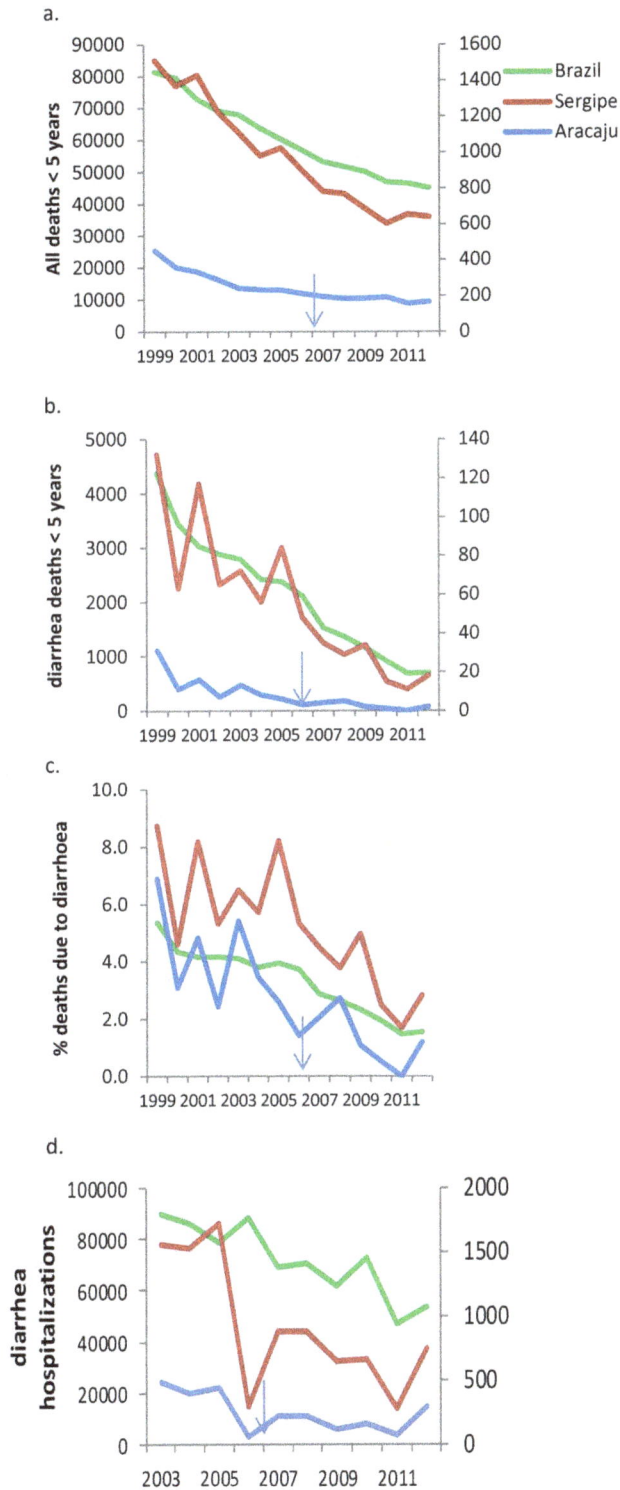

Figure 4. Childhood (<5 years old) all cause and diarrhea deaths and hospitalizations in Brazil, Sergipe and Aracaju City. Arrows illustrate the year of vaccine introduction.

Surveillance data confirm the long term decline in all cause and diarrhoea-specific childhood mortality [6,15], which have largely been attributed to improved accessibility to services, sanitation and public health interventions [15]. These trends are considerable confounders to assess changes occurring after vaccine introduc-

tion. We therefore have described whether the secular trends changed before and after vaccine introduction, and whether the proportion of all deaths that are due to diarrhoea changed before and after vaccine introduction. Both indicators suggest that the vaccine introduction was associated with statistically significant changes in the trends. Not only the number of diarrhoea deaths decreased more rapidly after vaccine introduction, but the proportion of diarrhoea became a smaller proportion of all deaths. Nationally, the proportion of deaths attributed to diarrhoea declined from 5.4% of all deaths in 1999 to 3.9% by 2005, but changed again from 3.9% in 2005 to 1.5% in 2012. The same pattern was observed for Sergipe, with a 36% reduction in the number of episodes between 1999 and 2005 and a 78% reduction after vaccine introduction, with the proportion of childhood deaths due to diarrhoea reducing from 8.2% in 2005 to 2.5% in 2012. The patterns therefore strongly suggest that these changes are due to the vaccine and the higher proportion of diarrhoea deaths in Sergipe is in agreement with previous data reporting a higher diarrhoea mortality in the Northeast of the country[6].

Data for diarrhoea-related hospitalizations were only available from 2002 and secular trends before vaccine introduction were less well documented. However the data suggests that changes in the number of hospitalizations before vaccine introduction were minimal. These trends had an evident change after vaccine introduction, with a 39.2% national reduction in diarrhoea-related hospitalization and an even larger 56.7% reduction in Sergipe. These data thus confirm that the vaccine is associated with significant reductions in hospitalizations and that these reductions were higher in a state where diarrhoea was a significant public health problem. Reductions in diarrhoea-related deaths and hospitalisations have been reported from Latin America [16], the United States [17], Europe [18,19] and Australasia [20] and interestingly these reductions have been higher than expected from previous impact models, which has been attributed to many cases being undetected before vaccine introduction and a sustained vaccine efficacy over several years [21].

Our hospital data show that the proportion of children with rotavirus infection has also decreased over the years, with a remarkable low proportion of cases having rotavirus in 2011. This low proportion was observed in both vaccinated and unvaccinated children and in infants and older children. Although counterintuitive, our findings are in agreement with reports demonstrating the significant herd protection of the vaccine [22,23], which is likely due to the reduced virus transmission in the environment and possibly vaccine strains spreading to unvaccinated children [24].

Our study also documents changes in the rotavirus genotypes. A high proportion of G2P[4] strains from 2006 to 2010 had been reported by us and others in Brazil and by countries that use the Rotarix vaccine in Australasia [20] and Europe [19,22,25]. We have however also observed further changes in 2011, when the G2P[4] became less frequent and other strains, such as G8[4], G8P[6] and G3P[8)] became more frequent. The G2P[4] decrease and the increase of other unusual G8 strains suggest that these changes may not be limited to the G2P[4] genotype. G8 is considered to have a bovine origin and is not included in the current vaccines [26] and has frequently been reported from African countries, where it accounts for about 12% of cases [27] and has recently been reported from Europe [28]. A further genotype increasingly isolated in 2011/12 was G3P[8]. This genotype has been reported with increased frequency in regions with a high coverage of RotaTeq [10], but it is also one of the five globally common rotavirus genotypes and its significance in the Brazilian context needs further study.

Table 2. Genotypes identified in children attending the emergency hospital with diarrhea (2006–2012).

	ELISA-positive/tested	Genotype	N	(%)
2006	18/73 (25%)	G2P[4]	16	(89)
		GNTP4	1	(6)
		G2PNT	1	(6)
2007	30/324 (9.3%)	G2P[4]	28	(93)
		GNTPNT	2	(7)
2008	77/416 (18.5%)	G2P[4]	77	(100)
2009	41/384 (10.7%)	G1P[8]	28	(68)
		G2P[4]	9	(22)
		G2P[4]P[8]	1	(2)
		G2PNT	2	(5)
		GNTPNT	1	(2)
2010	40/335 (11.9%)	G2P[4]	26	(65)
		G1P[6]	4	(10)
		G1P[4]	3	(8)
		G2P[6]	2	(5)
		G2P[4]P[8]	1	(3)
		G1P[8]	1	(3)
		G8P[4]	1	(3)
		G12P[8]	1	(3)
		G12P[4]	1	(3)
2011	8/207 (3.9%)	G2P4	2	(25)
		G3P[8]	2	(25)
		G8P[4]	2	(25)
		G2G8P[4]	1	(13)
		G2PNT	1	(13)
2012	13/70 (18.5%)	G8P[4]	7	(54)
		G8P[6]	2	(15)
		G1G2P[4]	2	(15)
		G3P[8]	1	(8)
		G8G2P[4]	1	(8)
All	227/1809 (12.5%)			

It is also interesting that despite the reduced mortality and hospitalizations, the proportion of diarrhea episodes classified as severe has increased over the years. This increase occurred both in vaccinated and unvaccinated children and in children with and without rotavirus. This might be an artefact caused by self-selection of patients, changes in service organization and provision and older children becoming more prominent because younger children are protected by the vaccine. In addition, other pathogens not included in this analysis (e.g. norovirus) may become more established and further studies are needed to establish if other pathogens may take the ecological niche of rotavirus.

Our study also has important limitations. The evaluation was partly conducted using data collected through surveillance systems, which are not devoid of problems. Surveillance is often based on sentinel sites that may change over time and become unrepresentative and incomplete data reporting may underestimate the mortality and hospitalizations attributed to diarrhoea. Furthermore, using all-cause diarrhoea as a marker for rotavirus diarrhoea could mask changes in the epidemiology of other pathogens. In addition, the hospital case series only recorded a

child as vaccinated if both doses of the vaccine were recorded, and not vaccinated if the child had received none or one vaccine dose. Labelling partially vaccinated children as unvaccinated could have reduced the number of episodes in the non-vaccinated group. However rotavirus infections were uncommon in all children and very few of the children receive only one dose of the vaccine, and for these reasons we believe this limitation is unlikely to modify the interpretation of the data. Furthermore, children admitted to the hospital outside working hours were assessed the following morning, but ambulatory children attending at night were missed. If attendance patterns and genotype distributions were associated with clinical severity, then this sampling strategy could have led to bias towards children with mild or severe presentations and the exclusion of children with moderate diarrhea and distortions in the genotype distribution.

Despite these shortcomings, similar approaches are being used to monitor vaccine efficacy elsewhere and African countries are preparing to use this method to monitor the vaccines when introduced on a large scale in the continent [29–31].

A further limitation is that our prospective data collection was based in one medical centre, receiving both self-selected and referred cases and therefore genotype representation is likely to be biased towards children with more severe episodes.

Despite these limitations, the data presented here add to the evidence of the growing public health impact of rotavirus vaccines in Brazil, with large reductions in the number of diarrhoea related childhood hospitalizations and deaths. Our data also provide new evidence that the predominance of the G2P[4] genotype in countries using the monovalent rotavirus vaccine is temporal and that other unusual genotypes may appear with time. Continued surveillance therefore is needed to document the continued effectiveness of the vaccines and the potential emergence of unusual rotavirus genotypes.

Acknowledgments

We thank Mr Genigesium Castro Junior from Aracaju Health Secretary for providing access to hospitalization data and Mr Dácio de Lyra Rabello Neto, CGIAE-DASIS-SVS, from the Ministry of Health for the data on 2012 mortality. We also thank Ms Fred Dove who for many years has conducted the rotavirus genotyping at the Institute of Infection and Global Health, UK. The study was jointly conceived by the late Professor Charles Anthony Hart and the authors and we honour his long lasting contribution to our work.

Author Contributions

Conceived and designed the experiments: RQG LEC. Performed the experiments: RQG AR RRR SSD NdaM VSS AdeJA MIG NC. Analyzed the data: RQG AdeJA LEC. Contributed reagents/materials/analysis tools: LEC RQG NC. Contributed to the writing of the manuscript: LEC RQG NC.

References

1. Ruiz-Palacios GM, Perez-Schael I, Velazquez FR, Abate H, Breuer T, et al. (2006) Safety and efficacy of an attenuated vaccine against severe rotavirus gastroenteritis. N Engl J Med 354: 11–22.
2. Vesikari T, Matson DO, Dennehy P, Van Damme P, Santosham M, et al. (2006) Safety and efficacy of a pentavalent human-bovine (WC3) reassortant rotavirus vaccine. N Engl J Med 354: 23–33.
3. (2013) Rotavirus vaccines WHO position paper: January 2013 - Recommendations. Vaccine 31: 6170–6171.
4. Gurgel RG, Bohland AK, Vieira SC, Oliveira DM, Fontes PB, et al. (2009) Incidence of rotavirus and all-cause diarrhea in northeast Brazil following the introduction of a national vaccination program. Gastroenterology 137: 1970–1975.
5. Correia JB, Patel MM, Nakagomi O, Montenegro FM, Germano EM, et al. (2010) Effectiveness of monovalent rotavirus vaccine (Rotarix) against severe diarrhea caused by serotypically unrelated G2P[4] strains in Brazil. J Infect Dis 201: 363–369.
6. Mendes PS, Ribeiro Hda C Jr, Mendes CM (2013) Temporal trends of overall mortality and hospital morbidity due to diarrheal disease in Brazilian children younger than 5 years from 2000 to 2010. J Pediatr (Rio J) 89: 315–325.
7. Gurgel RQ, Correia JB, Cuevas LE (2008) Effect of rotavirus vaccination on circulating virus strains. Lancet 371: 301–302.
8. Gurgel RQ, Cuevas LE, Vieira SC, Barros VC, Fontes PB, et al. (2007) Predominance of rotavirus P[4]G2 in a vaccinated population, Brazil. Emerg Infect Dis 13: 1571–1573.
9. Linhares AC, Stupka JA, Ciapponi A, Bardach AE, Glujovsky D, et al. (2011) Burden and typing of rotavirus group A in Latin America and the Caribbean: systematic review and meta-analysis. Rev Med Virol.
10. Matthijnssens J, Nakagomi O, Kirkwood CD, Ciarlet M, Desselberger U, et al. (2012) Group A rotavirus universal mass vaccination: how and to what extent will selective pressure influence prevalence of rotavirus genotypes? Expert Rev Vaccines 11: 1347–1354.
11. IBGE IBdGeEP (2010) Censo Demográfico 2010.
12. Nakagomi T, Nakagomi O, Takahashi Y, Enoki M, Suzuki T, et al. (2005) Incidence and burden of rotavirus gastroenteritis in Japan, as estimated from a prospective sentinel hospital study. J Infect Dis 192 Suppl 1: S106–110.
13. Lanata CF, Fischer-Walker CL, Olascoaga AC, Torres CX, Aryee MJ, et al. (2013) Global causes of diarrheal disease mortality in children <5 years of age: a systematic review. PLoS One 8: e72788.
14. Meloni A, Locci D, Frau G, Masia G, Nurchi AM, et al. (2011) Epidemiology and prevention of rotavirus infection: an underestimated issue? J Matern Fetal Neonatal Med 24 Suppl 2: 48–51.
15. Oliveira TC, Latorre Mdo R (2010) Trends in hospital admission and infant mortality from diarrhea: Brazil, 1995–2005. Rev Saude Publica 44: 102–111.
16. De Oliveira LH, Giglio N, Ciapponi A, Garcia Marti S, Kuperman M, et al. (2013) Temporal trends in diarrhea-related hospitalizations and deaths in children under age 5 before and after the introduction of the rotavirus vaccine in four Latin American countries. Vaccine 31 Suppl 3: C99–108.
17. Payne DC, Boom JA, Staat MA, Edwards KM, Szilagyi PG, et al. (2013) Effectiveness of pentavalent and monovalent rotavirus vaccines in concurrent use among US children <5 years of age, 2009–2011. Clin Infect Dis 57: 13–20.
18. Vesikari T, Uhari M, Renko M, Hemming M, Salminen M, et al. (2013) Impact and Effectiveness of RotaTeq(R) Vaccine Based on 3 Years of Surveillance Following Introduction of a Rotavirus Immunization Program in Finland. Pediatr Infect Dis J 32: 1365–1373.
19. Zeller M, Rahman M, Heylen E, De Coster S, De Vos S, et al. (2010) Rotavirus incidence and genotype distribution before and after national rotavirus vaccine introduction in Belgium. Vaccine 28: 7507–7513.
20. Dey A, Wang H, Menzies R, Macartney K (2012) Changes in hospitalisations for acute gastroenteritis in Australia after the national rotavirus vaccination program. Med J Aust 197: 453–457.
21. Rha B, Tate JE, Payne DC, Cortese MM, Lopman BA, et al. (2014) Effectiveness and impact of rotavirus vaccines in the United States −2006–2012. Expert Rev Vaccines 13: 365–376.
22. Paulke-Korinek M, Kundi M, Rendi-Wagner P, de Martin A, Eder G, et al. (2011) Herd immunity after two years of the universal mass vaccination program against rotavirus gastroenteritis in Austria. Vaccine 29: 2791–2796.
23. Yi J, Anderson EJ (2013) Rotavirus vaccination: short-term indirect herd protection, long-term uncertainty. Expert Rev Vaccines 12: 585–587.
24. Rivera L, Pena LM, Stainier I, Gillard P, Cheuvart B, et al. (2011) Horizontal transmission of a human rotavirus vaccine strain-a randomized, placebo-controlled study in twins. Vaccine 29: 9508–9513.
25. Matthijnssens J, Zeller M, Heylen E, De Coster S, Vercauteren J, et al. (2014) Higher proportion of G2P[4] rotaviruses in vaccinated hospitalised cases compared to unvaccinated hospitalised cases, despite high vaccine effectiveness against heterotypic G2P[4] rotaviruses. Clin Microbiol Infect.
26. Browning GF, Chalmers RM, Fitzgerald TA, Corley KT, Campbell I, et al. (1992) Rotavirus serotype G3 predominates in horses. J Clin Microbiol 30: 59–62.
27. Todd S, Page NA, Duncan Steele A, Peenze I, Cunliffe NA (2010) Rotavirus strain types circulating in Africa: Review of studies published during 1997–2006. J Infect Dis 202 Suppl: S34–42.
28. (2003) Rotavirus vaccines, an update. Wkly Epidemiol Rec 78: 2–3.
29. Pukuta ES, Esona MD, Nkongolo A, Seheri M, Makasi M, et al. (2014) Molecular surveillance of rotavirus infection in the democratic republic of the congo august 2009 to june 2012. Pediatr Infect Dis J 33: 355–359.
30. Abebe A, Teka T, Kassa T, Seheri M, Beyene B, et al. (2014) Hospital-based surveillance for rotavirus gastroenteritis in children younger than 5 years of age in Ethiopia: 2007–2012. Pediatr Infect Dis J 33 Suppl 1: S28–33.
31. Tsolenyanu E, Seheri M, Dagnra A, Djadou E, Tigossou S, et al. (2014) Surveillance for rotavirus gastroenteritis in children less than 5 years of age in Togo. Pediatr Infect Dis J 33 Suppl 1: S14–18.

13

Quantifying and Exploiting the Age Dependence in the Effect of Supplementary Food for Child Undernutrition

Milinda Lakkam[1], Stefan Wager[2], Paul H. Wise[3], Lawrence M. Wein[4]*

1 Institute for Computational and Mathematical Engineering, Stanford University, Stanford, California, United States of America, **2** Statistics Department, Stanford University, Stanford, California, United States of America, **3** School of Medicine, Stanford University, Stanford California, United States of America, **4** Graduate School of Business, Stanford University, Stanford, California, United States of America

Abstract

Motivated by the lack of randomized controlled trials with an intervention-free control arm in the area of child undernutrition, we fit a trivariate model of weight-for-age z score (WAZ), height-for-age z score (HAZ) and diarrhea status to data from an observational study of supplementary feeding (100 kCal/day for children with WAZ < -2.5) in 17 Guatemalan communities. Incorporating time lags, intention to treat (i.e., to give supplementary food), seasonality and age interactions, we estimate how the effect of supplementary food on WAZ, HAZ and diarrhea status varies with a child's age. We find that the effect of supplementary food on all 3 metrics decreases linearly with age from 6 to 20 mo and has little effect after 20 mo. We derive 2 food allocation policies that myopically (i.e., looking ahead 2 mo) minimize either the underweight or stunting severity – i.e., the sum of squared WAZ or HAZ scores for all children with WAZ or HAZ <0. A simulation study based on the statistical model predicts that the 2 derived policies reduce the underweight severity (averaged over all ages) by 13.6–14.1% and reduce the stunting severity at age 60 mo by 7.1–8.0% relative to the policy currently in use, where all policies have a budget that feeds $\approx 4\%$ of children. While these findings need to be confirmed on additional data sets, it appears that in a low-dose (100 kCal/day) supplementary feeding setting in Guatemala, allocating food primarily to 6–12 mo infants can reduce the severity of underweight and stunting.

Editor: C. Mary Schooling, CUNY, United States of America

Funding: Graduate School of Business, Stanford University and a B.C. and E.J. Eaves Stanford Graduate Fellowship. The funders had no role in study design, data collection and analysis, decision to publish, or preparation of the manuscript.

Competing Interests: The authors have declared that no competing interests exist.

* Email: lwein@stanford.edu

Introduction

With over 3 M deaths per year of children under 5 years attributable to undernutrition [1] and the level of food aid far less than required [2,3], it is vital to optimally allocate food to the appropriate children in the appropriate amounts. To address this problem in a rigorous manner requires knowledge about three key aspects [4]: (i) the evolution of weight and height (and perhaps disease) of children under 5 years in the absence of food aid; (ii) the impact that weight and height (and perhaps other factors such as age, sex and disease) have on morbidity and mortality, and (iii) the impact of supplementary or therapeutic food on weight and height (and perhaps other factors such as disease).

A bivariate statistical model of weight and height can be constructed from a longitudinal data set [4] to address (i), and logistic regression [4,5] or proportional hazards [6] models can estimate the impact of anthropometric measurements on mortality to address (ii). The ideal approach to (iii) would use longitudinal measurements of weight and height from a large randomized control trial with a control arm that does not receive any food. There appears to be only one study that possesses these characteristics for therapeutic food [7] and no studies involving supplementary feeding [8]. As a result, very little is known about how the impact of food on weight and height is influenced by a child's age, sex and pre-intervention weight, height and presence of disease, and the amount of therapeutic or supplementary food

consumed. Furthermore, the ethical issues inherent in using a control group that does not receive food suggests that there may not be any large randomized control trials with intervention-free arms performed in the future.

Consequently, the most promising approach to making headway on aspect (iii) is to jointly estimate aspects (i) and (iii) – i.e., fit a statistical model of weight and height in the presence of nonrandom food aid – using observational or dose-response studies of nutrition programs that do not include intervention-free control arms. In this study, we make a first step in this direction and analyze data from a nutrition program in Guatemala, where every child under 5 years in 17 villages has his weight, height and diarrhea status (the number of days in the previous week with diarrhea) measured every 2 mo, and children with weight-for-age z score (WAZ) less than -2.5 receive supplementary food of ≈ 100 kCal/day. We use the WAZ $= -2.5$ threshold to cast the nutrition program as a natural experiment – where children with WAZ just above -2.5 (who do not receive treatment) act as a control group for the children with WAZ just below -2.5 (who do receive treatment) – and analyze it via a regression discontinuity design [9], which is a design where the assignment of an intervention is based on the value of an observed covariate lying below (or above) a fixed threshold. By comparing observations that are just above and just below WAZ $= -2.5$, the regression discontinuity design allows us to estimate the average treatment effect. In econometrics, statistics and related fields, regression discontinuity designs have become the preferred approach for evaluating the effects of intervention in a setting such as ours, where randomization is not possible [9]. More specifically, a generalized additive model (GAM) [10] is used to predict future (i.e., 2 mo hence) WAZ, height-for-age z score (HAZ) and diarrhea status (because deaths from wasting do not occur in this setting, we focus on WAZ and HAZ instead of weight-for-height z score, WHZ) in terms of current and past values of (WAZ,HAZ,diarrhea) along with seasonal and age-interaction terms. This statistical model allows us to isolate how age influences the impact that supplementary food has on WAZ, HAZ and diarrhea status. We use these statistical results to derive 2 allocation policies that minimize the underweight (or stunting) severity, i.e., the sum of squared expected WAZ (or HAZ) scores among children with WAZ <0(or HAZ <0), 2 mo into the future. We build a simulation model based on our GAM that compares the derived allocation policies to the allocation policy that is currently used in the nutrition program in Guatemala, and to the counterfactual of no supplementary food.

Materials and Methods

Data

Our data set tracks 2125 children (1047 boys, 1078 girls) from 17 communities participating in a nutrition program in Guatemala from November 2009 to April 2012. Every 2 months, children from birth to age 60 mo had their WAZ, HAZ – both measured according to World Health Organization (WHO) child growth standards [11] – and the number of days with diarrhea in the previous week recorded. The nutrition program provided supplementary food to all children with WAZ < -2.5. Children over 12 mo received $\approx$100 kCal/day of Incaparina (a supplement made from maize and soy flours) and sugar, and children between 6–12 mo received half this amount and – for children with inadequate or no breastfeeding despite promoter efforts to support breastfeeding until at least 1 year of age –2 400-gm cans of powdered infant formula (Nestle NAN Pro 1 or 2, made of whey and casein milk proteins) per mo. The Stanford Institutional Review Board, which includes members with medical and social science expertise, and the Review Committee of the Hospital Obras Sociales de Monsignor Gregorio Schaffer, San Lucas Toliman reviewed and approved this study prior to study initiation. Informed consent in Spanish and/or the local indigenous language was obtained from a parent/guardian for all children at enrollment. All patient information was anonymized and de-identified prior to analysis.

Generalized Additive Model

For boys and girls, we build separate GAMs for the evolution of (W_t, H_t, D_t) for age t varying from 1 to 60 mo, which are the WAZ, HAZ and the number of days with diarrhea in the previous week for a child of age t mo (see Table 1 for a description of most of the variables). Define the Intention To Treat (ITT) indicator variable $I_t = 1$ if $W_t < -2.5$ and $I_t = 0$ otherwise, and let M_t be the month of the year when a child is of age t. Let $\hat{t} = (t - 31.76)/15.74$ be the standardized age, where 31.76 mo and 15.74 mo are the mean and standard deviation of the ages among all entries in the data set.

An analysis of GAM results with varying amounts of history suggests that we need to maintain 4 mo of history; i.e., if we are trying to estimate a child's $(W_{t+2}, H_{t+2}, D_{t+2})$ then we need to use (W_t, H_t, D_t) and $(W_{t-2}, H_{t-2}, D_{t-2})$. To ease the interpretation of our GAM coefficients, we let the response variables be

Table 1. The estimated parameters for boys from the GAM.

Variable	Description	Estimating $W_{t+2}-W_t$			Estimating $H_{t+2}-H_t$			Estimating D_{t+2}		
		Est.	S.E.	p	Est.	S.E.	p	Est.	S.E.	p
	Intercept	-0.230	0.018	0.000	-0.907	0.025	0.000	-0.751	0.081	0.000
W_t	WAZ	-0.095	0.007	0.000	0.124	0.009	0.000	-0.184	0.039	0.000
$W_t\hat{t}$	WAZ × age	0.014	0.006	0.026	-0.068	0.009	0.000	-0.056	0.036	0.115
$W_t - W_{t-2}$	WAZ increment	-0.256	0.011	0.000	-0.000	0.016	0.981	0.183	0.066	0.006
$(W_t - W_{t-2})\hat{t}$	WAZ incr. × age	-0.090	0.010	0.000	0.021	0.013	0.116	0.084	0.055	0.122
H_t	HAZ	0.038	0.006	0.000	-0.177	0.008	0.000	-0.007	0.033	0.835
$H_t\hat{t}$	HAZ × age	0.006	0.005	0.280	0.092	0.007	0.000	0.068	0.030	0.024
$H_t - H_{t-2}$	HAZ increment	-0.020	0.009	0.030	-0.205	0.013	0.000	0.063	0.053	0.236
$(H_t - H_{t-2})\hat{t}$	HAZ incr. × age	-0.007	0.008	0.375	-0.022	0.011	0.036	-0.041	0.042	0.337
D_t	Diarrhea	0.003	0.003	0.387	-0.003	0.004	0.429	0.102	0.014	0.000
$D_t\hat{t}$	Diarrhea × age	0.014	0.003	0.000	0.007	0.004	0.091	-0.021	0.013	0.100

For each variable, we give the estimated coefficient (Est.), the standard error (S.E.) and the p-value.

$(W_{t+2}-W_t, H_{t+2}-H_t, D_{t+2})$. We fit $W_{t+2}-W_t$ and $H_{t+2}-H_t$ by least squares and model D_t by a Poisson random variable. We let the link functions be the identity function for $W_{t+2}-W_t$ and $H_{t+2}-H_t$ and the natural logarithm for D_{t+2}. The predictor variables include the current values (W_t, H_t, D_t) and their age-interaction terms $(W_t\hat{t}, H_t\hat{t}, D_t\hat{t})$, the most recent increments $((W_t-W_{t-2}),(H_t-H_{t-2}))$ and their age interaction terms $((W_t-W_{t-2})\hat{t},(H_t-H_{t-2})\hat{t})$, as well as seasonal functions $(f_M^W(M_t), f_M^H(M_t), f_M^D(M_t))$ for the month of the year, age functions $(g^W(t), g^H(t), g^D(t))$ in the absence of supplementary food, and age functions $(g_I^W(t)I_t, g_I^H(t)I_t, g_I^D(t)I_t)$ due to the ITT. The seasonal functions are modeled as periodic cubic splines and the age functions are modeled as cubic smoothing splines. We denote the sample covariance matrix calculated from the residuals of the GAM by Σ. The 3 GAM equations are stated with their resulting coefficients in §1 of File S1.

To make the most use of the available data without imputing any missing data, we include every set of 3 consecutive measurements by assuming they occur at ages $t-2$, t and $t+2$ for some t. We also discard as outliers any z scores outside the range of $[-5,5]$.

Proposed Allocation Policies

Because of the difficulty of solving a dynamic program with a system state that is the joint population-wide probability density function (PDF) of (W_t, H_t, D_t), we derive 2 derived policies – referred to as the derived WAZ policy and the derived HAZ policy – that estimate every child's $(W_{t+2}, H_{t+2}, D_{t+2})$ given all the information known at age t, and minimizes the sum of $E[W_{t+2}]^2$ (or $E[H_{t+2}]^2$) over all children with $W_t < 0$ (or $H_t < 0$), subject to a constraint on the amount of supplementary food allocated. As in [12], this objective captures moderate and mild forms of undernutrition and also incorporates the fact that more severe undernutrition leads to more severe consequences; however, we use $E[W_{t+2}]^2$ rather than $E[W_{t+2}^2]$ so that the proposed policy is relatively simple.

Let $c_t = 0.5$ if $t \in [6,12]$ and $c_t = 1$ if $t > 12$, which represents the normalized amount of supplementary food consumed by a child at age t. The allocation policy that solves this constrained optimization problem prioritizes all children with $W_t < 0$ by $(E[W_{t+2}|I_t=1])^2 - E[W_{t+2}|I_t=0])^2)/c_t$ (with smaller values getting higher priority), and allocates the food until it is gone (§2 of File S1).

Simulation Model

The simulation model tracks 1 M children of each sex from age 6 to 60 mo. A child's initial (W_t, H_t, D_t) at 6 mo is randomly sampled with replacement from all children of the same sex in the data set when they were 6 mo. At each 2-mo time step, the values of $(W_{t+2}, H_{t+2}, D_{t+2})$ are calculated using the GAM and then adding an additive trivariate noise term that is normally distributed with mean zero and covariance matrix Σ (and rounding the value of D_{t+2} to the nearest integer).

We consider the 5 policies described in Table 2. All policies except the no food policy allocate the same amount of food, which is dictated by the amount of food allocated under the current policy (i.e., $W_t < -2.5$). This food budget is 1.2 (0.7) units of food per boy (girl) over a child's 27 feeding opportunities, which corresponds to 4.7% of children being fed at any given time. We do a 1-dimensional search for thresholds (for the quantities being prioritized in Table 2) for the simple WAZ policy and the 2 derived policies so that the amount of food allocated by these policies is equal to this food budget. The thresholds for the simple WAZ policy are -1.8 for boys (i.e., a boy under 2 yr receives food if $W_t < -1.8$) and -1.7 for girls, the thresholds for the derived WAZ policy are -0.082 for boys (i.e., a boy receives food if $(E[W_{t+2}|I_t=1])^2 - E[W_{t+2}|I_t=0])^2)/c_t < -0.082$) and -0.138 for girls, and the thresholds for the derived HAZ policy are -0.44 for boys and -0.56 for girls.

For each policy and various values of θ, we report $P(H_t < \theta)$ and $P(W_t < \theta)$ for all $t \in [6,60]$ mo. We also compute 2 variants of the severity index considered in [12], the average of $\sum_{t=6}^{60} W_t^2 I_{\{W_t < 0\}}/28$ over all children and the average of $H_{60}^2 I_{\{H_{60} < 0\}}$, where $I_{\{x\}}$ is the indicator function of the event x. These quantities are the average squared shortfalls below the reference median (i.e., zero) for WAZ averaged over all ages and for HAZ at age 60 mo. We refer to these measures as the underweight severity and the stunting severity, respectively.

Results

GAM Results

The GAM parameters are very similar for boys (Table 1) and girls (Table 1 of File S1), and the statistically significant parameters have the following interpretations. WAZ exhibits global mean reversion (i.e., heavier children tend to lose weight and lighter children tend to gain weight), which is more pronounced in younger children, and local mean reversion (i.e., children who have recently lost weight tend to gain it back and vice versa), which is more pronounced in older children. Taller children tend to gain weight although children who recently grew taller are less likely to gain weight. Current diarrhea status has no impact on weight gain overall, although older boys are more likely to gain weight after a diarrhea episode while younger boys are more apt to lose weight (this effect is not observed in girls). HAZ also exhibits global mean reversion that is more prominent in younger children and local mean reversion that is more prominent in older children, and the magnitude of global mean reversion for HAZ is larger than it is for WAZ. Heavier children are more apt to grow taller, an effect that is more evident in younger children. Current diarrhea status and recent weight gain are not associated with height gain. Diarrhea is reinforcing; i.e., current diarrhea tends to lead to future diarrhea. Lighter children and children who recently gained weight both tend to get more diarrhea, and the former effect is more pronounced in older girls than younger girls. Current height of boys has no overall impact on getting diarrhea, although taller girls are more likely to get diarrhea than shorter girls. Older tall children are more likely to get diarrhea than younger tall children.

Turning to the spline functions, which are also very similar for boys (Fig. 1) and girls (Fig. 1 of File S1), we see that low WAZ and high diarrhea prevalence are on very similar annual cycles (with November - April being the most severe months), while HAZ has a more rapid increase and lags slightly behind WAZ, peaking during August - November (Figs. 1a–c). In the absence of intervention, faltering in WAZ and HAZ occurs during the first 2 yr, at which point WAZ stabilizes and HAZ increases for boys (Figs. 1d–e); for girls, WAZ does not stabilize until ≈ 40 mo and HAZ begins to increase at 30 mo. The prevalence of diarrhea decreases with age (Fig. 1f). The effect of ITT (i.e., supplementary food) has a similar pattern for all 3 variables: the impact is beneficial (i.e., higher WAZ and HAZ, lower diarrhea) and linearly decreasing between 6 and 20 months, and thereafter has little or no effect (with the exception that ITT leads to an increase in diarrhea for older girls). ITT's effect on HAZ is twice as large as its effect on WAZ.

Table 2. Food allocation policies.

Name of Policy	Children Receiving Food	Severity Index	
		Underweight	Stunting
No Food	None	1.87	5.44
Current	$W_t < -2.5$	1.84	5.50
Simple WAZ	Under 2 yr and prioritized by W_t	1.77	5.35
Derived WAZ	Prioritized by $(E[W_{t+2}|I_t=1])^2 - E[W_{t+2}|I_t=0]^2)/c_t$	1.59	5.11
Derived HAZ	Prioritized by $(E[H_{t+2}|I_t=1])^2 - E[H_{t+2}|I_t=0]^2)/c_t$	1.58	5.06

A description of the food allocation policies and their severity indices for boys, which measure the average of squared shortfalls below the reference median (i.e., zero) for WAZ averaged over all 28 measured ages (underweight) and for HAZ at age 60 mo (stunting).

The covariance parameters are very similar for boys and girls (§1 of File S1), where weight gain and height gain are positively correlated, weight gain and diarrhea are negatively correlated, and height gain and diarrhea are the least correlated. The adjusted R^2 for $(W_{t+2} - W_t, H_{t+2} - H_t, D_t)$ are 0.151, 0.259 and 0.041 for boys, and 0.226, 0.309 and 0.052 for girls.

Food Allocation Results

The results for boys (Figs. 2–5) and girls (Figs. 2–5 of File S1) are very similar, aside from the fact that girls are less underweight than boys, and hence have a smaller food budget. Given the strong influence of age on the effect of intervention (Figs. 1g–i), it is not surprising that the two derived policies allocate much of the food to children <12 mo (Fig. 2). Consequently, the two derived policies reduce the far left tail of the HAZ and WAZ distributions between 6–12 mo (Figs. 3–4). Although some of this gain is dissipated through the next 4 years, these 2 policies still dominate the other policies throughout the first 5 years. The current policy incurs a significant increase in extreme underweight (WAZ < -3) during 12–30 mo because it fails to feed enough children <12 mo who are in danger of faltering. A similar outcome – but at WAZ < -2.5– is incurred by the simple WAZ policy for children during 20–24 mo.

The severity indices (Table 2 for boys, Table 2 of File S1 for girls) reveal that the derived HAZ policy achieves slightly smaller underweight and stunting severity indices than the derived WAZ policy, although both policies perform well on both measures relative to the other policies, and achieve a 13.6–14.1% reduction in WAZ severity and a 7.1–8.0% reduction in HAZ severity relative to the current policy. The performance gap between the 2 derived policies and the simple WAZ policy is 2–3 times larger than the gap between the simple WAZ policy and the no food policy. In our simulations, the current policy increases the HAZ severity index by 1.1% relative to the no food policy for boys, and increases it by 0.1% for girls. An examination of the stunting PDFs for the 5 policies (Fig. 5) reveals that the current policy reduces the number of children with $H_{60} \in [-3.5, -1]$, but increases the number of children with $H_{60} < -4$. This increase in the extreme tail occurs because there is a small group of children with WAZ values that are consistently < -2.5 and with very low HAZ levels, and ITT further lowers their HAZ levels during months 18–36 and 46–60 (although even at the lowest points in Fig. 1 h of -0.08 at 25 mo and -0.1 at 60 mo, children continue to grow taller under ITT). In contrast, the 2 derived policies reduce the number of children with $H_{60} < -2$ and move them to the $H_{60} > -2$ region.

Sensitivity Analysis

We perform a sensitivity analysis for boys to assess the robustness of our main result that the 2 derived policies outperform the current policy. We perform the following procedure 10^3 times: take a random sample with replacement of 1047 boys (which is the original sample size in the data set) from our data set, re-estimate the statistical model (i.e., get new values for the parameters in Table 1 and the functions in Fig. 1), use the statistical model to simulate 10^4 boys under the current policy and the derived WAZ policy (for all runs, the derived WAZ policy is based on the results in Table 1 and Fig. 1, not on the re-estimated model), and compute the percentage reduction in the two severity indices that the derived WAZ policy achieves relative to the current policy. The PDFs of the 10^3 percentage reductions (Figs. 6a–b) show that the derived WAZ policy achieves a mean percentage reduction of 14.7% for underweight severity and 7.6% for stunting severity relative to the current policy, and the percentage of times that the current policy performs better than the derived WAZ policy is 4.7% for underweight severity and 0.2% for stunting severity.

We perform an identical sensitivity analysis to assess whether the current policy reduces the underweight and stunting severities relative to the no food policy. We find that the current policy reduces underweight severity by 1.4% on average and reduces it 79.7% of the time, whereas the current policy increases stunting severity by 1.2% on average and increases it 90.6% of the time (Figs. 6c–d).

Discussion

Statistical Results

The similarity between some of our statistical results and the existing literature is reassuring, and provides some confidence in the remaining statistical results that have no counterpart in the literature. The patterns of growth faltering in Figs. 1d–e are similar to the patterns seen elsewhere [13], as are the decrease in diarrhea prevalence with age (Fig. 1f and [14]). Similarly, the seasonal patterns in Figs. 1a–c are not unlike those found in Malawi [15], and – as is typical in Latin America [16] – stunting is much more prevalent than underweight. Rearranging equations (13)-(16) in the Supporting Material of [4] shows that the model there, which is based on data from Bwamanda in the Democratic Republic of Congo [17], also exhibits global and local mean reversion; global mean reversion in HAZ data is also observed in [15].

Turning to the cross terms, we find that high weight leads to a future increase in HAZ, but that recent weight gain does not; the latter finding agrees with correlations derived in [15]. An analysis

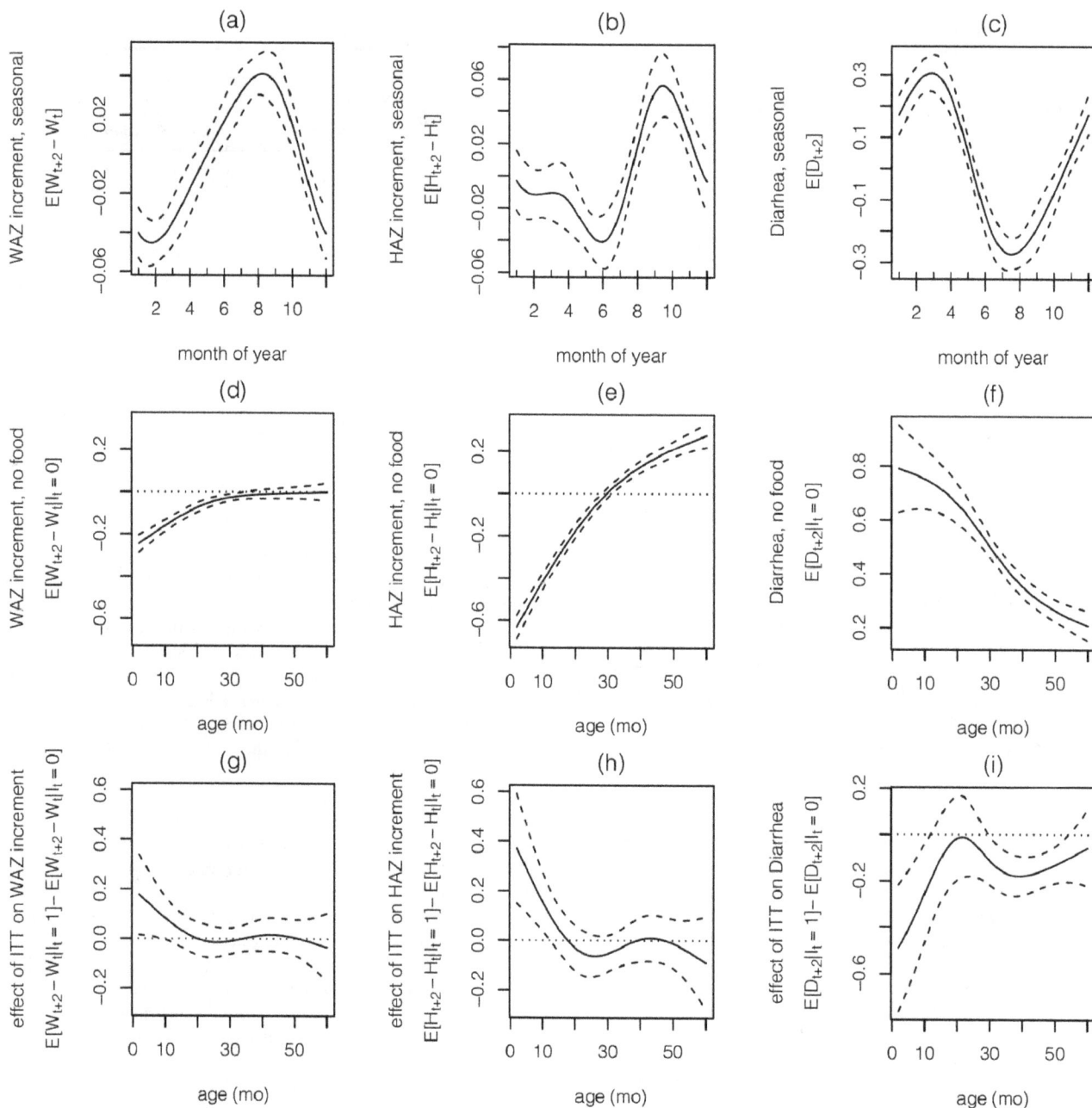

Figure 1. The estimated spline functions (and 95% confidence intervals) for boys from the GAM. The seasonal functions (**a**) $f_M^W(M_t)$, (**b**) $f_M^H(M_t)$ and (**c**) $f_M^D(M_t)$ for WAZ and HAZ increments and diarrhea. The age functions in the absence of supplementary food (**d**) $g^W(t)$, (**e**) $g^H(t)$ and (**f**) $g^D(t)$ for WAZ and HAZ increments and diarrhea. The age functions due to ITT (**g**) $g_I^W(t)$, (**h**) $g_I^H(t)$ and (**i**) $g_I^D(t)$ for WAZ and HAZ increments and diarrhea.

of WHZ (rather than WAZ) and HAZ find that both low WHZ and a recent drop in WHZ lead to future reductions in HAZ [18].

Our statistical results provide limited evidence to support the fact that diarrhea can reduce nutritional status. The lack of significance of the D_t coefficient in predicting future WAZ or HAZ gain may be because most of the catch-up growth occurs before the next visit. In addition, the coefficient of $D_t\hat{i}$ in the WAZ equation for boys is consistent with the observation that infants take longer to catch up in weight than older children [19]. Although our model predicts that underweight children are more apt to get diarrhea, which is consistent with earlier results [20,21],

the same is not true of stunted children (in fact, taller girls are more likely to get diarrhea than shorter girls in our model); some of the anticipated effect (i.e., stunted children are more likely to get diarrhea) may be partially masked by the age dependence (i.e., the value of the $H_t\hat{i}$ coefficient) and the 2-mo follow-up period. In any case, diarrhea is very difficult to predict and the only factors that play a strong role are seasonality, being underweight, and currently having diarrhea, which collectively suggest environmental and microbiome causes.

Our most intriguing statistical result is the strong dependence of age on the impact of intervention (Figs. 1g–i). Considerable

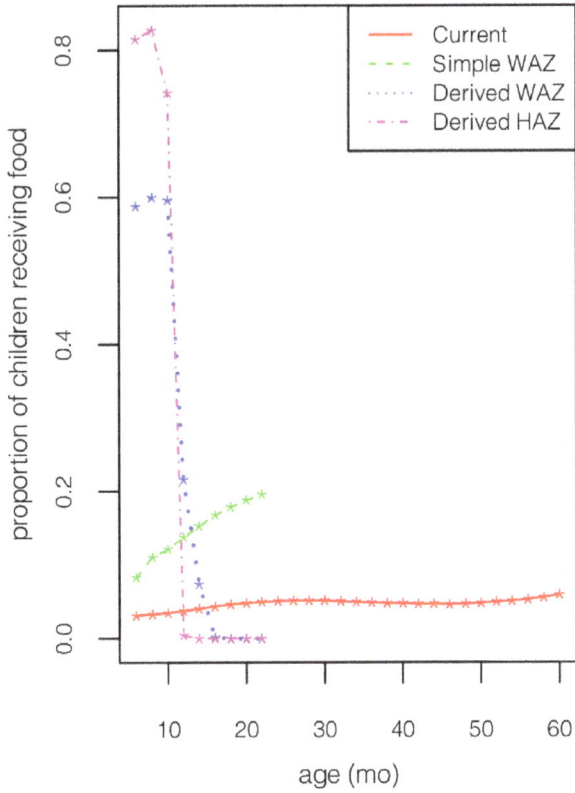

Figure 2. The proportion of boys by age who receive food under the various allocation policies.

after age 3. A meta-analysis in Web Appendix 4 of [24] suggests that linear growth during 6–12 mo is larger than during 12–18 mo in populations with average per capita income >$1/day, but is smaller for incomes <$1/day. Fig. 1 h is not inconsistent with this observation because the income in Guatemala is >$1/day.

The magnitude of the seasonality in Figs. 1a-b and of the global and local mean reversion (Table 1) implies that approaches that ignore these factors can lead to misleading estimates – and systematic overestimates in the case of global mean reversion – of the increase in weight and height that is due to supplementary feeding.

Food Allocation Results

The 2 derived policies anticipate growth faltering and exploit the age dependence in the impact of intervention by front-loading much of the intervention on infants (Fig. 2), who gain a substantial head start relative to the current policy (Figs. 3–4). Although some of the gap disappears by the time children reach age 5 years (perhaps partly due to global mean reversion), much of the improvement remains intact at age 5. The derived policies are fairly simple to implement, although they do require knowledge of a child's height and weight from his previous visit.

Due to the very limited amount of food distributed by the current policy ($\approx$4% of children receive food at any point in time) and the fact that many more children are stunted than underweight, the improvements achieved by the 2 derived policies are modest when measured by stunting (HAZ < -2), but are more pronounced for severe stunting (HAZ < -3) and in the extreme left tail of the HAZ distribution (Fig. 4).

Because of the reinforcing cross terms – i.e., large HAZ leads to future increases in WAZ and large WAZ leads to future increases in HAZ – and the similar age dependence in how intervention increases WAZ and HAZ, the 2 derived policies have very similar performance with respect to reducing the severity of underweight and stunting.

There has been increasing focus on the lifetime effects of stunting [25], and in Latin America, where severe wasting is rare and stunting is prevalent, reducing stunting is one of the primary goals of supplementary feeding programs. To this end, we note that our model predicts that the current policy – because it allows some underweight, stunted children to become very severely

evidence has been amassed about the importance of nutrition in the first 1000 days (from conception to 24 mo) [1,22], and Figs. 1g-i can be viewed as a refinement of this principle. Our age-dependent results are similar to those in an earlier study in Guatemala [23], which found that – after controlling for diarrhea, previous height and weight, sex, home diet and socioeconomic status – height gain and weight gain due to supplemental food decreased throughout the first 3 years of life and had little effect

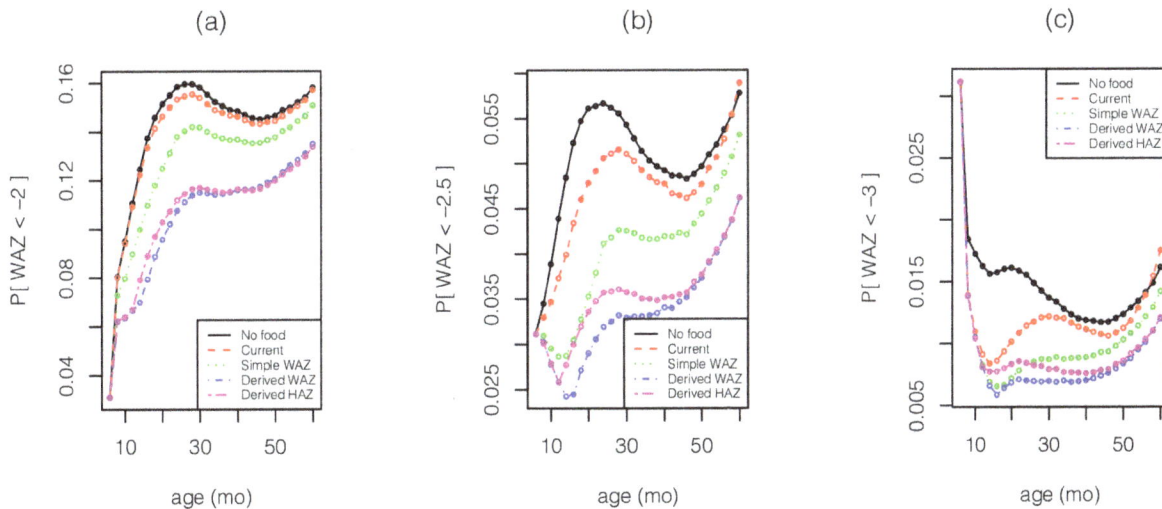

Figure 3. For boys, the left tails, $P(\text{WAZ} < \theta)$ for θ equals (a) -2, (b) -2.5, (c) -3 vs. age under the various policies.

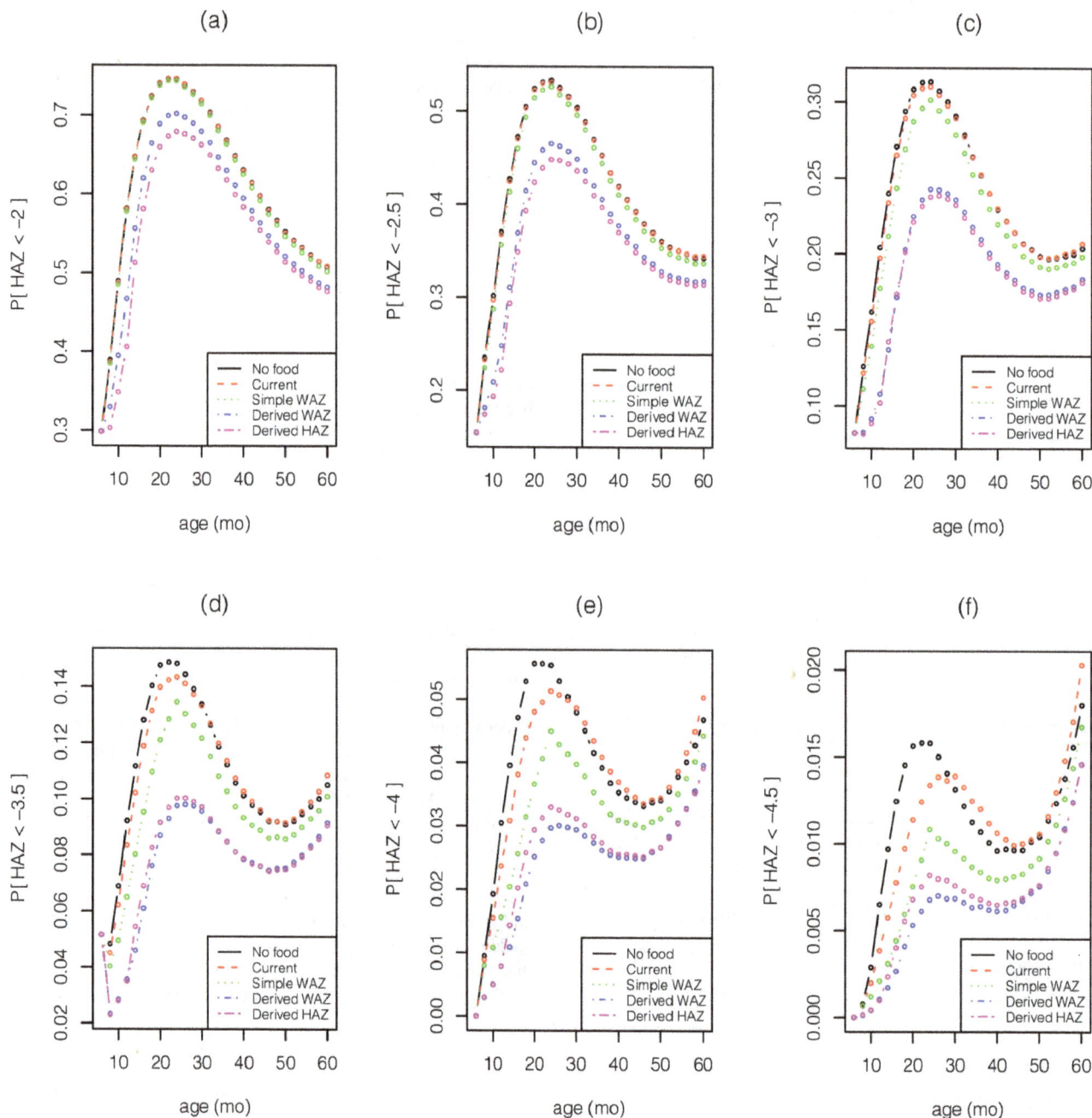

Figure 4. For boys, the left tails, P(HAZ $< \theta$) for θ equals (a) −2, (b) −2.5, (c) −3, (d) −3.5, (e) −4, (f) −4.5 vs. age under the various policies.

stunted (Fig. 5b) – has a slightly higher severity of stunting than the no food policy (Fig. 6d). This result is driven by the fact that ITT leads to a slight decrease in HAZ in our model during months 18–36 and 46–60 (Fig. 1h); it is not clear whether this effect is real (albeit small), or is caused by overshooting of the cubic spline in Fig. 1h. In contrast, despite the wide confidence intervals in Figs. 1g–i, our sensitivity analysis (Figs. 6a–b) suggests that our main result – i.e., that the 2 derived policies outperform the current policy – is somewhat robust.

There has also been concern about the long-term cardiovascular risks associated with catch-up growth in early childhood [26]. While this remains an important issue, particularly for rapid

weight gain among infants born at low birth weight, the immediate mortality and developmental risks associated with serious childhood malnutrition would seem to warrant monitored nutritional supplementation.

Limitations of Analysis

Aside from the obvious shortcoming that our analysis is based on data from a non-randomized study, there are 2 major limitations in our data set. The first is that health promoters in the Guatemala nutrition program had discretion to feed sick children, and hence ITT did not exactly coincide with the actual receipt of food. We use ITT so as not to be biased by the behavior

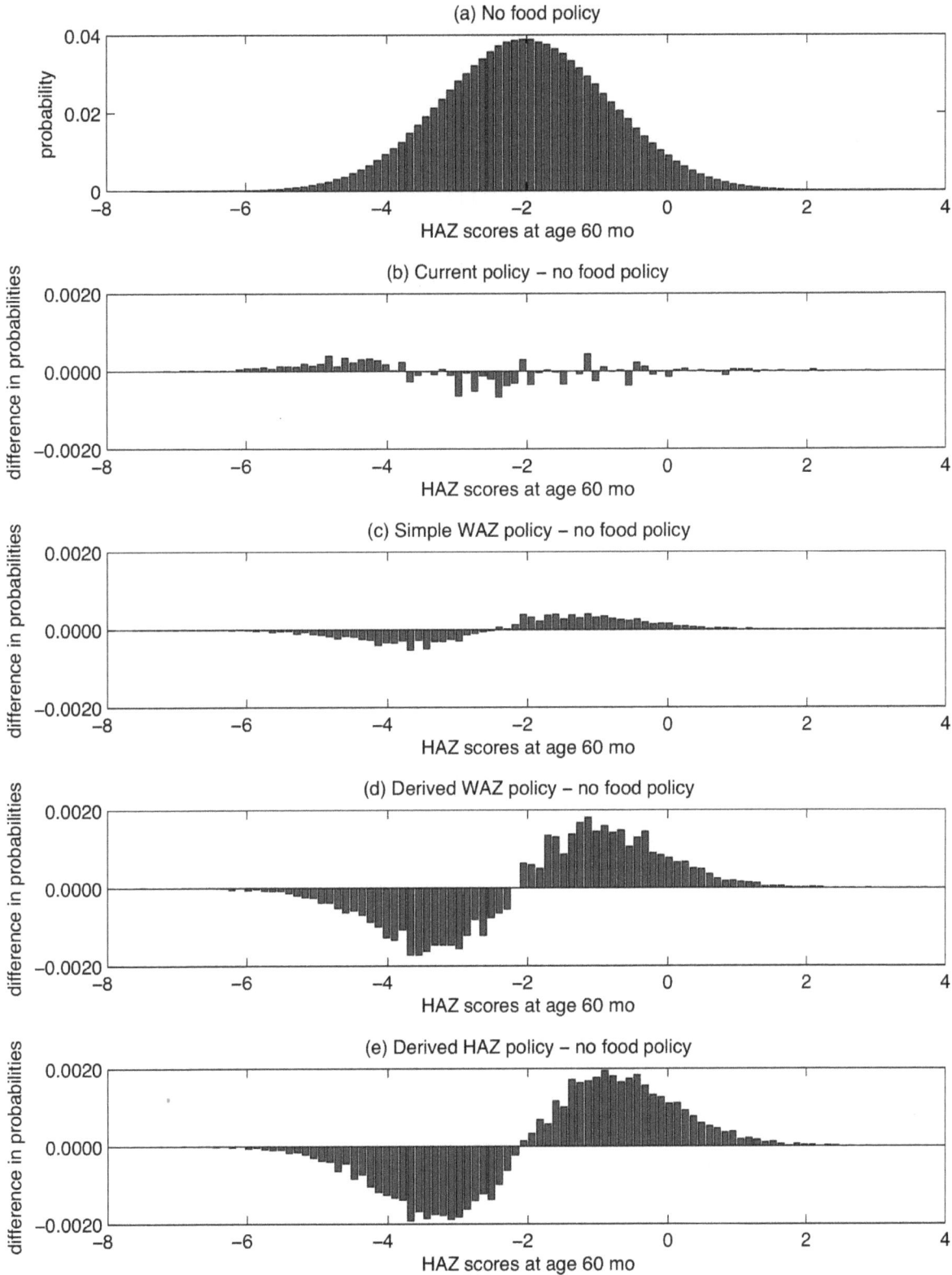

Figure 5. For boys, (a) the PDF for HAZ at age 60 mo, and (b)-(e) the difference in PDFs for HAZ at age 60 mo between 2 policies.

of health promoters. Note that if the health promoters were not given discretion to feed sick children, there may have been an incentive to alter WAZ data (e.g., change −2.3 to −2.6 so as to feed a sick child). The second limitation in our data set is the

amount of missing data. While children were supposed to see a health promoter every 2 mo, the actual time between consecutive visits in the data set was 1 mo, 2 mo, 3 mo, 4 mo and >4mo with probabilities 0.094, 0.638, 0.122, 0.121 and 0.024, respectively.

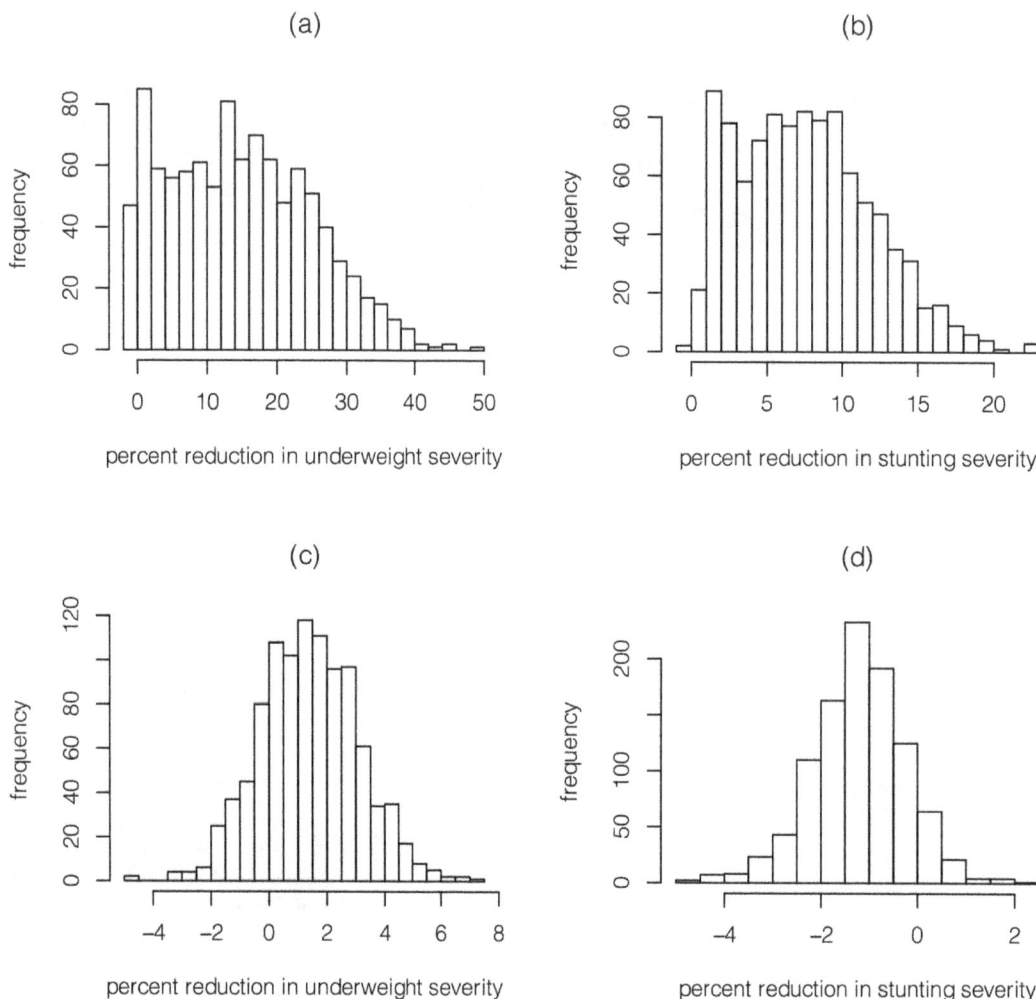

Figure 6. For boys, the PDFs of the percent reduction of the severity indices of (a)-(b) the derived WAZ policy relative to the current policy, and (c)-(d) the current policy relative to the no food policy.

With respect to estimating the impact of ITT and its age interaction, the primary concern with our assumption that consecutive visits are exactly 2 mo is if ITT causes children to visit more or less frequently relative to no ITT. To assess this issue, we re-ran the GAM with the same predictor variables as before but now with the time until the next visit as the response variable. The overall mean effect of ITT was very close to zero (see Fig. 6 of File S1, which is the analogue to Figs. 1g-i in the main text) and the 3 p-values for the cubic spline were 0.91, 0.88 an 0.96.

There are other aspects that could be investigated: estimating the variance of ITT, the interaction of diarrhea and z scores (e.g., a $D_t W_t$ interaction term could address whether diarrhea lowers future weight gain only when current WAZ is low [19]), and whether ITT is a function of D_t [19]. However, we note that our qualitative conclusions would not change even if diarrhea was omitted from the model. Also, the data used here are not well suited to estimate the influence that pre-intervention (WAZ,HAZ) levels have on the impact of intervention because of the lack of intervention-free children with low WAZ and because of the presence of global mean reversion, which may have a similar effect (Fig. 2 in [27]).

The age dependence in the impact of treatment should not be extrapolated to other settings, other doses or other undernutrition

thresholds without performing similar statistical analyses of other longitudinal data sets. It should be noted that the community health system within which the nutritional surveillance and supplementation program is embedded also provides basic preventive and therapeutic health services, including routine antihelminthic medication for children greater than 2 years of age and when needed, referral to local and regional, clinical facilities. In addition, identification of malnutrition and the provision of supplementation may elevate the nutritional needs of the child in question and result indirectly in a relative reallocation of some family resources to the child. This in turn could modify the impact of supplementation on growth in different cultural or resource settings. It may be the case that 100 kCal/day is an insufficient dose – particularly after taking into account the possibility of food sharing within families – to improve the nutritional status of children over 2 years old, but that larger doses are sufficient. Similarly, even at the current dose, our findings should not be extrapolated to thresholds other than WAZ = −2.5. It is possible that age-specific treatment effects differ by level of undernutrition. In particular, children >20 mo may respond more to supplementary feeding when their initial undernutrition levels are more severe, because of the developmental delays associated with undernutrition. If so, regression discontinuity around a more extreme threshold might have yielded flatter estimated age functions in Figs. 1g–i.

Conclusion

Fitting a trivariate statistical model of WAZ, HAZ and diarrhea to a longitudinal data set from a nutritional program in Guatemala generates results that reinforce and quantify relationships that are already known, and identify new relationships, including a strong age dependence in the impact of supplementary food on WAZ, HAZ and diarrhea, with the benefits decreasing from 6 mo to 20 mo old and staying at a small level between 20 and 60 mo old. Our statistical results highlight the danger of ignoring seasonality and global and local mean reversion when estimating the impact of supplementary food. The food allocation policies derived here perform better than the current policy: by allocating much of the food to infants, the derived policies reduce the underweight severity by 13.6–14.1% and the stunting severity by 7.1–8.0% relative to the current policy, despite using a budget that allocates food to only 4.7% of the children at any time under the current policy. This result should not be extrapolated to other geographical regions, to doses other than 100 kCal/day, or to undernutrition thresholds other than WAZ = −2.5. To confirm this result,

the derived policies should be compared to the current policy or the simple WAZ policy in a randomized study. More generally, given the paucity of randomized controlled trials with intervention-free control groups, our statistical approach has the potential to uncover new knowledge from observational studies pertaining to therapeutic and supplementary food for children, and our optimization approach allows this knowledge to be leveraged to improve nutritional status in a budget-constrained setting.

Acknowledgments

We thank Mike Baiocchi and Jeremy Goldhaber-Fiebert for helpful conversations. We also wish to thank Dr. Rafael Tun, Jos Vicente Macario Cosigu, and Dominga Pic Salazar for coordination of the community health worker and nutrition program.

Author Contributions

Conceived and designed the experiments: SW LMW. Performed the experiments: ML SW. Analyzed the data: ML SW LMW. Contributed reagents/materials/analysis tools: PHW. Wrote the paper: LMW.

References

1. Black RE, Victora CG, Walker SP, Bhutta ZA, Christian P, et al. (2013) Maternal and child undernutrition and overweight in low-income and middle-income countries. Lancet 382: 427–451.
2. Horton S, Shekar M, McDonald C, Mahal A, Krystene Brooks J (2010) Scaling up nutrition: What will it cost? Washington, DC: World Bank.
3. Shoham J, Dolan C, Gostelow L (2013) The management of acute malnutrition at scale: a review of donor and government financing arrangements. Technical report, Humanitarian Practice Network, Overseas Development Institute.
4. Yang Y, Van den Broeck J, Wein LM (2013) Ready-to-use food-allocation policy to reduce the effects of childhood undernutrition in developing countries. PNAS 110: 4545–4550.
5. Garenne M, Maire B, Fontaine O, Briend A (2006) Distributions of mortality risk attributable to low nutritional status in niakhar, senegal. J Nutrition 136: 2893–2900.
6. McDonald CM, Olofin I, Flaxman S, Fawzi WW, Spiegelman D, et al. (2013) The effect of multiple anthropometric deficits on child mortality: Meta-analysis of individual data in 10 prospective studies from developing countries. Am J Clinical Nutrition 97: 896–901.
7. Isanaka S, Nombela N, Djibo A, Poupard M, Van Beckhoven D, et al. (2009) Effective of preventive supplementation with ready-to-use therapeutic food on the nutritional status, mortality and morbidity of children aged 6 to 60 months in niger. JAMA 301: 277–285.
8. Dewey KG, Yang Z, Boy E (2009) Systematic review and meta-analysis of home fortification of complementary foods. Maternal Child Nutrition 5: 283–321.
9. Imbens GW, Lemieux T (2008) Regression discontinuity designs: A guide to practice. J Econometrics 142: 615–635.
10. Hastie TJ, Tibshirani RJ (1990) Generalized additive models, volume 43. CRC Press.
11. De Onis M, Garza C, Onyango AW, Borghi E (2007) Comparison of the who child growth standards and the cdc-2000 growth charts. J Nutrition 137: 144–148.
12. Bhagowalia P, Chen SE, Masters WA (2011) Effects and determinants of mild underweight among preschool children across countries and over time. Economics Human Biology 9: 66–77.
13. Victora CG, de Onis M, Hallal PC, Blössner M, Shrimpton R (2010) Worldwide timing of growth faltering: revisiting implications for interventions. Pediatrics 125: e473–e480.

14. Walker CLF, Rudan I, Liu L, Nair H, Theodoratou E, et al. (2013) Global burden of childhood pneumonia and diarrhoea. Lancet 381: 1405–1416.
15. Maleta K, Virtanen SM, Espo M, Kulmala T, Ashorn P (2003) Seasonality of growth and the relationship between weight and height gain in children under three years of age in rural malawi. Acta Paediatrics 92: 491–497.
16. Victora CG (1992) The association between wasting and stunting: An international perspective. J Nutrition 122: 1105–1110.
17. Van den Broeck JV, Eeckels R, Vuylsteke J (1993) Influence of nutritional status on child mortality in rural zaire. Lancet 341: 1491–1495.
18. Richard SA, Black RE, Gilman RH, Guerrant RL, Kang G, et al. (2012) Childhood infection malnutrition network: Wasting is associated with stunting in early childhood. J Nutrition 142: 1291–1296.
19. Dewey KG, Mayers DR (2011) Early child growth: How do nutrition and infection interact. Maternal Child Nutrition 7: 129–142.
20. Yoon PW, Black RE, Moulton LH, Becker S (1997) The effect of malnutrition on the risk of diarrheal and respiratory mortality in children less than 2 y of age in cebu, phillipines. Am J Clinical Nutrition 65: 1070–1077.
21. Caulfield LE, de Onis M, Blossner M, Black RE (2004) Undernutrition as an underlying cause of child deaths associated with diarrhea, pneumonia, malaria, and measles. Am J Clinical Nutrition 80: 193–198.
22. Adair LS, Fall CHD, Osmond C et al (2013) Associations of linear growth and relative weight gain during early life with adult health and human capital in countries of low and middle income: Findings from five birth cohort studies. Lancet 382: 525–534.
23. Schroeder DG, Martorell R, Rivera JA, Ruel MT, Habicht JP (1995) Age differences in the impact of nutritional supplementation on growth. The Journal of nutrition 125: 1051S–1059S.
24. Bhutta ZA, Ahmed T, Black RE, Cousens S, Dewey K, et al. (2008) What works? interventions for maternal and child undernutrition and survival. Lancet 371: 417–440.
25. Victora CG, Adair C L Fall, Hallal PC, Martorell R, Richter L, et al. (2008) Maternal and child undernutrition: Consequences for adult health and human capital. Lancet 371: 340–357.
26. Singhal A, Lucas A (2004) Early origins of cardiovascular disease: Is there a unifying hypothesis? Lancet 363: 1642–1645.
27. Singh AS, Kang G, Ramachandran A, Sarkar R, Peter P, et al. (2010) Locally made ready-to-use therapeutic food for treatment of malnutrition: A randomized control trial. Indian Pediatrics 47: 679–686.

14

Ebola Outbreak Response; Experience and Development of Screening Tools for Viral Haemorrhagic Fever (VHF) in a HIV Center of Excellence Near to VHF Epicentres

Rosalind Parkes-Ratanshi[1]*, Ali Elbireer[1,2], Betty Mbambu[1], Faridah Mayanja[1], Alex Coutinho[1], Concepta Merry[1,3,4]

1 Infectious Diseases Institute, Makerere College of Health Sciences, Kampala, Uganda, 2 Johns Hopkins University, School of Medicine, Baltimore, Maryland, United States of America, 3 Trinity College Dublin, Dublin, Ireland, 4 Northwestern University, Chicago, Illinois, United States of America

Abstract

Introduction: There have been 3 outbreaks of viral hemorrhagic fever (VHF) in Uganda in the last 2 years. VHF often starts with non-specific symptoms prior to the onset of haemorrhagic signs. HIV clinics in VHF outbreak countries such as Uganda see large numbers of patients with HIV 1/2 infection presenting with non-specific symptoms every day. Whilst there are good screening tools for general health care facilities expecting VHF suspects, we were unable to find tools for use in HIV or other non-acute clinics.

Methods: We designed tools to help with communication to staff, infection control and screening of HIV patients with non-specific symptoms in a large HIV clinic during the outbreaks in Uganda. We describe our experiences in using these tools in 2 Ebola Virus Disease outbreaks in Uganda.

Results: During the Ebola Virus Disease (EVD) outbreaks, enhanced infection control and communication procedures were implemented within 24 hours of the WHO/Ministry of Health announcement of the outbreaks. During course of these outbreaks the clinic saw 12,544 patients with HIV 1/2 infection, of whom 3,713 attended without an appointment, suggesting new symptoms. Of these 4 were considered at risk of EVD and seen with full infection procedures; 3 were sent home after further investigation. One patient was referred to the National Referral Hospital VHF unit, but discharged on the same day. One additional VHF suspect was identified outside of a VHF outbreak; he was transferred to the National Referral Hospital and placed in isolation within 2 hours of arriving at the HIV clinic.

Discussion: Use of simple screening tools can be helpful in managing large numbers of symptomatic patients attending for routine and non-routine medical care (including HIV care) within a country experiencing a VHF outbreak, and can raise medical staff awareness of VHF outside of the epidemics.

Editor: Jens H. Kuhn, Division of Clinical Research, United States of America

Funding: These authors have no support or funding to report.

Competing Interests: The authors have declared that no competing interests exist.

* Email: rratanshi@idi.co.ug

Introduction

Viral hemorrhagic fevers (VHFs) refer to a group of illnesses that are caused by viruses of diverse families, including Lassa fever, Rift Valley Fever, marburg viruses, and ebola viruses [1,2]. VHF's characteristically lead to overall vascular system damage and often accompanied by hemorrhage (bleeding). VHF have high case fatality rate (between 25–100% [3]) and spread easily (in an outbreak in Zaire up 25% of cases were health care workers [4]). Providing care to VHF suspects without adequate infection control processes can cause extreme anxiety [5]. Exposure to VHF patients often results in health care workers being quarantined, which can be frightening and unpleasant [6]. VHF outbreaks provoke widespread national and international interest, often with dramatic media reporting [7]. Therefore, health care workers in VHF areas are usually very aware of health professional fatalities in previous outbreaks, through both media reports and peer to peer communication [8,9]. Therefore providing medical care in any setting near to a VHF outbreak is stressful for health care workers [10–12]. Consequently, managing this anxiety and stress in health care workers, whilst continuing to provide a comprehensive service is essential in maintaining an effective health care service during a VHF outbreak.

The initial symptoms and signs of VHF are often non-specific, including fever, rash and vomiting, prior to emergence of a more haemorrhagic pattern [13–16]. In Sub-Saharan African countries, where there is a high burden of infectious disease, non-specific symptoms are commonly seen in many patients without VHF attending health care facilities, especially in those presenting with malaria [17,18] and complications of HIV [19]. This means that during a VHF outbreak there are many people attending health care facilities near to the epicenter who may have similar symptoms to those with VHF, but who are not exposed or infected. In Uganda there are about 438,000 people who regularly access care and treatment for HIV1/2 infection, and many of them attend clinic every month [20]. Therefore, up to 20,000 patients attend for HIV 1/2 related care every day across the country. Missed appointments and especially HIV drug treatment interruptions may adversely affect the health of HIV infected patients. Health centres distant from a VHF epicenter in Angola saw reduced attendance of patients for other causes during the VHF outbreak [21], suggesting that patients also suffer from anxiety during VHF outbreaks and have been found to exhibit altered health seeking behaviours. Ensuring that patients attend for their HIV appointments is vital for good HIV care and treatment, and therefore reassurance to patients during a VHF outbreak is another priority for maintaining good clinical services.

In 2012 Uganda experienced 3 separate outbreaks of viral haemorrhagic fever; two Ebola Virus Disease (EVD) outbreaks [22] and one Marburg Virus Disease (MVD) outbreak. The Adult Infectious Disease clinic (AIDC) at the Infectious Diseases Institute (IDI) in Kampala sees up to 500 patients with HIV 1/2 infection per day. During the recent VHF outbreaks in Uganda it was essential to protect and reassure both the health care workers and patients as much as possible, whilst maintaining routine clinical services for all patients. However, whilst good tools were available for VHF treatment centres [1,23], we were unable to find any readily available tools or literature that would assist us to deal with a large and often symptomatic HIV clinic population during a VHF outbreak. Therefore, the IDI team developed 3 tools; an action plan for staff and management, a screening tool for symptomatic patients, and a laboratory information leaflet to assist guide and assist health care workers to continue routine clinic activities as safely as possible. In this article we present these tools and our experience with using them.

Methods

The Adult Infectious Disease Clinic (AIDC) at the Infectious Diseases Institute is located within the Mulago National Referral Hospital Complex, Kampala. Between July –September 2012 there were 9925 patients infected with HIV 1/2 registered at the clinic and there were an average of 465 patients seen per day. Patients are seen on appointment (scheduled) or if they are unwell (unscheduled). Between 29th July and 4th October 2012 in Kibale District Western Uganda and 17th November and 30th November 2012 in Luweero District, Central Uganda, there were 2 outbreaks of EVD virus. Between 22nd October and 23rd November 2012 there was a MVD outbreak in South West Uganda. The AIDC clinic is located approximately 206 km, 64 km and 404 km miles respectively from these 3 VHF outbreaks (figure 1). 41% of the AIDC patients live outside of Kampala, and many travel from across the country for their HIV care in the AIDC clinic. During each VHF outbreak both suspected and confirmed VHF patients travelled to Kampala and sought care at the National Referral

Hospital and from other health care providers. Therefore, there was a credible risk of VHF suspects attending for care at the AIDC.

As details of the first outbreak emerged, the clinic management team looked for tools which we could use for information and patient screening in our clinic. The CDC/WHO Infection Control document for VHF in African settings was used as a reference, but this was not specific for an HIV out-patient setting [23]. Therefore we produced and distributed our own tools on 30th July 2012. The first tool (figure 2) was an action plan developed to establish the process of our response to the epidemic, and was circulated to all staff and IDI senior management, along with the CDC Ebola leaflet for background information[24]. As per the action plan, we met to discuss with situation with all staff, and to give them concise and scientific information on the virus.

During each outbreak we identified an infection control nurse to be stationed at the clinic entrance. Her role was to perform triage of patients and to encourage standard infection control procedures such as hand-washing. She was responsible for ensuring that there were adequate hand washing facilities and supplies. All staff and patients were requested to wash their hands before and after entering the clinic. At entrances where soap and water were not available, alcohol gel was used. All staff were reminded to wash hands or use alcohol gel in between patients. The infection control nurse also gave twice daily health talks to patients in the waiting area, and answered questions related to VHF. This nurse also performed a basic triage of unwell patients with respect to haemorrhagic symptoms, and discussed all potential cases with a senior staff member before they were allowed to enter the main clinical unit. Any VHF suspects were directly referred to the National Referral Hospital Ebola unit and not admitted to the AIDC clinic. These activities were continued until Ministry of Health announcements stating the end of the outbreak.

Symptomatic patients are seen and managed in a designated 'urgent care' area of the clinic. This is an isolated area, where patients can be seen and can wait apart from other patients. During the VHF outbreaks the staff working in this area were provided with additional protective clothing. All clinic doctors were provided with screening tool (figure 3) for use for all patients who had attended for an unscheduled visit, and any patients with scheduled appointments who reported symptoms suggestive of VHF not identified by the infection control nurse. The tool was reproduced and made available in all clinical rooms. The tool was mainly based on symptoms, and included a points system, where 2 or more symptoms or any sign, or one symptom in a patient having been to an outbreak area highlighted the patient as a possible VHF suspect. These were then discussed with a senior doctor for advice on referral to the VHF unit at the National Hospital. Cardinal signs of haemorrhagic necessitated an immediate referral to the National Hospital. A senior doctor visits the urgent care team frequently to provide support and advice, and this support was increased during the outbreaks. For this study we have reviewed the screening tools filled and the urgent care admissions list to find those considered to be possible VHF suspects during the study period.

The internationally accredited IDI Core laboratory processes an average of 600 samples a day from over 40 sites around the country. The third tool was an information leaflet distributed to all lab staff and to all staff who were taking and dealing with blood and other samples (Figure 4).

Staff taking blood samples and working in the lab received sensitization on how to take samples, to manage samples and to dispose of samples in a safe manner.

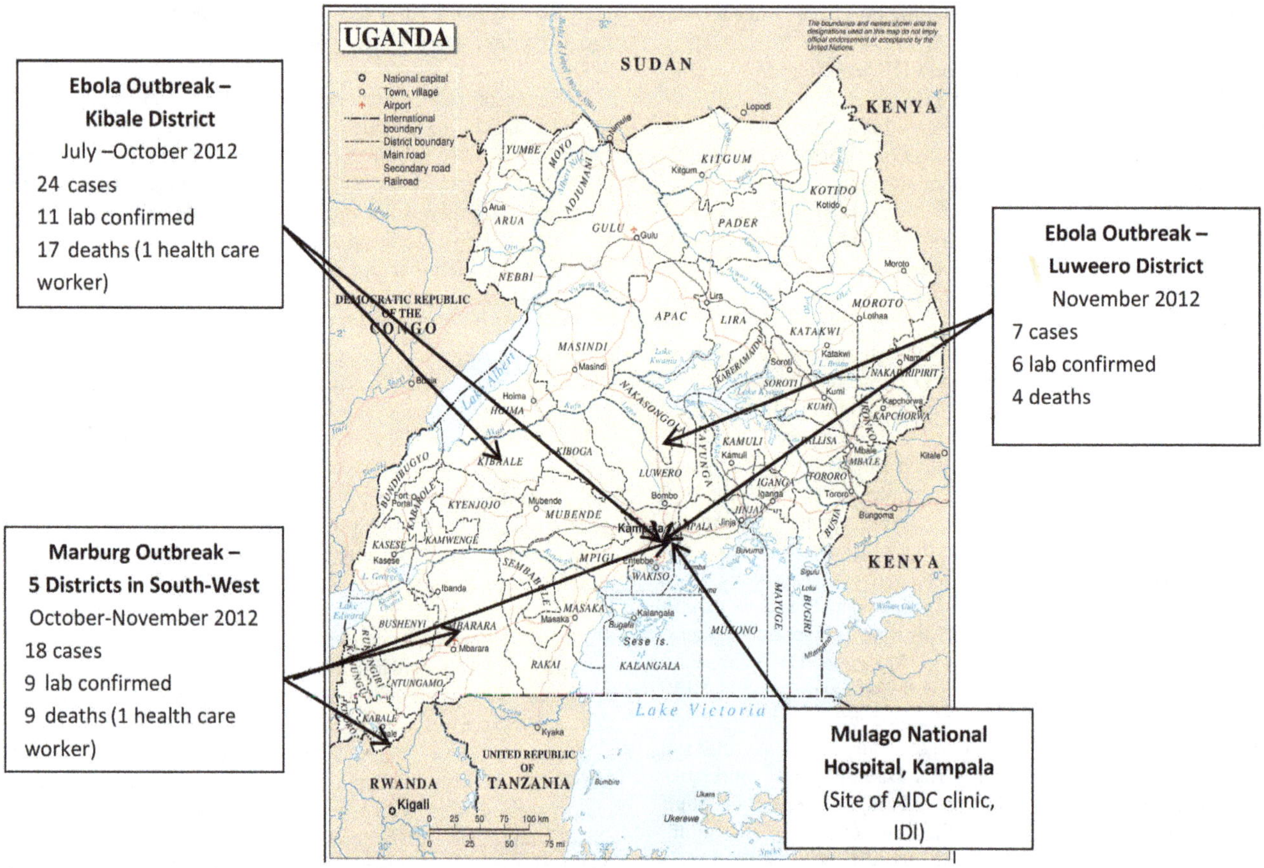

Figure 1. Map of VHF outbreaks in Uganda July 2012–June 2013.

Ethical considerations

This process was approved by the Institutional Review Board. The study and use of data was reviewed and approved by the Scientific Review Board of the Infectious Diseases Institute, the Institutional Review Board of Makerere University and the Uganda National Council of Science and Technology. Individual written patient consent was waived by these ethical and review committees since data was collected for routine clinical care and unique identifiers are removed for operational research purposes.

Results

Outbreak 1 – Ebola Virus Disease Outbreak, Kibale (29th July 2012 to 4th October 2012)

We developed the first draft of the tools within 24 hours of the WHO and Uganda Ministry of Health (MoH) announcements. The action plan was initiated and the screening tool was first distributed to staff on 30th July 2012. The screening tool was then refined and re-circulated on 31st July 2012. Over the 67 days of this outbreak, we saw 9458 patients in the clinic and of these 3077 were unscheduled appointments. The laboratory processed about 38,000 samples. The AIDC clinical team identified 2 possible suspects. Case 1 was female patient identified by the infection control nurse. She reported to the infection control nurse with a history of haematuria and diarrhea. She had not travelled to the VHF epicenter area and had not cared for patients from that area. The patient was seen in the urgent care isolation zone, with barrier nursing. Detailed further history revealed dysuria and diarrhea. She was afebrile and urine analysis was normal. She received

ciprofloxacin and paracetamol and was discharged home. Case 2 was a female patient with fecal blood who had not been identified by the infection control nurse or the doctor, but reported bloody diarrhea to a counsellor, in the clinic. The counselor requested she see a doctor but the patient absconded from the clinic. She was contacted by telephone by a clinic doctor later that day and gave a 3 month history of altered bowel habit, with some per rectal bleeding, not consistent with an acute infection. This was worse after taking her ART. She had not travelled to the epicenter area and had not cared for patients from that area. VHF was ruled out on clinical history and was encouraged to come back for further investigations of her chronic problem. Case 3 had fever, headache, abdominal pain, and an itchy skin rash. She was afebrile, and she was treated for a non-specific rash with prurigo. She was treated with cetirizine, hydrocortisone cream and magnesium suspension for gastritis. She was discharged home that day.

Outbreak 2 - Ebola Virus Disease (EVD) Outbreak, Luweero (17th November and 30th November 2012)

We instigated the process 24 hours before the WHO and MoH announcements (due to information received from Mulago Hospital) and an updated screening form were circulated to staff on 16th November 2012 (figure 2 shows the response times in this outbreak). Over the 13 days of this outbreak we saw 3086 patients with HIV 1/2 infection in the clinic, and 636 had unscheduled appointments. The lab processed about 7,200 samples. We identified one possible suspect (case 4) who had a rash, fever, and diarrhea and was from Luweero district. This patient was

Plan for infection control at AIDC in case of major or potentially severe communicable disease outbreaks

Background

The purpose of this document is to plan activities in the case of a communicable disease outbreak (including but not limited to Ebola Virus Disease, Marburg Virus Disease) in Uganda.

Strategy

The strategy in this situation is to protect staff and patients as much as possible and safely refer possible cases, without causing undue panic.

Objectives

The specific objectives are;

1) To ensure general infection control practices are in place
2) To add disease specific infection control policies if necessary
3) To identify and refer possible cases to the National centre as swiftly and calmly as possible
4) To keep all staff and SMT aware of the situation regularly
5) To liaise with Mulago National Referral Hospital, Ministry of Health, CDC, WHO and other partners as necessary

Abbreviations

HOD – Head of Department
PCT – Prevention, Care and Treatment program
PNO- Principle Nursing Officer
ED – Executive Director
MO – Medical officer
PMO – Principle Medical Officer
Mulago – National Referral Hospital, Mulago Complex

AIDC- Adult infectious diseases clinic
SMT- Senior Management team
SMO- Senior Medical Officer
MOH – Ministry of Health
CDC – Centres for Disease Control
WHO – World Health Organisation
BOD – Board of Directors

Specific Activities

Activity	Person responsible	Timeline	Dates Completed during second outbreak
1. Sensitize staff on issue and current situation	Deputy HOD PCT	Daily if necessary	16.11.12
2. Identify lead nurse and SMO to take these activities forward	PNO, Clinic manager	Day 1	
3. Ensure infection control measures in place a. Soap, water and hand towels (disposable) in each clinic room b. Soap, water and hand towels (disposable) at clinic entrance c. Gloves and disposable aprons in each clinic room d. Full gown and mask available in urgent care in case of high suspicion who needs transfer to Mulago	Head of nursing	Daily	16.11.12
4. Sensitization of staff and friends without causing undue panic • Posters on hand washing in each room/ waiting area • Health talks to friends • Distribution of info leaflet to staff • No hand shaking policy	Clinic manager / head of counseling	Ongoing	16.11.12
5. Liaise with MOH/Mulago staff to see where to refer patients and offer support	HOD PCT	Day 1 and ongoing	19.11.12
6. Stop all unnecessary field visits of IDI staff (research and outreach) to epidemic areas	Head of research/ Head of outreach	Ongoing	NA at present
7. To liaise with CDC/ WHO to seek advice and offer support where appropriate	ED /HOD PCT	Day 1 and ongoing	
8. Enhanced surveillance at AIDC a. Nurse at entrance to encourage hand washing and look for sentinel signs b. Doctors to fill proforma for all urgent care patients to screen for those infected c. Named SMO or higher to be consulted on all suspected cases	Clinic manager/PMO	Daily	16.11.12
9. Liaise with Outreach team to discuss procedures at other sites where IDI work	HOD PCT and HOD outreach	As necessary	19.11.12
10. SMT members to be informed of procedures / plans. (IDI BOD to be informed at discretion of ED)	HOD PCT	As necessary	19.11.12

References

1. Infection Control for Viral Haemorrhagic Fevers in the African Health care setting CDC WHO 1998

2. Ebola Hemorrhagic Fever Information Packet. CDC. 2009

3. www.cdc.gov/ncidod/dvrd/spb/mnpages/dispages/ebola.htm

Figure 2. Plan for infection control at AIDC in case of major or potentially severe communicable disease outbreaks.

given metronidazole and ciprofloxacin and transferred to the VHF unit at Mulago Hospital. Full infection control procedures were followed by staff handling the patient, and in handling laboratory samples. The patient was discharged from the VHF unit later in the day with no definite diagnosis. Laboratory samples were disposed of as per the protocol. Staff received counseling, but were not quarantined as they had no direct contact with body fluids. During the second outbreak we were contacted by another HIV service provider and research clinic working within the Mulago Hospital Complex, who requested our tools for use in their clinic.

Outbreak 3 - Marburg Virus Disease Outbreak, South West Uganda (22nd October-23rd November 2012)

The process was not fully implemented as there were no reported suspects reaching Kampala, and the outbreak was mainly confined to the South West of Uganda.

Form for assessment in urgent care for haemorrhagic fevers

Name of Patient _____ AIDC number _____ DOB _____

Symptoms

Does the patient have fever?   Yes/No

Does the patient have a headache?   Yes/No

Does the patient have joint pain or muscle aches?   Yes/No

Does the patient have a sore throat?   Yes/No

Does the patient have diarrhoea/ vomiting or stomach pain?   Yes/No

How long has the patient had these symptoms?   _____

How many symptoms? _____

Signs

Does the patient have red eyes?   Yes/No

Does the patient have a rash?   Yes/No

Does the patient have hiccups?   Yes/No

High suspicion signs

Does the patient have bleeding eyes or mouth or other bleeding? Yes/No

If yes send directly to National Referral Hospital Mulago A &E (regardless of other symptoms/geography)

Geography

Has the patient been to Luweero in the last 3 weeks?   Yes/No

If yes, where and when _____

Has the friend worked or been in Mulago hospital in the last 3 weeks? Yes/No

Please discuss with PNO, HOD PCT, HOD research, or Team leader doctors if

1) Patient has 2 or more symptoms
2) Patient has ANY sign
3) Patient has 1 symptom and has been to W Uganda or Mulago

Decision _____ Senior Clinician name _____

Figure 3. Form for assessment in urgent care for haemorrhagic fevers.

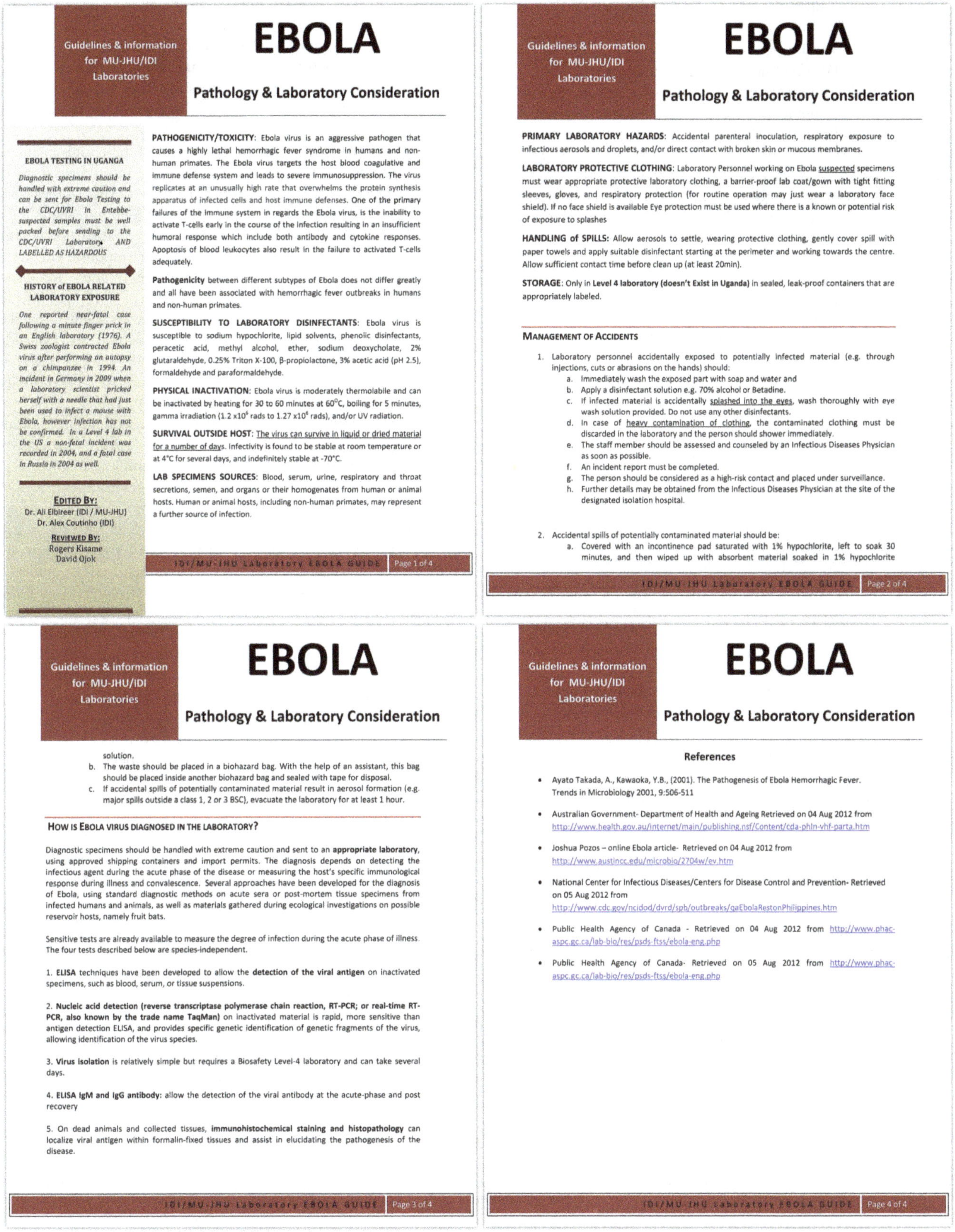

Guidelines & information for MU-JHU/IDI Laboratories

EBOLA

Pathology & Laboratory Consideration

EBOLA TESTING IN UGANGA

Diagnostic specimens should be handled with extreme caution and can be sent for Ebola Testing to the CDC/UVRI in Entebbe- suspected samples must be well packed before sending to the CDC/UVRI Laboratory AND LABELLED AS HAZARDOUS

HISTORY of EBOLA RELATED LABORATORY EXPOSURE

One reported near-fatal case following a minute finger prick in an English laboratory (1976). A Swiss zoologist contracted Ebola virus after performing an autopsy on a chimpanzee in 1994. An incident in Germany in 2009 when a laboratory scientist pricked herself with a needle that had just been used to infect a mouse with Ebola, however infection has not be confirmed. In a Level 4 lab in the US a non-fetal incident was recorded in 2004, and a fatal case in Russia in 2004 as well.

EDITED BY:
Dr. Ali Elbireer (IDI / MU-JHU)
Dr. Alex Coutinho (IDI)

REVIEWED BY:
Rogers Kisame
David Ojok

PATHOGENICITY/TOXICITY: Ebola virus is an aggressive pathogen that causes a highly lethal hemorrhagic fever syndrome in humans and non-human primates. The Ebola virus targets the host blood coagulative and immune defense system and leads to severe immunosuppression. The virus replicates at an unusually high rate that overwhelms the protein synthesis apparatus of infected cells and host immune defenses. One of the primary failures of the immune system in regards the Ebola virus, is the inability to activate T-cells early in the course of the infection resulting in an insufficient humoral response which include both antibody and cytokine responses. Apoptosis of blood leukocytes also result in the failure to activated T-cells adequately.

Pathogenicity between different subtypes of Ebola does not differ greatly and all have been associated with hemorrhagic fever outbreaks in humans and non-human primates.

SUSCEPTIBILITY TO LABORATORY DISINFECTANTS: Ebola virus is susceptible to sodium hypochlorite, lipid solvents, phenolic disinfectants, peracetic acid, methyl alcohol, ether, sodium deoxycholate, 2% glutaraldehyde, 0.25% Triton X-100, β-propiolactone, 3% acetic acid (pH 2.5), formaldehyde and paraformaldehyde.

PHYSICAL INACTIVATION: Ebola virus is moderately thermolabile and can be inactivated by heating for 30 to 60 minutes at 60°C, boiling for 5 minutes, gamma irradiation (1.2 x10^6 rads to 1.27 x10^6 rads), and/or UV radiation.

SURVIVAL OUTSIDE HOST: The virus can survive in liquid or dried material for a number of days. Infectivity is found to be stable at room temperature or at 4°C for several days, and indefinitely stable at -70°C.

LAB SPECIMENS SOURCES: Blood, serum, urine, respiratory and throat secretions, semen, and organs or their homogenates from human or animal hosts. Human or animal hosts, including non-human primates, may represent a further source of infection.

IDI/MU-JHU Laboratory EBOLA GUIDE | Page 1 of 4

Guidelines & information for MU-JHU/IDI Laboratories

EBOLA

Pathology & Laboratory Consideration

PRIMARY LABORATORY HAZARDS: Accidental parenteral inoculation, respiratory exposure to infectious aerosols and droplets, and/or direct contact with broken skin or mucous membranes.

LABORATORY PROTECTIVE CLOTHING: Laboratory Personnel working on Ebola suspected specimens must wear appropriate protective laboratory clothing, a barrier-proof lab coat/gown with tight fitting sleeves, gloves, and respiratory protection (for routine operation may just wear a laboratory face shield). If no face shield is available Eye protection must be used where there is a known or potential risk of exposure to splashes

HANDLING of SPILLS: Allow aerosols to settle, wearing protective clothing, gently cover spill with paper towels and apply suitable disinfectant starting at the perimeter and working towards the centre. Allow sufficient contact time before clean up (at least 20min).

STORAGE: Only in **Level 4 laboratory (doesn't Exist in Uganda)** in sealed, leak-proof containers that are appropriately labeled.

MANAGEMENT OF ACCIDENTS

1. Laboratory personnel accidentally exposed to potentially infected material (e.g. through injections, cuts or abrasions on the hands) should:
   a. Immediately wash the exposed part with soap and water and
   b. Apply a disinfectant solution e.g. 70% alcohol or Betadine.
   c. If infected material is accidentally splashed into the eyes, wash thoroughly with eye wash solution provided. Do not use any other disinfectants.
   d. In case of heavy contamination of clothing, the contaminated clothing must be discarded in the laboratory and the person should shower immediately.
   e. The staff member should be assessed and counseled by an Infectious Diseases Physician as soon as possible.
   f. An incident report must be completed.
   g. The person should be considered as a high-risk contact and placed under surveillance.
   h. Further details may be obtained from the Infectious Diseases Physician at the site of the designated isolation hospital.

2. Accidental spills of potentially contaminated material should be:
   a. Covered with an incontinence pad saturated with 1% hypochlorite, left to soak 30 minutes, and then wiped up with absorbent material soaked in 1% hypochlorite

IDI/MU-JHU Laboratory EBOLA GUIDE | Page 2 of 4

Guidelines & information for MU-JHU/IDI Laboratories

EBOLA

Pathology & Laboratory Consideration

solution.
   b. The waste should be placed in a biohazard bag. With the help of an assistant, this bag should be placed inside another biohazard bag and sealed with tape for disposal.
   c. If accidental spills of potentially contaminated material result in aerosol formation (e.g. major spills outside a class 1, 2 or 3 BSC), evacuate the laboratory for at least 1 hour.

HOW IS EBOLA VIRUS DIAGNOSED IN THE LABORATORY?

Diagnostic specimens should be handled with extreme caution and sent to an **appropriate laboratory**, using approved shipping containers and import permits. The diagnosis depends on detecting the infectious agent during the acute phase of the disease or measuring the host's specific immunological response during illness and convalescence. Several approaches have been developed for the diagnosis of Ebola, using standard diagnostic methods on acute sera or post-mortem tissue specimens from infected humans and animals, as well as materials gathered during ecological investigations on possible reservoir hosts, namely fruit bats.

Sensitive tests are already available to measure the degree of infection during the acute phase of illness. The four tests described below are species-independent.

1. **ELISA** techniques have been developed to allow the **detection of the viral antigen** on inactivated specimens, such as blood, serum, or tissue suspensions.

2. **Nucleic acid detection (reverse transcriptase polymerase chain reaction, RT-PCR; or real-time RT-PCR, also known by the trade name TaqMan)** on inactivated material is rapid, more sensitive than antigen detection ELISA, and provides specific genetic identification of genetic fragments of the virus, allowing identification of the virus species.

3. **Virus isolation** is relatively simple but requires a Biosafety Level-4 laboratory and can take several days.

4. **ELISA IgM and IgG antibody:** allow the detection of the viral antibody at the acute-phase and post recovery

5. On dead animals and collected tissues, **immunohistochemical staining and histopathology** can localize viral antigen within formalin-fixed tissues and assist in elucidating the pathogenesis of the disease.

IDI/MU-JHU Laboratory EBOLA GUIDE | Page 3 of 4

Guidelines & information for MU-JHU/IDI Laboratories

EBOLA

Pathology & Laboratory Consideration

References

- Ayato Takada, A., Kawaoka, Y.B., (2001). The Pathogenesis of Ebola Hemorrhagic Fever. Trends in Microbiology 2001, 9:506-511
- Australian Government- Department of Health and Ageing Retrieved on 04 Aug 2012 from http://www.health.gov.au/internet/main/publishing.nsf/Content/cda-phln-vhf-parta.htm
- Joshua Pozos – online Ebola article- Retrieved on 04 Aug 2012 from http://www.austincc.edu/microbio/2704w/ev.htm
- National Center for Infectious Diseases/Centers for Disease Control and Prevention- Retrieved on 05 Aug 2012 from http://www.cdc.gov/ncidod/dvrd/spb/outbreaks/qaEbolaRestonPhilippines.htm
- Public Health Agency of Canada - Retrieved on 04 Aug 2012 from http://www.phac-aspc.gc.ca/lab-bio/res/psds-ftss/ebola-eng.php
- Public Health Agency of Canada- Retrieved on 05 Aug 2012 from http://www.phac-aspc.gc.ca/lab-bio/res/psds-ftss/ebola-eng.php

IDI/MU-JHU Laboratory EBOLA GUIDE | Page 4 of 4

Figure 4. Laboratory Information -Ebola.

Post outbreak experiences (1st December 2012–1st July 2013)

During the 6 months following the outbreaks in Uganda, 10306 patients visited IDI (6032 unscheduled appointments). Clinic staff identified one VHF suspect (case 5) outside of a known outbreak in mid-2013. The patient presented with headache, fever, and diarrhea. He had epistaxis, hematemesis and bloody diarrhea. On examination he had hyperemic conjunctiva. He was found to have a thrombocytopenia with a platelet count of 114×10^3/uL. This patient was admitted to the National Referral Hospital within 2 hours of being seen in the clinic. The patient was isolated on the ward, and hospital staff treated the patient as VHF suspect. Senior clinic staff were notified immediately. No staff member was exposed to patient fluids. Urgent communication to lab staff ensured that blood samples taken by staff were handled safely. The MOH national VHF response team was notified and he was tested by the MOH team for VHF within 24 hours of admission. The case was VHF serology negative. No definite diagnosis was found.

(Table 1 summarizes clinical information on all suspects seen)

Discussion

The VHF outbreaks in Uganda have caused a considerable amount of anxiety for both patients and staff in our large HIV clinic. In order to manage this anxiety and reduce the risk of occupational exposure in our clinic while providing an uninterrupted service we have designed and implemented easy to use tools in our clinic for use in VHF outbreaks. The action plan enabled us to communicate with staff within the clinic and in outreach projects around the country, as quickly and early as possible, in order to provide valuable information and to reduce anxiety. In both outbreaks we managed to communicate important information to staff within 48 hours of the announcements.

The use of an objective point based screened tool enabled us to continue to see a high number of HIV patients, often with vague symptoms, in a safe and effective manner in an out-patient HIV clinic which was not a VHF receiving centre. Our main objective was to provide a sensitive tool for identifying possible VHF suspects within a population of patients with HIV in order to refer them to a designated VHF clinic. Therefore, our tool was purposefully less specific than the WHO screening tools to be used in VHF centres, for instance, whilst we asked about symptoms, the questions we asked about exposure were limited to being in the

geographical area, and did not go into details about contact with patients/attendance at burials etc. This did increase the number of "possible" suspects that were highlighted to a senior doctor, but our experience was that this was manageable number and that it was important to have a more sensitive tool that could be a primary screening, prior to more intensive screening by the VHF receiving centre.

The lessons learnt from the development of these tools included that having access to tools to follow also helped to reduce stress of the staff, as they were able to perform their normal duties with reassurance that not every patient they encountered might have VHF. During the second outbreak we were able to update the existing screening form very quickly and our response was more rapid and coordinated. Additionally the use of these tools has sensitized our staff on the symptoms and signs of VHF, and how to identify a possible suspect quickly. This was highlighted by the identification and rapid management of a possible suspect outside of a known outbreak. Whilst the IDI laboratory employs universal precautions at all times, management of suspected VHF samples requires a higher level of caution. The laboratory document enabled laboratory staff to understand what additional precautions they needed to take, and consequently to reduce anxiety by providing a procedure for management of samples.

Whilst our tool is "ideal" for our clinical environment, it does have to be adapted to each outbreak. What is "ideal" for us may not work in other clinics with different models of care e.g. nurse led services, services without an "urgent care" area. Perhaps the WHO or local Ministries of Health in countries at risk of outbreak could consider making these tools or adapted versions of these tools available for other out-patient clinic settings with high patient loads. Whilst our experience suggests that the action plan and the screening tools are easily understandable to staff, we did find that with multiple experiences we became quicker at implementing our response. Therefore, we think that health facilities may consider simple training programme or staff sensitization prior to an outbreak, which might also help health care workers to become familiar with the tools and to implement them quickly if an outbreak occurs.

Conclusions

We believe that these tools/response aids may serve an unmet need in countries which suffer relatively frequent VHF outbreaks

Table 1. Summary of VHF suspect characteristics.

Patient	Age and Sex	Cd4 count	ART regimen	Symptoms	Possible exposure	Outcome
Case 1	46, F	592 (21%)	TDF/3TC/LPR-RIT	Dysuria, haematuria, diarrhea. No fever	Nil known	Treated for bacterial gastro-enteritis/UTI as outpatient with Ciprofloxacin
Case 2	42, F	196 (8%)	AZT/3TC/Nevirapine	Abdominal pain and diarrhoea after taking drugs	Nil known	Drug side effect – monitored as out patient
Case 3	35, F	492 (23%)	AZT/3Tc/Nevirapine	Headache, Abdominal pain, Rash	Nil known	PPE and gastritis – treated with cetirizine, hydrocortisone and magnesium suspension
Case 4	42, M	139 (13%)	TDF/3TC/EFV	Fever, joint pain, sore throat, diarrhoea	From district containing epicentre (Luweero)	Given treatment for bacterial gastroenteritis with ciprofloxacin/metronidazole. Transferred to National Referral Hospital VHF unit for investigation but discharged
Case -5	35,M	237 (17%)	Nil	Fever, headache, bloody diarrhoea, epistaxis, heamatemasis	Outside of known outbreak	Transferred to National Referral Hospital VHF unit

and have a high HIV prevalence. We would encourage other HIV clinics or clinics with a high turnover of patients, who work in areas of potential VHF outbreaks to consider a risk management strategy, with readily available and objective assessment tools, which can be activated quickly during a similar emergence outbreak situation.

Acknowledgments

We would like to acknowledge the patients (our "friends" as they are called) who regularly attend the AIDC at the Infectious Diseases Institute. We would also like to thanks the staff at the AIDC, who tirelessly care for the patients in the clinic. We would especially like to thank the doctors and nurses who work in the urgent care area during the outbreaks.

Author Contributions

Conceived and designed the experiments: RPR CM FM BM AE. Performed the experiments: RPR FM BM. Analyzed the data: RPR. Contributed reagents/materials/analysis tools: CM AE. Wrote the paper: RPR FM AE AC CM BM.

References

1. Centers for Disease C Viral hemorrhagic fevers. Available: http://wwwcdcgov/ncidod/dvrd/spb/mnpages/dispages/vhf.htm:.
2. WHO Hemorrhagic Fevers, Viral.Available: http://wwwwhoint/topics/haemorrhagic_fevers_viral/en/.
3. Feldmann H, Geisbert TW (2011) Ebola haemorrhagic fever. Lancet 377: 849–862.
4. Sanchez AKT, Rollin PE, Peters CJ, Nichol ST, Khan AS, et al. (1995) Reemergence of Ebola virus in Africa. Emerging Infectious Diseases 1: 96–97.
5. Locsin RC, Matua AG (2002) The lived experience of waiting-to-know: Ebola at Mbarara, Uganda—hoping for life, anticipating death. J Adv Nurs 37: 173–181.
6. Bitekyerezo M, Kyobutungi C, Kizza R, Mugeni J, Munyarugero E, et al. (2002) The outbreak and control of Ebola viral haemorrhagic fever in a Ugandan medical school. Trop Doct 32: 10–15.
7. Mwesiga A (2011) Reporting epidemics: newspapers, information dissemination and the story of Ebola in the Ugandan district of Luweero. Pan Afr Med J 9: 43.
8. Green A (2012) Uganda battles Marburg fever outbreak. Lancet 380: 1726.
9. Kinsman J (2012) "A time of fear": local, national, and international responses to a large Ebola outbreak in Uganda. Global Health 8: 15.
10. Hewlett BL, Hewlett BS (2005) Providing care and facing death: nursing during Ebola outbreaks in central Africa. J Transcult Nurs 16: 289–297.
11. Raabe VN, Mutyaba I, Roddy P, Lutwama JJ, Geissler W, et al. (2010) Infection control during filoviral hemorrhagic fever outbreaks: preferences of community members and health workers in Masindi, Uganda. Trans R Soc Trop Med Hyg 104: 48–50.
12. Borchert M, Mutyaba I, Van Kerkhove MD, Lutwama J, Luwaga H, et al. (2011) Ebola haemorrhagic fever outbreak in Masindi District, Uganda: outbreak description and lessons learned. BMC Infect Dis 11: 357.
13. Mupere E, Kaducu OF, Yoti Z (2001) Ebola haemorrhagic fever among hospitalised children and adolescents in northern Uganda: epidemiologic and clinical observations. Afr Health Sci 1: 60–65.
14. Shoemaker T, MacNeil A, Balinandi S, Campbell S, Wamala JF, et al. (2012) Reemerging Sudan Ebola virus disease in Uganda, 2011. Emerg Infect Dis 18: 1480–1483.
15. Roddy P, Howard N, Van Kerkhove MD, Lutwama J, Wamala J, et al. (2012) Clinical manifestations and case management of Ebola haemorrhagic fever caused by a newly identified virus strain, Bundibugyo, Uganda, 2007–2008. PLoS One 7: e52986.
16. Jeffs B (2006) A clinical guide to viral haemorrhagic fevers: Ebola, Marburg and Lassa. Trop Doct 36: 1–4.
17. Mbonye AK, Magnussen P (2010) Symptom-based diagnosis of malaria and its implication on antimalarial drug use in pregnancy in Central Uganda: results from a community trial. Int J Adolesc Med Health 22: 257–262.
18. Ndyomugyenyi R, Magnussen P, Clarke S (2007) Diagnosis and treatment of malaria in peripheral health facilities in Uganda: findings from an area of low transmission in south-western Uganda. Malar J 6: 39.
19. Wakeham K, Harding R, Bamukama-Namakoola D, Levin J, Kissa J, et al. (2010) Symptom burden in HIV-infected adults at time of HIV diagnosis in rural Uganda. J Palliat Med 13: 375–380.
20. UNAIDS (2013) Uganda AIDSinfo. Available: http://wwwunaidsorg/en/regionscountries/countires/uganda/: Accessed 2013 Jul 11.
21. Roddy P, Marchiol A, Jeffs B, Palma PP, Bernal O, et al. (2009) Decreased peripheral health service utilisation during an outbreak of Marburg haemorrhagic fever, Uige, Angola, 2005. Trans R Soc Trop Med Hyg 103: 200–202.
22. (2012) Outbreak news. Ebola haemorrhagic fever, Uganda - update. Wkly Epidemiol Rec 87: 493.
23. WHO CfDCa (1998) Infection Control for Viral Haemorrhagic Fevers in the African Health care setting. Available: http://wwwwhoint/csr/resources/publications/ebola/WHO_EMC_ESR_98_2_EN/en/:.
24. Control CfD (2009) Ebola Hemorrhagic Fever Information Packet. http://wwwcdcgov/vhf/ebola/Ebola-FactSheetpdf.

15

Epidemiology of Pathogenic Enterobacteria in Humans, Livestock, and Peridomestic Rodents in Rural Madagascar

DeAnna C. Bublitz[1,2¤], Patricia C. Wright[1,3], Jonathan R. Bodager[4], Fidisoa T. Rasambainarivo[1], James B. Bliska[1,2], Thomas R. Gillespie[1,4,5*]

1 Centre ValBio, Ranomafana, Madagascar, 2 Department of Molecular Genetics and Microbiology, Center for Infectious Diseases, Stony Brook University, Stony Brook, New York, United States of America, 3 Department of Anthropology, Stony Brook University, Stony Brook, New York, United States of America, 4 Department of Environmental Health, Rollins School of Public Health, Emory University, Atlanta, Georgia, United States of America, 5 Department of Environmental Sciences and Program in Population Biology, Ecology, and Evolution, Emory University, Atlanta, Georgia, United States of America

Abstract

Background: Among the families of enteric bacteria are globally important diarrheal agents. Despite their potential for zoonotic and environmental transmission, few studies have examined the epidemiology of these pathogens in rural systems characterized by extensive overlap among humans, domesticated and peridomestic animals. We investigated patterns of infection with Enterotoxigenic *Escherichia coli*, *Shigella* spp., *Salmonella enterica*, *Vibrio cholerae*, and *Yersinia* spp. (*enterocolitica*, and *pseudotuberculosis*) in Southeastern Madagascar where the potential for the aforementioned interactions is high. In this pilot project we conducted surveys to examine behaviors potentially associated with risk of infection and if infection with specific enterobacteria species was associated with diarrheal disease.

Methodology/Principal Findings: PCR was conducted on DNA from human, livestock, and rodent fecal samples from three villages. Overall, human prevalence was highest (77%), followed by rodents (51%) and livestock (18%). Rodents were ~2.8 times more likely than livestock to carry one of the bacteria. The incidence of individual species varied between villages, with the observation that, *E. coli* and *Shigella* spp. were consistently associated with co-infections. As an aggregate, there was a significant risk of infection linked to a water source in one village. Individually, different pathogens were associated with certain behaviors, including: those who had used medication, experienced diarrhea in the past four weeks, or do not use toilets.

Conclusions/Significance: Different bacteria were associated with an elevated risk of infection for various human activities or characteristics. Certain bacteria may also predispose people to co-infections. These data suggest that a high potential for transmission among these groups, either directly or via contaminated water sources. As these bacteria were most prevalent in humans, it is possible that they are maintained in humans and that transmission to other species is infrequent. Further studies are needed to understand bacterial persistence, transmission dynamics, and associated consequences in this and similar systems.

Editor: Ulrike Gertrud Munderloh, University of Minnesota, United States of America

Funding: This study was supported by the Jim and Robin Herrnstein Foundation, Stony Brook University, and the Emory University Global Health Institute. Research reported in this publication that was performed by DeAnna Bublitz was supported by the National Institute of Allergy and Infectious Diseases of the National Institutes of Health under Award Number T32AI007539 (awarded to James Bliska). The content is solely the responsibility of the authors and does not necessarily represent the official views of the National Institutes of Health. The funders had no role in study design, data collection and analysis, decision to publish, or preparation of the manuscript.

Competing Interests: The authors have declared that no competing interests exist.

* Email: thomas.gillespie@emory.edu

¤ Current address: Host-Parasite Interactions Section, Laboratory of Intracellular Parasites, Rocky Mountain Laboratories, National Institute of Allergy and Infectious Diseases, Hamilton, Montana, United States of America

Introduction

Enteric diseases are a leading cause of illness and death in the developing world. Gastric infections and diarrhea are estimated to account for 2.2 million global mortalities annually. Diarrheal pathogens present an exceptional threat to children under 5, for whom nearly 15% of all deaths can be attributed to diarrhea, making it the second leading cause of death for infants worldwide [1,2]. Additionally, disease caused by these infections results in years of life lost due to malnutrition and stunted growth, both physical and cognitive [2]. These infections are especially prevalent in the developing world, particularly Africa, where infection-related diarrhea accounts for as much as 8.5% of all fatalities [3]. A recent 3-year study evaluating over 9000 children with moderate to severe diarrhea in Africa and Asia found that Enterotoxigenic *E. coli* and *Shigella* were two of the four most common causes of infection. *V. cholerae* was also identified as a significant cause of diarrhea in certain sites [4].

The source of these pathogens can be varied, though the interplay among humans, companion and food animals, and peridomestic animals is increasingly being recognized as a key interface for disease transmission [5–7]. As human populations grow they are increasingly pressed into higher density living. The same is true for the agriculture and livestock needed to support these communities. Moreover, in poorer communities there is a greater incidence of peridomestic rodents living in and around homes and food sources [8,9]. Residing in closer quarters creates a greater chance for the transmission of infectious diseases between humans, livestock, and rodents [5]. Numerous epidemics and pandemics have been linked to the cycle of transmission from livestock and humans including avian flu, Nipah virus, and swine flu [10–12]. Rodents present a similar risk as they can be the source of a wide range of diseases including tularemia, *Cryptosporidium* spp., *Campylobacter jejuni*, and hantavirus [7]. Furthermore, rodents are host to parasites such as ticks and fleas that can perpetuate the cycle of other pathogens like Lyme disease and plague [13,14]. Despite the high potential for zoonotic transmission, these interactions among humans, livestock, and peridomestic animals are still relatively understudied.

Madagascar is a nation of ~22 million people. While efforts have been made to improve living conditions for the people of Madagascar, only ~50% of the population is using improved water sources and less than 20% have access to improved sanitation facilities [15]. Diarrheal diseases cause approximately 37% of all infection and parasite-related deaths each year in this country [16]. A recent study investigating diarrheal disease in Madagascar found that nearly 50% of children under 5 tested positive for pathogenic intestinal microorganisms and roughly 10% of this age group died from diarrhea-related illness [15,17].

Much of the Malagasy population is rural and relies on livestock and rice farming for subsistence. Anthropogenic disturbance associated with agricultural practices and timber harvesting has led to nearly 90% of Madagascar's forest being lost [18,19]. Habitat loss and fragmentation can be devastating to biodiversity and endemic species but creates ideal spaces for invasive and generalist species such as introduced rodents [20–23]. Disruption of the natural environment coupled with high-density living presents an increased chance for contact with rodents and thus, the potential for disease transmission to both humans and livestock. Hantavirus, which can be transmitted as an aerosol from rodent urine, becomes more prevalent with habitat disturbance [7,21,22]. In regions where sanitation infrastructure is lacking, these interactions are all the more likely, exacerbating one's risk of infection with a zoonotic or waterborne pathogen [1,24]. In addition, zoonotic *Yersinia pestis*, the causative agent of plague, is endemic to Madagascar. It is estimated that 40% of the population is exposed to *Y. pestis*, which can be carried by rats and transmitted via aerosol or flea bites, resulting in severe and often fatal illness [25,26]. However, as this is not typically an enteric pathogen it is not covered in this study.

This pilot project was undertaken to look at the prevalence of five pathogenic enterobacteria: Enterotoxigenic *Escherichia coli* (ETEC), *Shigella* spp. (*flexneri* and *dysenteriae*), *Salmonella enterica*, *Vibrio cholerae*, and *Yersinia* spp. (*enterocolitica*, and *pseudotuberculosis*) in humans, livestock, and rodents. These groups were sampled from three villages near Ranomafana National Park: Ambatolahy (Amb), Ambodiaviavy (Avy), and Ankialo (Ank), in Southeastern Madagascar. The work herein estimates prevalence levels for these five bacteria in the above mentioned sample groups and looks at the relative risk association to various activities to identify potential

sources or patterns of transmission. As humans interact with, and alter, their environment it becomes increasingly important to understand the risks in regards to pathogen transmission to and from all potential hosts and their environment. Our results highlight a little studied facet of disease ecology in Madagascar and suggest a relationship between humans, livestock, and rodents in propagating zoonotic and waterborne pathogens.

Methods

Ethics Statement

All protocols, including obtaining oral consent from participants, were reviewed and approved by the Ministry of Health of the government of Madagascar, the Stony Brook University Internal Review Board and Institutional Animal Care and Use Committee. As approved by the Stony Brook Internal Review Board, oral informed consent of participants was obtained prior to specimen collection and survey. In the case of minors, a parent or guardian provided informed consent. Given the low literacy rate of the population being studied, we opted for oral consent administered and recorded on the survey sheets by the native interpreter conducting the interview. All participants were anonymously given unique identifiers. Permits were not required for sample collection from the animals in this study. All cows and pigs sampled were handled according to the guidelines of the National Veterinary Services Laboratories (Publication N231597), USDA, Fort Collins, Colorado. Rodents were handled following protocols outlined by the CDC [27]. No endangered species were involved in this study.

Study Site

The study took place in and around Ranomafana National Park, Madagascar, (located 47°18′ 40 to 47°37′E and 21°2′ to 21°25′S) a 43,500 hectare World Heritage Site well known for its high levels of species endemism and diversity [28,29]. Three communities located on the edge of the park were selected as the focus of this study: Ambodiaviavy (Avy, population = 363), Ankialo (Ank, population = 361), and Ambatolahy (Amb, population = 256). The communities are located in different areas of the park and have distinct cultural practices. The study population included several peridomestic rodents (*Rattus rattus*, *Mus musculus*), bovine (*Bos indicus*), porcine (*Sus domesticus*), and humans.

Sample collection and surveys

In June and July 2011, household and individual surveys were administered in the three communities: Avy (n = 65, total households = 10), Ank (n = 70, total households = 10), and Amb (n = 47, households = 10). A cluster sampling method was used: in each village, ten households were selected and every person inhabiting a selected household was surveyed. Participants were chosen independent of age, sex, or symptoms, but some were selected based on livestock ownership. Surveys were comprehensive with inquiries of demographic information, health status, hygiene, medication usage, water usage, and exposure to livestock and wildlife (70 questions for individual survey and 40 variables for the household survey). Potential behaviors associated with risk for diarrheal disease and infection with enterobacteria were queried in both surveys. Trained local field assistants administered all surveys in the local language (Malagasy) in order to reduce survey bias. Data were recorded on paper forms, answers were converted from "Yes/Always," "Sometimes," or "No/Never," to a 2, 1, or 0, respectively. These numbers were entered into Microsoft Excel spreadsheets with the associated behavior, and reviewed for accuracy. Fisher's exact test using Prism 6 (Graphpad, La Jolla,

CA) was used to analyze associations and calculate confidence intervals (CI) and relative risk (RR) between survey responses and infection status.

All survey participants were asked to provide a fecal specimen for examination of diarrheal pathogens and 89% complied. Concurrently, domesticated animals of participants (bovine and porcine) were sampled and baited rodent live-traps were set inside participant homes overnight. The following morning, fecal specimens were collected from trapped peridomestic rodents. All of the traps were washed thoroughly with 10% bleach solution between uses. Human volunteers were instructed to wash their hands prior to collecting fecal samples in sealable plastic bags that were collected the same or the next day. Given that we did not have access to a clinic and were limited in time at each village, we cannot assure 100% sterile transfer of the samples from the participants into the bags. Fresh fecal matter from livestock was collected from the rectum using a non-sterile latex glove, or from the ground if defecation was observed. For the latter, only fecal material that had not directly been in contact with the ground was collected. All samples were moved to a field laboratory as soon as possible (Amb and Avy) or processed on site (Ank). Approximately one milliliter of feces from each sample was homogenized with an equal volume of RNAlater nucleic acid stabilizing buffer (Ambion, Life Technologies, Grand Island, NY) and stored at −20°C at CentreValBio until transport to the United States.

Molecular methods

Total nucleic acid was extracted from fecal specimens (n = 278) preserved in RNAlater using the FastDNA SPIN Kit for Soil (MP Biomedicals, LLC, Solon, OH), following the manufacturer-recommended procedures. Using PCR, we screened the samples for ETEC, *S. enterica*, *Shigella* spp. (*flexneri* and *dysenteriae*), *V. cholerae*, and *Yersinia* spp. We chose to amplify the gene *yadA* in *Yersinia* as it is similar in *enterocolitica*, and *pseduotuberculosis* species and could be used to screen for both simultaneously [30]. The *yadA* primers should generate a product of 849 bp with *Y. enterocolitica* serogroup 03/09 strains, a product of 759 bp ith *Y. enterocolitica* serogroup 08 strains, and 681 bp product with *Y. pseudotuberculosis* (including the positive control strain used). Likewise, the *invA* gene in *S. enterica* was used for its conserved nature across serovars [31]. A portion of the ipaH gene was amplified to detect *Shigella flexneri* and *dysenteriae*. For positive controls in the PCR reactions, *V. cholerae*, ETEC, and *S. flexneri* strains were obtained from American Type Culture

Collection (ATCC, Manassas, VA). The 32777 strain in the Bliska Laboratory collection was used as a positive control for *Y. pseudotuberculosis*. The *S. enterica* serovar 14028 positive control strain was obtained from the laboratory of Dr. Adrianus van der Velden (Both: Stony Brook University, Stony Brook, NY). All positive control strains are listed in Table 1. Genomic DNA was isolated from each of the strains using a DNeasy kit (Qiagen, Valencia, CA) according to the manufacturer's protocol. All primers are listed in Table 1 and detect previously described genes for each bacterial species [26,31,32]. The primers were synthesized by Eurofilms MWG Operon (Stony Brook University, Stony Brook, NY). PCR was conducted on 2.0 μl of DNA sample using 0.5 μmol of each primer (Table 1) in 25 μl of Platinum PCR mix (Invitrogen, Life Technologies, Grand Island, NY). As a negative control, the same PCR reaction was run using water to confirm that there was no contamination of the reagents. Additionally, all of the primers were tested on all of the positive control strains to test for cross-reactivity and none was found. The amplification setting was as previously described; sensitivity of detection for each pathogen is listed in Table 1 [32].

Results

For this pilot study a cluster sampling method was used: in each village, ten households were selected and every person inhabiting a selected household was surveyed. Participants were chosen independent of age, sex, or symptoms. Participating households were selected at random except that preference was given to households owning livestock. Overall, 304 fecal samples were tested (humans = 163, cattle = 58, pigs = 18, and rodents = 65). Of the species sampled, humans had the highest overall prevalence of infection (77%, CI = 0.70–0.83), followed by rodents (51%, CI = 0.38–0.63), then livestock (18%, CI = 0.10–0.29) (Table 2). When looking at the prevalence of each pathogen individually, there was variability among villages. Among humans, *Shigella* spp. was the predominant pathogen detected in Amb (64%, CI = 0.48–0.77), while ETEC was the dominant bacterium found in human samples from Avy and Ank (69%, CI = 0.55–0.80 and 57%, CI = 0.43–0.70, respectively) (Table 3).

In regards to livestock, ETEC and *S. enterica* were the only enterobacteria detected in samples from Amb and Avy, while *Shigella* spp., *V. cholerae*, as well as the previous two, were found in samples from Ank (Table 3). These pathogens were more prevalent in pigs than cattle (67%, CI = 0.41–0.87 and 3%,

Table 1. Bacterial strains (positive controls), target genes, and primers* used in this study.

Genus and Species (ATCC #)	Target Gene	PCR primers (5'-3')	Product Size	Sensitivity (cells)
Enterotoxigenic *E. coli* serotype O78:H11 (35401)	Enterotoxin (LT) gene	f - GAGACCGGTATTACAGAAATC r - GAGGTGCATGATGAATCCAG	117 bp	40
Shigella flexneri serotype 2b (12022)	ipah	f - CTTGACCGCCTTTCCGATAC r - CAGCCACCCTCTGAGAGTA	610 bp	5×10[4]
Salmonella enterica serovar Typhimurium (14028)	invA	f - TATCGCCACGTTCGGGCAA r - TCGCACCGTCAAAGGAACC	275 bp	40
Vibrio cholerae (14035)	ctxA	f - GGCAGATTCTAGACCTCCT r - TCGATGATCTTGGAGCATTC	563 bp	40
Yersinia pseudotuberculosis serogroup O1 (32777)	yadA	f - CTTCAGATACTGGTGTCGCTGT r - ATGCCTGACTAGAGCGATATCC	681 bp (849[a], 751[b])	Unknown

*All primer sequences and sensitivities obtained from Wang et al. (1997) except *Yersinia* obtained from Thoerner et al. (2003).
[a]Product size with *Y. enterocolitica* serogroup 03 or 09 strains.
[b]Product size with *Y. enterocolitica* serogroup 08 strains.

Table 2. Prevalence of Enterobacteriaceae infection by subject and location.

Host	Location							
	Ambatolahy		Ambodiaviavy		Ankialo		All Villages	
	+/Total	Prevalence	+/Total	Prevalence	+/Total	Prevalence	+/Total	Prevalence
Human	43/47	0.91	42/58	0.72	41/58	0.71	126/163	0.77
Cattle	0/14	0.00	2/17	0.12	0/27	0	2/58	0.03
Pig	4/4	1.00	1/1	1.00	7/13	0.54	12/18	0.67
Rodent	12/33	0.36	10/14	0.71	11/18	0.61	33/65	0.51

CI = 0.004–0.12, respectively). Overall, few livestock tested positive for any of the target pathogens (Amb = 14%, Avy = 11%, Ank = 15%).

Except for *Yersinia*, all target species were detected in rodent samples, though *V. cholerae* was only found in rodent samples from Avy (Table 3). The occurrence of infection in rodents was 36% (CI = 0.20–0.55) in Amb, 71% (CI = 0.42–0.92) in Avy, and 61% (CI = 0.36–0.83) in Ank (Table 2). However, it should be noted that fewer rodents were sampled in either Avy or Ank versus Amb (n = 14, 18, and 33, respectively).

As depicted in Table 2, prevalence of enterobacteria infection was markedly higher for residents of Amb. This was linked to an increased risk association of having one or more of the pathogens for the residents of Amb vs. the residents of Avy or Ank (RR = 1.279, p = 0.0066) (Table 4). However, when broken down by pathogen, there was a reduced risk of *V. cholerae* and ETEC infection in Amb (*V. cholerae* RR = 0.0840, p = 0.0003; *E. coli* RR = 0.6762, p = 0.0229). Conversely, there was a higher risk of infection with these two pathogens in Avy (*V. cholerae* RR = 3.26, p = 0.0003; ETEC RR = 1.366, p = 0.0313). There was an elevated chance of *Shigella* spp. infection in Amb (RR = 1.575, p = 0.0092) compared to the other two villages, with a dramatically reduced risk in Ank (RR = 0.438, p<0.0001). Lastly, there was a higher prevalence of *Yersinia* spp. in humans from Amb versus Avy or Ank (RR = 2.241, p = 0.0344)(Table 4). All but one sample yielded a product of 681 bp in size indicating that *Y. pseudotuberculosis* is likely the species present. The one outlier was 759 bp suggesting infection with *Y. enterocolitica*.

Given that 77% of humans tested were found to be carrying at least one of these pathogens, we wanted to examine the prevalence of co-infections in this population. In Amb, none of the bacteria were significantly linked to one another while samples from Avy and Ank both showed patterns of co-infection (Table 5). In Avy, 86% of ETEC and 97% of *Shigella* spp. positive samples were also positive for one of the other bacteria tested, of which ETEC co-infection with *Shigella* spp was the most common (Prevalence = 75%, p<0.0001) (Table 5). While in Ank, *S. enterica* and *Shigella* spp. were both equally associated with co-infection with 100% of those infected with either pathogen testing positive for at least one other enterobacteria (p = 0.0029) and 60% of those were co-infections of *Shigella* spp. and *S. enterica* (p = 0.0011) (Table 5). *Shigella* spp. was also significantly linked to infection with *Yersinia* spp. in Ank (p = 0.0338). Overall, co-infections involving ETEC or *Shigella* spp. were most common at a prevalence of 74% and 91% respectively, across all three villages. ETEC co-infections with *Shigella*/EIEC was the most common with 55% of total ETEC infections co-occurring with *Shigella* spp. (p = 0.0276) (Table 5).

Broadly, none of the potential risk factors that we analyzed, including age, sex, working in fields, washing hands or boiling water, were significantly associated with an increased risk of infection in humans (Table 4). While there was no overall risk tied to fetching water from an open vs. a closed source in the three villages combined (RR = 0.8503, p = 0.1387), there was a substantial increase in risk of infection linked to collecting water from a closed source in Avy (RR = 2.174, p = 0.0041). Additionally, infection with ETEC was significantly linked to fetching water from a closed source (RR = 1.977, p = 0.0087). However, other activities, such as having experienced diarrhea within the four weeks prior to the survey, or tending livestock were not connected to an amplified risk of infection when all pathogens are considered as an aggregate (Table 4).

Certain factors and activities were associated with an elevated risk of infection when the pathogens are evaluated individually. There was an increased risk of *Shigella* spp. for individuals 15 years

Table 3. Incidence of each Enterobacteriaceae species in humans, livestock, and rodents by village.

| Pathogen | Ambatolahy | | | | | | | |
| | Human | | Livestock* | | Rodent | | |
	+/Total	Prevalence	+/Total	Prevalence	+/Total	Prevalence
E. coli	20/47	0.43	4/29	0.14	10/33	0.30
Shigella spp.	30/47	0.64	0/29	0.00	4/33	0.12
S. enterica	15/47	0.32	0/29	0.00	6/33	0.18
V. cholerae	1/47	0.02	0/29	0.00	0/33	0.00
Yersinia spp.	13/47	0.28	0/29	0.00	0/33	0.00

| | Ambodiaviavy | | | | | | |
| | Human | | Livestock* | | Rodent | | |
	+/Total	Prevalence	+/Total	Prevalence	+/Total	Prevalence
E. coli	40/58	0.69	2/18	0.11	8/14	0.57
Shigella spp.	32/58	0.55	0/18	0.00	5/14	0.36
S. enterica	9/58	0.16	2/18	0.11	6/14	0.43
V. cholerae	10/58	0.17	0/18	0.00	2/14	0.14
Yersinia spp.	8/58	0.14	0/18	0.00	0/14	0.00

| | Ankialo | | | | | | |
| | Human | | Livestock* | | Rodent | | |
	+/Total	Prevalence	+/Total	Prevalence	+/Total	Prevalence
E. coli	33/58	0.57	6/40	0.15	8/18	0.44
Shigella spp.	15/58	0.26	6/40	0.15	10/18	0.56
S. enterica	15/58	0.26	6/40	0.15	5/18	0.28
V. cholerae	10/58	0.17	1/40	0.03	0/18	0.00
Yersinia spp.	6/58	0.10	0/40	0.00	0/18	0.00

*Cattle and pigs.

of age or under in Amb (RR = 1.655, p = 0.0355) while this group carried a greater risk of infection by ETEC in Avy (RR = 1.450, p = 0.0487) (Table 6). In Avy there was also a modest association between infection with ETEC and individuals who did not boil their water (RR = 1.447, p = 0.0487) as well as those who had used medication (RR = 1.826, p = 0.0348) or experienced diarrhea (RR = 1.513, p = 0.0438) in the past four weeks. Of those who had used medication, over 76% had used antibiotics (antibacterial, -protozoal, and – helmintic), 78% had used anti-inflammatories, and 52% had used both. There was a 3.8 and 4.5 times greater risk of infection with *V. cholerae* in Amb and Ank, respectively, for individuals who reported never using a toilet (Amb p = 0.022; Ank p = 0.0318). Lastly, when all three villages were combined, males were 2.14 times more likely to be infected with *S. enterica* (p-0.016). Additionally, people who never used a toilet carried a greater risk of infection with *Yersinia* spp. (RR = 3.575, p = 0.0013). Importantly, having suffered from diarrhea in the past four weeks was significantly associated with infection with *V. cholerae* (RR = 2.622, p = 0.0156) (Table 6).

Rodents tested had a greater risk of carrying one of these bacteria compared to livestock. With roughly equal numbers of samples, the RR of a rodent testing positive for one of the infectious agents was 2.756 times greater than that of the livestock tested (RR = .3628, p<0.0001). There was also a modest positive association between rodents in Amb and carrying at least one of the five pathogens as compared to rodents in Avy or Ank (RR

= 0.5541, p = 0.0259). Additionally, there was no associated risk for humans having touched rodents by their tail (RR = 1.083, p = 0.4369) (Table 4). All of the significant findings have been summarized in Table 7.

Discussion

This study evaluated the prevalence of five pathogenic bacteria in humans, livestock, and rodents from three villages in Madagascar. Of the three sample groups, humans carried the highest prevalence (77%) followed by rodents (51%), and livestock (18%). The incidence of each pathogen varied from village to village with people from Amb carrying the greatest RR of infection (Table 4). Additionally, the distribution of the bacteria was different in livestock versus rodents with rodents testing positive for more of the pathogens and having a greater overall RR than livestock in all three villages (Table 4).

For many parts of the world, such as Madagascar, enteric pathogens are a major source of illness and death [1,2,15,17]. The impact of humans on their environment and the implications of those alterations on disease transmission are becoming more and more clear. Madagascar is an island with incredible species diversity across all taxa, of which a majority are endemic [33,34]. This country has also seen drastic changes to the original environment for agriculture and resource extraction, leading to fragmenting or clearing nearly 90% of the original forestland

Table 4. Risk factors for infection with Enterobacteriaceae in people living in villages in Southeast Madagascar.

Variable	n*	RR	95% CI lower	95% CI upper	p
Age (≤15)	162	1.079	0.898	1.297	0.486
Sex (male vs. female)	162	1.036	0.875	1.227	0.7103
Amb vs. Ank or Avy	**163**	**1.279**	**1.107**	**1.477**	**0.0066**
Avy vs. Amb or Ank	163	0.9052	0.7519	1.09	0.3292
Ank vs. Amb or Avy	163	0.8732	0.7221	1.056	0.1715
Amb vs. Ank or Avy *V. cholerae*	**163**	**0.0841**	**0.0118**	**0.5988**	**0.0003**
Amb vs. Ank or Avy *E. coli*	**163**	**0.6762**	**0.4716**	**0.9696**	**0.0229**
Amb vs. Ank or Avy *Shigella* spp.	**163**	**1.575**	**1.158**	**2.144**	**0.0092**
Amb vs. Ank or Avy *Yersinia* spp.	**163**	**2.241**	**1.144**	**4.389**	**0.0344**
Avy vs. Amb or Ank *V. cholerae*	**163**	**3.26**	**1.682**	**6.321**	**0.0003**
Avy vs. Amb or Ank *E. coli*	**163**	**1.366**	**1.057**	**1.766**	**0.0313**
Ank vs. Amb or Avy *Shigella* spp.	**163**	**0.438**	**0.2754**	**0.6966**	**<0.0001**
Collects water from an open source (vs. closed well or pump)	119	0.8503	0.6876	1.052	0.1387
Avy only - collects water from open source	**38**	**2.174**	**1.146**	**4.122**	**0.0041**
Boils water	163	0.9678	0.8197	1.143	0.7126
Washes hands prior to eating	163	0.9385	0.7664	1.149	0.8016
Uses a toilet	163	1.119	0.9441	1.327	0.449
Works in agricultural fields	153	0.9744	0.7503	1.266	1
Tends livestock	144	0.9198	0.7601	1.113	0.4386
Contact with rodents	151	1.083	0.911	1.288	0.4369
Experienced diarrhea (vs. no diarrhea) in past 4 Weeks	159	1.114	0.9155	1.357	0.4453
Experienced diarrhea with blood (vs. no blood) in past 4 weeks	25	0.7719	0.3409	1.748	0.4217
Used medicine (traditional or commercial) in past 4 Weeks	163	1.064	0.8684	1.303	0.5279
Rodents vs. livestock	**rodent-65 livestock-76**	**2.756**	**1.622**	**4.684**	**<0.0001**

*Total n varies due to incomplete notation on some surveys or respondents do not participate in the given activity (e.g. tend livestock).
Bold = statistically significant associations.

[18,19,34]. Overall, zoonotic pathogens account for nearly 61% of the organisms infectious to humans and 75% of emerging pathogens in the last decade [35]. While populations of humans, livestock, and rodents have been living together for thousands of years, these alterations to the landscape and ecology of Madagascar are an opportunity for new interactions between these populations, and potentially the transmission of zoonoses or waterborne pathogens.

This pilot study focused on the villages of Ambatolahy, Ambodiaviavy, and Ankialo near Ranomafana National Park in Southeastern Madagascar. Our results demonstrated that humans accounted for the greatest number of positive samples as compared to livestock or rodents (Table 2). Of the five pathogens tested, ETEC was the most prevalent in humans and livestock. When broken down by village, ETEC was also the dominant pathogen detected in human samples from Avy and Ank, while *Shigella* spp. was the predominant bacterium found in Amb (Table 3). It should be noted that Enteroinvasive *E. coli* (EIEC) strains can also have and express the toxin encoded by the ipaH gene. Having used the ipaH gene to screen for *Shigella* spp. it is also possible that the bacteria detected were EIEC. However, the disease caused by EIEC is nearly identical to Shigellosis and still presents an equal threat to the health of these communities [36]. This would be an important avenue to follow up on with

sequencing of the samples to establish which species are present in these populations.

Globally, information about multiple enterobacteria infections is lacking, as such, this study also examined the prevalence of co-infections in humans. ETEC and *Shigella* spp. were predominantly associated with co-infections with 74% of ETEC and 91% of *Shigella* spp. infected samples testing positive for at least one other enterobacteria species (Table 5). These same pathogens were also the most prevalent individually in Amb and Avy while in Ank, *S. enterica* and *Shigella* spp. were present in equal amounts and both linked to co-infection in that village (Table 3, 5). Given that the numbers were identical for *S. enterica* and *Shigella* spp.in Ank, it was impossible to tease apart which might be the predisposing factor.

The percent of people infected with multiple pathogens was higher than reported rates from similar studies in Brazil and India [37–39]; however, the populations these previous studies sampled tended to be urban and in very different geographical locations than Madagascar. Co-infections in children under five in Madagascar were assessed in a recent report; however, they only documented co-infections between bacteria and parasites or viruses [17]. Given the paucity of data on rates of co-infection with multiple enterobacteria, it is difficult to say whether our data are within the expected range, and certainly this is an area needing further investigation. Furthermore, follow up work should be done to determine if the different co-infection profile of Ank is tied to its

Table 5. Prevalence of Enterobacteriaceae co-infections in humans from villages in Southeastern Madagascar.

	Ambodiaviavy				
	E. coli			*Shigella* spp.	
	Prevalence	p		Prevalence	p
Shigella spp.	0.75	<0.0001		N/A	N/A
S. enterica	0.23	0.0454		0.25	0.0333
V. cholerae	0.48	0.0022		0.56	<0.0001
Yersinia spp.	0.20	0.0484		0.25	0.0063
All enterics	0.86	<0.0001		0.97	<0.0001
	Ankialo				
	Shigella spp.			*S. enterica*	
	Prevalence	p		Prevalence	p
Shigella spp.	N/A	N/A		0.60	0.0011
S. enterica	0.60	0.0011		N/A	N/A
Yersinia spp.	0.27	0.0338		N/A	N/A
All enterics	1.00	0.0029		1.00	0.0029
	All Villages				
	E. coli			*Shigella* spp.	
	Prevalence	p		Prevalence	p
Shigella spp.	0.55	0.0276		N/A	N/A
S. enterica	0.30	0.0413		0.38	0.0001
V. cholerae	0.26	0.0148		0.31	0.0002
Yersinia spp.	N/A	N/A		0.25	0.0109
All enterics	0.74	0.0010		0.91	<0.0001

more remote location or other variations in behavior or activities from that of the people in Avy or Amb.

We attempted to identify potential risk factors amongst humans for infection with enteric pathogens. People in Amb were significantly more likely to be infected than people in Avy or Ank (Table 4). Water contamination is a notable source of these pathogens [1,40]. Given the high proportion of open water sources used by the subjects of this study, it was unexpected that there was no significant correlation between fetching water from a closed vs. an open source and their infection status (Table 4). Surprisingly, in the village of Avy, there was a substantial risk associated with people who fetched water from a closed source as opposed to the open sources and ETEC was implicated as the responsible agent (Table 4, 5). These data suggest that one or more of the pumps may be contaminated. It would be insightful to test the pump water directly and determine which families use which pump to see if there is a pattern of bacterial contamination and infection. This finding highlights the importance of these types of studies as follow-up analysis can be focused on areas of interest, such as these pumps.

In addition to the contaminated water source, there was a greater RR for infection with ETEC for people in Avy who reported not boiling their water (Table 5). Interestingly, people that reported always boiling their water before consumption were not at a reduced risk for infection by these bacteria (Table 4). There are several possible explanations. For one, there could be survey bias in that people felt pressure to report that they always boil water when in fact, they do not. This is a risk when having surveys administered in person rather than with complete anonymity. However, given the lower level of literacy and the need for explanation of certain questions, we felt the best way to conduct the surveys was with a native interpreter. Alternatively, coupled with the data from the open versus closed sources of water, this may not be a significant cause of disease transmission overall.

Other factors linked to infection were being under the age of 15 or male. People in Avy who had used medication, either traditional or commercial, in the past four weeks carried a greater risk of infection by ETEC. This finding could be due to several factors. There were a high number of people using either antibiotics (anti-bacterial, -protozoal, and- helmintic) or anti-inflammatories, often times both. It is possible that anti-inflammatory use may hinder the immune response making people susceptible to infection. Moreover, antibiotic misuse may mean a diagnosed infection was not cleared completely. These data could also be indicative of the more worrying trend of antibiotic-resistant bacteria which is well documented in developing nations, due in part to misuse of antibiotics [41,42]. Further studies are warranted to sequence the strains and whether genes associated with antibiotic resistance are present in these bacteria. Individuals who reported never using toilets had a greater RR of carrying either *V. cholerae* or *Yersinia* spp. Hygiene and sanitation are critical indicators of health [1,3,40]. Developing countries tend to have limited sanitation facilities and also have higher rates of infection with various enteric pathogens [40]. While Madagascar has made significant improvements in this area there is still work

Table 6. Risk factors for infection with individual Enterobacteriaceae species in people living in villages in Southeast Madagascar.

Ambatolahy

Variable	Pathogen	n*	RR	95% CI lower	95% CI upper	p
Age (≤15)	Shigella spp.	47	1.655	1.031	2.658	0.0355
Does not use a toilet	Yersinia spp.	47	3.818	1.019	14.30	0.022

Ambodiaviavy

Variable	Pathogen	n*	RR	95% CI lower	95% CI upper	p
Age (≤15)	E. coli	58	1.45	1.014	2.073	0.0487
Collects water from an closed source (pump, well)	E. coli	58	1.977	1.044	3.744	0.0087
Used medicine (traditional or commercial) in past 4 Weeks	E. coli	58	1.826	0.9169	3.637	0.0348
Does not boil water	E. coli	57	1.447	1.027	2.04	0.0478
Experienced diarrhea (vs. no diarrhea) in past 4 Weeks	E. coli	58	1.513	1.148	1.994	0.0438

Ankialo

Variable	Pathogen	n*	RR	95% CI lower	95% CI upper	p
Does not use a toilet	V. cholerae	58	4.543	1.680	12.28	0.0318

All Villages

Variable	Pathogen	n*	RR	95% CI lower	95% CI upper	p
Sex (male vs. female)	S. enterica	162	2.14	1.145	4.000	0.016
Uses a toilet	Yersinia spp.	163	3.575	1.868	6.843	0.0013
Experienced diarrhea (vs. no diarrhea) in past 4 Weeks	V. cholerae	163	2.622	1.393	4.934	0.0156

*Total n varies due to incomplete notation on some surveys or respondents do not participate in the given activity.

that needs to be done in providing facilities and changing behavior [15].

Lastly, in Avy, infection with ETEC was significantly associated with having suffered from diarrhea in the past 4 weeks. However, when all villages were factored together, *V. cholerae* was associated with participants having reported diarrhea in the past four weeks (Table 6). Both pathogens are known to cause diarrhea and depending on the study referenced, the location, and the population tested, both have been pointed to as leading causes of infection and disease [4,17,39]. Overall, a relatively low association of diarrhea with positive infection status is not surprising. Many of these pathogens can be carried in an asymptomatic state and people often suffer from diarrhea less upon subsequent infections with these enteric pathogens. Asymptomatic carriers can facilitate spread, especially in regions lacking adequate sanitation infrastructure. Meanwhile, repeated infections, especially in children have negative implications on their general health, growth and susceptibility to other infections [43–54]. Our study further confirms the role these pathogens play in causing disease in people and are perhaps where future attention should be focused as far as vaccine and treatment efforts.

All livestock species demonstrated relatively low prevalence of all five target pathogens, and there was no correlative risk for people who reported tending livestock vs. those who did not (Table 2 and 4). However, it should be noted that pigs carried a significantly higher risk of harboring one of these bacteria over cattle. This is especially pertinent as pigs have played a key role in other epidemics and pandemics, such as swine flu and Nipah virus [11,12].

While infection prevalence was relatively low for livestock, rodents had a nearly 2.8 times higher risk of carrying one of the pathogenic intestinal microorganisms over livestock. Moreover, rodents had the second highest overall prevalence at 51% (Table 2). Rodents are common in human and fragmented environments presenting a great opportunity for diseases to move between them, humans, and domestic animals [7,55]. Peridomestic rodents living in close quarters with human environments are known sources of various diseases including: hantavirus, *Salmonella* spp., *Campylobacter jejuni*, *Giardia* spp. and *Cryptosporidium* spp. [7] [21] However, there was no link between humans having reported touching rodents and an elevated risk of being infected. This could be due to underreporting of contact with rodents or contact people are unaware of, such as while sleeping or rodent fecal matter in their food. Given that *Yersinia pestis* is endemic to Madagascar, exposure to rodents and the fleas they carry is a serious risk for plague in addition to other diseases [25,26]. Enteric *Yersinia* spp. were detected in humans in all three villages; however, none of the cattle or pigs, the most likely source of enteric *Yersinia*, that we tested were found to carry the bacteria. The lack of positive livestock samples could indicate that there is another animal reservoir for enteric *Yersinia*. Regardless, there were positive samples, indicating that enteric *Yersinia* spp., especially *Y.*

Table 7. Summary of significant findings for infection with Enterobacteriaceae in human, livestock, and rodent populations.

Ambatolahy

Increased risk of *E. coli*, *Shigella* spp., *V. cholerae*, and *Yersinia* spp.

Increased risk for people 15 years or younger

Increased risk for people who did not use a toilet

Ambodiaviavy

Increased risk of *E. coli* and *V. cholerae*

Increased risk for people collecting water from an open source

Increased risk for people 15 years or younger

Increased risk for people who used medicine in past four weeks

Increased risk for people who did no boil their water

Increased risk for people who experienced diarrhea in past four weeks

Co-infection association between *E. coli* and *Shigella* spp.

Ankialo

Increased risk of *Shigella* spp.

Increased risk for people who did not use a toilet

Co-infection association between *S. enterica* and *Shigella* spp.

Co-infection association between *Shigella* spp. and *Yersinia* spp.

Additional risk factors (across all villages)

Higher prevalence of bacteria in rodents vs. livestock

Higher prevalence of bacteria in pigs vs. cattle

Males at higher risk for *S. enterica* than females

People who used a toilet at higher risk for *Yersinia* spp.

People who experienced diarrhea in past four weeks at higher risk for *V. cholerae*

pseudotuberculosis, persist in the human population in this region of Madagascar and make follow-up studies to sequence the present strains important.

There are many variables to consider when dissecting the lifecycle and transmission routes of a pathogen. As we expand our understanding of emerging infectious diseases it becomes increasingly clear that the way humans interact with their environment has profound effects on the dispersal of zoonotic pathogens [5,18,55–59]. This report points to areas for further study, namely water sources and human behavior that may account for the infection status of the human volunteers. Moreover, these data emphasize that humans, livestock, and rodents are all potential sources of pathogenic bacteria and as these groups interact more, the possibility for transmission increases, as does the likelihood of transmission to wildlife such as lemurs [18]. Understanding the host-origin and the subsequent dissemination of a disease at the human-livestock-wildlife interface can aid in combating the spread of these agents. Our work has shed light on the prevalence of various pathogenic bacteria in the human, livestock, and rodent populations in Southeastern Madagascar. More generally, this work has highlighted the complexity of these studies and that generalizations cannot always be drawn even from relatively related populations. What may be a risk factor in one village may not be for another nearby. It is important to take into account the individual as well as the population in studies such as these. Hopefully these findings will help in implementing preventative measures for people, their companion animals and livestock, and peridomestic rodents. More broadly, this work helps to expand our knowledge of disease transmission so that we can better combat these illnesses and enhance the quality of life for these people and others in similar settings.

Acknowledgments

We are grateful for logistical and infrastructural support from MICET, particularly director Benjamin Andriamihaja, the administration and support personnel of the Centre ValBio, Madagascar National Parks, Ian Fried, and Emilie Redwood. We would also like to thank Dr. Martha Furie and Dr. Jorge Benach for the generous use of their laboratory space at Stony Brook University and for helping to make this work possible.

Author Contributions

Conceived and designed the experiments: TRG PCW DCB. Performed the experiments: TRG DCB PCW JRB FTR JBB. Analyzed the data: TRG DCB. Contributed reagents/materials/analysis tools: TRG JBB PCW. Wrote the paper: TRG DCB JBB.

References

1. WHO/UNICEF (2000) Global Water Supply and Sanitation Assessment 2000 Report. Switzerland: WHO/UNICEF. Available: http://www.who.int/water_sanitation_health/monitoring/jmp2000.pdf. Accessed 2013 October 10.
2. Johansson EW, Wardlaw T (2009) Diarrhoea: Why children are still dying and what can be done. Switzerland: UNICEF and WHO. Available: http://www.who.int/maternal_child_adolescent/documents/9789241598415/en/. Accessed 2013 October 10.
3. Family and Community Health Unit, Water Sanitation and Health Unit, and WHO (2013) Water-related diseases. Available: http://www.who.int/water_sanitation_health/diseases/diarrhoea/en/. Accessed 2013 October 10.
4. Kotloff KL, Nataro JP, Blackwelder WC, Nasrin D, Farag TH, et al. (2013) Burden and aetiology of diarrhoeal disease in infants and young children in developing countries (the Global Enteric Multicenter Study, GEMS): a prospective, case-control study. Lancet 382: 209–222.
5. Daszak P, Cunningham AA, Hyatt AD (2000) Emerging infectious diseases of wildlife–threats to biodiversity and human health. Science 287: 443–449.
6. Rabinowitz P, Conti L (2013) Links among human health, animal health, and ecosystem health. Annu Rev Public Health 34: 189–204.
7. Meerburg BG, Singleton GR, Kijlstra A (2009) Rodent-borne diseases and their risks for public health. Crit Rev Microbiol 35: 221–270.
8. Calderon G, Pini N, Bolpe J, Levis S, Mills J, et al. (1999) Hantavirus reservoir hosts associated with peridomestic habitats in Argentina. Emerg Infect Dis 5: 792–797.
9. Katakweba AAS, Mulungu LS, Eiseb SJ, Mahlaba TaA, Makundi RH, et al. (2012) Prevalence of heamoparasites, leptospires and coccolbacilli with potential for human infection in the blood of rodents and shrews from selected localities in Tanzania, Namibia and Swaziland. African Zoology 47: 119–127.
10. Chen Y, Liang W, Yang S, Wu N, Gao H, et al. (2013) Human infections with the emerging avian influenza A H7N9 virus from wet market poultry: clinical analysis and characterisation of viral genome. Lancet 381: 1916–1925.
11. Daszak P, Zambrana-Torrelio C, Bogich TL, Fernandez M, Epstein JH, et al. (2013) Interdisciplinary approaches to understanding disease emergence: the past, present, and future drivers of Nipah virus emergence. Proc Natl Acad Sci U S A 110 Suppl 1: 3681–3688.
12. Garten RJ, Davis CT, Russell CA, Shu B, Lindstrom S, et al. (2009) Antigenic and genetic characteristics of swine-origin 2009 A(H1N1) influenza viruses circulating in humans. Science 325: 197–201.
13. Radolf JD, Caimano MJ, Stevenson B, Hu LT (2012) Of ticks, mice and men: understanding the dual-host lifestyle of Lyme disease spirochaetes. Nat Rev Microbiol 10: 87–99.
14. Chouikha I, Hinnebusch BJ (2012) Yersinia–flea interactions and the evolution of the arthropod-borne transmission route of plague. Curr Opin Microbiol 15: 239–246.
15. WHO/DFID-AHP (2013) Madagascar: health profile. Available: http://www.who.int/countries/mdg/en/. Accessed 2013 October 10.
16. World Health Organization DoMaHI (2011) Global Burden of Disease and Death Estimates. Available: www.who.int/gho/mortality_burden_disease/

global_burden_disease_death_estimates_sex_2008.xls. Accessed 2013 October 10.

17. Randremanana R, Randrianirina F, Gousseff M, Dubois N, Razafindratsimandresy R, et al. (2012) Case-control study of the etiology of infant diarrheal disease in 14 districts in Madagascar. PLoS One 7: e44533.

18. Junge RE, Barrett MA, Yoder AD (2011) Effects of anthropogenic disturbance on indri (Indri indri) health in Madagascar. Am J Primatol 73: 632–642.

19. Harper GJ, Steininger MK, Tucker CJ, Juhn D, Hawkins F (2007) Fifty years of deforestation and forest fragmentation in Madagascar. Env Conserv 34: 325–333.

20. With KA (2004) Assessing the risk of invasive spread in fragmented landscapes. Risk Anal 24: 803–815.

21. Dearing MD, Dizney L (2010) Ecology of hantavirus in a changing world. Ann N Y Acad Sci 1195: 99–112.

22. Mills JN (2006) Biodiversity loss and emerging infectious disease: An example from the rodent-borne hemorrhagic fevers. Biodiversity 7: 9–17.

23. Goodman SM (2003) Rattus on Madagascar and the dilemma of protecting the endemic rodent fauna. Conserv Bio 9: 450–453.

24. Laudisoit A, Leirs H, Makundi RH, Van Dongen S, Davis S, et al. (2007) Plague and the human flea, Tanzania. Emerg Infect Dis 13: 687–693.

25. Chanteau S, Ratsitorahina M, Rahalison L, Rasoamanana B, Chan F, et al. (2000) Current epidemiology of human plague in Madagascar. Microbes Infect 2: 25–31.

26. Hinnebusch BJ (2005) The evolution of flea-borne transmission in Yersinia pestis. Curr Issues Mol Biol 7: 197–212.

27. Mills JN, Childs JE, Ksiazek TG, Peters CJ (1995) Methods for trapping and sampling small mammals for virologic testing. Department of Health and Human Services, Public Health Service, CDC. Available: http://www.cdc.gov/hantavirus/pdf/rodent_manual.pdf. Accessed 2013 October 10.

28. Wright PC (1992) Primate Ecology, Rainforest Conservation, and Economic Development: Building a National Park in Madagascar. Evol Anthro 1: 25–33.

29. Wright PC (1997) The future of biodiversity in Madagascar: A view from Ranomafana National Park. In: Patterson B, Goodman, SM, editors.Natural Change and Human Impact in Madagascar.Washington D. C.: Smithsonian University Press. pp. 381.

30. Thoerner P, Bin Kingombe CI, Bogli-Stuber K, Bissig-Choisat B, Wassenaar TM, et al. (2003) PCR detection of virulence genes in Yersinia enterocolitica and Yersinia pseudotuberculosis and investigation of virulence gene distribution. Appl Environ Microbiol 69: 1810–1816.

31. Rahn K, De Grandis SA, Clarke RC, McEwen SA, Galan JE, et al. (1992) Amplification of an invA gene sequence of Salmonella typhimurium by polymerase chain reaction as a specific method of detection of Salmonella. Mol Cell Probes 6: 271–279.

32. Wang RF, Cao WW, Cerniglia CE (1997) A universal protocol for PCR detection of 13 species of foodborne pathogens in foods. J Appl Microbiol 83: 727–736.

33. IUCN (2009) IUCN statement on Madagascar. Available: http://www.iucn.org/?2995/IUCN-statement-on-Madagascar. Accessed 2013 October 10.

34. Ganzhorn JU, II LPP, Schatz GE, Sommer S (2001) The biodiversity of Madagascar: one of the world's hottest hotspots on its way out. Oryx 35: 346–348.

35. WHO/DFID-AHP (2006) The control of neglected zoonotic diseases. Switzerland: WHO/DFID-AHP. Available: http://www.who.int/zoonoses/Report_Sept06.pdf. Accessed 2013 October 10.

36. van den Beld MJ, Reubsaet FA (2012) Differentiation between Shigella, enteroinvasive Escherichia coli (EIEC) and noninvasive Escherichia coli. Eur J Clin Microbiol Infect Dis 31: 899–904.

37. Lindsay B, Ramamurthy T, Sen Gupta S, Takeda Y, Rajendran K, et al. (2011) Diarrheagenic pathogens in polymicrobial infections. Emerg Infect Dis 17: 606–611.

38. Gomes TA, Rassi V, MacDonald KL, Ramos SR, Trabulsi LR, et al. (1991) Enteropathogens associated with acute diarrheal disease in urban infants in Sao Paulo, Brazil. J Infect Dis 164: 331–337.

39. Nair GB, Ramamurthy T, Bhattacharya MK, Krishnan T, Ganguly S, et al. (2010) Emerging trends in the etiology of enteric pathogens as evidenced from an active surveillance of hospitalized diarrhoeal patients in Kolkata, India. Gut Pathog 2: 4.

40. Prüss-Üstün A, Bos R, Gore F, Bartram J (2008) Safer water, better health: costs, benefits and sustainability of interventions to protect and promote health. Geneva: World Health Organization. Available: http://www.who.int/water_sanitation_health/publications/safer_water/en/. Accessed 2013 October 10.

41. Okeke IN, Aboderin OA, Byarugaba DK, Ojo KK, Opintan JA (2007) Growing problem of multidrug-resistant enteric pathogens in Africa. Emerg Infect Dis 13: 1640–1646.

42. Hart CA, Kariuki S (1998) Antimicrobial resistance in developing countries. BMJ 317: 647–650.

43. Brunkard JM, Newton AE, Mintz E (2014) Cholera. In: CDC and Brunette GW, editors.CDC Health Information for International Travel 2014.New York, NY: Oxford University Press. pp. 158–160.

44. Bronze MS, Greenfield RA (2005) Biodefense: principles and pathogens. Wymondham, England: Horizon Bioscience.

45. Centers for Disease Control and Prevention (1982) Epidemiologic notes and reports outbreak of Yersinia enterocolitica – Washington state. Morbidity and Mortality Weekly Report.pp. 562–564.

46. Chapman PA, Siddons CA (1996) A comparison of immunomagnetic separation and direct culture for the isolation of verocytotoxin-producing Escherichia coli O157 from cases of bloody diarrhoea, non-bloody diarrhoea and asymptomatic contacts. J Med Microbiol 44: 267–271.

47. Cohen D, Block C, Green MS, Lowell G, Ofek I (1989) Immunoglobulin M, A, and G antibody response to lipopolysaccharide O antigen in symptomatic and asymptomatic Shigella infections. J Clin Microbiol 27: 162–167.

48. Gaudio PA, Sethabutr O, Echeverria P, Hoge CW (1997) Utility of a polymerase chain reaction diagnostic system in a study of the epidemiology of shigellosis among dysentery patients, family contacts, and well controls living in a shigellosis-endemic area. J Infect Dis 176: 1013–1018.

49. Gordon MA, Graham SM, Walsh AL, Wilson L, Phiri A, et al. (2008) Epidemics of invasive Salmonella enterica serovar enteritidis and S. enterica Serovar typhimurium infection associated with multidrug resistance among adults and children in Malawi. Clin Infect Dis 46: 963–969.

50. Harris JB, LaRocque RC, Chowdhury F, Khan AI, Logvinenko T, et al. (2008) Susceptibility to Vibrio cholerae infection in a cohort of household contacts of patients with cholera in Bangladesh. PLoS Negl Trop Dis 2: e221.

51. Nuorti JP, Niskanen T, Hallanvuo S, Mikkola J, Kela E, et al. (2004) A widespread outbreak of Yersinia pseudotuberculosis O:3 infection from iceberg lettuce. J Infect Dis 189: 766–774.

52. Perron GG, Quessy S, Letellier A, Bell G (2007) Genotypic diversity and antimicrobial resistance in asymptomatic Salmonella enterica serotype Typhimurium DT104. Infect Genet Evol 7: 223–228.

53. Qadri F, Saha A, Ahmed T, Al Tarique A, Begum YA, et al. (2007) Disease burden due to enterotoxigenic Escherichia coli in the first 2 years of life in an urban community in Bangladesh. Infect Immun 75: 3961–3968.

54. Qadri F, Svennerholm AM, Faruque AS, Sack RB (2005) Enterotoxigenic Escherichia coli in developing countries: epidemiology, microbiology, clinical features, treatment, and prevention. Clin Microbiol Rev 18: 465–483.

55. Lohmus M, Albihn A (2013) Gastrointestinal Pathogens in Rodents Overwintering in Human Facilities around Uppsala, Sweden. J Wildl Dis 49: 747–749.

56. Gillespie TR, Chapman CA, Grenier EC (2005) Effects of logging on gastrointestinal parasite infections and infection risk in African primates. J App Ecol 42: 699–707.

57. Gillespie TR, Greiner EC, Chapman CA (2005) Gastrointestinal parasites of the colobus monkeys of Uganda. J Parasitol 91: 569–573.

58. Hale CR, Scallan E, Cronquist AB, Dunn J, Smith K, et al. (2012) Estimates of enteric illness attributable to contact with animals and their environments in the United States. Clin Infect Dis 54 Suppl 5: S472–479.

59. Johnston AR, Gillespie TR, Rwego IB, McLachlan TL, Kent AD, et al. (2010) Molecular epidemiology of cross-species Giardia duodenalis transmission in western Uganda. PLoS Negl Trop Dis 4: e683.

16

Psychiatric Symptoms in Patients with Shiga Toxin-Producing *E. coli* O104:H4 Induced Haemolytic-Uraemic Syndrome

Alexandra Kleimann[1][*][ɔ], Sermin Toto[1][ɔ], Christian K. Eberlein[1], Jan T. Kielstein[2], Stefan Bleich[1], Helge Frieling[1][¶], Marcel Sieberer[1][¶]

1 Department of Psychiatry, Social Psychiatry and Psychotherapy, Hannover Medical School, Hannover, Germany, 2 Department of Nephrology and Hypertension, Hannover Medical School, Hannover, Germany

Abstract

Background: In May 2011 an outbreak of Shiga toxin-producing enterohaemorrhagic *E. coli* (STEC) O104:H4 in Northern Germany led to a high number of in-patients, suffering from post-enteritis haemolytic-uraemic syndrome (HUS) and often severe affection of the central nervous system. To our knowledge so far only neurological manifestations have been described systematically in literature.

Aim: To examine psychiatric symptoms over time and search for specific symptom clusters in affected patients.

Methods: 31 in-patients suffering from *E. coli* O104:H4 associated HUS, were examined and followed up a week during the acute hospital stay. Psychopathology was assessed by clinical interview based on the AMDP Scale, the Brief Symptom Inventory and the Clinical Global Impressions Scale.

Results: At baseline mental disorder due to known physiological condition (ICD-10 F06.8) was present in 58% of the examined patients. Patients suffered from various manifestations of cognitive impairment (n = 27) and hallucinations (n = 4). Disturbances of affect (n = 28) included severe panic attacks (n = 9). Psychiatric disorder was significantly associated with higher age (p<0.0001), higher levels of C-reactive protein (p<0.05), and positive family history of heart disease (p<0.05). Even within the acute hospital stay with a median follow up of 7 days, symptoms improved markedly over time (p <0.0001).

Conclusions: Aside from severe neurological symptoms the pathology in *E.coli* O104:H4 associated HUS frequently includes particular psychiatric disturbances. Long term follow up has to clarify whether or not these symptoms subside.

Editor: Holger Rohde, Universitätsklinikum Hamburg-Eppendorf, Germany

Funding: This work was funded by the research budget of the Department of Psychiatry, Socialpsychiatry and Psychotherapy, Hannover Medical School, Hannover, Germany. The funding department as an institution had no role in study design, data collection and analysis, decision to publish, or preparation of the manuscript.

Competing Interests: The authors have declared that no competing interests exist.

* Email: kleimann.alexandra@mh-hannover.de

ɔ These authors contributed equally to this work.

¶ These authors also contributed equally to this work.

Introduction

From May to July 2011 an outbreak of Shiga toxin-producing enterohaemorrhagic *Escherichia coli* (STEC) O104:H4 infections in Northern Germany occurred. Of the 3.186 reported STEC-patients 845 (22%) presented with haemolytic-uraemic syndrome. Ninety percent of the affected patients were adults [1]. According to the German STEC-HUS registry 69% of all HUS patients presented with neurological symptoms like headache or visual disturbances or neurological signs ranging from tremor and aphasia to delirium, coma and seizures [2]. One explanation for this unusual high incidence of neurological symptoms/signs was the increased virulence of the outbreak-strain O104:H4, which combined virulence factors of typical enteroaggregative and Shiga toxin-producing E. coli and showed an unusual age distribution of the affected patients as STEC-HUS usually occurs in pre-school children, were it shows lower rates of central nervous system (CNS) involvement. [3]

In the majority of cases infection with Shiga toxin-producing *Escherichia coli* leads to watery diarrhoea followed by bloody diarrhoea and abdominal cramps due to colitis [4]. These symptoms can be followed by the haemolytic-uraemic syndrome, which is defined by the sudden onset of microangiopathic haemolytic anaemia, thrombocytopenia and acute kidney injury [5]. In severe cases of HUS patients can also show CNS pathology associated with worse outcome. CNS pathology sometimes occurs before the onset of the haemolytic-uraemic syndrome and shows different manifestations that range from lethargy to seizures and coma [6] [7].

Little is known about the mechanisms causing CNS pathology. In infection with STEC different cytotoxins, Shiga toxin 1 and Shiga toxin 2, play a crucial role in systemic disease. The subunit StxB of Shiga toxin 2 is able to bind to glycolipid receptor, globotriaosylceramide (Gb3), on the cell membrane of target cells. Subunit StxA inhibits protein synthesis within the target cell, leading to its apoptosis [8]. Gb3 expressing cells have been found in the glomerular endothelium and neurons of different animals, in rabbits they determine the localization of pathological lesions [9]. Obata et al localized Gb3 on neurons and vascular endothelial cells within the human CNS [10]. Autopsy of the human CNS showed oedema, hypoxic-ischemic changes, microthrombosis and microhaemorrhages [11]. Former MRI studies in affected humans showed abnormal findings in up to 50% of patients, especially in the basal ganglia, but also in almost every other structure of the central nervous system. These lesions could not be correlated with the variety of clinical symptoms, severity of disorder or outcome, suggesting that the Shiga toxin could also have a direct effect on the central nervous system [3] [12].

In all previous outbreak reports on STEC-HUS specific psychiatric symptoms were not reported. None of the reports used a structured psychiatric evaluation of patients, neither during the acute phase nor during follow up.

The aim of our analysis was to conduct a structured psychiatric evaluation of patients suffering from STEC-HUS amidst the 2011 outbreak in our tertiary care center. Furthermore we were trying to substantiate suspected specific psychiatric symptom clusters suggested by the treating physicians and whenever possible perform a short term follow up during the hospital stay.

Materials and Methods

Ethics Statement

This study was performed in accordance with the Declaration of Helsinki.

Data were obtained during psychiatric consultation service and have been analysed retrospectively and anonymously. Results of blood samples, obtained in clinical indication, have been analysed retrospectively as well. The examinations were part of clinical routine treatment and patients gave their verbal informed consent to be examined. Therefore no written informed consent was given by the participants and all data were anonymized and de-identified prior to analysis. All 52 STEC-HUS in-patients treated at the Hannover Medical School participated in a study on the German outbreak of E. Coli O104:H4 [2]. Approval for this analysis was obtained from the Ethics Committee of the Hannover Medical School, Permit Number: 1106–2011.

Study design and patients

During the German outbreak of E. Coli O104:H4 from May to July 2011 32 out of 52 STEC- HUS in-patients at our tertiary care hospital received psychiatric consultation service examinations. Systematic psychiatric consultation was initiated after various psychiatric symptoms were noted in many patients by their treating doctors. Due to the lack of data on psychiatric symptoms in infection with E. Coli O104:H4 all patients received a structured psychiatric consultation as well as follow up examinations.

One of the 32 screened patients was excluded from the analysis as criteria for HUS were not met. All interviews were conducted by experienced psychiatrists, trained for the assessment of the study. The first interview with the patient was performed after a median of 7 days (range 2 to 23 days) after the onset of diarrhoea.

The second interview was performed 7 days later (range 7 to 9 days).

Assessment of baseline data included demographic data like qualification and marital status, psychiatric and medical history, family medical history, present medication, treatment with plasma exchange or dialysis and laboratory results. Afterwards psychopathology was rated using the 115-item Association for Methodology and Documentation in Psychiatry (AMDP) scale. Assessment of global psychological distress and psychopathology with respect to the past seven days was performed using the Brief Symptom Inventory (BSI). Severity of psychiatric symptoms was conducted using the Clinical Global Impressions Scale (CGI). At follow up examination present medication and again psychopathology, severity of psychiatric symptoms and global psychopathological distress was examined using the AMDP scale, the CGI and the BSI (past seven days). Additionally patients' charts, clinical progress documentation and third party informations (physicians, nurses) were collected at baseline and follow up to gain more information about psychopathological abnormalities. 22 Patients completed both assessments, 9 only participated at baseline visit and were discharged before the conduction of the second interview.

Definition of STEC-HUS and severity of illness

Infection with E. coli O104:H4 was confirmed by either positive stool cultures and/or presence of Shiga toxin, confirmed either by ELISA or PCR. HUS was defined according to the Robert-Koch-Institute (the national level health authority) definition if at least two out of three criteria were fulfilled: (i) thrombocytopenia (< 150×10^9/L), (ii) microangiopathic haemolytic anaemia lactate dehydrogenase (LDH>240 U/L and haemoglobin <12.0 g/dL), and (iii) acute kidney injury according to the AKIN definition [13] [14].

Severity of illness was assessed through lowest platelet count, highest peak of C-reactive Protein (CRP) and haemolytic activity, which was defined through highest peak of lactate dehydrogenase (LDH) and minimum haemoglobin level.

Psychiatric Assessment

AMDP scale. The AMDP scale was developed in Europe by the Association for Methodology and Documentation in Psychiatry (AMDP) in order to standardize the assessment of psycho-pathological symptoms [15]. It is based on a semi-structured interview method and consists of 115 items. Each psychiatric symptom is scored from 0 (not at all), one (mild), two (moderate) to three (severe). The AMDP system is the most commonly used and best known psychiatric documentation system in the German-speaking area and has been translated into many other languages [16]. Several studies reported that it has moderate to high interrater reliability for most symptoms and that it can be considered a well-established test with good to very good reliability and validity [17].

Brief Symptom Inventory. The BSI was derived from the Symptom Check-List-90-revised (SCL-90-R) and has been used extensively in diverse populations as a screening instrument for global psychological distress [18]. It is a 53-item self-administered questionnaire that uses five-point Likert scales and measures nine dimensions: somatisation (SOM), obsessive-compulsive (O-C), depression (DEP), anxiety (ANX), interpersonal sensitivity (I-S), hostility (HOS), phobic anxiety (PHO), paranoid ideation (PAR), and psychoticism (PSY). Items of the BSI are assessed using a 5-point scale ranging from 'not at all' (0) to 'extremely' (4). Patients rate their symptoms with respect to the last seven days. In addition, the inventory comprises three general distress measures:

Table 1. Frequency of abnormalities within the AMDP-Scale and other psychiatric findings.

Psychiatric Symptom	Baseline (%)	Follow up (%)
Disorders of consciousness	11 (35.9)	4 (18.2)
Disturbances of orientation	12 (39.1)	5 (22.7)
Disturbances of attention and memory	27 (88)	18 (81.9)
Dyscalculia	6 (19.4)	1 (4.5)
Formal disorders of thought	24 (78.2)	17 (77.3)
Phobias and Compulsions	13 (42.4)	7 (31.9)
Delusions	6 (19.4)	2 (9.1)
Disorders of perception	8 (26)	4 (18.2)
Disorders of ego	5 (16.3)	4 (18.2)
Disturbances of affect	27 (88)	17 (77.4)
Panic attacks	9 (29.0)	9 (40.9)
Disorders of drive and psychomotility	26 (84.8)	10 (45.5)
Circadian disturbances	3 (9.7)	5 (22.7)
Other disturbances	19 (61.3)	11 (50.0)
Organic psychiatric disorder (F06.8)	18 (58.1)	9 (40.9)

The General Severity Index (GSI) quantifies severity of illness and is used for outcome measurements. The Positive Symptom Distress Index (PSDI) is designed to measure the intensity of symptoms and the Positive Symptom Total (PST) reports the number of symptoms.

Scores are interpreted by comparison to age-appropriate norms. Normative data are available for both clinical and non-clinical samples of adolescents (over 13 years) and adults. The BSI demonstrated strong internal consistency reliability and a strong correlation with the SCL-90-R [19] [20]. Convergent validity was examined in various studies. Studies also showed a good reliability for the German version of the BSI which was used in this study [21].

Clinical Global Impressions scale. The Clinical Global Impressions scale is commonly used to measure symptom severity

(CGI-S), improvement (CGI-I) and efficacy of treatments in treatment studies of patients with mental disorders [22]. It is based on external rating. The severity of mental illness is rated on the following seven-point scale: 1 = normal, not at all ill; 2 = borderline mentally ill; 3 = mildly ill; 4 moderately ill; 5 markedly ill; 6 severely ill; 7 among the most extremely ill patients. Improvement, in this study assessed after one week, also can be rated on a seven-point scale: 1 = very much improved; 2 = much improved; 3 = minimally improved; 4 = no change; 5 = minimally worse; 6 = much worse; 7 = very much worse. In this observational study the Clinical Global Impression-Efficacy Index has not been used.

Statistical analysis

Deviation from normal distribution was tested using the Kolmogorov–Smirnov test. Correlation analysis between continuous data was then performed using Pearson's test. Between group comparisons (presence of psychiatric disorder vs. healthy) were performed using t-tests for continuous data and Chi squared or Fisher's exact test for categorical data. For not normally distributed data non-parametric Mann-Whitney U-test was used.

BSI data were compared with a healthy control group (German reference population). For comparement scores from all scales were transformed into t-values (mean = 50; SD = 10). These were calculated according to age and gender specific German norm groups. Between group analyses were performed using two way Analysis of Variance (ANOVA) and Bonferroni's *post-hoc* test when appropriate. Considering the significant correlation between age and presence of psychiatric disorder (p<0.0001) a receiver operating characteristic (ROC) - analysis and calculation of Youden's Index (Sensitivity + Specificity − 1) has been performed.

Results are presented as means (SD). P-values of less than 0.05 (two-tailed) were considered significant. Analysis was performed using the Statistical Package for the Social Sciences (SPSS™) for Windows 16.0.2 (SPSSInc., Chicago,IL) and most data are presented using Graph Pad Prism 5 (Graph Pad Inc., San Diego, CA).

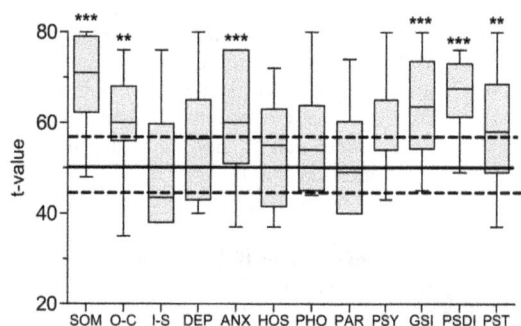

Figure 1. BSI t-values at baseline. Figure 1 shows the results of the Brief Symptom Inventory at baseline as boxplots. Results are compared to a healthy cohort which is marked by horizontal lines (t = 50, SD = 10). The horizontal line inside the "box" represents the median. The boundaries of the "box" indicate the 25th and 75th percentiles; the whiskers indicate the largest and smallest observed values. P-values given in the figure are derived from Bonferroni's *post hoc* test after two way ANOVA (cases vs controls): **P<0.01 ***P<0.001.

Table 2. Sample characteristics and differences between patients with or without organic psychiatric disorder at baseline.

Characteristics, mean (SD)	No diagnosis of organic psychiatric disorder	F06.8	p-value
Age, years	22 (13.4)	47 (15.3)	<0.0001
Women, n (%)	8 (61.5)	14 (77.8)	0.326
Hight, cm	170 (8)	172 (7)	0.951
Weight, kg	68 (12.2)	75 (14.3)	0.118
Duration of Diarrhoea, days	6 (5.1)	7 (5)	0.630
Duration of HUS, days	8 (2.9)	8 (5)	0.371
Duration of Dialysis, days	4.5 (4.3)	6 (5.2)	0.527

P-values are from Student's T-test except for gender, which is from Chi-squared test.

Results

Sample characteristics

All 31 patients at baseline and 22 of them at follow up have been included in analysis. The following data describe the sample characteristics at baseline: Women comprised 71% of the sample. Median age was 40 years (SD 19.2) and ranged from 18 to 81 years. Median duration of diarrhoea was 7 days (SD 5) and of associated HUS 8 days (SD 4.5).

Assessed previous illnesses included prior renal disease (n = 0), smoking (n = 1; type 2), diabetes (n = 1), hyperlipidemia (n = 2) and elevated arterial blood pressure (n = 5). Only one patient reported a history of psychiatric disorder (Panic disorder).

Frequency and characterization of psychiatric symptoms

Table 1 shows frequency of psychopathological abnormalities on the AMDP scale at baseline and follow up. Aggregation of collected data and clinical psychiatric examination revealed that an organic psychiatric disorder (ICD-10 F06.8) was confirmed in 58% of patients. On the CGI only 7 patients (22.6%) were rated as not psychiatric ill, meaning that even more patients suffered from psychopathological abnormalities, though diagnosis criteria for a psychiatric disorder were not fulfilled. At baseline 88% of patients showed disturbances of affect. Mostly feelings of anxiety and panic attacks were reported. Some patients suffered from 10 panic attacks daily. Anxiety was often reported as generalized without obvious specific causes. The second most observed abnormalities were disturbances of attention and memory (88%). These mostly included concentration and attention deficits which were associated with slow and stiff thinking (formal disorders of thought: 78.2%). Four patients suffered from vivid hallucinations. As an illustrating example a patient reported he was seeing different people in his room and described the surrounding as if he was travelling in a train. He reported knowing that these scenic hallucinations could not be real and memorized them in detail after recovery. No patient reported or showed signs of suicidal tendencies.

Brief Symptom Inventory

To confirm the findings in the AMDP-Scale in a self-reported instrument, patients completed the BSI. As some patients could not read due to visual disturbances or poor concentration in a few cases questions were read to them. Fig. 1 shows the results of the two way ANOVA analysis comparing patients with an age and gender matched healthy control group (t = 50). Post-hoc analyses show that the clinical sample significantly differs from the healthy controls.

Laboratory results

There was no statistically significant difference in the levels of lowest platelet count or minimum haemoglobin between healthy and psychiatric affected patients. Presence of psychiatric disorder at baseline and follow-up was significantly associated with higher peak CRP ($p<0.05$). Presence of psychiatric disorder at follow up was also associated with higher levels of peak LDH ($p<0.05$).

Other correlations and significant findings

Psychopathological abnormalities started between 0 to 10 days after onset of HUS (median 1.5 d, SD 2.9), 50% of patients developed symptoms within 24 h of HUS onset.

Table 2 and 3 provide details of the sample characteristics and their correlation with the presence of psychiatric disorder. Fisher's

Table 3. Family history of illness and risk factors in patients with or without organic psychiatric disorder.

Characteristics	No diagnosis of organic psychiatric disorder (%)	F06.8 (%)	p-value
Hypertension	0 (0.0)	5 (27.8)	0.058
Family history of ...			
Mental disorders	5 (38.5)	6 (33.3)	0.768
Drug addiction	3 (23.1)	3 (16.7)	0.656
Heart disease	3 (23.1)	11 (61.1)	< 0.05
Cancer	7 (53.8)	9 (50)	0.961

P-values are from Chi-squared test, except for high blood pressure and heart disease, which are from Fisher's exact test. Results for other risk factors (diabetes, hyperlipidaemia, nephrological illness) are not shown due to small amount.

Table 4. Age and organic psychiatric disorder.

Age	No diagnosis of organic psychiatric disorder	F06.8	p-value (Fisher's test)
< 30 years	12	1	
			<0.0001
> 30 years	1	17	

Dichotomized age groups show a high predictive value for presence of organic psychiatric disorder. Youden's index value is 1.87.

test showed statistically significant results according to age (p< 0.0001) and family history of heart disease (p<0.05). ROC-analysis and calculation of Youdens's Index for age younger/older than 30.5 years is shown in Table 4. The observed significance with higher age was also found investigating single items like anxiety (p<0.0001), panic attacks (p<0.005) or slow thinking (p< 0.0001).

Statistical analysis showed no significant difference between treatment with different types of medication like antibiotics (n = 6), eculizumab (n = 12), anticoagulants (n = 24) or antiepileptics (n = 19) and severity, outcome or presence of psychiatric disorder at baseline or in the completer-group.

Course of the disease

According to the CGI scale patients significantly improved over time (p<0.0001). Evaluation of the CGI revealed that at follow up 50% of patients scored 1, meaning "much improved". In only one patient the condition remained unchanged and none showed signs of worsening. However, 9 patients remained with the diagnosis of an organic psychiatric disorder. Fig. 2 shows the *post hoc* analysis of the BSI with all completers between baseline and follow-up.

Discussion

To our knowledge, we here report the first systematic psychometric analysis of CNS involvement in adult patients with STEC-HUS. Thirty-one in-patients with *E.coli* O104:H4 STEC-HUS during the 2011 German outbreak were studied. The majority of patients (58%) met the ICD-10 criteria for a mental disorder due to a known physical condition. Given that nine patients were already discharged at the follow up exam the frequency of psychiatric symptoms/diagnosis could be even higher.

Presence of psychiatric disorder at baseline was related to age or family history of heart disease, as well as higher CRP levels. CRP levels are known to be increased in patients suffering from depression or anxiety disorders [23]. The strong bidirectional connection between cardiovascular diseases and depression has been examined in various studies, but there are no previous data on susceptibility for psychiatric disorders concerning family history of heart disease [24].

Interestingly neither laboratory and other demographic data than age, nor the prescribed medication were related to the psychiatric symptoms.

The rapid onset of psychiatric symptoms, which occurred within 24 h after diagnosis of HUS in half of the patients, as well as their improvement over time correspond with recently published data from neurological examinations [25]. Our observation that higher age could be a risk factor for development of psychiatric symptoms is in line with a reported significance between higher age and a low score in the Mini-Mental State Examination of affected patients with HUS [26]. Interestingly, this association was not found for other neurological deficits but is stable in our exact analysis of different symptoms (anxiety only, panic attacks only etc.). From the view of a toxin-mediated hypothesis of CNS involvement in STEC-HUS older patients could be more often affected due to a higher vulnerability or weakening of the blood-brain barrier [27]. The ability of Shiga toxin to cross the blood-brain barrier has already been shown in the rat [28]. A recent publication focussing on the neurologic examination reported an elevated albumin ratio in the cerebrospinal fluid (CSF) of four out of five STEC-HUS affected patients. The authors interpreted these findings as a possible sign of blood-CSF barrier dysfunction [29]. Additionally age was also reported to be the overriding risk factor for death in the German STEC-HUS registry [30]. The significant correlation of psychiatric disorder in patients with higher peak CRP but not

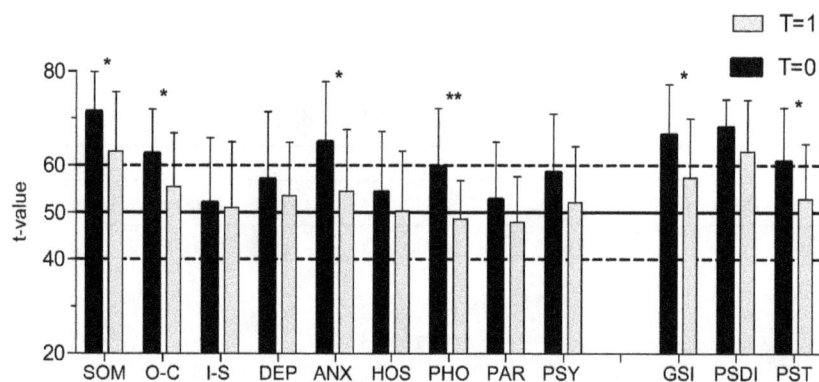

Figure 2. BSI t-values at follow up compared to baseline. BSI t-values of completers at follow up (t = 1) compared to baseline (t = 0). Healthy cohort is marked by horizontal lines (t = 50, SD = 10). Numbers given in the figure represent mean (SD). P-values given in the figure are derived from Bonferroni's *post hoc* test after two way ANOVA (follow up vs baseline): *P<0.05 **P<0.01.

with lowest haemoglobin or lowest platelet count contributes to the thesis that CRP could be a better fitting laboratory marker of CNS complications in STEC-HUS then the usual indicators for the degree of progression in HUS [31]. Also, an interesting recently published laboratory finding is the alteration of circulating microRNAs (mi-R 126) in STEC-HUS patients with moderate to severe CNS involvement compared to patients with HUS only [32].

The majority of affected patients suffered from anxiety symptoms and/or cognitive dysfunction. At first sight the anxiety syndrome of affected patients could be interpreted as a reaction due to suffering from a life-threatening epidemic disease. Clinical interview on the other hand revealed that most patients were not able to indicate the reason of their anxiety. Anxiety was described as a generalized state of affect, mixed with free floating anxiety and panic attacks up to 10 times daily. The mixture of generalized anxiety and panic attacks is typical for organic anxiety syndromes (ICD-10 F06.4) [33]. Interestingly, some of the patients suffering from panic attacks also reported recurring chest pain. The phobic scale within the BSI could represent sickness behavior and impairment due to diarrhoea and HUS. Specific phobias were negated.

Dysfunction of memory and disturbances of thought mainly included slow thinking and poor concentration. For instance, some patients were not able to read more than a few sentences. Seven patients reported severe dyscalculia.

In contrast to the various neurological findings in CNS pathology, observed psychiatric disturbances were relatively specific. Still, making a precise distinction between neurological and psychiatric symptoms is complicated as both are a sign of CNS affection and long term observations could help in making a more precise distinction.

Focussing on the psychiatric part, the question if a special circuit or anatomical structure is affected predominantly should be considered. Tironi-Farinati et al. showed that intraventricular injection of Shiga toxin 2 causes dendritic abnormalities in rat brains and increases the expression of Gb3 [34]. They also reported a localization of Gb3 expressing cells in the CA1 region of the hippocampus and the striatum of rats. Another recent study conducted by Meuth et al. showed neuronal expression of Gb3 and dose dependent neuronal cytotoxity of Shiga toxin 2 on thalamic neurons and astrocytes of female rats, fitting to recently published research showing symmetric MRI alterations in the lateral thalamus and brainstem (50%) of affected patients [7] [35].

Involvement of the hippocampus and/or thalamus could possibly explain anxiety, panic attacks and disturbances of memory and attention [36] [37]. These questions remain unanswered, as our report only allows a description of psychiatric symptoms, but is not suitable to establish causality.

Beside the possible scientific value of accurate psychiatric examinations, these findings could also be clinically important, as only few patients received a sufficient symptomatic treatment such as benzodiazepines to lower severe anxiety. Though the course of the disease seems to be benign, due to lack of long-term data we cannot exclude the possibility of vulnerable patients developing disorders afterwards. In our outpatient clinic two patients asked for consultancy weeks after discharge.

Limitations

First this study is limited by its open design and the single center setting, both limitations owed to the acute onset of the crisis making a proper planned randomized multi-center evaluation impossible. Given that the so far largest report on STEC-HUS in adults before the described outbreak involved 22 patients the assessment of 31 patients is rather high [38]. Still, the sample size is small and does not allow interpretations beyond a descriptive level. It is possible that moderate effects of medication or correlation with more laboratory findings only gain statistical significance in a larger cohort.

Second a major limitation of this study is the lack of long-term follow up data and its retrospective design. Though our analysis showed healing tendency for psychiatric disorders it is possible that patients suffer from residual symptoms or new psychiatric disturbances. Thus, there is a great need for further studies on long-term outcome. Third, continuous observation could reveal more data about correlations with other systemical abnormalities, especially neurological deficits, impact on outcome and more specific laboratory results.

Implications

CNS involvement in patients with *Escherichia coli* O104:H4 associated haemolytic uraemic syndrome shows high rates of psychiatric affection with a probably benign course of psychiatric disorder. A higher sensitivity for psychiatric disturbances could be important for an optimized disease severity based treatment approach of *Escherichia coli* O104:H4- associated haemolytic uraemic syndrome. Further studies are needed to assess potential long-term sequelae of STEC-HUS and investigate the underlying mechanisms of these symptoms.

Author Contributions

Conceived and designed the experiments: MS CKE ST. Performed the experiments: MS CKE ST AK. Analyzed the data: AK HF JTK. Wrote the paper: AK HF. Treatment of STEC-HUS patients: JTK. Critical revision of the manuscript for important intellectual content: SB JTK CKE MS ST HF.

References

1. Frank C, Werber D, Cramer JP, Askar M, Faber M, et al. (2011) Epidemic profile of shiga-toxin producing Escherichia coli O104:H4 outbreak in Germany. N Engl J Med 365: 1771–1780.

2. Kielstein JT, Beutel G, Fleig S, Steinhoff J, Meyer TN, et al. (2012) Best supportive care and therapeutic plasma exchange with or without eculizumab in shiga-toxin-producing E. coli O104:H4 induced haemolytic-uraemic syndrome: An analysis of the German STEC-HUS registry. Nephrol Dial Transplant 27: 3807–3815.

3. Nathanson S, Kwon T, Elmaleh M, Charbit M, Launay EA, et al. (2010) Acute neurological involvement in diarrhea-associated hemolytic uremic syndrome. Clin J Am Soc Nephrol 5: 1218–1228.

4. Andreoli SP, Trachtman H, Acheson DW, Siegler RL, Obrig TG (2002) Hemolytic uremic syndrome: Epidemiology, pathophysiology, and therapy. Pediatr Nephrol 17: 293–298.

5. Proulx F, Seidman EG, Karpman D (2001) Pathogenesis of shiga toxin-associated hemolytic uremic syndrome. Pediatr Res 50: 163–171.

6. Hamano S, Nakanishi Y, Nara T, Seki T, Ohtani T, et al. (1993) Neurological manifestations of hemorrhagic colitis in the outbreak of Escherichia coli O157:H7 infection in Japan. Acta Paediatr 82: 454–458.

7. Magnus T, Rother J, Simova O, Meier-Cillien M, Repenthin J, et al. (2012) The neurological syndrome in adults during the 2011 northern German E. coli serotype O104:H4 outbreak. Brain 135: 1850–1859.

8. Mallard F, Antony C, Tenza D, Salamero J, Goud B, et al. (1998) Direct pathway from early/recycling endosomes to the golgi apparatus revealed through the study of shiga toxin B-fragment transport. J Cell Biol 143: 973–990.

9. Zoja C, Corna D, Farina C, Sacchi G, Lingwood C, et al. (1992) Verotoxin glycolipid receptors determine the localization of microangiopathic process in rabbits given verotoxin-1. J Lab Clin Med 120: 229–238.

10. Obata F, Tohyama K, Bonev AD, Kolling GL, Keepers TR, et al. (2008) Shiga toxin 2 affects the central nervous system through receptor globotriaosylceramide localized to neurons. J Infect Dis 198: 1398–1406.

11. Siegler RL, Pavia AT, Christofferson RD, Milligan MK (1994) A 20-year population-based study of postdiarrheal hemolytic uremic syndrome in Utah. Pediatrics 94: 35–40.
12. Donnerstag F, Ding X, Pape L, Bultmann E, Lucke T, et al. (2012) Patterns in early diffusion-weighted MRI in children with haemolytic uraemic syndrome and CNS involvement. Eur Radiol 22: 506–513.
13. Robert-Koch-Institut (2011) Ausbruchs-Falldefinition für EHEC- und HUS-fälle im Rahmen des Ausbruchs im Frühjahr 2011 in Deutschland. 2013.
14. Mehta RL, Kellum JA, Shah SV, Molitoris BA, Ronco C, et al. (2007) Acute kidney injury network: Report of an initiative to improve outcomes in acute kidney injury. Crit Care 11: R31.
15. Pietzcker A, Gebhardt R, Strauss A, Stockel M, Langer C, et al. (1983) The syndrome scales in the AMDP-system. Mod Probl Pharmacopsychiatry 20: 88–99.
16. Moller HJ (2009) Standardised rating scales in psychiatry: Methodological basis, their possibilities and limitations and descriptions of important rating scales. World J Biol Psychiatry 10: 6–26.
17. Renfordt E, Busch H, von Cranach M, Gulbinat W, Tegeler J (1983) Particular aspects of the interrater reliability of the AMDP psychopathology scale. Mod Probl Pharmacopsychiatry 20: 125–142.
18. Derogatis LR, Melisaratos N (1983) The brief symptom inventory: An introductory report. Psychol Med 13: 595–605.
19. Piersma HL, Reaume WM, Boes JL (1994) The brief symptom inventory (BSI) as an outcome measure for adult psychiatric inpatients. J Clin Psychol 50: 555–563.
20. Recklitis CJ, Rodriguez P (2007) Screening childhood cancer survivors with the brief symptom inventory-18: Classification agreement with the symptom checklist-90-revised. Psychooncology 16: 429–436.
21. Franke H (2000) BSI. Brief Symptom Inventory - deutsche Version. Manual. Göttingen: Beltz.
22. Guy W (1976) Clinical global impressions. ECDEU Assessment Manual for Psychopharmacology National Institute of Mental Health, Rockville, MD; revised.
23. Duivis HE, Vogelzangs N, Kupper N, de Jonge P, Penninx BW (2010) Differential association of somatic and cognitive symptoms of depression and anxiety with inflammation: findings from the Netherlands Study of Depression and Anxiety (NESDA). J Am Coll Cardiol. 29;56(1):31–7.
24. Nemeroff CB, Goldschmidt-Clermont PJ (2012) Heartache and heartbreak—the link between depression and cardiovascular disease. Nat Rev Cardiol 9(9):526–39.
25. Greinacher A, Friesecke S, Abel P, Dressel A, Stracke S, et al. (2011) Treatment of severe neurological deficits with IgG depletion through immunoadsorption in patients with Escherichia coli O104:H4-associated haemolytic uraemic syndrome: A prospective trial. Lancet 378: 1166–1173.
26. Weissenborn K, Donnerstag F, Kielstein JT, Heeren M, Worthmann H, et al. (2012) Neurologic manifestations of E coli infection-induced hemolytic-uremic syndrome in adults. Neurology 79: 1466–1473.
27. Dankbaar JW, Hom J, Schneider T, Cheng SC, Lau BC, et al. (2009) Age- and anatomy-related values of blood-brain barrier permeability measured by perfusion-CT in non-stroke patients. J Neuroradiol 36: 219–227.
28. Lucero MS, Mirarchi F, Goldstein J, Silberstein C (2012) Intraperitoneal administration of shiga toxin 2 induced neuronal alterations and reduced the expression levels of aquaporin 1 and aquaporin 4 in rat brain. Microb Pathog 53: 87–94.
29. Skripuletz T, Wurster U, Worthmann H, Heeren M, Schuppner R, et al. (2013) Blood-cerebrospinal fluid barrier dysfunction in patients with neurological symptoms during the 2011 northern German E. coli serotype O104:H4 outbreak. Brain.
30. German EHEC-HUS Registry (2011) The German 2011 epidemic of shiga toxin-producing E. coli—the nephrological view. Nephrol Dial Transplant 26: 2723–2726.
31. Teramoto T, Fukao T, Hirayama K, Asano T, Aoki Y, et al. (2009) Escherichia coli O-157-induced hemolytic uremic syndrome: Usefulness of SCWP score for the prediction of neurological complication. Pediatr Int 51: 107–109.
32. Lorenzen JM, Menne J, Schmidt BM, Schmidt M, Martino F, et al. (2012) Circulating microRNAs in patients with shiga-toxin-producing E. coli O104:H4 induced hemolytic uremic syndrome. PLoS One 7: e47215.
33. World Health Organization. World health organization: The ICD-10 classification of mental and behavioral disorders. Clinical descriptions and diagnostic guidelines. Geneva, world health organization, 1992
34. Tironi-Farinati C, Loidl CF, Boccoli J, Parma Y, Fernandez-Miyakawa ME, et al. (2010) Intracerebroventricular shiga toxin 2 increases the expression of its receptor globotriaosylceramide and causes dendritic abnormalities. J Neuroimmunol 222: 48–61.
35. Meuth SG, Gobel K, Kanyshkova T, Ehling P, Ritter MA, et al. (2012) Thalamic involvement in patients with neurologic impairment due to shiga toxin 2. Ann Neurol .
36. McGaugh JL (2000) Memory—a century of consolidation. Science 287: 248–251.
37. Gross CT, Canteras NS (2012) The many paths to fear. Nat Rev Neurosci 13: 651–658.
38. Dundas S, Murphy J, Soutar RL, Jones GA, Hutchinson SJ, et al. (1999) Effectiveness of therapeutic plasma exchange in the 1996 Lanarkshire escherichia coli O157:H7 outbreak. Lancet 354: 1327–1330.

17

Chloride Secretion Induced by Rotavirus is Oxidative Stress-Dependent and Inhibited by *Saccharomyces boulardii* in Human Enterocytes

Vittoria Buccigrossi[1], Gabriella Laudiero[1], Carla Russo[1], Erasmo Miele[1], Morena Sofia[1], Marina Monini[2], Franco Maria Ruggeri[2], Alfredo Guarino[1]*

1 Department of Translational Medical Science, Section of Pediatrics, University of Naples "Federico II", Naples, Italy, **2** Department of Veterinary Public Health & Food Safety, Viral Zoonoses Unit, Istituto Superiore di Sanità Rome – Italy, Rome, Italy

Abstract

Rotavirus (RV) infection causes watery diarrhea via multiple mechanisms, primarily chloride secretion in intestinal epithelial cell. The chloride secretion largely depends on non-structural protein 4 (NSP4) enterotoxic activity in human enterocytes through mechanisms that have not been defined. Redox imbalance is a common event in cells infected by viruses, but the role of oxidative stress in RV infection is unknown. RV SA11 induced chloride secretion in association with an increase in reactive oxygen species (ROS) in Caco-2 cells. The ratio between reduced (GSH) and oxidized (GSSG) glutathione was decreased by RV. The same effects were observed when purified NSP4 was added to Caco-2 cells. N-acetylcysteine (NAC), a potent antioxidant, strongly inhibited the increase in ROS and GSH imbalance. These results suggest a link between oxidative stress and RV-induced diarrhea. Because *Saccharomyces boulardii* (Sb) has been effectively used to treat RV diarrhea, we tested its effects on RV-infected cells. Sb supernatant prevented RV-induced oxidative stress and strongly inhibited chloride secretion in Caco-2 cells. These results were confirmed in an organ culture model using human intestinal biopsies, demonstrating that chloride secretion induced by RV-NSP4 is oxidative stress-dependent and is inhibited by Sb, which produces soluble metabolites that prevent oxidative stress. The results of this study provide novel insights into RV-induced diarrhea and the efficacy of probiotics.

Editor: Ravi Jhaveri, University of North Carolina School of Medicine, United States of America

Funding: This work was supported in part by Biocodex Laboratories, Gentilly, France. The funders had no role in study design, data collection and analysis, decision to publish, or preparation of the manuscript. No additional external funding was received for this study.

* E-mail: alfguari@unina.it

Introduction

Rotavirus (RV) infection is the most frequent and severe form of acute gastroenteritis in infants and children worldwide and frequently requires hospitalization [1,2]. Up to 40% of hospitalized children under 5 years of age with diarrhea are infected with RV [3,4]. In developing regions, acute diarrhea still represents a leading cause of childhood mortality, second only to pneumonia, and RV is the most common agent [1,5]. RV immunization has been identified as a major priority for the health of children by authoritative institutions [6]. No specific therapy is available, but selected probiotics, including *Saccharomyces boulardii* (Sb), reduce the severity and duration of diarrhea.

RV infects mature enterocytes of the small intestinal villi, inducing broad functional and structural damage [7]. In human enterocytes, RV diarrhea is the result of a sequence of combined secretory and osmotic mechanisms, including overstimulation of intestinal ion transepithelial secretion and intestinal damage, leading to malabsorption and osmotic diarrhea [8,9]. Non-structural protein 4 (NSP4) plays a key role in secretory diarrhea. NSP4 is produced by RV and induces diarrhea in mice through the release of intracellular stores of calcium from enterocytes [10].

RV was recently shown to induce early, NSP4-dependent ion secretion [9,11].

Redox imbalance is a common event in cells infected by viruses, but its role in RV diarrhea remains unclear. Oxidants, such as H_2O_2, induce anion secretion in selected segments of the intestinal tract, such as the rat ileum and colon [12,13], and in an intestinal cell model [13,14], but there is no evidence that oxidative stress induced by viral infections is linked with intestinal ion secretion. Redox imbalance is generally derived from a decrease in antioxidant enzyme levels, the depletion of cellular antioxidant defenses, and enhanced production of reactive oxygen species (ROS), leading to the rapid killing of infected cells and the release of viral particles [15–17]. A previous study reported that the oxidative/antioxidative profile is altered in gut homogenates from RV-infected mice, indicating oxidative stress [18]. In addition, RV induces a strong increase in mitochondrial superoxide dismutase expression [19]. Therefore, in this study, we investigated the involvement of oxidative stress in RV-induced diarrhea and the direct role of NSP4, if any.

Sb, a probiotic yeast, reduces diarrheal duration and the severity of RV gastroenteritis in children [20] and is recommended as an adjunct to oral rehydration solution by guidelines of authoritative institutions [21,22].

In vitro and *in vivo* studies indicate that Sb exerts an antidiarrheal effect by acting on the resident microflora and inducing an anti-inflammatory effect [23]. The stimulation of brush border disaccharidases (e.g., lactase, sucrase) has been proposed as an additional mechanism to explain the antidiarrheal activity of this yeast [24]. None of these proposed mechanisms is consistent with the rapid efficacy observed in acute gastroenteritis, which is more consistent with a direct interaction of Sb with enterocytes and/or the virus than with modifications of intestinal microecology or immune regulation. It is becoming clear that several intestinal effects of probiotics are not associated with the direct interaction between the microorganisms and intestinal epithelial cells but are induced by soluble mediators released by the probiotics in the surrounding medium [25,26]. The effects exerted on target cells by these released metabolic products have been designated the "postbiotic effect" [27]. Therefore, in the present study, we also investigated the effects of Sb-conditioned medium on RV-induced enterotoxic effects in our experimental model.

Materials and Methods

Intestinal Cell Line

Caco-2 cells were used as previously described [28]. Caco-2 cells were grown in Dulbecco's modified Eagle minimum essential medium (DMEM; Life Technologies Italia, Monza, Italy) with a high glucose concentration (4.5 g/L) at 37°C in a 5% CO_2 atmosphere. The medium was supplemented with 10% fetal bovine serum (FBS, Life Technologies Italia, Monza, Italy), 1% non-essential amino acids, penicillin (50 mU/mL), and strepto-mycin (50 µg/mL).

Virus strain and infection protocol. The simian rotavirus strain SA11 (RV) was used as previously described [9]. Briefly, the virus was activated with 20 µg/mL trypsin for 30 min at 37°C. The viral suspension was added to the apical side of cell monolayers. After 60 min, the cells were washed and incubated in FBS-free medium for the indicated time periods after infection.

Purification of BacNSP4SA11

Sf9 cell monolayers (2×10^7 cells) grown in Sf900 medium (Life Technologies Italia, Monza, Italy) in 175 cm^2 flasks were infected with the recombinant baculoviruses BacNSP4SA11 (moi 10). When a cytopathic effect was observed, the recombinant protein was harvested from the cells lysed with lysis buffer (50 mM NaH_2PO_4, 10 mM imidazole, 300 mM NaCl, pH 8.0,, 1% Triton X-100, and 0.1% Protease Inhibitor Cocktail (Sigma-Aldrich S.r.l. Milan, Italy). The lysates were clarified by centrifugation at 22,000 g at 4°C for 5 min and purified by affinity chromatography using Ni-NTA agarose colums (Qiagen), following the manufacturer's instructions. After 3 washes (with 50 mM NaH_2PO_4, 20 mM imidazole, 300 mM NaCl, pH 8.0), the His-tagged proteins were eluted in 400 µL of elution buffer (50 mM NaH_2PO_4, 250 mM imidazole, 300 mM NaCl, pH 8.0) and dialyzed against PBS. The purified 21–28 kDa HisNSP4 proteins, which corresponded to glycosylated NSP4, were visualized by SDS-PAGE and western blotting using a monoclonal anti poly-histidine antibody (Fig. S1). Protein concentration was quantified using the Bradford reagent (Bio-Rad, Milan, Italy) and several 0.2 mg/ml stock solutions were prepared.

An histidine-tagged HEV major ORF2 capsid protein of a swine hepatitis E virus (HEV) strain, expressed and purified as reported above for NSP4, was used as irrelevant control protein

(Ruggeri F.M. unpublished). Then, we tested the effects of this protein in experiments on intestinal ion transport.

ROS Production

ROS production was measured by 7′-dichlorofluorescein diacetate (DCFH-DA) spectrofluorometry. After stimulation, cells were exposed to 20 DCFH-DA (D6665; Sigma-Aldrich, St. Louis, MO for 30 minutes at 37°C in the dark. Intracellular ROS production was measured in a fluorometer (SFM 25; Kontron Instruments, Japan).

DCF Fluorescence Imaging

Caco-2 cells were grown on glass cover slips for 3 days and were then fixed and permeabilized with paraformaldehyde (4%) and Triton (0.2%) for 30 min at 4°C. The cells were then incubated with 20 µM DCF-HA for 30 min at 37°C in the dark. Fluorescence images from multiple fields were obtained using a Nikon Eclipse e 80i microscope. The images were analyzed using NiS Elements D imaging software (Nikon Instruments Inc., NY, USA).

GSH Assay

Intracellular levels of reduced (GSH) and oxidized glutathione (GSSG) were measured as described by Allen et al. [29] with a few modifications. Proteins were precipitated with 1% sulfosalicylic acid, and the supernatants were used to measure, in parallel, total and reduced glutathione. GSSG was determined by subtracting GSH from total glutathione. The GSH and GSSG contents were normalized for protein content and expressed as % of total glutathione.

Ion Transport Studies

Ion transport experiments were performed in Ussing chambers (WPI, Sarasota, FL) as previously described [30]. Ion secretion was studied in Ussing chambers by monitoring increases in short-circuit current (Isc), as an indication of active, luminally directed anion secretion. Maximal changes in short circuit current (delta Isc) were recorded as an indicator of mucosal ion secretion. Neutralization experiments were performed using specific anti-NSP4 polyclonal antibodies. NSP4 (200 ng/ml) was incubated at 37°C for 1 hour with the antibodies (10 µg/ml) and then added to Caco-2 cells in Ussing chambers. The same concentration of preimmune antibodies was incubated with NSP4 and used as controls.

In experiments performed to investigate the role of Cl^- in the electrical response, Cl^- was substituted with SO_4^- at an equimolar concentration. To investigate in greater detail the role of Cl^- in the electrical effect of NSP4, we used CaCCinh-A01 to inhibit TMEM16 channels [11]. Cells were incubated with CaCCinh-A01 (30 µmol/L), and electrical parameters were monitored. To investigate the role of Ca^{2+} in the effects of NSP4 Caco-2 cells were mounted in Ussing chambers with Ca^{2+}-free Ringer and NSP4 was added 30 min later. Parallel monolayers BAPTA-AM with Ca^{2+}-free Ringer alone or NSP4 served as controls.

Transepithelial Resistance Measurement

The transepithelial resistance of cell monolayers grown on filters was measured using a Millicel-ERS resistance monitoring appa-ratus (Merck Millipore, Billerica, MA). The resistance was expressed in Ohms/cm^2. Transepithelial resistance was measured at 24, 48, and 72 h after the specific stimulations.

A

B

C

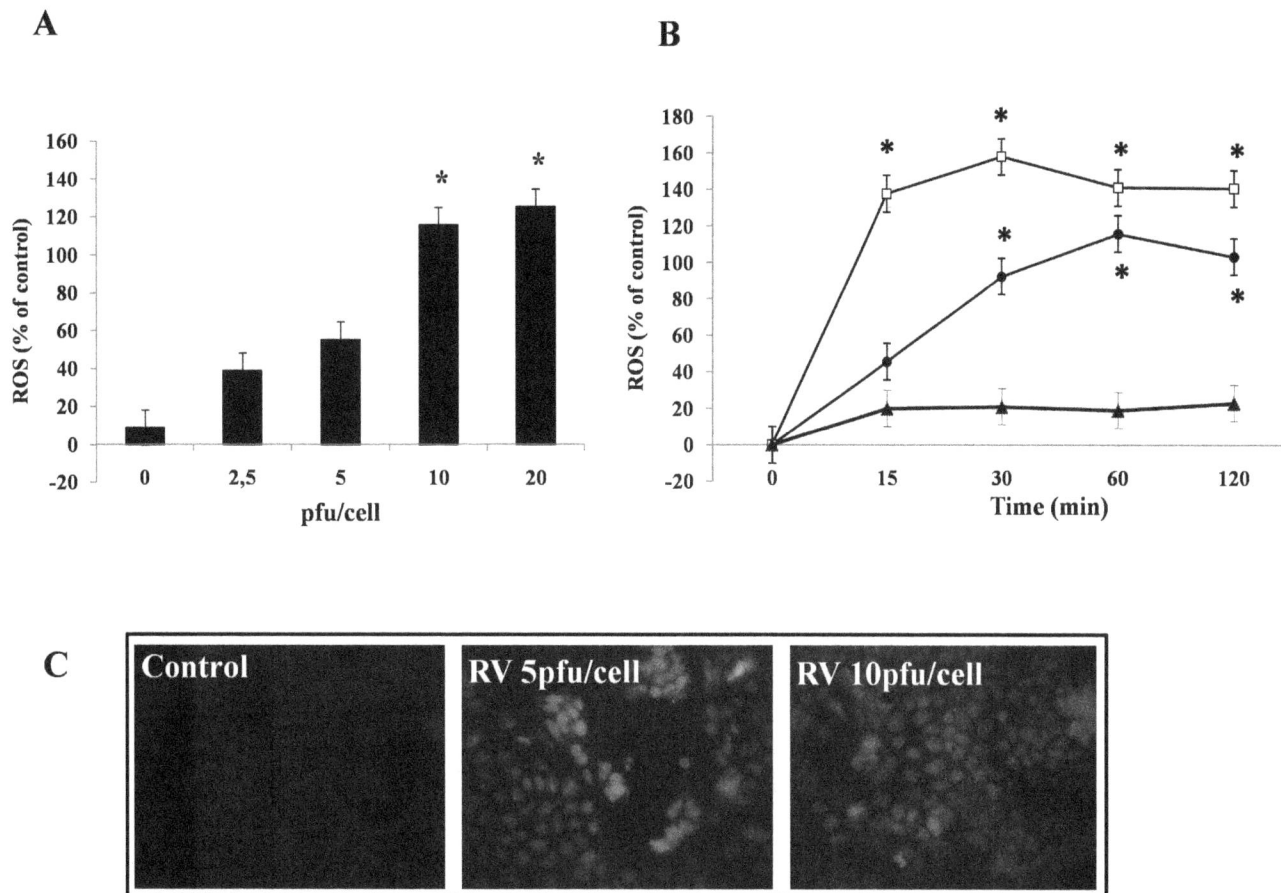

Figure 1. RV induces ROS generation in a dose- and time-dependent manner. Caco-2 cells were exposed to increasing dose of RV for 1 h (A) and to 10 pfu/cell for 15, 30 60 and 120 min post-infection (B). Intracellular ROS levels were evaluated by the DCFH-DA fluorometric method. RV (●), untreated cells as a negative control (▲), and H_2O_2 as a positive control (□). The data are representative of 3 separate experiments. *$p < 0.05$ vs. 0 pfu/cell or time 0. (C) Immunofluorescent staining of ROS by DCFH-DA after 1 hour post-RV infection was compared with that in untreated cells (control). Representative staining is shown at 1 h post-exposure. Magnification: 200X.

Preparation of Sb Culture Supernatant

Lyophilized Sb (Biocodex, Gentilly, France) was cultured in RPMI 1640 cell culture medium (100 mg/mL) for 24 h at 37°C. The cell-free culture supernatant (SbS) was obtained by centrifugation and passage of the Sb culture through a 0.22-mm filter. All studies were performed using SbS directly on Caco-2 cells.

Human Intestinal Organ Culture

Biopsies from the distal part of the duodenum were obtained from 2 children seen at the Department of Pediatrics who underwent endoscopy for intestinal disorders. All biopsies were from macroscopically normal areas, and intestinal histology was subsequently reported to be normal. Organ culture was performed in DMEM with a high glucose concentration (4.5 g/L) supplemented with 0.5% FCS, 1% non-essential amino acids, 2% penicillin (50 mU/mL), and streptomycin (50 mg/mL) and incubated in 5% CO_2/95% air for 1 h before treatment. Experiments were performed by adding RV (50 pfu/5 mm^2) for 2 h to maximize the effect before spontaneous tissue disruption. Specimens were exposed to RV alone or were preincubated with SbS (2 h) and then homogenized in lysis buffer 100 mM Tris-HCl pH 7.5, 300 mM NaCl, 2% NP40, 1% Na deoxycholic acid, 0.2% SDS, 100 μg/mL PMSF, 5 μg/mL aprotinin, 1 μg/mL leupeptin, 0.7 μg/mL pepstatin). The GSH/GSSG ratio was determined as

described above for cells. The experiments with human specimens were conducted with the understanding and written consent of each child's parents, and the study methodologies conformed to the standards set by the Declaration of Helsinki.

Ethics Statement

The study protocol (2008-001349-24) was approved by the Ethics Committee of the School of Medicine, University of Naples "Federico II" Italy. A written informed consent was obtained, for each enrolled child from the parents.

Results

RV Induces Intestinal Epithelial Oxidative Stress and Impairs Antioxidant Defenses

To determine if RV alters the enterocyte oxidative state, we measured the intracellular levels of ROS and glutathione in Caco-2 cells. ROS levels progressively increased in cells exposed to increasing virus dose, with a maximal effect at 10–20 pfu/cell (Fig. 1A). Because ROS generation is usually rapid following a toxic stimulus, we performed time-course experiments in Caco-2 cells infected with RV for 15 up to 120 min. An increase in ROS was evident as early as 15 min after RV infection and reached its maximum level at 60 min (Fig. 1B). Intracellular ROS induction

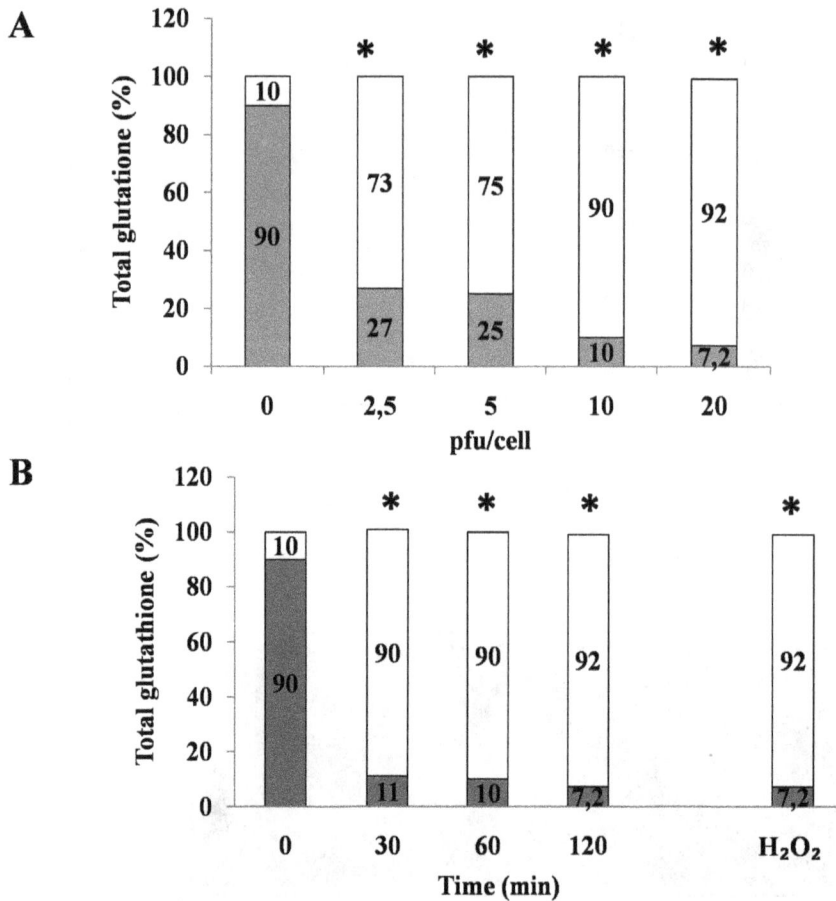

Figure 2. RV induces changes in intracellular antioxidant defenses. Caco-2 cells were exposed to different doses of RV for 1 h (A) and to 10 pfu/cell for 30, 60, and 120 min (B), and the ratio of GSH (grey) and GSSG (white) was evaluated. H_2O_2 was used as a positive control. the data are representative of 3 separate experiments. *$p < 0.05$ vs. 0 pfu/cell or time 0.

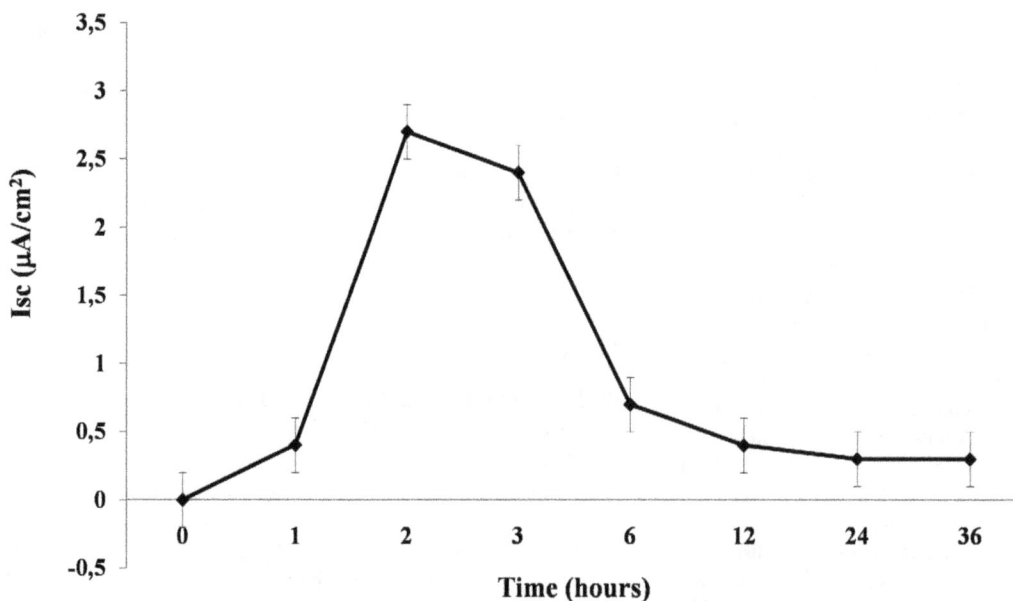

Figure 3. Rotavirus infection induces early chloride secretion. Caco-2 cell monolayers were infected with RV at 10 pfu/cell, and the Isc was evaluated in Ussing chambers. The data are representative of 3 separate experiments. *$p < 0.05$ vs. time 0.

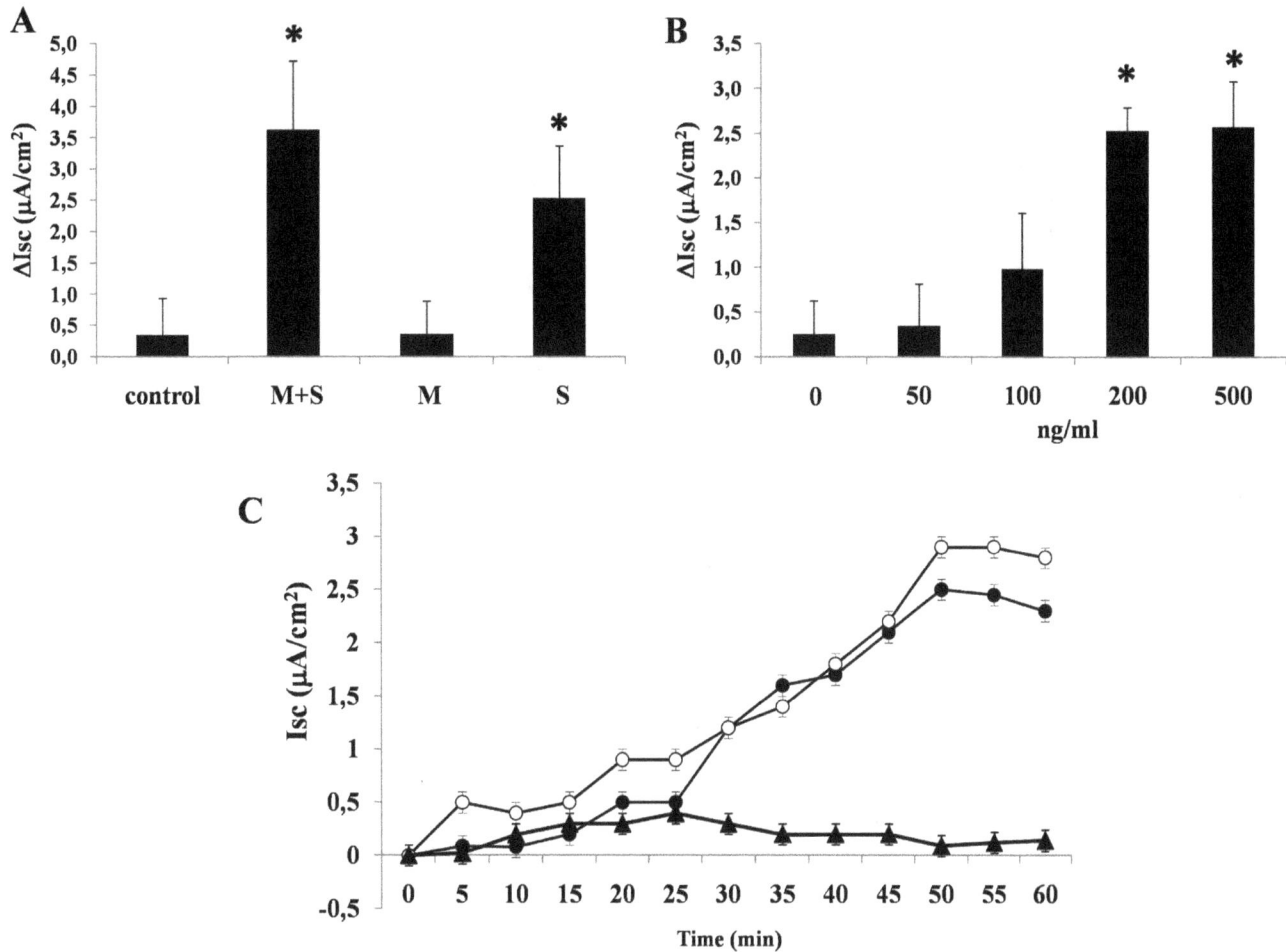

Figure 4. NSP4 induces chloride secretion in intestinal epithelial cells. (A) NSP4 (200 ng/mL) was added to the mucosal (M) or serosal (S) side or both (M+S) of Caco-2 cell monolayers for 1 hour, and the Isc was measured to evaluate chloride secretion. The maximal Isc shown was measured at 50 min time point. (B) NSP4 induced an increase in the Isc in a dose-dependent manner. The maximal Isc shown was measured at 50 min time point. (C) Caco-2 cells were infected with RV 10 pfu/cell (○) or exposed to NSP4 at 200 ng/ml (●) and Isc was measured for 1 hours every 5 minutes. A Isc similar increase was observed in RV infected cells and in virus-free cells exposed to NSP4. An histidine-tagged HEV ORF2 capsid protein was used as negative control (▲). The data are representative of 3 separate experiments. *p<0.05 vs. control or 0 ng/mL.

was confirmed by the increase in the green signal of DCF-DA by fluorescent microscopy in cells exposed to RV for 1 hour (Fig. 1C).

We next investigated whether RV-induced ROS generation was associated with a decrease in antioxidant defenses by measuring glutathione, a major intracellular ROS scavenger. Glutathione protects cells against oxidative stress, and the intracellular proportions of GSH and GSSG are approximately 80−90% GSH and 10−20% GSSG under in uninfected cells. The GSH/GSSG ratio was reversed in RV-infected Caco-2 cells: 10% GSH and 90% GSSG. The effect peaked at 10–20 pfu/cell and was already evident as early as 15 min after infection (Fig. 2A and B).

The addition of RV to Caco-2 cell monolayers resulted in an increase in the short circuit current (Isc) consistent with anion secretion (Fig. 3). The increase in the Isc was statistically significant at 1 h after infection, reached a peak after 2 h, and then slowly decreased. At 12 h after infection, electrical evidence of active ion secretion was no longer detected (Fig. 3).

NSP4 Induces an Enterotoxic but not a Cytotoxic Effect in Caco-2 Cells

Because we previously observed that antibodies against NSP4 effectively inhibited the enterotoxic but not the cytotoxic effect of RV [9], we exposed Caco-2 cells to pure NSP4. NSP4 induced a significant increase in the Isc in the Ussing chamber experiments, consistent with electrogenic fluid secretion in Caco-2 cell monolayers (Fig. 4). The effect was dose-dependent and was observed when the viral protein was added to the serosal but not the mucosal side of the Caco-2 cell monolayers (Fig. 4A and B). The enterotoxic effect was evident as early as 30 min after the addition of purified NSP4 and reached a peak at approximately 50 min, after which the Isc value remained constant for 10–15 min (Fig. 4C). The pattern of the effect was similar to that previously observed in cells exposed to supernatants of RV-infected enterocytes [9]. To determine whether the enterotoxic effect was specific, we preincubated NSP4 with specific antibodies and then added the solution to Caco-2 cells in Ussing chambers. Specific antibodies significantly inhibited the electrical effect of NSP4 (NSP4 2,57±0,31 vs NSP4 with Ab 0,74±0,42; p<0.05).

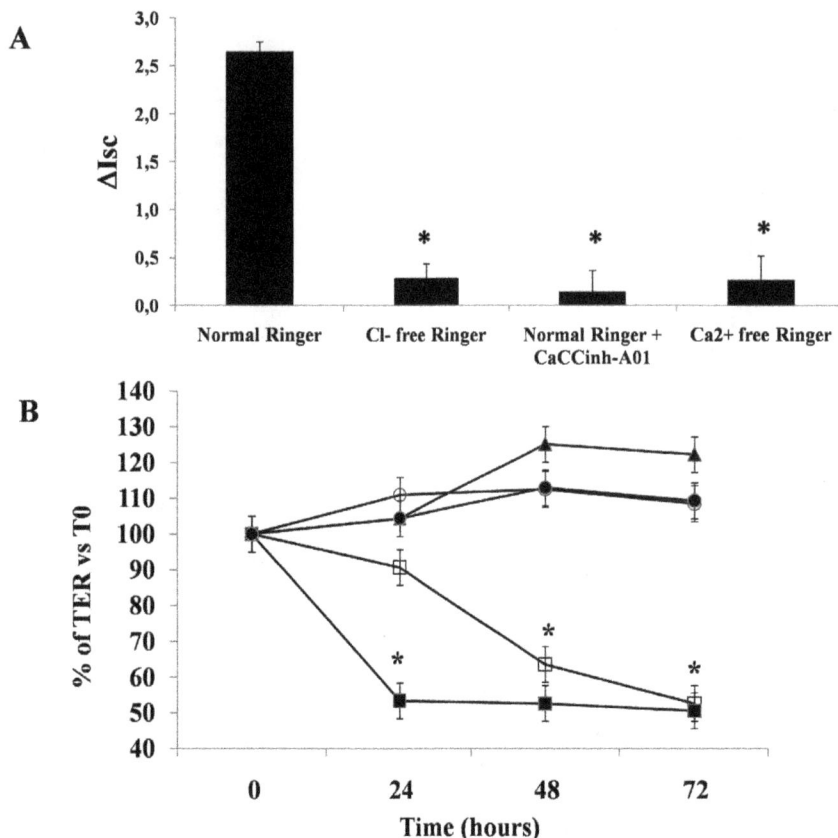

Figure 5. Modifications of Isc by NSP4 in various experimental conditions. (A) Changes in the Isc induced by pure NSP4 under various experimental conditions. The Isc was measured after the addition of NSP4 (200 ng/ml) in normal Ringer's solution, chloride-free Ringer's solution, Ringer's solution supplemented with CaCCinh-A01 or Ca^{2+} free Ringer. Isc changes were measured after 50 min of stimulation. The data are representative of 3 separate experiments. *$p<0.05$ vs. normal Ringer's solution. (B) The effect of NSP4 on intestinal epithelial integrity. The cytotoxic effect of NSP4 was evaluated by measuring TEER in Caco-2 cells. Cell monolayers were exposed to NSP4 at the serosal (●) or mucosal (○) side, to RV (□) and H_2O_2 (■) as positive controls, or to vehicle as a negative control (▲). The data are representative of 3 separate experiments. *$p<0.05$ vs. time 0.

Incubation with preimmune antibodies had no effect on NSP4-induced increase in Isc (data not shown). To determine whether the electrical effect was caused by anion secretion rather than cation absorption, we performed the same experiments using Cl^- free Ringer's solution. In the absence of Cl^-, the electrical effect was virtually abolished. Thus, the effect of NSP4 on the Isc was entirely due to transepithelial Cl^- secretion (Fig. 5A). We also added NSP4 at concentrations capable of eliciting the maximal secretory response (200 ng/mL) to Caco-2 cells in the presence of the TMEM16 channel inhibitor CaCCinh-A01. CaCCinh-A01 completely inhibited the secretory effect of NSP4 (Fig. 5A). To investigate the involvement of intracellular Ca^{2+} in the enterotoxic effects, cell monolayers were mounted in Ussing chambers with Ca^{2+} free-Ringer as described in the Materials and Methods. The subsequent addition of NSP4 resulted in a reduced increase in the Isc compared to NSP4 alone (Fig. 5A).

In our experimental model, NSP4 did not affect epithelial integrity as judged by TEER measurements. By contrast, TEER decreased in cells infected by RV (Fig. 5B).

To determine if NSP4 induces oxidative stress, we stimulated Caco-2 cells with enterotoxin, and ROS levels were determined. As shown in Fig. 6, the addition of purified NSP4 induced ROS production in a time-dependent manner that virtually overlapped that observed for chloride secretion in Ussing chambers. These data demonstrate that the enterotoxic effect of RV diarrhea is

directly and exclusively induced by NSP4 and is closely linked with ROS production.

Oxidative Stress and Chloride Secretion Induced by RV and NSP4 are Strongly Inhibited by Pretreatment with Antioxidants

To explore the relationship between oxidative stress and the enterotoxic effect induced by viral infection at the intestinal level, we preincubated Caco-2 cells with the antioxidant NAC. Pretreatment with NAC (5 mM for 24 hours) completely inhibited the RV-induced increase in ROS (Fig. 7A) and preserved the normal GSH/GSSG ratio (Fig. 7B). To further investigate the role of the redox imbalance induced by RV in chloride secretion, we performed experiments under conditions of oxidative stress prevention. Pretreatment with NAC (5 mM for 24 hours) completely prevented intestinal chloride secretion (Fig. 8A), suggesting that redox imbalance is a major mechanism in RV-induced secretory diarrhea.

To determine if oxidative stress is also involved in NSP4-induced chloride secretion, Caco-2 cells were pretreated with NAC and then stimulated with the viral enterotoxin. Under these conditions, the enterotoxic effect of NSP4 was strongly inhibited (Fig. 8B). NAC did not reduce the cAMP- or Ca^{2+}-mediated chloride secretion induced by Forkolin and Carbachol (Fig. S2

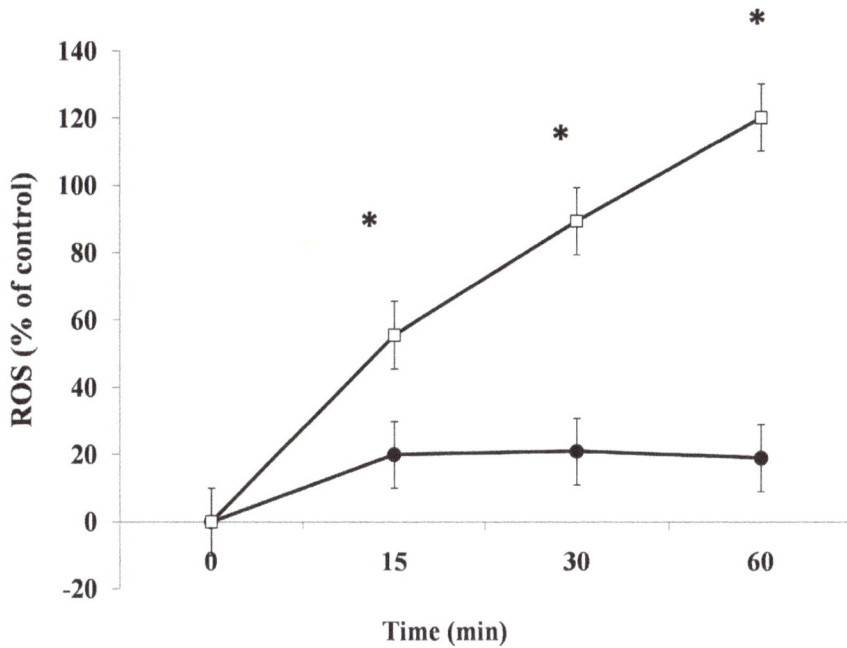

Figure 6. NSP4 induces time-dependent generation of ROS. Caco-2 cells were exposed to 200 ng/ml NSP4 (□) for 15, 30, and 60 min, and ROS intracellular levels were evaluated by the DCFH-DA fluorometric method and compared to a negative control (●). The data are representative of 3 separate experiments. *p<0.05 vs. time 0.

A

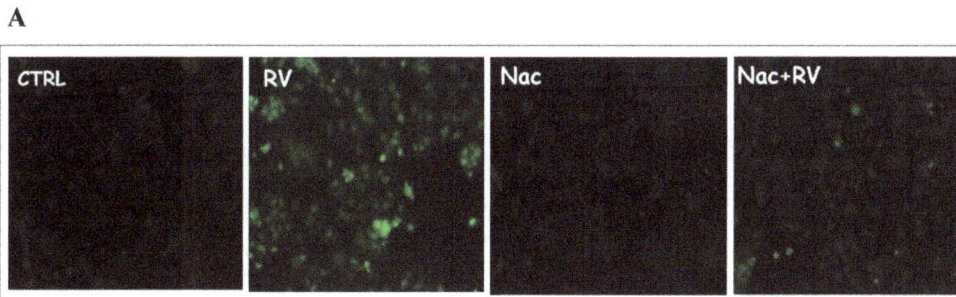

B

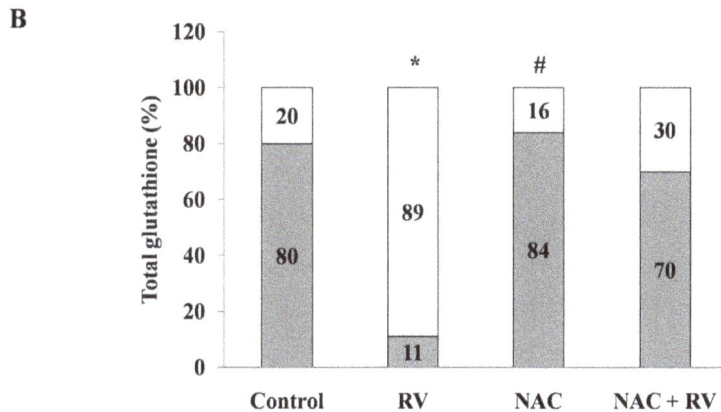

Figure 7. The effect of NAC on RV-induced oxidative stress in Caco-2 cells. (A) The addition of NAC (5 mM for 24 hours) to RV-infected cells completely inhibited ROS generation as shown by a representative staining at 1 h post-infection. Magnification: 200X. The data are representative of 3 separate experiments with 3–4 replicates for each experimental condition. (B) Effect of NAC (5 mM for 24 hours) on the RV-induced GSH/GSSG imbalance. The data are presented as the percent of GSH (grey) and GSSG (white) vs. total glutathione. The data are representative of 3 separate experiments. *p<0.05 vs. control; #p<0.05 vs. RV.

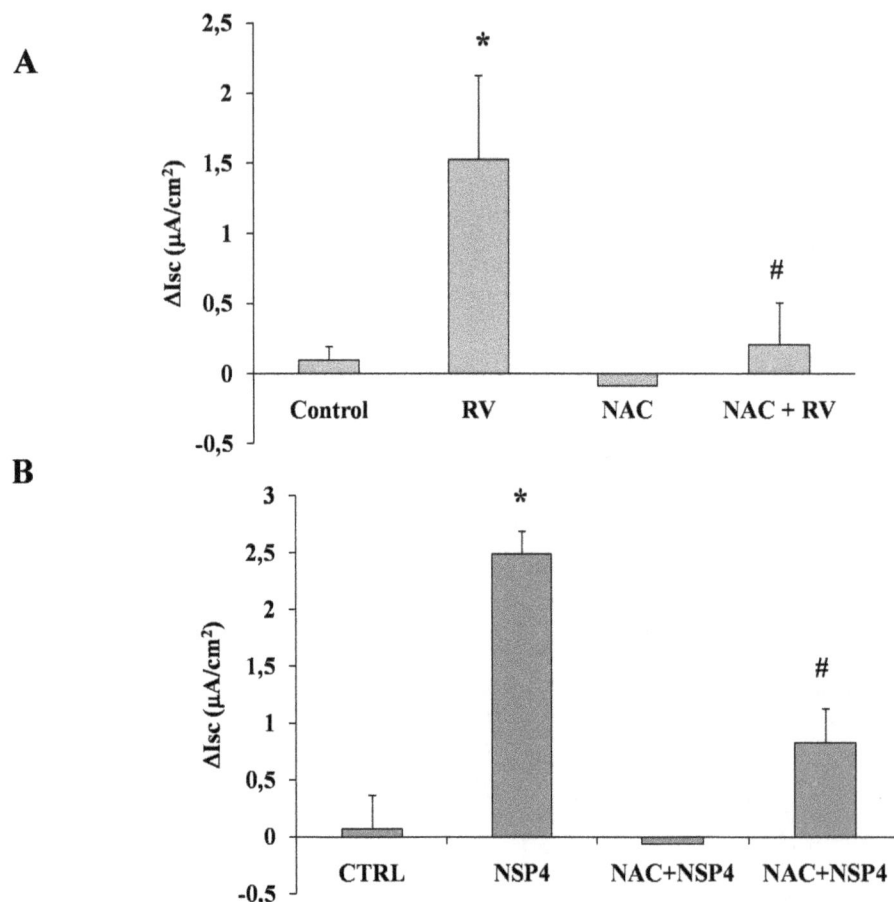

Figure 8. The effect of NAC on chloride secretion induced by RV and NSP4. (A) The addition of NAC (5 mM for 24 hours) to RV-infected cells completely inhibited the Isc induced by RV. (B) Pretreatment with NAC (5 mM for 24 hours) strongly inhibited the Isc increase induced by NSP4. The data are representative of 3 separate experiments. *p<0.05 vs. control; #p<0.05 vs. RV or NSP4.

panel A) suggesting that NAC effect is not direct on these second messengers.

SbS Prevents RV-induced Enterotoxic Effects and Oxidative Stress in Caco-2 Cells and Cultured Human Small Intestinal Mucosa

To evaluate the effects of the probiotic Sb, which has been shown to be highly clinically effective, in our experimental model of RV-induced diarrhea *in vitro*, we added SbS to Caco-2 cells during the pre-infection phase and 2 h after RV infection (10 pfu/cell), then measured the Isc. SbS substantially reduced chloride secretion (Fig. 9A). This effect was observed when SbS was added before but not after virus infection. ROS levels and the GSH/GSSG ratio were evaluated in time-course experiments. The increase in ROS induced by RV was strongly inhibited in cells exposed to SbS compared to infected controls. The maximal effect was observed at 60 min (Fig. 9B). In addition, SbS reduced the GSH/GSSH imbalance at 30 min and restored the redox equilibrium to the same levels as in the control at 120 min after infection (Fig. 9C).

Organ culture experiments were performed to compare the results obtained using Caco-2 cells with those in human tissue. Intestinal specimens were obtained from 2 children undergoing upper gastrointestinal endoscopy. After stimulation with RV (50 pfu/5 mm^2) in the presence or absence of SbS, we evaluated the GSH/GSSG ratio. The GSH/GSSG ratio decreased upon

RV exposure in intestinal biopsies exposed to RV for 1 h, confirming the oxidative stress pattern observed in Caco-2 cells. When SbS was preincubated for 30 min before RV infection, the ratio for both biopsies was similar to that observed in the controls, confirming that SbS prevented the GSH/GSSG imbalance induced by RV in human intestinal epithelia (Fig. 10).

Again, SbS did not reduce the cAMP- or Ca^{2+}-mediated chloride secretion induced by Forkolin and Carbachol (Fig. S2 panel B) suggesting that SbS effect is not direct on these second messengers.

Discussion

NSP4 plays a substantial role in RV diarrhea. Since the first description of the NSP4 enterotoxin, a number of hypotheses have been proposed regarding its role in chloride secretion. The chloride secretory response is regulated by a phospholipase C-dependent calcium signaling pathway that is induced by NSP4 [31], and NSP4 plays a key role in ion secretion in human-derived enterocytes [9]. Ousingsawat et al. demonstrated that NSP4 modulates multiple pro-secretory pathways to induce diarrhea by activating the recently identified Ca^{2+}-activated Cl$^-$ channel TMEM16A and inhibiting Na$^+$ absorption by the epithelial Na$^+$ channel ENaC and the Na$^+$/glucose cotransporter SGLT1 [11]. We have now characterized the effects of NSP4 on ion secretion. The addition of NSP4 to Caco-2 cell monolayers resulted in the

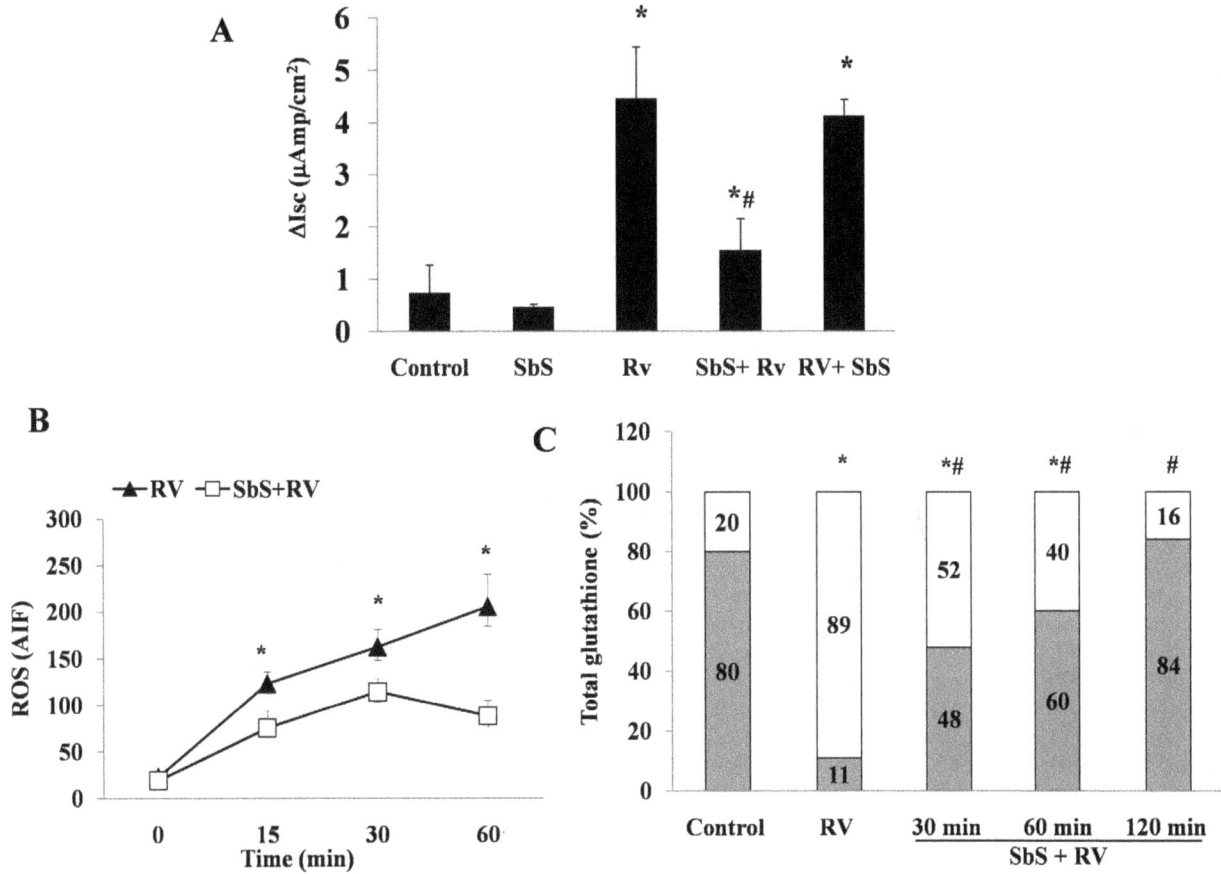

Figure 9. The effect of SbS on RV-induced chloride secretion and oxidative stress in Caco-2 cells. (A) The Isc, (B) ROS levels, and (C) the GSH/GSSG ratio were evaluated in RV-infected Caco-2 cells (10 pfu/cell) with (□) or without the addition of SbS (▲). The data are representative of 3 separate experiments. (A) *p<0.05 vs. control; #p<0.05 vs. RV. (B) *p<0.05 vs. SbS+RV. (C) *p<0.05 vs. control; #p<0.05 vs. RV.

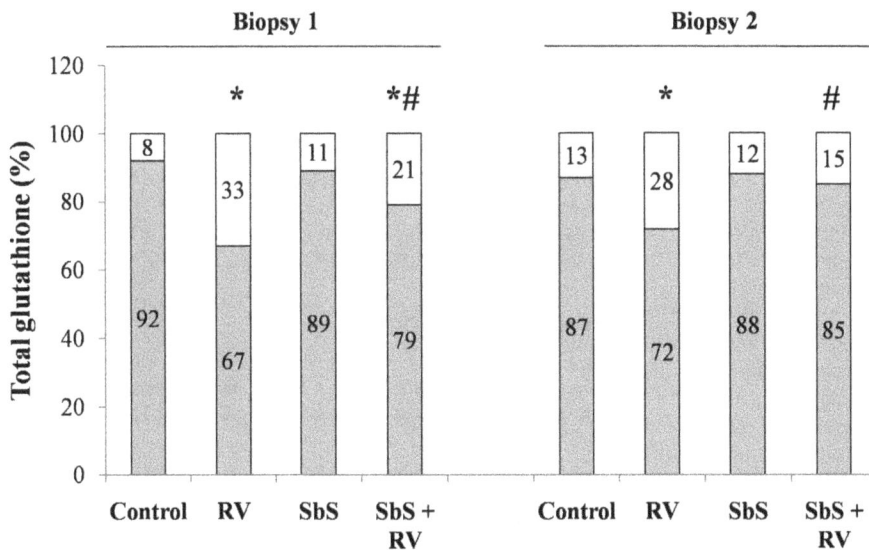

Figure 10. Antioxidant defenses in RV-infected human intestinal mucosa. Duodenal mucosal specimens were infected with RV (50 pfu/ 5 mm^2) alone or in combination with SbS in an *ex vivo* organ culture model, and the GSH (grey)/GSSG (white) ratio was evaluated. *p<0.05 vs. control; #p<0.05 vs. RV.

same electrical effect observed in Caco-2 cells infected with RV. Our results indicate that NSP4 exerts a polar effect in Caco-2 cells due to its interaction with the basolateral but not the apical cell membrane, suggesting that *in vivo* the viral protein acts when the epithelial integrity is damaged, thereby permitting contact of NSP4 with the basolateral side. It is possible that the decrease in short circuit current at later time points be due to disrupted tight junctions. However, the earlier secretion occur to be indeed directly by NSP4. In addition, the abrogation of the electrical response in the absence of Ca^{2+} or blocking TMEM16A channels, confirm the Ca^{2+} dependence as mechanism involved in the secretory effect. In addition, purified NSP4 induces ROS generation and GSH/GSSH imbalance with the same pattern as RV, further linking NSP4-induced oxidative stress to chloride secretion.

In gut homogenates of RV-infected mice, the oxidative/antioxidative profile is altered, indicating the presence of oxidative stress [18]. This effect was observed at a late stage of infection and might have been due to a decrease in glutathione recycling and/or production of glutathione-synthesizing enzymes. Our data provide clear evidence for a link between oxidative stress and RV-induced chloride secretion, which is the main mechanism of RV diarrhea.

Exogenous redox stressors induce chloride secretion depending on the site of action [32]. Our results demonstrate that the direct interaction between NSP4 and enterocytes leads to active chloride secretion, in agreement with a previous study in which intraperitoneal injection of NSP4 induced diarrhea in mouse pups [33]. Morris et al. demonstrated that the RV nonstructural glycoprotein NSP4 acts as a viral enterotoxin, inducing Ca^{2+}-dependent Cl^- secretion through Ca^{2+} release from intracellular stores in mice [33].

Our results provide further compelling evidence for this mechanism in human enterocytes. A previous study reported that infected Caco-2 cells maintain redox balance during RV infection [19]. The authors concluded that cell destruction caused by RV was likely not associated with oxidative damage to cellular components [19], suggesting that RV infection does not induce oxidative stress, enabling the accumulation of viral particles before cell destruction and virus release. The main difference with our results is in the timing of the observed effects, the sequence of which was clearly described in our original experimental model [9]. In particular, Gac et al. [19] evaluated oxidative stress at late time points post-infection, such as 48 and 72 h, whereas our findings indicate that RV induces an early increase in ROS production and a decrease in the GSH/GSSG ratio that is already detectable in the first hours following virus entry, suggesting that oxidative stress is a very early event.

There is consistent evidence that specific probiotic strains reduce the duration of RV diarrhea. However, the mechanisms of action of these probiotics are still unclear. Changes in the global structure of intestinal microflora, support of intestinal barrier function, stimulation of the immune response, and a number of other mechanisms have all been claimed as explanations of the efficacy against gastroenteritis. Sb has been shown to be highly effective against RV diarrhea in clinical trials [34,35]. In our RV experimental model, SbS prevented RV-induced ROS production, increased antioxidant defenses, and reduced chloride

secretion. The effect was observed using yeast-conditioned medium, suggesting that factor(s) secreted by the yeast were active in our system and induced a direct antisecretory effect, illustrating the so-called postbiotic effect of probiotics [36]. Sb-secreted factors were previously reported to be effective in the inhibition of proinflammatory cytokines [23]. In our experimental model, Sb inhibited RV-induced chloride secretion as a consequence of oxidative stress. A direct action on the enterocyte, with direct evidence of a consistent reduction of chloride flux from the serosal to luminal side, is in agreement with the rapid efficacy of Sb against diarrhea [20]. It is, therefore, a logical hypothesis that the protective effect against oxidative stress is the main mechanism underlying the clinical efficacy of Sb.

In conclusion, using a validated model of RV infection in human enterocytes, we demonstrated for the first time that RV induces chloride secretion through the generation of ROS, which a direct effect of NSP4. In addition, we determined that the supernatant of a culture of Sb acts on the glutathione-based defense system to limit chloride secretion. These results, which were obtained in an *in vitro* model of human-derived enterocytes and were replicated in human tissue, show a direct link between viral infection and the generation of oxidative stress, opening novel strategies to inhibit watery diarrhea induced by RV. These data also provide a new explanation for the high efficacy of Sb against childhood diarrhea observed in clinical trials. Specifically, taken together, these results demonstrate that the chloride secretion induced by the RV protein NSP4 is oxidative stress-dependent and inhibited by the postbiotic effect of Sb in human enterocytes.

Supporting Information

Figure S1 Purification of NSP4. A) Western blot analysis of Sf9 infected with the recombinant baculoviruses BacNSP4SA11. NSP4SA11 (a) were observed as different glycosylated states (21–28 kDa) or the dimeric protein (50 kDa). Uninfected Sf9 cells were used as a negative control (b). B) Purification of BacNSP4SA11: (Ft) eluate, (W1/W2) washing buffer, (E1, E2, E3, E4) eluate fractions. C) SDS-PAGE analysis followed by Coomassie staining of NSP4SA11 protein purified from SF9 infected cells with the recombinant baculoviruses BacNSP4SA11 (+). SF9 uninfected cell lysates are also shown as control (−).

Figure S2 Control experiments. A) Caco-2 cells were preincubated with NAC and then stimulated with Theofilline (5 mM) or Carbachol (1 μM) and Isc was measured in Ussing chambers. B) Caco-2 cells were preincubated with SbS and then stimulated with Theofilline (5 mM) or Carbachol (1 μM) and Isc was measured in Ussing chambers. *$p < 0.05$ vs CTRL.

Author Contributions

Conceived and designed the experiments: VB GL MM FMR AG. Performed the experiments: VB GL CR MS MM. Analyzed the data: VB. Contributed reagents/materials/analysis tools: EM MM FMR. Wrote the paper: VB AG.

References

1. Parashar UD, Burton A, Lanata C, Boschi-Pinto C, Shibuya K, et al. (2009) Global mortality associated with rotavirus disease among children in 2004. J Infect Dis 200: S9–S15. Available: http://www.ncbi.nlm.nih.gov/pubmed/19817620. Accessed 2 September 2011.

2. Albano F, Bruzzese E, Bella A, Cascio A, Titone L, et al. (2007) Rotavirus and not age determines gastroenteritis severity in children: a hospital-based study.

Eur J Pediatr 166: 241–247. Available: http://www.ncbi.nlm.nih.gov/pubmed/16941130. Accessed 5 September 2012.

3. Forster J, Guarino A, Parez N, Moraga F, Román E, et al. (2009) Hospital-based surveillance to estimate the burden of rotavirus gastroenteritis among European children younger than 5 years of age. Pediatrics 123: e393–400. Available: http://www.ncbi.nlm.nih.gov/pubmed/19254975. Accessed 6 November 2011.

4. Parashar UD, Gibson CJ, Bresee JS, Glass RI (2006) Rotavirus and severe childhood diarrhea. Emerg Infect Dis 12: 304–306. Available: http://www.pubmedcentral.nih.gov/articlerender.fcgi?artid = 3373114&tool = pmcentrez& rendertype = abstract. Accessed 26 July 2012.

5. Tanaka G, Faruque ASG, Luby SP, Malek MA, Glass RI, et al. (2007) Deaths from rotavirus disease in Bangladeshi children: estimates from hospital-based surveillance. Pediatr Infect Dis J 26: 1014–1018. Available: http://www.ncbi.nlm.nih.gov/pubmed/17984808. Accessed 6 September 2012.

6. Guarino A, Winter H, Sandhu B, Quak SH, Lanata C (2012) Acute gastroenteritis disease: Report of the FISPGHAN Working Group. J Pediatr Gastroenterol Nutr 55: 621–626. Available: http://www.ncbi.nlm.nih.gov/pubmed/22983379. Accessed 4 February 2013.

7. Hagbom M, Sharma S, Lundgren O, Svensson L (2012) Towards a human rotavirus disease model. Curr Opin Virol 2: 408–418. Available: http://www.ncbi.nlm.nih.gov/pubmed/22722079. Accessed 24 July 2012.

8. Field M (2003) Intestinal ion transport and the pathophysiology of diarrhea. J Clin Invest 111: 931–943. doi:10.1172/JCI200318326.Worldwide.

9. De Marco G, Bracale I, Buccigrossi V, Bruzzese E, Canani RB, et al. (2009) Rotavirus induces a biphasic enterotoxic and cytotoxic response in human-derived intestinal enterocytes, which is inhibited by human immunoglobulins. J Infect Dis 200: 813–819. Available: http://www.ncbi.nlm.nih.gov/pubmed/19604044. Accessed 5 August 2011.

10. Ball JM, Tian P, Zeng CQ, Morris AP, Estes MK (1996) Age-dependent diarrhea induced by a rotaviral nonstructural glycoprotein. Science 272: 101–104. Available: http://www.ncbi.nlm.nih.gov/pubmed/8600515. Accessed 6 September 2012.

11. Ousingsawat J, Mirza M, Tian Y, Roussa E, Schreiber R, et al. (2011) Rotavirus toxin NSP4 induces diarrhea by activation of TMEM16A and inhibition of Na+ absorption. Pflügers Arch Eur J Physiol 461: 579–589. Available: http://www.ncbi.nlm.nih.gov/pubmed/21399895. Accessed 30 June 2011.

12. Grisham MB, Gaginella TS, von Ritter C, Tamai H, Be RM, et al. (1990) Effects of neutrophil-derived oxidants on intestinal permeability, electrolyte transport, and epithelial cell viability. Inflammation 14: 531–542. Available: http://www.ncbi.nlm.nih.gov/pubmed/2174408. Accessed 3 February 2012.

13. Tamai H, Gaginella TS, Kachur JF, Musch MW, Chang EB (1992) Ca-mediated stimulation of Cl secretion by reactive oxygen metabolites in human colonic T84 cells. J Clin Invest 89: 301–307. Available: http://www.pubmedcentral.nih.gov/articlerender.fcgi?artid = 442848&tool = pmcentrez& rendertype = abstract.

14. Nguyen TD, Canada AT (1994) Modulation of human colonic T84 cell secretion by hydrogen peroxide. Biochem Pharmacol 47: 403–410. Available: http://www.ncbi.nlm.nih.gov/pubmed/8304984. Accessed 3 February 2012.

15. Hosakote YM, Liu T, Castro SM, Garofalo RP, Casola A (2009) Respiratory syncytial virus induces oxidative stress by modulating antioxidant enzymes. Am J Respir Cell Mol Biol 41: 348–357. Available: http://www.pubmedcentral.nih.gov/articlerender.fcgi?artid = 2742754&tool = pmcentrez&rendertype = abstract. Accessed 16 November 2011.

16. Ivanov A V, Smirnova O a, Ivanova ON, Masalova O V, Kochetkov SN, et al. (2011) Hepatitis C virus proteins activate NRF2/ARE pathway by distinct ROS-dependent and independent mechanisms in HUH7 cells. PLoS One 6: e24957. Available: http://www.pubmedcentral.nih.gov/articlerender.fcgi?artid = 3172309 &tool = pmcentrez&rendertype = abstract. Accessed 16 November 2011.

17. Agrawal L, Louboutin J-P, Reyes B a S, Van Bockstaele EJ, Strayer DS (2011) HIV-1 Tat neurotoxicity: A model of acute and chronic exposure, and neuroprotection by gene delivery of antioxidant enzymes. Neurobiol Dis: 1–14. Available: http://www.ncbi.nlm.nih.gov/pubmed/22036626. Accessed 16 November 2011.

18. Sodhi CP, Katyal R, Rana SV, Attri S S V. (1996) Study of oxidative-stress in rotavirus infected infant mice. Indian J Med Res 104: 245–249.

19. Gac M, Bigda J, Vahlenkamp TW (2010) Increased mitochondrial superoxide dismutase expression and lowered production of reactive oxygen species during rotavirus infection. Virology 404: 293–303. Available: http://www.ncbi.nlm.nih.gov/pubmed/20538313. Accessed 23 September 2011.

20. Corrêa NBO, Penna FJ, Lima FMLS, Nicoli JR, Filho L a P (2011) Treatment of Acute Diarrhea With Saccharomyces boulardii in Infants. J Pediatr Gastroenterol Nutr 53: 497–501. Available: http://www.ncbi.nlm.nih.gov/pubmed/21734600. Accessed 16 November 2011.

21. Pieścik-Lech M, Shamir R, Guarino A, Szajewska H (2013) Review article: the management of acute gastroenteritis in children. Aliment Pharmacol Ther 37: 289–303. Available: http://www.ncbi.nlm.nih.gov/pubmed/23190209. Accessed 10 January 2013.

22. Guarino A, Lo Vecchio A, Canani RB (2009) Probiotics as prevention and treatment for diarrhea. Curr Opin Gastroenterol 25: 18–23. Available: http://www.ncbi.nlm.nih.gov/pubmed/19114770. Accessed 13 August 2012.

23. Pothoulakis C (2009) Review article: Anti-inflammatory mechanisms of action of Saccharomyces boulardii. Aliment Pharmacol Ther 30: 826–833. doi:10.1111/j.1365-2036.2009.04102.x.Review.

24. Buts J-P, De Keyser N (2010) Transduction pathways regulating the trophic effects of Saccharomyces boulardii in rat intestinal mucosa. Scand J Gastroenterol 45: 175–185. Available: http://www.ncbi.nlm.nih.gov/pubmed/19958054. Accessed 23 September 2011.

25. Chen X, Kokkotou EG, Mustafa N, Bhaskar KR, Sougioultzis S, et al. (2006) Saccharomyces boulardii Inhibits ERK1/2 Mitogen-activated Protein Kinase Activation Both in Vitro and in Vivo and Protects against Clostridium difficile Toxin. J Biol Chem 281: 24449–24454. doi:10.1074/jbc.M605200200.

26. Rooj AK, Kimura Y, Buddington RK (2010) Metabolites produced by probiotic Lactobacilli rapidly increase glucose uptake by Caco-2 cells. BMC Microbiol 10: 16. Available: http://www.pubmedcentral.nih.gov/articlerender.fcgi?artid = 2835675&tool = pmcentrez&rendertype = abstract. Accessed 7 March 2013.

27. Tsilingiri K, Barbosa T, Penna G, Caprioli F, Sonzogni A, et al. (2012) Probiotic and postbiotic activity in health and disease: comparison on a novel polarised ex-vivo organ culture model. Gut 61: 1007–1015. Available: http://www.ncbi.nlm.nih.gov/pubmed/22301383. Accessed 19 November 2012.

28. Buccigrossi V, Laudiero G, Nicastro E, Miele E, Esposito F, et al. (2011) The HIV-1 Transactivator Factor (Tat) Induces Enterocyte Apoptosis through a Redox-Mediated Mechanism. PLoS One 6: e29436. Available: http://www.pubmedcentral.nih.gov/articlerender.fcgi?artid = 3246489&tool = pmcentrez&rendertype = abstract. Accessed 8 February 2012.

29. Allen S, John S, Tara F, Jessica G, Paula D (2001) A kinetic microassay for glutathione in cells plated on 96-well microtiter plates. Methods cell Sci 22: 305–312.

30. Canani RB, Cirillo P, Mallardo G, Buccigrossi V, Secondo A, et al. (2003) Effects of HIV-1 Tat protein on ion secretion and on cell proliferation in human intestinal epithelial cells. Gastroenterology 124: 368–376. Available: http://www.ncbi.nlm.nih.gov/pubmed/12557143. Accessed 5 August 2011.

31. Lorrot M, Vasseur M (2007) How do the rotavirus NSP4 and bacterial enterotoxins lead differently to diarrhea? Virol J 4: 31. Available: http://www.pubmedcentral.nih.gov/articlerender.fcgi?artid = 1839081&tool = pmcentrez&rendertype = abstract. Accessed 7 September 2012.

32. Schultheiss G, Hennig B, Diener M (2008) Sites of action of hydrogen peroxide on ion transport across rat distal colon. Br J Pharmacol 154: 991–1000. Available: http://www.pubmedcentral.nih.gov/articlerender.fcgi?artid = 2451038 &tool = pmcentrez&rendertype = abstract. Accessed 3 February 2012.

33. Morris AP, Scott JK, Ball JM, Zeng CQ, Wanda K, et al. (1999) NSP4 elicits age-dependent diarrhea and Ca2+− mediated I-influx into intestinal crypts of CF mice. Am J Physiol Gastrointest Liver Physiol 277: G431–G444.

34. Guarino A, Lo Vecchio A, Berni Canani R (2009) Probiotics as prevention and treatment for diarrhea. Curr Opin Gastroenterol 25: 18–23.

35. Dylag M, Szajewska H, Sko A (2007) Meta-analysis: Saccharomyces boulardii for treating acute diarrhoea in children. Aliment Pharmacol Ther: 257–264. doi:10.1111/j.1365-2036.2006.03202. x.

36. Tsilingiri K, Rescigno M (2013) Postbiotics: what else? Benef Microbes 4: 101–107. Available: http://www.ncbi.nlm.nih.gov/pubmed/23271068. Accessed 7 March 2013.

18

Post-Discharge Mortality in Children with Severe Malnutrition and Pneumonia in Bangladesh

Mohammod Jobayer Chisti[1,2], Stephen M. Graham[2,3]*, Trevor Duke[2], Tahmeed Ahmed[1], Abu Syed Golam Faruque[1], Hasan Ashraf[1], Pradip Kumar Bardhan[1], Abu S. M. S. B. Shahid[1], K. M. Shahunja[1], Mohammed Abdus Salam[1]

1 International Centre for Diarrhoeal Disease Research, Bangladesh, Dhaka, Bangladesh, 2 Centre for International Child Health, The University of Melbourne Department of Paediatrics and Murdoch Childrens Research Institute, Royal Children's Hospital, Melbourne, Australia, 3 International Union Against Tuberculosis and Lung Disease, Paris, France

Abstract

Background: Post-discharge mortality among children with severe illness in resource-limited settings is under-recognized and there are limited data. We evaluated post-discharge mortality in a recently reported cohort of children with severe malnutrition and pneumonia, and identified characteristics associated with an increased risk of death.

Methods: Young children (<5 years of age) with severe malnutrition (WHO criteria) and radiographic pneumonia on admission to Dhaka Hospital of icddr,b over a 15-month period were managed according to standard protocols. Those discharged were followed-up and survival status at 12 weeks post-discharge was determined. Verbal autopsy was requested from families of those that died.

Results: Of 405 children hospitalized with severe malnutrition and pneumonia, 369 (median age, 10 months) were discharged alive with a follow-up plan. Of these, 32 (8.7%) died in the community within 3 months of discharge: median 22 (IQR 9–35) days from discharge to death. Most deaths were reportedly associated with acute onset of new respiratory or gastrointestinal symptoms. Those that died following discharge were significantly younger (median 6 [IQR 3,12] months) and more severely malnourished, on admission and on discharge, than those that survived. Bivariate analysis found that severe wasting on admission (OR 3.64, 95% CI 1.66–7.97) and age <12 months (OR 2.54, 95% CI 1.1–8.8) were significantly associated with post-discharge death. Of those that died in the community, none had attended a scheduled follow-up and care-seeking from a traditional healer was more common (p<0.001) compared to those who survived.

Conclusion and Significance: Post-discharge mortality was common in Bangladeshi children following inpatient care for severe malnutrition and pneumonia. The underlying contributing factors require a better understanding to inform the potential of interventions that could improve survival.

Editor: Susanna Esposito, Fondazione IRCCS Ca' Granda Ospedale Maggiore Policlinico, Università degli Studi di Milano, Italy

Funding: This research study was funded by the Dhaka Hospital of International Centre for Diarrhoeal Disease Research, Bangladesh (ICDDR, B; grant no Gr-00233) and its donors, which provide unrestricted support to ICDDR, B for its operations and research. Current donors providing unrestricted support include: Australian Agency for International Development, Government of the People's Republic of Bangladesh, Canadian International Development Agency, Swedish International Development Cooperation Agency, and the Department for International Development, United Kingdom. The funders had no role in study design, data collection and analysis, decision to publish, or preparation of the manuscript.

Competing Interests: The authors have declared that no competing interests exist.

* Email: steve.graham@rch.org.au

Introduction

Malnutrition is recognized as a major underlying risk factor for death in children with common infections causing global child mortality such as pneumonia, diarrhea and sepsis [1,2]. Furthermore, these infectious diseases further increase the high risk of mortality that is reported in children with severe malnutrition managed as inpatients in resource-poor settings of Africa and Asia [3–7]. Malnutrition is also a consistent risk factor for post-discharge death in common childhood illnesses in high-mortality settings, including studies from Bangladesh of children hospitalized with diarrhea [8–10]. However, there are limited data available from studies that have followed severely malnourished children following discharge from inpatient facilities. Currently, these data are all from settings in sub-Saharan Africa [5,11,12] and previous studies have not reported post-discharge death in children with severe malnutrition and pneumonia.

Bangladesh has high rates of childhood malnutrition. A UNICEF report published in 2013 reported that 36% of Bangladeshi children had moderate or severe wasting and that 41% had moderate or severe stunting in the period 2007 to 2011 [13]. We recently undertook a study to determine bacterial and mycobacterial aetiology of pneumonia in children with severe malnutrition admitted to the Dhaka Hospital of the International Centre for Diarrhoeal Disease Research, Bangladesh (icddr'b) in Dhaka, Bangladesh [14]. The aim of this analysis was to report inpatient and early post-discharge mortality in this same cohort of children with severe malnutrition and radiological pneumonia, and to identify characteristics associated with an increased risk of death following discharge.

Materials and Methods

Ethics statement

The study (protocol number: PR-10067) was approved by the Research Review Committee (RRC) and the Ethical Review Committee (ERC) of icddr,b. Written informed consent was obtained from parents or attending guardians of all the participating children.

Study setting and design

This was a prospective study cohort study that included young children (0–59 months of age) with severe malnutrition, respiratory symptoms and radiological pneumonia as previously described in detail [14]. In brief, eligible children admitted to the Dhaka Hospital of icddr,b between April 2011 and June 2012 were enrolled following informed consent. Demographic, contact details (phone and address) and clinical data were collected prospectively on standardized data collection proforma. Radiographs were interpreted independently by a radiologist and a study pediatrician (MJC). Radiological pneumonia was defined as the presence of end-point consolidation or other (non-end-point) infiltrate in lungs according to the WHO radiological classification of pneumonia [15]. Severe malnutrition was defined in children as severe wasting [z score for weight for height <-3 of the median of the WHO anthropometry] or severe underweight [z score for weight for age <-4 of the median of the WHO anthropometry], or the presence of nutritional edema. Clinical management was according to standardized guidelines with regards to antibiotics, detection and management of hypoxemia and hypoglycemia, fluid management and nutritional support [14,16].

Once children were considered to have shown clinical improvement for pneumonia and stabilized, they were transferred to the nutritional rehabilitation unit (NRU) for ongoing care before hospital discharge and were managed according to standard guidelines [6]. During the NRU stay, mothers are taught to prepare high energy food from locally available and culturally acceptable foodstuffs, and advised to provide such food once discharged. The decision to discharge is normally based on the criteria used by the NRU staff, i.e. weight gain of $>15\%$ of admission weight (after resolution of edema in those with nutritional edema). However, many children are discharged before these criteria are reached and are discharged "on risk bond". The main reason is request for early discharge by the mother because of pressure from the child's father or grandparents for the mother (and child) to return home once the child is thought to be no longer acutely ill. No additional nutritional supplements such as Ready-to-Use Therapeutic Food (RUTF) are provided on discharge.

The primary outcome for analysis was survival status at 3 months post-discharge. Secondary outcomes included the type and duration of new symptoms associated with those that died as reported by verbal autopsy and the proportion of those discharged that were lost-to-follow-up.

Follow-up procedure

All of the enrolled children that survived hospitalization were requested to attend follow-up for 3 months post-discharge as per routine follow-up by NRU. This included children that were discharged either as left against medical advice or those discharged "on risk bond" from the NRU. Follow-up was planned weekly for the first 2 weeks following discharge and monthly thereafter until the following criteria are met: weight for length ≥-1 z score and/ or weight for age ≥-2 z score. Routine follow-up included measurement of nutritional parameters and vital signs, as well as assessment for and management of any intercurrent illness. Neither additional nutritional supplements such as RUTF nor support for transport costs were provided at follow-up visits.

There were 86 children discharged that had been diagnosed with tuberculosis, of which 27 were microbiologically confirmed [14]. It was planned that all children discharged receiving anti-tuberculosis treatment were followed until completion of the course i.e. for 6 months.

For this study, all care-givers were provided instructions verbally in local language regarding follow-up. They were requested to return to the hospital at 12 weeks following discharge but advised that if their children developed any symptoms or signs of illness at any time prior to this, then they should either return to the hospital or consult with a study physician by mobile phone at any time. The phone numbers of the study physicians were provided during discharge and all caregivers had access to mobile phones. No funding was provided for potential phone call costs. If any of the caregivers did not attend the 12-week post-discharge follow-up, the study staff attempted to contact them via mobile phone. If any of the care-givers could not be contacted by mobile phone or still did not attend the follow-up after contact by mobile phone, then research assistants visited their home to ensure follow-up. Study participants were defined as "lost to follow-up" if research assistants visited the given address on at least two separate occasions and failed to identify them.

Verbal autopsy was requested when possible for those children that were identified as having died during the follow-up period. Verbal autopsy procedure followed the WHO standard questionnaire [17]. Information obtained included the presence and duration of symptoms prior to death as well as treatment sought. Interviews were undertaken by the study physicians at icddr'b for the majority that were willing to attend, otherwise the interview was performed by mobile phone (n = 4).

Data analysis

All data were entered into SPSS for Windows (version 15.0; SPSS Inc, Chicago) and Epi-Info (version 6.0, USD, Stone Mountain, GA). Follow-up was planned prospectively and ethically approved. However, the primary objective of this study that determined sample size was to determine prevalence of sepsis and tuberculosis, as previously reported [14]. We used this sample of patients to determine characteristics associated with post-discharge death. Differences in proportions were compared by the Chi-square test. Differences of means were compared by Student's t-test for normally distributed data and Mann-Whitney test was used for comparison of data that were not normally distributed. Strength of association was determined by calculating odds ratio (OR) and their 95% confidence intervals (CIs). Two pragmatic categorical variables (age and severity of malnutrition on admission) were identified based on previous literature [8] and univariate analysis of the dataset for bivariate analysis using logistic regression.

Results

A total of 405 children with severe malnutrition and radiological pneumonia were enrolled at admission and have been described previously [14]. Of these, 35 (8.6%) died as inpatients and 1 patient absconded without follow-up arranged. Figure 1 illustrates a flowchart from admission to follow-up showing that 369 children were discharged with a follow-up plan, including 29 that left against medical advice prior to planned discharge. The median (IQR) age in months of these 369 children was 10 (5, 18) months. The median (IQR) duration of inpatient care before transfer to the NRU for the 340 survivors that were discharged was 6 (4, 10) days, and was of similar duration for the 29 that left against medical advice - 8 (4, 9) days. Of those transferred to the NRU, the majority were discharged early "on risk bond". Only 43 (13%) remained at the NRU until they reached the standard discharge criteria and median (IQR) duration of hospital stay for these was 18 (12,22) days which compared to only 5 (4,8) days for the remaining 297 that were discharged early.

At 3 months post-discharge, 32 (8.7%) children were known to have died in the community. None of those that died attended any follow-up visit. A further 54 (15%) of the 369 children discharged were lost-to follow-up with no knowledge of outcomes at 3 months post-discharge – Figure 1. Table 1 lists and compares patient characteristics on admission that were associated with known death following discharge and compared to those known to have survived. The features of the 54 children that were lost-to-follow-up but with unknown outcomes are also listed.

Compared to survivors, those that died post-discharge were younger [median (IQR): 6.5 (3, 12) months], more severely malnourished on admission and more commonly had a previous admission for pneumonia (Table 1). On bivariate analysis, severe wasting on admission (OR 3.64 [95% CI 1.66–7.97], p = 0.001) and age <12 months (OR 2.54 [95% CI 1.1–8.8], p = 0.03) were significantly associated with post-discharge death. Those that died post-discharge were also significantly more malnourished at discharge than those that survived. There was no significant difference in changes to nutritional parameters (by z score) from admission to discharge between those that died and survivors. Post-discharge death was more common in those that were discharged early "on risk bond" from the NRU than those that

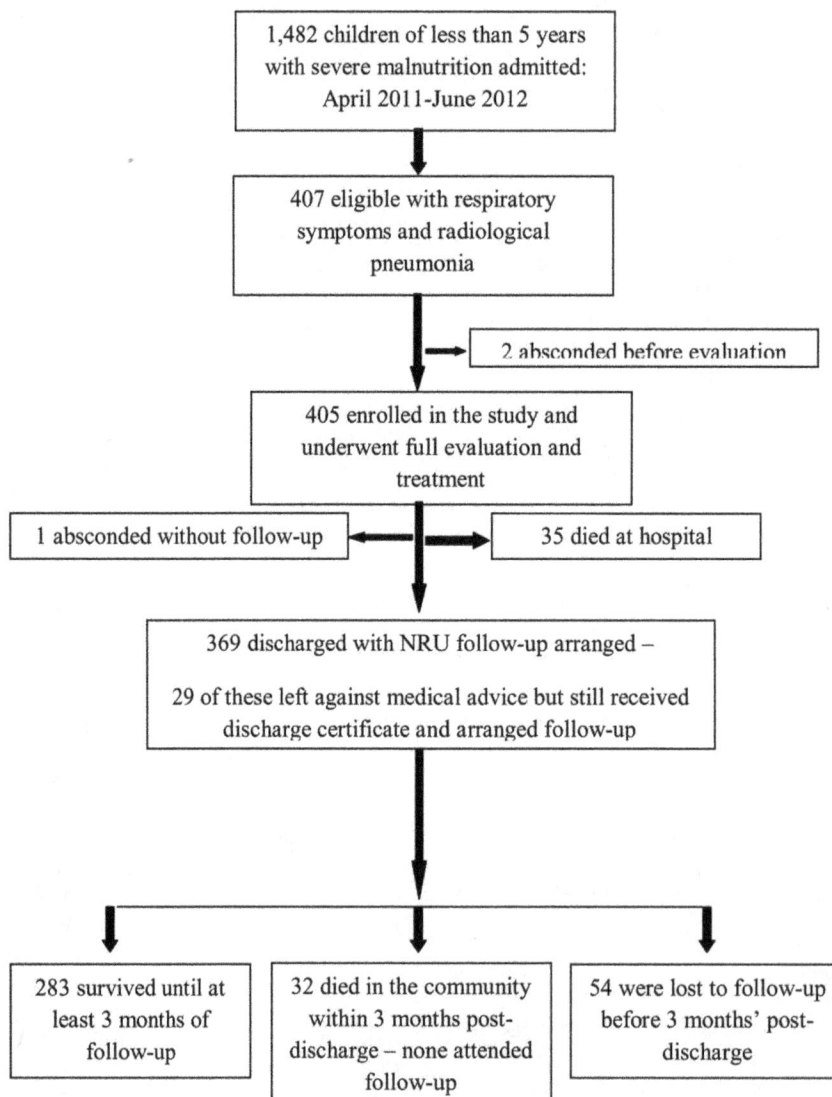

Figure 1. Flowchart of study subjects from admission until final follow-up.

Table 1. Characteristics of severely malnourished children (<5 years) with pneumonia who died within 3 months following discharge compared to those known to have survived evaluating known risk factors for outcome such as age, severity of malnutrition and severity of pneumonia.

Characteristics	Deaths (N = 32) N (%)	Survivors (N = 283) N (%)	LTFU (n = 54) N (%)	Unadjusted OR (95% CI)
On admission				
Age in months: median (IQR)*	6 (3,12)	10 (5, 18)	12 (5, 21)	
Age less than 12 months	23 (72)	157 (56)	27 (50)	2.05 (0.9–4.9)
Male	15 (47)	160 (57)	31 (57)	0.68 (0.3–1.5)
Live outside Dhaka district	10 (31)	60 (21)	9 (17)	1.69 (0.7–4.0)
Poor socio-economic condition - income <125 USD per month	25 (78)	235 (83)	51 (94)	0.73 (0.3–2.0)
History of previous pneumonia prior to present episode*	6 (19)	18 (6)	4 (7)	3.4 (1.1–10.2)
Severe wasting* (z score <−4 weight-for-height/length)	20 (63)	107 (38)	23 (43)	2.74 (1.2–6.2)
Severe underweight* (z score <−5 weight-for-age)	22 (69)	124 (44)	22 (41)	2.82 (1.2–6.7)
Nutritional edema	3 (9)	12 (4)	1 (2)	2.34 (0.5–9.6)
Lower chest wall in-drawing	12 (38)	116 (41)	15 (28)	0.86 (0.4–1.9)
Hypoxemia (arterial oxygen saturation <90% in room air)	3 (9)	22 (8)	2 (4)	1.23 (0.3–4.7)
Confirmed TB	3 (9)	16 (6)	8 (15)	1.74 (0.4–6.9)
Clinical TB – not confirmed	1 (3)	50 (18)	8 (15)	0.15 (0.01–1.1)
On discharge				
Duration of hospital stay in days: median (IQR)	7 (4, 11)	6 (4, 10)	6 (3, 9)	
Left against medical advice*	8 (25)	21 (7)	0 (0)	4.16 (1.5–11.3)
Severe wasting* (z score <−4 weight-for-height/length)	14 (45)	55 (20)	15 (28)	3.40 (1.5–7.8)
Severe underweight* (z score <−5 weight-for-age)	18 (56)	84 (30)	18 (33)	3.05 (1.4–6.8)

*P value significant (<0.05) for comparison of deaths vs. survivors.
LTFU = lost-to follow-up; OR = Odds ratio; CI = Confidence interval; IQR = Interquartile range.

were discharged once NRU criteria were met with only 1 death in the latter group (P = 0.25).

The median time gap between discharge and death was 22 (9, 35) days. Most deaths occurred within 1 month following discharge and 34% before the first scheduled follow-up visit (Table 2). Characteristics of these early post-discharge deaths such as age and nutritional status were similar to those that died later than two weeks post-discharge (data not shown). There were 86 children discharged receiving anti-tuberculosis treatment [14]. Four of these died within the 3 month follow-up period of which 3 had microbiologically confirmed tuberculosis and the other had clinically diagnosed tuberculosis that was not confirmed microbiologically. Death was recorded more significantly commonly in those that left against medical advice (8 or 28% died of 29) compared to those that were discharged according to usual protocol (24 or 7% of 340) – odds ratio 23.6 (95% CI 9.4–59); P< 0.0001.

Clinical findings from those that had verbal autopsy responses available are shown in Table 2. These findings suggest that deaths usually followed acute lower respiratory tract infections or acute gastroenteritis. Of the 32 deaths, 14 were receiving treatment from a traditional healer compared to only 1 of the 283 survivors at 12

weeks' post-discharge: unadjusted odds ratio 56.2 (95% CI 15.1–229); P<0.001. Although all the care givers had the access to mobile phone (their own or their relatives), none (0%) of the care givers among the deaths had consulted with study physicians using their mobile phone whereas 115 (41%) of 283 survivors consulted the study physicians by phone (p<0.001).

Discussion

This study provides original data reporting a high mortality within 3 months of discharge of Bangladeshi children following hospitalization with severe malnutrition and pneumonia. The reported post-discharge mortality of 8.7% is similar to the inpatient mortality for this group, and most of the post-discharge deaths occurred within 1 month following discharge. Previous studies from urban and rural Bangladesh have reported similar or higher post-discharge mortality in children hospitalized with diarrhea, with severe malnutrition recognized as a risk factor for death [9,10]. Pneumonia is known to be a common co-morbidity in children with severe malnutrition that is associated with inpatient death [4]. We provide original data of post-discharge outcomes in this group.

Table 2. Characteristics of post-discharge deaths: timing of death and verbal autopsy findings.

Time of death after discharge n = 32		
Timing of death post-discharge	**N (%)**	**Cumulative**
Death during weeks 1–2	11 (34%)	34%
Death during weeks 3–4	8 (25%)	59%
Death during month 2	9 (28%)	87%
Death during month 3	4 (13%)	100%
Caregiver providing verbal autopsy n = 32		
Mother	18 (56%)	
Father	7 (22%)	
None available*	7 (22%)	
Verbal autopsy findings n = 25		
Place of death		
Home	20 (80%)	
At other hospital (local)	4 (16%)	
On the way to hospital	1 (4%)	
Reported symptoms (new onset)	**N (%)**	**Duration in days (median, IQR)**
Cough	21 (84%)	5 (3, 7)
Difficulty breathing	18 (72%)	2.5 (2, 4)
Fever	14 (56%)	3.5 (2, 5)
Watery diarrhea	14 (56%)	3 (1.8, 4)
Vomiting	11 (44%)	2 (1, 3)
Abdominal distension	8 (32%)	2 (1.3, 2)
Poor feeding	12 (48%)	3 (2, 5)
White patches on tongue (oral thrush)	4 (16%)	5 (3.5, 6.5)
Treatment		
History of taking treatment during illness	13 (52%)	
Any documentation of treatment	7 (28%)	

*For the 7 deaths without verbal autopsy information, deaths were confirmed by relatives or neighbors when given home address was visited, but the family had moved house and were unable to be contacted or declined further contact with the study team.

While studies directly reporting post-discharge mortality of children with severe malnutrition are surprisingly limited [10–12], there are data from recent intervention studies in populations of children with severe malnutrition that do follow such children once discharged to the community for home-based management. A recent study that included 393 HIV-uninfected Malawian children with severe malnutrition and with a very low rate of defaulting reported 44 (11%) deaths within 3 months [5]. In another study in Malawi evaluating home-based RUTF, the proportion of those with WHO-defined severe malnutrition that died among the non-intervention group was 6.2% [18]. However, that study population was somewhat different to the one reported here in that it only included children older than 10 months and excluded those who had evidence of systemic infection or severe edema at enrolment.

Admission characteristics that were associated with post-discharge mortality included young age and severity of malnutrition, consistent with previous observations of post-discharge mortality in children [8,9,19]. Previous hospitalization for pneumonia and having congenital heart disease were also significantly associated with mortality but the numbers for each of these groups were small. Severity of malnutrition on discharge was associated with poor outcome as was leaving against medical advice. The symptoms present prior to death reported at verbal autopsy suggested recent respiratory or gastrointestinal infection are these symptoms are similar to those reported in previous studies [5,10,18].

None of these findings are surprising as young and severely malnourished children are well recognized as being particularly vulnerable to new infections causing severe disease and associated with poor outcomes [8]. Many of these children at discharge were still malnourished and so likely to have persistent and profound immunodeficiency [20]. In addition, they would have frequent exposure to infection, community-acquired upon return to home-based care as well as being at risk from nosocomial infections acquired during the inpatient stay in a crowded hospital.

The study also highlighted potential problems relating to access to care when this particularly vulnerable population developed new symptoms following discharge. Most died at home within one month of discharge with no contact with the hospital staff despite the recent offer of support and advice via mobile phones. It appeared that many sought treatment elsewhere including often with traditional healers. Care seeking with traditional healers has previously been reported as associated with an increased risk of death in children at-risk for severe and rapid-onset disease such as in this population [21,22].

Our study has a number of important limitations. Primary outcome of survival status at 3 months was not known for 15% of those discharged. The HIV status of the study participants was not known despite this being an important risk factor for a poor outcome in African studies [5]. However, it is unlikely to be an important confounder in this population given that Bangladesh has a very low HIV prevalence among the adult population reported as <0.1% in 2011 [13]. The reported pattern of illness prior to death relied on verbal autopsy which has recognized limitations [23]. Analysis of post-discharge mortality and determinants of risk were not the primary outcomes of this study that determined sample size [14]. Finally, the study does not represent post-discharge mortality among malnourished children that have received complete "nutritional rehabilitation" because most of the study participants were discharged before they met the NRU's criteria for discharge.

Despite the limitations, this study highlights the potential of a number of interventions that could improve post-discharge mortality in this population. As noted above, most of these children were discharged for home-based care before they met the nutritional criteria set by the NRU. It was reported that the main reason for this was pressure from the family who requested discharge once the child had apparently recovered from pneumonia. However, many of these children were still severely malnourished at discharge and it was observed that this was significantly associated with a poor outcome. Clearly, these children would still be profoundly immunosuppressed and vulnerable to severe infection at the time of discharge. A recent small study from the same institution reported a lower post-discharge death rate (2.8%) at 6-month follow-up among 180 Bangladeshi children with severe malnutrition that had completed full protocol of nutritional rehabilitation [24]. However, the challenge may not be simply to seek to prolong the stay in the NRU until criteria are met as this does have some negative risks as well such as nosocomial infection, overcrowding of the NRU and poor compliance by families. Rather, it may be possible to better select those that would benefit from ongoing care in the NRU, and to improve home-based care to those that are discharged for home-based care.

Two potential options for home-based care that have received recent attention are to provide additional nutritional support as a form of RUTF and/or to provide preventive therapy to reduce the risk of severe infections such as cotrimoxazole preventive therapy (CPT). An intervention study that compared home-based RUTF to standard care in Malawian children with severe malnutrition reported significantly fewer deaths and less relapse among those receiving home-based RUTF at 2 month follow-up [18]. Reported illness of fever, cough and diarrhea were also all significantly less frequent in those that received RUTF. The benefit included those that were still severely malnourished by WHO criteria. CPT is widely recommended for HIV-infected children (and oncology patients) because it improves survival and reduces the incidence of serious infections such as invasive bacterial disease and *Pneumocystis* pneumonia [25,26]. Future studies, such as recently undertaken in Kenya [27] need to clarify if CPT provides post-discharge benefit for HIV-uninfected children with severe malnutrition. Attempts to influence the gut biome using probiotics have not been beneficial in one recently published study [5]. More intensive follow-up with ready access to health care advice such as by using mobile phones has shown benefit in previous studies [28]. It is likely that different settings may require different solutions given the many potential determinants of mortality in this population. It is also difficult to determine the generalizability of the findings of this study.

In conclusion, post-discharge mortality is common among severely malnourished children with pneumonia and most of these deaths occur within one month of discharge. Risk factors for death include young age and severity of malnutrition and verbal autopsy suggests that death is preceded by recent respiratory or gastrointestinal infection, consistent with limited data from previous studies. There are a number of interventions that could potentially reduce post-discharge mortality in this population but a better understanding of the determinants of poor outcome and evidence from clinical studies are required.

Acknowledgments

We gratefully acknowledge these donors for their support and commitment to icddr,b's research efforts. We would like to express our sincere thanks to all physicians, clinical fellows, nurses, members of feeding team and cleaners of the hospital for their invaluable support and contribution during patient enrollment and data collection.

Author Contributions

Conceived and designed the experiments: MJC SMG TD TA ASGF HA PKB KMS ASMSBS MAS. Performed the experiments: MJC SMG TD TA KMS ASMSBS MAS. Analyzed the data: MJC SMG TD TA ASGF HA PKB KMS ASMSBS MAS. Contributed reagents/materials/analysis tools: KMS ASMSBS. Contributed to the writing of the manuscript: MJC SMG TD TA ASGF HA PKB KMS ASMSBS MAS. Designed the software used in analysis: MJC KMS. Defended institutional review board (Research Review Committee and Ethical Review Committee): MJC MAS.

References

1. Walker CL, Rudan I, Liu L, Nair H, Theodoratou E, et al. (2013) Global burden of childhood pneumonia and diarrhoea. Lancet 381: 1405–1416.

2. Bejon P, Mohammed S, Mwangi I, Atkinson SH, Osier F, et al. (2008) Fraction of all hospital admissions and deaths attributable to malnutrition among children in rural Kenya. Am J Clin Nutr 88: 1626–1631.

3. Roy SK, Buis M, Weersma R, Khatun W, Chowdhury S, et al. (2011) Risk factors of mortality in severely-malnourished children hospitalized with diarrhoea. J Health Popul Nutr 29: 229–235.

4. Chisti MJ, Tebruegge M, La Vincente S, Graham SM, Duke T (2009) Pneumonia in severely malnourished children in developing countries - mortality risk, aetiology and validity of WHO clinical signs: a systematic review. Trop Med Int Health 14: 1173–1189.

5. Kerac M, Bunn J, Seal A, Thindwa M, Tomkins A, et al. (2009) Probiotics and prebiotics for severe acute malnutrition (PRONUT study): a double-blind efficacy randomised controlled trial in Malawi. Lancet 374: 136–144.

6. Ahmed T, Ali M, Ullah MM, Choudhury IA, Haque ME, et al. (1999) Mortality in severely malnourished children with diarrhoea and use of a standardised management protocol. Lancet 353: 1919–1922.

7. Brewster DR, Manary MJ, Graham SM (1997) Case management of kwashiorkor: an intervention project at seven nutrition rehabilitation centres in Malawi. Eur J Clin Nutr 51: 139–147.

8. Wiens MO, Pawluk S, Kissoon N, Kumbakumba E, Ansermino JM, et al. (2013) Pediatric post-discharge mortality in resource poor countries: a systematic review. PLoS One 8: e66698.

9. Roy SK, Chowdhury AK, Rahaman MM (1983) Excess mortality among children discharged from hospital after treatment for diarrhoea in rural Bangladesh. Br Med J (Clin Res Ed) 287: 1097–1099.

10. Islam MA, Rahman MM, Mahalanabis D, Rahman AK (1996) Death in a diarrhoeal cohort of infants and young children soon after discharge from hospital: risk factors and causes by verbal autopsy. J Trop Pediatr 42: 342–347.

11. Reneman L, Derwig J (1997) Long-term prospects of malnourished children after rehabilitation at the Nutrition Rehabilitation Centre of St Mary's Hospital, Mumias, Kenya. J Trop Pediatr 43: 293–296.

12. Hennart P, Beghin D, Bossuyt M (1987) Long-term follow-up of severe protein-energy malnutrition in Eastern Zaire. J Trop Pediatr 33: 10–12.

13. Marais BJ (2010) Does finding M. Tuberculosis in sputum always equal tuberculosis disease? Am J Respir Crit Care Med 181: 195–196; author reply 196–197.

14. Chisti MJ, Graham SM, Duke T, Ahmed T, Ashraf H, et al. (2014) A Prospective Study of the Prevalence of Tuberculosis and Bacteraemia in Bangladeshi Children with Severe Malnutrition and Pneumonia Including an Evaluation of Xpert MTB/RIF Assay. PLoS One 9: e93776.

15. Cherian T, Mulholland EK, Carlin JB, Ostensen H, Amin R, et al. (2005) Standardized interpretation of paediatric chest radiographs for the diagnosis of pneumonia in epidemiological studies. Bull World Health Organ 83: 353–359.

16. World Health Organization (2013) Pocket book for hospital care of children: guidelines for the management of common childhood illnessess Geneva: World Health Organization.

17. World Health Organization (2007) International Standard Verbal Autopsy Questionnaire. In The 2007 WHO Verbal Autopsy Instrument. 20–33.

18. Ciliberto MA, Sandige H, Ndekha MJ, Ashorn P, Briend A, et al. (2005) Comparison of home-based therapy with ready-to-use therapeutic food with standard therapy in the treatment of malnourished Malawian children: a controlled, clinical effectiveness trial. Am J Clin Nutr 81: 864–870.

19. Veirum JE, Sodeman M, Biai S, Hedegard K, Aaby P (2007) Increased mortality in the year following discharge from a paediatric ward in Bissau, Guinea-Bissau. Acta Paediatr 96: 1832–1838.

20. Waterlow JC, Alleyne GA (1971) Protein malnutrition in children: advances in knowledge in the last ten years. Adv Protein Chem 25: 117–241.

21. Mercer A, Haseen F, Huq NL, Uddin N, Hossain Khan M, et al. (2006) Risk factors for neonatal mortality in rural areas of Bangladesh served by a large NGO programme. Health Policy Plan 21: 432–443.

22. D'Souza RM (2003) Role of health-seeking behaviour in child mortality in the slums of Karachi, Pakistan. J Biosoc Sci 35: 131–144.

23. Qureshi JS, Samuel JC, Mulima G, Kakoulides S, Cairns B, et al. (2014) Validating a verbal autopsy tool to assess pre-hospital trauma mortality burden in a resource-poor setting. Trop Med Int Health.

24. Ashraf H, Alam NH, Chisti MJ, Mahmud SR, Hossain MI, et al. (2012) A follow-up experience of 6 months after treatment of children with severe acute malnutrition in Dhaka, Bangladesh. J Trop Pediatr 58: 253–257.

25. Chintu C, Bhat GJ, Walker AS, Mulenga V, Sinyinza F, et al. (2004) Co-trimoxazole as prophylaxis against opportunistic infections in HIV-infected Zambian children (CHAP): a double-blind randomised placebo-controlled trial. Lancet 364: 1865–1871.

26. World Health Organization (2006) Guidelines on cotrimoxazole prohylaxis for HIV-related infections among children, adolescents and adults in resource-limited settings: recommendations for a public health approach. HIV/AIDS Programme, World Health Organization, geneva.

27. Chang AB, Redding GJ, Everard ML (2008) Chronic wet cough: Protracted bronchitis, chronic suppurative lung disease and bronchiectasis. Pediatr Pulmonol 43: 519–531.

28. Zurovac D, Sudoi RK, Akhwale WS, Ndiritu M, Hamer DH, et al. (2011) The effect of mobile phone text-message reminders on Kenyan health workers' adherence to malaria treatment guidelines: a cluster randomised trial. Lancet 378: 795–803.

19

Bacterial Etiologies of Five Core Syndromes: Laboratory-Based Syndromic Surveillance Conducted in Guangxi, China

Baiqing Dong[1]¶, Dabin Liang[2]¶, Mei Lin[2]*, Mingliu Wang[2], Jun Zeng[2], Hezhuang Liao[2], Lingyun Zhou[2], Jun Huang[2], Xiaolin Wei[3], Guanyang Zou[4], Huaiqi Jing[5]

1 Department of Emergency Response, Guagnxi Zhuang Autonomous Region Health Bureau, Nanning, Guangxi, China, 2 Divsion of Bacterial Infectious Disease Control, Guagnxi Zhuang Autonomous Region Center for Disease Prevention and Control, Nanning, Guangxi, China, 3 School of Public Health and Primary Care, Chinese University of Hong Kong, Hong Kong, China, 4 COMDIS Health Services Delivery Research Consortium, China Program, Nuffield Centre for International Health and Development, University of Leeds, Shenzhen, China, 5 National Institute for Communicable Disease Control and Prevention, Chinese Center for Disease Control and Prevention, Beijing, China and State Key Laboratory for Infectious Disease Prevention and Control, Collaborative Innovation Center for Diagnosis and Treatment of Infectious Diseases, Beijing, China

Abstract

Background: Under the existing national surveillance system in China for selected infectious diseases, bacterial cultures are performed for only a small percentage of reported cases. We set up a laboratory-based syndromic surveillance system to elucidate bacterial etiologic spectrum and detect infection by rare etiologies (or serogroups) for five core syndromes in the given study area.

Methods: Patients presenting with one of five core syndromes at nine sentinel hospitals in Guagnxi, China were evaluated using laboratory-based syndrome surveillance to elucidate bacterial etiologies. We collected respiratory and stool specimens, as well as CSF, blood and other related samples for bacterial cultures and pulse field gel electrophoresis (PFGE) assays.

Results: From February 2009 to December 2011, 2,964 patients were enrolled in the study. Etiologies were identified in 320 (10.08%) patients. *Streptococcus pneumonia* (37 strains, 24.18%), *Klebsiella pneumonia* (34, 22.22%), *Pseudomonas aeruginosa* (19, 12.42%) and *Haemophilus influenza* (18, 11.76%) were the most frequent pathogens for fever and respiratory syndrome, while *Salmonella* (77, 81.05%) was most often seen in diarrhea syndrome cases. *Salmonella paratyphi A* (38, 86.36%) occurred in fever and rash syndrome, with *Cryptococcus neoformans* (20, 35.09%), *Streptococcus pneumonia* (5, 8.77%), *Klebsiella pneumonia* (5, 8.77%),*streptococcus suis* (3, 5.26%) and *Neisseria meningitides group B* (2, 3.51%) being the most frequently detected in encephalitis-meningitis syndrome. To date no pathogen was isolated from the specimens from fever and hemorrhage patients.

Conclusions: In addition to common bacterial pathogens, opportunistic pathogens and fungal infections require more attention. Our study contributes to the strengthening of the existing national surveillance system and provides references for other regions that are similar to the study area.

Editor: Xue-jie Yu, University of Texas Medical Branch, United States of America

Funding: BQD received funding by the Chinese Center for Disease Control and Prevention (2009ZX10004203-003) (http://www.chinacdc.cn/). The Chinese Center for Disease Control and Prevention played a role in study design. ML received the funding by the Department of Science and Technology of the Guangxi Zhuang Autonomous Region, China (2012GXNSFAA053159) (http://www.gxst.gov.cn/). The Department of Science and Technology of Guangxi has no role in study design, data collection and analysis, decision to publish or preparation of the manuscript.

Competing Interests: The authors have declared that no competing interests exist.

* Email: gxlinmei@126.com

¶ BQD and DBL are co-first authors on this work.

Introduction

Since 2003, a real-time web-based disease surveillance system was developed to monitor 39 notifiable diseases in China. This system was based on the existing reporting system for selected infectious diseases established in the 1950s [1]. This system consists of a 5-level reporting network that ranges from township, county, prefecture, province and finally to the national level. Infectious diseases can be reported to the Central Data Bank in China Center for Disease Control and Prevention (or CDC) whenever they are detected at hospitals in any of these five levels. Besides the above-mentioned 39 known diseases, pneumonia of unknown cause is required to be reported through the system. This

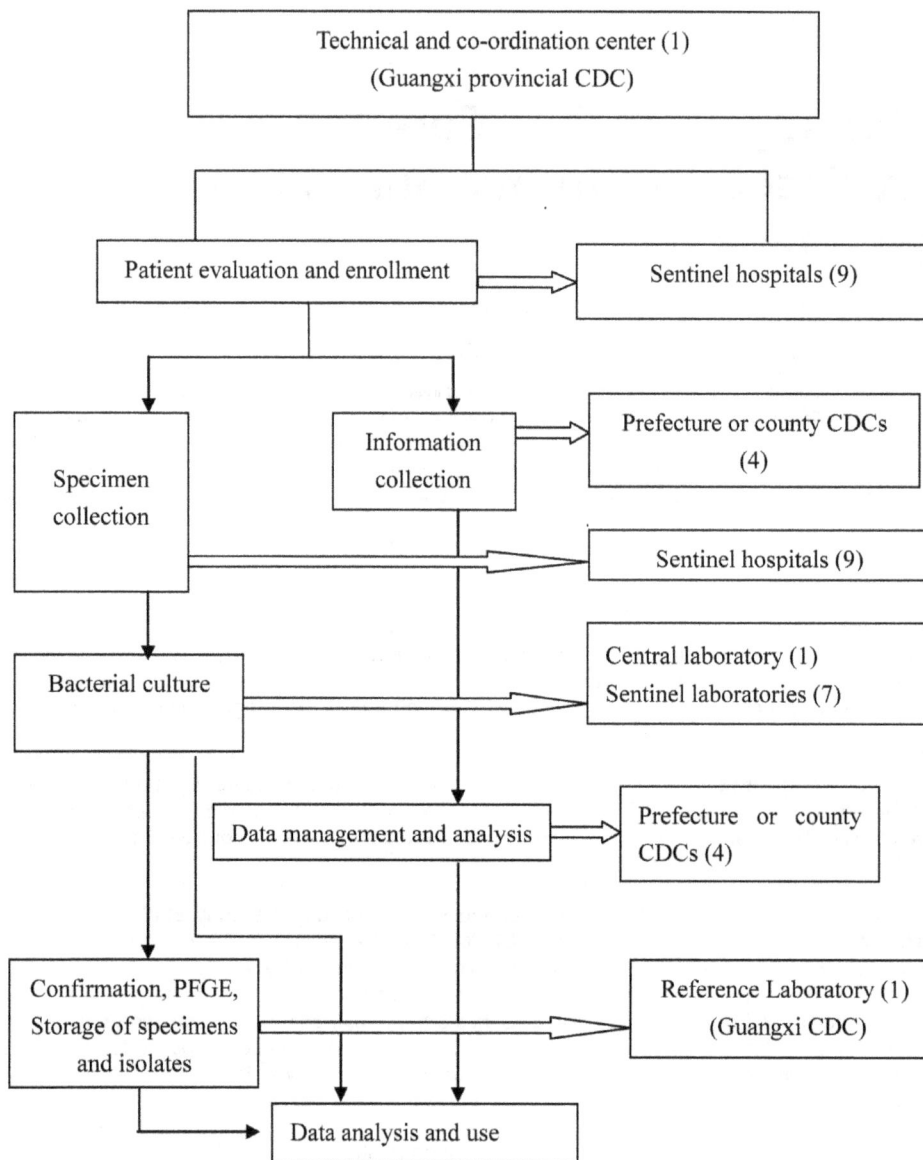

Figure 1. Surveillance network for the five core syndromes.

surveillance system makes timely nation-wide disease reporting and early outbreak detection possible.

Nevertheless, the national surveillance system does have limitations. Under this system, reported cases of bacterial infection were determined mainly by clinical features without accompanying laboratory confirmation, since bacterial culture is not routinely performed for suspected infection cases in hospitals. As a result, defining an overall picture of the etiological spectrum is difficult. In addition, the national system merely includes commonly known diseases and pneumonia of unknown cause, and does not consider rare or emerging diseases that present with other syndromes.

Besides the national infectious disease surveillance system, more specific surveillance activities were conducted to explore the prevalence and etiology of bacterial infectious diseases [2], [3]. But these previous surveillance efforts were aimed at a single syndrome or pathogen.

Currently, limited data exist for the integrated surveillance of various syndrome etiologies in China. In 2011 a systematic

surveillance network was set up in Guangxi, China to monitor mainly fever and respiratory, diarrhea, fever and rash, fever and hemorrhage and encephalitis-meningitis syndromes. With signs and syndromes as a starting point, clinical information and specimens can be collected at the early stages of these diseases. Use of syndromic surveillance can determine the etiological spectrum of infectious diseases through multiple-etiology testing on such specimens. This paper aims to explore bacterial etiology spectra for five core syndromes: fever and respiratory, diarrhea, fever and rash, fever and hemorrhage and encephalitis-meningitis under a laboratory-based syndromic surveillance system. Results from our study will contribute to the strengthening of the existing national surveillance system and provide references for other settings that are similar to the study area on strategy development for vaccine introduction and infectious disease surveillance, as well as on bacterial etiology study.

Materials and Methods

Set-up of the surveillance network

The Guangxi Zhuang Autonomous Region (or Guangxi) is one of the provincial administrative regions in China, and is located in the southwestern region of the nation. Guangxi had a population of 48,160,001 at the end of 2009 and is divided into 14 areas called "prefecture-level-city" (or prefecture). Each prefecture is composed of a number of counties (including counties, districts and county-level cities). There are 119 counties in Guangxi.

A total of 12 counties/districts in 4 prefectures located in southern, central or northern Guangxi were selected as surveillance sites. There were 6 districts in the Nanning prefecture and 1 county in the Beihai prefecture located in southern Guangxi. Meanwhile, central Guangxi was represented by 4 districts/counties of the Guiguang prefecture and in northern Guangxi 1 county of the Guilin Prefecture was included. The health facilities in these selected sites were experienced in bacterial disease surveillance and capable of conducting such systematic surveillance.

The surveillance network consisted of the provincial CDC, 1 prefecture CDC, 3 County CDCs, 9 sentinel hospitals (2 provincial level, 4 prefecture-level and 3 county-level), 1 central laboratory (provincial level) and 7 surveillance laboratories (affiliated with the sentinel hospitals) (Figure 1). The physicians at the sentinel hospitals evaluated cases and enrolled eligible cases that met the case definitions into the surveillance network. Relevant information and clinical specimens from the enrolled cases were collected. The CDC health workers regularly visited the sentinel hospitals to search for cases meeting the surveillance definition according to the standard operational procedures of this surveillance network.

The surveillance for encephalitis-meningitis syndrome covered the period from February 2009 to December 2011. For the remaining 4 syndromes, the study period was from June 2010 to December 2011.

Case Definitions

Patients presenting to the sentinel hospitals who met any of the following definitions [4] were enrolled in the surveillance system:

- Fever and respiratory syndrome: including upper respiratory infection (URI) and pneumonia. URI was characterized as fever with axillary temperature $\geq 37.3°C$, weakness, headache, cough, sore throat or muscle pain. Pneumonia cases with inflammation in the end-expiratory airway, pulmonary alveolus and pulmonary interstitium that was characterized as fever, cough and accompanied by polypnea, tachypnea with positive chest radiological findings were also included.

- Diarrhea syndrome: passage of three or more loose, liquid, bloody, purulent or mucoid stools in any 24-hour period.

- Fever and rash syndrome: fever with axillary temperature $\geq 37.3°C$ lasting more than 1 day and rash presenting on the skin. Suspected cases of typhoid and paratyphoid fever in endemic areas were also enrolled.

- Fever and hemorrhage syndrome: fever with axillary temperature $\geq 37.3°C$ and hemorrhage in the skin, mucosa or other parts of the body.

- Encephalitis-meningitis syndrome: Fever, headache, vomiting, accompanied by altered consciousness or meningeal irritation, including various central nervous system symptoms.

Specimen Collection

Appropriate clinical specimens were collected from patients enrolled with the five core syndromes:

- Specimens collected for fever and respiratory syndrome included a blood specimen, one throat swab and a sputum specimen. A pleural effusion specimen, a bronchoalveolar lavage fluid specimen and a nasopharyngeal aspirate specimen were collected as needed.

- A stool specimen was collected for each eligible case with diarrhea syndrome.

- Specimens collected for fever and rash syndrome included a blood specimen and one throat swab. A stool specimen and pus specimen from the skin were collected as needed.

- A blood specimen was collected for each eligible case with fever and hemorrhage syndrome. An exudate specimen from the skin and a cerebrospinal fluid specimen (CSF) were collected as needed.

- A blood and CSF specimen were collected for cases with encephalitis-meningitis syndrome.

Data collection and Analysis

Standardized case information forms were used to collect information on identification, epidemiology, clinical features, laboratory analysis and clinical specimens of enrollees with the five core syndromes.

To measure the prevalence of laboratory-confirmed bacterial infection, the percentage of positive cultures was calculated by specimens and syndromes. To characterize the bacterial spectrum, the proportions were calculated for each key etiology isolated from the five syndromes. To analyze the epidemiologic link between cases with identical pulsed field gel electrophoresis (PFGE) patterns, we compared the information for demography, clustering, addresses, sentinel hospitals and date of specimen collection. Data were analyzed using SPSS 13.0. A chi-square test was performed to test for statistical differences in bacterial culture results between genders, locations and ages. A P value <0.05 was considered statistically significant.

Laboratory Testing

Bacterial culturing of clinical specimens was performed according to routine operational procedures [5] (Table 1). Bacterial identification was done using the API biochemical identification system (bioMérieux, Marcy-l'Etoile, France) according to the manufacturer's guidelines.

Opportunistic pathogens were considered clinically significant if the organisms grew dominantly on culture media or the same organisms were detected from more than 2 cultures or from different types of samples. And the results were reported when supported by both laboratory data and clinical data.

PFGE was performed with the NotI restriction enzyme (Invitrogen) according to the standard operating procedure for Pulsenet (Pulsenet International) PFGE of *Escherichia coli* O157: H7, *E. coli* NON-0157 (STEC), *Salmonella* serotypes, *Shigella sonnei* and *Shigella flexner*. Plugs were submitted to electrophoresis using CHEF Mapper equipment (BioRad). The Lambda PFGE marker (Biolabs) was used in each assay. Images of the pulsetypes were uploaded and analyzed using BioNumerics software, Version 5.1 (Applied Maths).

Table 1. Methods of bacterial culture for five core syndromes.

Specimen	Enrichment			Culture/subculture			Syndrome	Bacterial pathogens detected
	Media	Conditions	Length of Incubation	Media*	Conditions	Length of Incubation		
Blood	Aerobic Blood culture bottle	5%CO$_2$,35°C	Day 1,2,4,7	Blood and chocolate agar	5%CO$_2$,35°C	for up to 48 hours	Encephalitis-meningitis	N.meningitidis, H.influenzae, Staphylococci, Streptococci, E. coli, Cryptococcus, others (Corynebacterium, K.pneumonia, M.luteus, H.alvei, Salmonella, S.maltophilia)
	Aerobic Blood culture bottle	5%CO$_2$,35°C	Day 1,2,4,7	Blood and chocolate agar	5%CO$_2$,35°C	for up to 48 hours	Fever and rash	S.typhi, S.paratyphi A
	Aerobic Blood culture bottle	5%CO$_2$,35°C	Day 1,2,4,7	Blood and chocolate agar	5%CO$_2$,35°C	for up to 48 hours	Fever and hemorrhage	S.suis
	Aerobic Blood culture bottle	5%CO$_2$,35°C	Day 1,2,4,7	Blood and chocolate agar	5%CO$_2$,35°C	for up to 48 hours	Fever and respiratory	Streptococci, Staphylococci, K.pneumoniae, P.aeruginosa, H.influenzae, others (Candida, E.coli, Acinetobacter, B.cepacia, S.maltophilia, S.marcescens, C.meningosepticum, O.anthropi, P.fluorescens, E.aerogenes, E.cloacae)
Sputum	Not needed	/	/	Chocolate, MacConkey and blood agar	5%CO$_2$,35°C	18–24 h	Fever and respiratory	Streptococci, Staphylococci, K.pneumoniae, P.aeruginosa, H.influenzae, others (Candida, E.coli, Acinetobacter, B.cepacia, S.maltophilia, S.marcescens, C.meningosepticum, O.anthropi, P.fluorescens, E.aerogenes, E.cloacae)
Nasopharyngeal aspirate	Not needed	/	/	Chocolate, MacConkey and blood agar	5%CO$_2$,35°C	for up to 48 hours	Fever and respiratory	Streptococci, Staphylococci, K.pneumoniae, P.aeruginosa, H.influenzae, others (Candida, E.coli, Acinetobacter, B.cepacia, S.maltophilia, S.marcescens, C.meningosepticum, O.anthropi, P.fluorescens, E.aerogenes, E.cloacae)
Bronchoalveolar lavage fluid	Not needed	/	/	Chocolate, MacConkey and blood agar	5%CO$_2$,35°C	for up to 48 hours	Fever and respiratory	Streptococci, Staphylococci, K.pneumoniae, P.aeruginosa, H.influenzae, others (Candida, E.coli, Acinetobacter, B.cepacia, S.maltophilia, S.marcescens, C.meningosepticum, O.anthropi, P.fluorescens, E.aerogenes, E.cloacae)
Pleural effusion	Not needed	/	/	Blood and chocolate gar	5%CO$_2$,35°C	for up to 48 hours	Fever and respiratory	Streptococci, Staphylococci, K.pneumoniae, P.aeruginosa, H.influenzae, others (Candida, E.coli, Acinetobacter, B.cepacia, S.maltophilia, S.marcescens, C.meningosepticum, O.anthropi, P.fluorescens, E.aerogenes, E.cloacae)

Table 1. Cont.

Specimen	Enrichment			Culture/subculture			Syndrome	Bacterial pathogens detected
	Media	Conditions	Length of Incubation	Media*	Conditions	Length of Incubation		
Throat swab	Not needed	/	/	Chocolate, MacConkey and blood agar	5%CO2,35°C	18–24 h	Fever and respiratory	Streptococci, Staphylococci, K.pneumoniae, P.aeruginosa, H.influenzae, others (Candida, E.coli, Acinetobacter, B.cepacia, S.maltophilia, S.marcescens, C.meningosepticum, O.anthropi, P.fluorescens, E.aerogenes, E.cloacae)
	Not needed	/	/	Chocolate, MacConkey and blood agar	5%CO2,35°C	18–24 h	Fever and rash	Streptococcus
Stool	Not needed	/	/	MacConkey, SSagar,XLD agar	35°C	18–24 h	Diarrhea	E.coli, Shigella, Salmonella
	APW	35°C	18–24 h	MacConkey agar	35°C	18–24 h	Diarrhea	P.shigelloides
	APW	35°C	18–24 h	Ampicillin MacConkey agar	35°C	18–24 h	Diarrhea	Aeromonas
	APW	35°C	18–24 h	TCBS	35°C	18–24 h	Diarrhea	Pathogenic Vibrios
	SBG	35°C	18–24 h	Chromogenic Salmonella agar	35°C	18–24 h	Diarrhea	Salmonella
	PBS	4°C	10 days	CIN	25°C	3 days	Diarrhea	Yersinia
	Not needed	/	/	CCDA	Microaerophilic, 42°C	3–5 days	Diarrhea	Campylobacter
	Not needed	/	/	Blood agar	35°C	18–24 h	Fever and rash	S.typhi, S.paratyphi A, others(S.maltophilia)
Cerebrospinal fluid	Not needed	/	/	Chocolate, MacConkey and blood agar	5%CO2,35°C	for up to 48 hours	Encephalitis-meningitis	N.meningitidis, H.influenzae, Staphylococci, Streptococci, E.coli, Others(K.pneumoniae, P.aeruginosa, Salmonella)
	Not needed	/	/	Chocolate, MacConkey and blood agar	5%CO2,35°C	for up to 48 hours	Fever and hemorrhage	S.suis
Pus	Not needed	/	/	Blood agar	5%CO2,35°C	for up to 48 hours	Fever and rash	Streptococcus, others (S.aureus)
Exudate	Not needed	/	/	Hottinger's Agar	28°C	for up to 48 hours	Fever and hemorrhage	Y.pestis

*APW Alkaline Peptone Water.
SBG Selenite brilliant green sulfa enrichment broth.
PBS Phosphate buffered saline.
CIN Ccefsulodin-irgasan-novobiocin agar.
SS Salmonella-Shigella agar.
XLD Xylose lysine desoxycholate agar.
TCBS Thiosulfate citrate bile salts sucrose agar.
CCDA Charcoal cefoperazone deoxycholate agar.

Table 2. Positive Cultures by specimen type for five core syndromes.

Syndrome	Specimen	No. tested	No. positive	% Positive
Fever and Respiratory	Sputum	700	103	14.71
	Throat/nasal swab	832	22	2.64
	Blood	1342	26	1.94
	Pleural effusion	9	1	11.11
	Bronchoalveolar lavage fluid	14	1	7.14
	Nasopharyngeal aspirate	11	0	0.00
Diarrhea	Stool	942	95	10.08
Fever and rash	Blood	379	40	10.55
	Stool	7	1	14.29
	Throat swab	239	1	0.42
	Pus	5	2	40.00
Fever and hemorrhage	Blood	114	0	0.00
	Exudate	2	0	0.00
Encephalitis-meningitis	Blood	694	25	3.60
	CSF	617	32	5.19
Total		5907	349	5.91

Quality Assurance and Control

Standard operational procedures (SOPs) for the surveillance were formulated and SOP training was given to standardize the surveillance activities. Health staff at the CDCs visited the sentinel hospitals and sentinel laboratories every other week to assure the quality of case evaluation, data collection, specimen collection and testing. The completed case information forms were reviewed by specific data managers for completeness and logic errors. Proficiency tests were performed in sentinel laboratories at irregular intervals.

Ethical Considerations

The study protocol was reviewed and approved by the Ethics Committee of Guangxi Zhuang Autonomous Region in January 2009. Signed informed consent was obtained from all study participants. For patients <18 years of age, a written consent form was signed by a parent or legal guardian.

Results

Demographics of Enrolled Patients

A total of 2,964 enrollees were evaluated from February 2009 to December 2011. Of these, 1,832 (61.81%) were male and 1,132 (38.19%) were female; 1,421 (47.94%) lived in urban areas and 1,543 (52.06%) in rural areas. The median age of the patients enrolled was 4 years (range, 0 to 119 years). Of these, 905 (30.53%) were patients with fever and respiratory syndrome, 939 (31.68%) with diarrhea syndromes, 319 (10.76%) with fever and rash syndrome, 111 (3.74%) with fever and hemorrhage syndrome and 690 (23.28%) with encephalitis/meningitis syndrome.

Positive Culture by Specimen Type

Of 5,907 specimens collected from 2,964 enrollees, 349 (5.91%) produced positive cultures for bacterial etiologies. For fever and respiratory syndrome, pathogens were isolated from 14.71% of the sputum specimens. For diarrhea syndrome, 10.08% of the stool specimens were culture positive. For fever and rash syndrome,

10.55% of blood specimens were culture positive. For encephalitis-meningitis syndrome, pathogens were isolated from 3.60% of blood specimens and 5.19% of CSF specimens. No pathogen was isolated for fever and hemorrhage syndrome (Table 2).

Culture Positive by five Core Syndromes

Bacterial pathogens were isolated from 320 (10.80%) cases out of 2,964 enrollees with one of the five core syndromes.

Pathogens were isolated from 140 (15.47%) out of 905 patients with fever and respiratory syndrome. Significantly higher positive rates were observed in patients living in rural areas (22.38%) compared to those in urban areas (11.05%) (P = 0.000), in males (17.29%) than in females (12.15%) (P = 0.041), and in patients aged 0~10 years (19.11%) than in patients >10 years (9.57%) (P = 0.000).

Pathogens were isolated from 93 (9.90%) out of 939 patients with diarrhea syndrome. No statistically significant differences in positive rates were observed between patients living in rural areas (9.22%) and urban areas (10.22%) (P = 0.643), between males (9.46%) and females (10.60%) (P = 0.568), between patients aged 0~10 years (8.54%) and >10 years of age (10.59%) (P = 0.320).

Pathogens were isolated from 42 (13.17%) out of 319 patients with fever and rash syndrome. Significantly higher positive rates were observed in patients living in urban areas (33.94%) than in rural areas (2.38%) (P = 0.000), in females (18.38%) than males (9.29%) (P = 0.018), and in patents >10 years of age (17.65%) than those aged 0~10 years (3.06%) (P = 0.000).

For encephalitis-meningitis syndrome pathogens were isolated from 45 (6.52%) out of 690 patients. No significant difference in positive rates was observed between patients living in rural areas (5.96%) and urban areas (9.71%) (P = 0.603), males (6.90%) and females (5.88%) (P = 0.156). Higher positive rates were found in children aged 0~10 years (4.04%) than patients >10 years of age (9.86%) (P = 0.002) (Table 3).

Table 3. Culture positive by five core syndromes.

	Fever and respiratory		Diarrhea		Fever and rash		Encephalitis-meningitis	
	Cases tested	No.positive (%)	Cases tested	No.positive (%)	Cases tested	No.positive (%)	Cases tested	No.positive (%)
Location								
urban	552	61(11.05)	646	66(10.22)	109	37(33.94)	103	10(9.71)
rural	353	79(22.38)	293	27(9.22)	210	5(2.38)	587	35(5.96)
X^2		21.132		0.227		62.53		2.017
P		0		0.634		0		0.156
Gender								
Male	584	101(17.29)	571	54(9.46)	183	17(9.29)	435	30(6.90)
Female	321	39(12.15)	368	39(10.60)	136	25(10.38)	255	15(5.88)
X^2		4.193		0.326		5.642		0.271
P		0.041		0.568		0.018		0.603
Age								
0–10 years	560	107(19.11)	623	66(10.59)	98	3(3.06)	396	16(4.04)
>10 years	345	33(9.57)	316	27(8.54)	221	39(17.65)	294	29(9.86)
X^2		14.864		0.987		12.634		9.386
P		0		0.32		0		0.002
Total	905	140(15.47)	939	93(9.90)	319	42(13.17)	690	45(6.52)

*To date no bacterial pathogen has been detected from specimens of fever and hemorrhage syndrome.

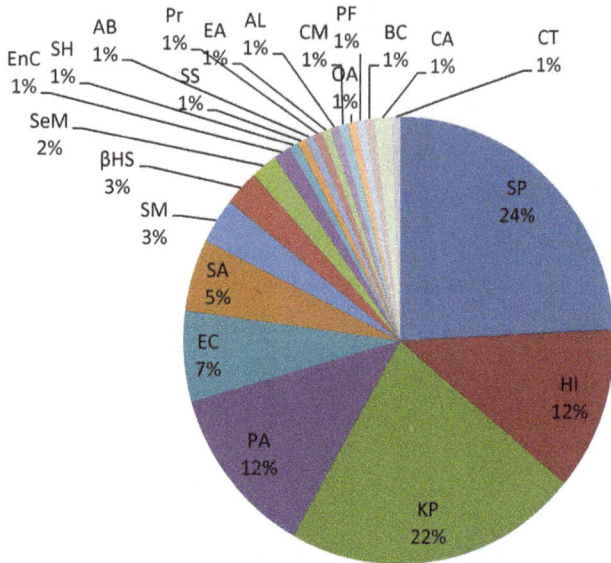

Figure 2. Etiological distribution of fever and respiratory syndrome in Guangxi, China, 2009–2011. Of 153 etiologies cultured from specimens of fever and respiratory syndromes: *Streptococcus pneumonia*(SP, 37 strains), *Haemophilus influenza*(HI,18), *Klebsiella pneumonia*(KP,34), *Pseudomonas aeruginosa*(PA,19), *Escherichia coli*(EC, 10), *Staphylococcus aureus*(SA,8), *Stenotrophomonas maltophilia*(SM,5), *β-hemolytic streptococcus*(βHS,4), *Serratia marcescens*(SeM,3), *Enterobacter cloacae*(EnC,2), *Staphylococcus hominis*(SH,1), *Staphylococcus saprophyticus*(SS,1), *Acinetobacter baumannii* (AB,1), *Proteus*(Pr,1), *Enterobacter aerogenes* (EA,1), *Acinetobacter lwoffii*(AL,1), *Chryseobacterium meningosepticum*(CM,1), *Ochrobactrum anthropic*(OA,1), *Pseudomonas fluorescens*(PF,1), *Burkholderia cepacia*(BC,1), *Candida albicans*(CA,2), *Candida tropicalis*(CT,1).

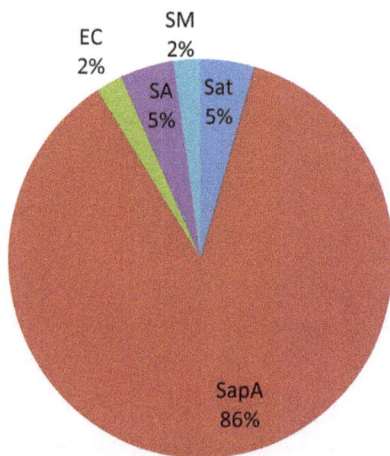

Figure 3. Etiological distribution of diarrhea syndrome in Guangxi, China, 2009–2011. Of 95 etiologies cultured from specimens of diarrhea syndromes: *Salmonella*(Sa,77), *Salmonella-typhi*(Sat,1), *Pathogenic Escherichia coli*(PE,3), *Enterotoxigenic Escherichia coli*(ETEC,1), *Campylobacter jejuni*(CJ,3), *Yersinia enterocolitica* (YE,1), *Yersinia pseudotuberculosis*(YP,2), *Plesiomonas shigelloides*(PS,1), *Aeromonas*(Ae,6).

Streptococcus pneumonia (37, 24.18%), followed by *Klebsiella pneumonia* (34 strains, 22.22%), *Pseudomonas aeruginosa* (19, 12.42%) and *Haemophilus influenza* (18, 11.76%) (Figure 2).

Of 95 (27.22%) pathogens isolated from diarrhea syndrome specimens, pathogenic bacteria and opportunistic pathogens accounted for 90.53% and 9.47%, respectively. The most frequently isolated pathogens were *non-typhoidal Salmonella* (77,

Etiologic Spectrum

Of 153 (43.84%) etiologies cultured from specimens of fever and respiratory syndromes, pathogenic bacteria, opportunistic pathogens and fungus accounted for 35.95%, 62.09% and 1.96%, respectively. The most frequently isolated pathogens were

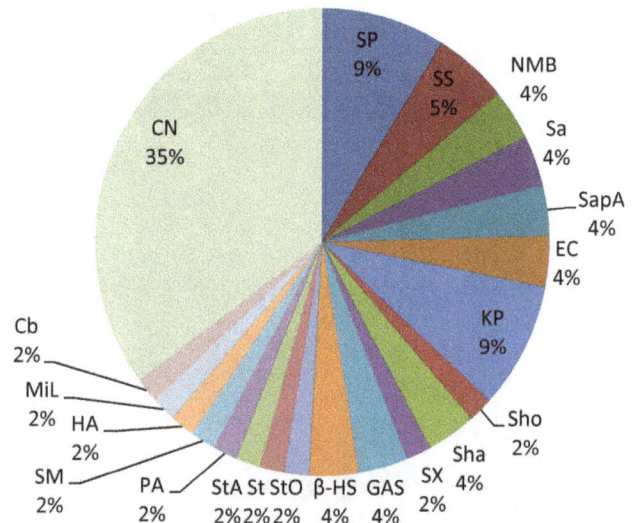

Figure 4. Etiological distribution of fever and rash syndrome in Guangxi, China, 2009–2011. Of 44 etiologies cultured from specimens of fever and rash syndromes: *Salmonella paratyphi A* (SapA,38 strains), *Salmonella-typhi* (Sat,2), *Escherichia coli*(EC,1), *Staphylococcus aureus* (SA,2), *Stenotrophomonas maltophilia*(SM,1).

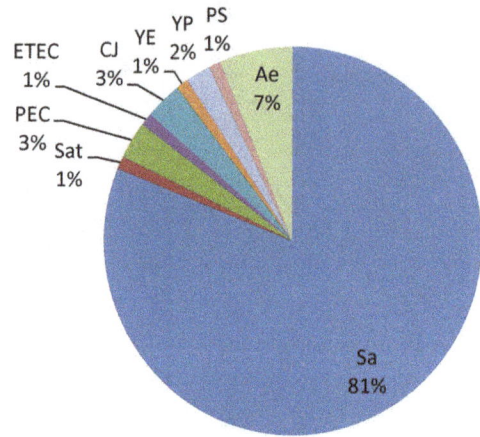

Figure 5. Etiological distribution of encephalitis-meningitis syndrome in Guangxi, China, 2009–2011. Of 57 etiologies cultured from specimens of encephalitis-meningitis syndromes: *Streptococcus pneumonia*(SP,5), *Streptococcus suis*(SS,3), *Neisseria meningitidis serogroup B*(NMB,2), *Salmonella*(Sa,2), *Salmonella paratyphi A*(SapA,2), *Escherichia coli* (EC,2), *Klebsiella pneumonia*(KP,5), *Staphylococcus hominis*(Sho,1), *Staphylococcus haemolyticus*(Sha, 2), *Staphylococcus xylosus*(SX ,1), *Group A streptococcus*(GAS,2), *β-hemolytic streptococcus* (β-HS, 2), *Streptococcus oralis*(StO, 1), *Streptococcus*(St,1), *Streptococcus agalactiae* (StA,1), *Pseudomonas aeruginosa* (PA,1), *Stenotrophomonas maltophilia*(SM,1), *Hafinia alvei*(HA,1), *Micrococcus luteus*(MiL,1), *Corynebacterium*(Cy,1), *Cryptococcus neoformans*(CN,20).

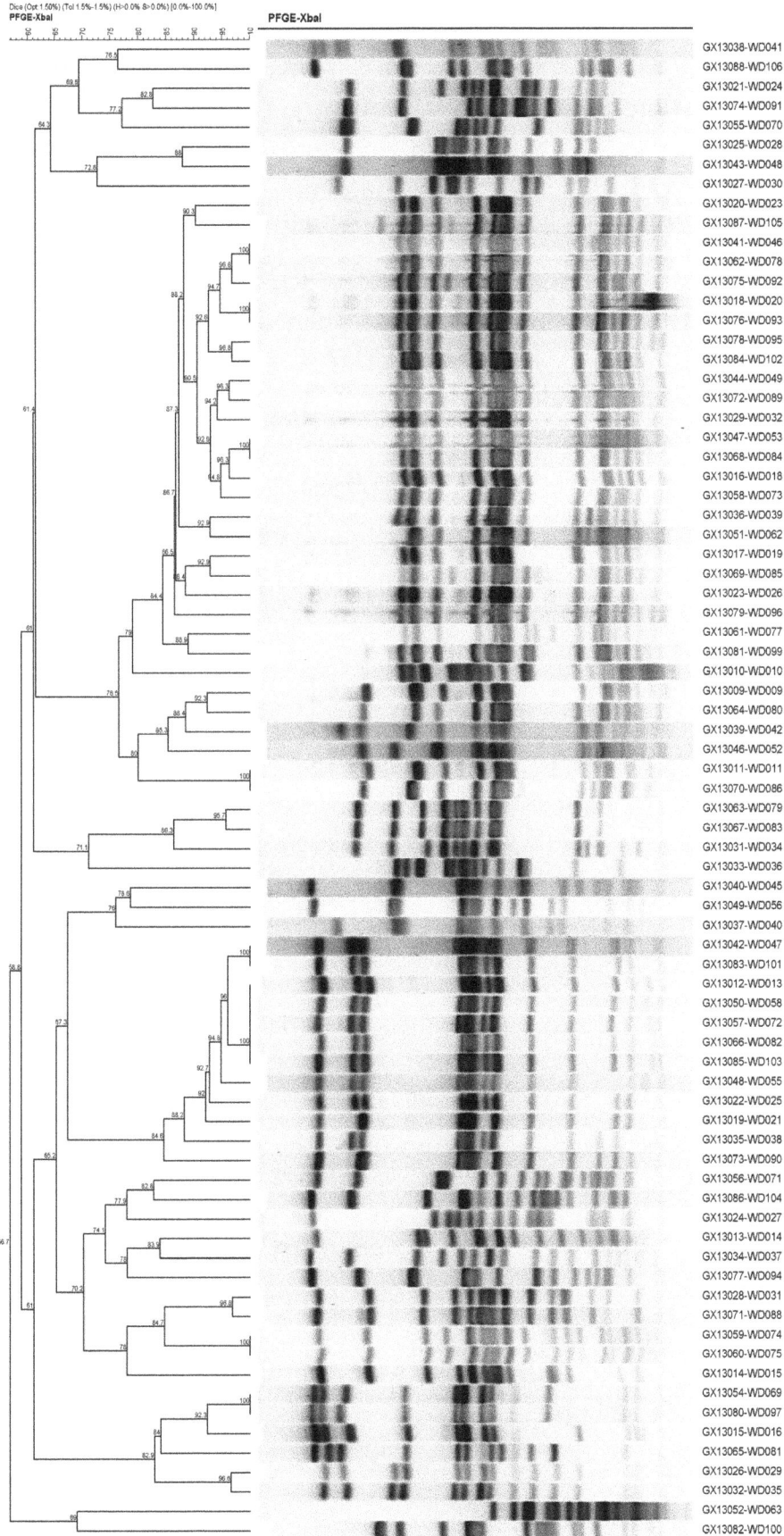

Figure 6. Comparison of PFGE patterns for isolates with high similarity.

81.05%), *Aeromonas* (6, 6.32%), *Pathogenic Escherichia coli* (6, 6.32%),and *Campylobacter jejuni* (3, 3.16%) (Figure 3).

Of 44 (12.61%) isolates cultured from specimens of fever and rash syndrome, pathogenic bacteria and opportunistic pathogens accounted for 93.18% and 4.55% of the isolates, respectively. The most frequently isolated pathogen was *Salmonella typhi A* (38, 86.36%), which was detected in cases caused by an outbreak of this syndrome (Figure 4).

Of 57 (16.33%) isolates cultured from specimens of encephalitis-meningitis syndrome, pathogenic bacteria, opportunistic pathogens and fungus accounted for 31.58%, 33.33% and 35.09%, respectively. *Cryptococcus neoformans* was the most frequently isolated pathogen (20, 35.09%), followed by *Streptococcus pneumonia* (5, 8.77%), *Klebsiella pneumonia* (5, 8.77%),*Streptococcus suis* (3, 5.26%) and *Neisseria meningitides* group B (2, 3.51%) (Figure 5).

To date no bacterial pathogen has been detected from specimens of fever and hemorrhage syndrome.

PFGE Analysis

A total of 112 strains of *Salmonella* were isolated in this surveillance system, making it the most commonly detected bacterial pathogen at present. PFGE assays indicated that these 112 *Salmonella* isolates were clustered in several pulsotypes. Figure 6 shows that identical PFGE patterns were observed in WD046 and WD078, WD020 and WD093, WD053 and WD084, WD011 and WD086, WD047 and WD101, (WD013, 058, 072, 082) and WD103, WD074 and WD075, WD069 and WD097.

Epidemiologic investigations conducted on those patients who had identical pulsotypes showed no obvious epidemiological links.

Discussion

Under the present surveillance system, a total of 349 (5.91%) pathogen isolates were detected from 5,907 specimens collected from eligible cases of five core syndromes. In this study the pathogenic spectrum of five core syndromes in China was characterized for the first time.

The surveillance findings showed that the predominant pathogens attributing to fever and respiratory syndrome were *Klebsiella pneumonia*, *Haemophilus influenza* and *Staphylococcus aureus*, which was similar to previous reports from other countries [6]. Although vaccination against *Haemophilus influenzae* type b *(Hib)* has remarkably reduced the incidence of this disease in industrialized countries, the global burden of this disease remains high [7]. In China, *Hib* was one of the most important pathogens that caused pneumonia in children [8], although the disease burden of this pathogen is unclear and the currently reported incidence is believed to be an underestimate [9].

Under the surveillance system described here, *Salmonella* predominated in pathogens isolated from eligible cases of diarrhea syndrome. Previous surveillance conducted by various areas of China showed that *Salmonella* is one of the most important pathogens causing diarrhea [10], [11]. As such, more attention to the public health importance of *Salmonella* is needed due to its high infection rate and capacity to cause wide-spread infection. *Campylobacter jejuni* is a frequently reported pathogen that causes diarrhea worldwide. The findings of a twelve-year surveillance in Israel showed that the annual incidence rate of *C. jejuni* infection episodes increased from 24.59 to 70.54/100,000 cases during the period between 1999 and 2010 [12]. This organism is one of the most common causes of Guillain–Barré syndrome (GBS) [13], which may lead to severe signs and syndromes and can be life-threatening [14].

For encephalitis-meningitis syndrome, the most frequently detected organisms were *Cryptococcus neoformans*, *Streptococcus species* and *Staphylococcus species*, which was similar to findings obtained in Malawi [15]. However, a study in Italy showed that *Listeria monocytogenes* and *Neisseria meningitides* were the most common pathogens that caused meningitis in that country [16]. Meningitis caused by *C. neoformans* may lead to high morbidity and mortality [17] and is a common form of meningitis in immunocompromised patients [18] such as HIV/AIDS patients, as well as in long-term antimicrobial users. The HIV epidemic and increasing use of immunosuppressive therapies are believed to have contributed to the rising incidence of infections caused by *C. neoformans* [19]. Guangxi is one of the provinces in China with the most severe HIV epidemic and the most rapid increase in newly reported HIV-positive cases in recent years [20]. This may contribute to high proportion of *C. neoformans* detected in the study area.

Streptococcus pneumoniae is the most common cause of community-acquired pneumonia, meningitis and bacteremia in children and adults [21]. The incidence of pneumococcal diseases had significantly decreased in high-income countries as routine use of the pneumococcal conjugate vaccines [22]. Yet the high cost is an obstacle to introduction of these vaccines in resource-poor settings [23]. As a result, pneumococcal diseases remain important public health problems in low and middle income countries [24].

Streptococcus suis infections are a global problem in the swine industry [25] and can also cause severe invasive infection in humans who have close contact with infected pigs or contaminated pork [26]. In recent years, the number of reported *S. suis* infections in humans has increased significantly [27].

Following the introduction of the meningococcal vaccine, the incidence of meningococcal meningitis has been as low as 0.15/100,000 during the past decade in Guangxi. However, the case-fatality rate is still as high as 16.59% in this province. Under the surveillance system described here, serogroup B was isolated, which was rarely reported as compared to A and C during the past 10 years in Guangxi [28]. Serogroup B has now become the main causative agent in Europe and South America [29], since routine vaccination with serogroup C vaccines has drastically reduced the incidence of disease caused by this serogroup. In the absence of satisfactory vaccine against serogroup B meningococcal meningitis [30], a future epidemic outbreak caused by this serogroup could thus bring new challenges to disease control efforts in Guangxi and elsewhere.

In China, most previous investigations and laboratory testing on rash illness were aimed mainly at viral diseases [31], [32] and orientia tsutsugamushi [33], such that there was little information concerning other bacterial diseases. While the surveillance system described here attempted to reveal the bacterial pathogenic spectrum of fever and rash syndrome, limited bacterial pathogens (mainly *Salmonella paratyphi A*) were detected. As such, continuous surveillance will be needed to further explore the etiologic spectrum in Guangxi.

In this study no bacterial pathogen was detected from specimens of fever and hemorrhage syndrome. The infections causing hemorrhage syndrome were mainly reported in northern China rather than southern China and few cases of hemorrhage due to bacterial pathogens were previously reported by the routine surveillance system in Guangxi. This low incidence may be due to the low prevalence of these diseases or because testing for the bacterial pathogens was not routinely performed.

In addition to the common pathogenic bacteria found under the surveillance system described here, opportunistic pathogens have also drawn attention. Opportunistic pathogens have accounted for two-thirds of the pathogens for fever and respiratory syndrome, and one-third of meningitis syndrome. Echoing findings were noted in Kenya, where 35.29% of the bacterial pathogens were opportunistic pathogens in non-HIV patients with acute respiratory infection [34]. For meningitis, the proportion of opportunistic pathogens measured in Guangxi was higher than for Ghana (8.58%) [35]. A high proportion of opportunistic pathogens may be due to immunodeficiency [36], overuse of antimicrobials [37], increasing use of immunosuppressive therapies or nosocomial infection [38].

Under the present surveillance system, lower positive culture rates were found in sputum (14.71%), stool (10.08%) and blood (1.94%–10.55) specimens. The positive culture rate for sputum specimens was lower than the 27.5% [39] reported in Romania. For stool specimens, the rate in Guangxi was lower than that in Iran (45.6%) [40]. For blood specimens of respiratory infection patients, the positive culture rate was also lower when compared with findings from Thailand (9.2%) [41]. The positive rate (4.93%) for CSF culture in Guangxi was similar to that observed in Africa (3.3%–7%) [35], [42]. Antibiotic use outside hospitals without a medical prescription is very common in China and may affect the growth of bacteria in cultured specimens. The differences in positive rates might also be due to the changing pathogenic spectrum of infections. Previous research showed that the proportion of respiratory infection caused by bacteria has decreased, while the infection caused by viruses,mycoplasma and chlamydia has obviously increased [43], [44]. Viruses were also found to be the most important etiology of diarrhea [45].

In the surveillance system described here, *Salmonella* was selected for PFGE analysis, since for this pathogen sufficient numbers of strains have been collected to allow clustering analysis. Although a number of strains were found to have identical PFGE patterns, no epidemiological links were found between those patients infected with the identical strains. The strains with identical PFGE patterns were detected from patients living in different part of the city, by different sentinel hospitals and at different time points. There was no other case with similar syndromes reported for the patients enrolled in the same period. While no evidence showed that clustering of cases infected with *Salmonella* occurred, risk factors for infection still widely exist in this environment. Therefore, close monitoring is needed to avoid outbreaks caused by common factors (e.g. water or food contamination).

The surveillance system set up in Guangxi was an active syndromic surveillance based on laboratory findings that allowed the timely detection of bacterial infections with laboratory conformation. This system complements the national surveillance system, allowed the bacterial spectrum of infectious disease to be characterized, and infections caused by rare or newly emerging

etiologies (or serogroups) to be identified. Moreover, implementation of this system allowed the disease control agencies to systematically monitor important pathogens which were not routinely detected in this area such as *Hib* and *Campylobacter jejuni* and to further study the etiologies using additional molecular biology assays. Implementation of such systems can also improve the detection sensitivity of pathogen such as *Streptococcus suis*, since cultures of this pathogen have been routinely performed on suspected cases of meningitis even without obtaining relevant epidemiologic information (e.g. frequent exposure to sick pigs or pork).

Implementation of an effective laboratory-based surveillance system requires close collaboration between the CDC system and the hospital system. Yet, it is still challenging to maintain a quality mechanism for public health surveillance due to insufficient understanding and lack of motivation from hospital staff. As such, strengthened cooperation between the CDC system and the hospital system, together with continuous training and education are needed to sustain the five-syndrome surveillance system in Guangxi.

Limitations

The current surveillance system has not included viral pathogens and we can only obtain the bacterial spectrum without understanding the patterns of viral infection for the five core syndromes. Using the surveillance system described here, viral etiologies can be included to make the findings of the study more complete and valuable.

To date we can only characterize the PFGE patterns for *Salmonella* rather than other pathogens detected in our study. PFGE analysis has not been performed on those isolates because the number of the remaining strains is insufficient for performing clustering analysis. As the surveillance continues, we will conduct the PFGE analysis on the remaining pathogen isolates when sufficient number of strains is collected.

Acknowledgments

We are grateful to the clinicians and nurses at the sentinel hospitals in Guangxi, China for their assistance in enrolling and sampling patients. We thank the laboratory technicians of sentinel laboratories and the health staffs of the sentinel Centers for Disease Prevention and Control for the conduct of the work performed in support of this surveillance method.

Author Contributions

Conceived and designed the experiments: BQD ML HQJ. Performed the experiments: ML DBL MLW JZ HZL LYZ JH. Analyzed the data: DBL HZL LYZ JH. Contributed reagents/materials/analysis tools: HQJ. Wrote the paper: BQD DBL ML MLW JZ HZL LYZ JH XLW GYZ.

References

1. Wang LD, Wang Y, Jin SG, Wu ZY, Chin DP, et al. (2008) Emergence and control of infectious diseases in China. The Lancet 372: 1598–1605.
2. Li Y, Yin Z, Shao Z, Li M, Liang X, et al. (2014) Population-based Surveillance for Bacterial Meningitis in China, September 2006–December 2009. Emerg Infect Dis 20: 61–69. doi: 10.3201/eid2001.120375.
3. Ran L, Wu S, Gao Y, Zhang X, Feng Z, et al. (2011) Laboratory-based surveillance of nontyphoidal Salmonella infections in China. Foodborne Pathog Dis 8: 921–927.
4. World Health Organization (2008) Communicable disease alert and response for mass gatherings: key considerations. Geneva: World Health Organization Press. 119p.
5. Murray PR, Baron EJ, Pfaller MA, Tenover FC, Yolken RH (1999) Manual of Clinical Microbiology. Washington DC: ASM Press. 1773p.
6. Charles PG, Whitby M, Fuller AJ, Stirling R, Wright AA, et al. (2008) The Etiology of community-acquired pneumonia in Australia: Why Penicillin plus

doxycycline or a macrolide is the most appropriate therapy. Clin Infect Dis 46: 1513–1521.
7. Peltola H (2000) Worldwide Haemophilus influenzae type b disease at the beginning of the 21st century: global analysis of the disease burden 25 years after the use of the polysaccharide vaccine and a decade after the advent of conjugates. Clin Microbiol Rev 13: 302–317.
8. Zhang Q, Guo Z, MacDonald NE (2011) Vaccine preventable community-acquired pneumonia in hospitalized children in Northwest China. Pediatr Infect Dis J. 30: 7–10. doi: 0.1097/INF.0b013e3181ec6245.
9. Levine OS, Liu G, Garman RL, Dowell SF, Yu S, et al. (2000) Haemophilus influenzae type b and Streptococcus pneumoniae as causes of pneumonia among children in Beijing, China. Emerg Infect Dis. 6: 165–70.
10. Zhu M, Cui S, Lin L, Xu B, Zhao J, et al. (2012) Analysis of the aetiology of diarrhoea in outpatients in 2007, Henan province, China. Epidemiol Infect. 141: 540–8. doi: 10.1017/S0950268812000970.

11. Qu M, Deng Y, Zhang X, Liu G, Huang Y, et al. (2012) Etiology of acute diarrhea due to enteropathogenic bacteria in Beijing, China. J Infect. 65: 214–22. doi: 10.1016/j.jinf.2012.04.010.

12. Weinberger M, Lerner L, Valinsky L, Moran GJ, Nissan I, et al. (2013) Increased incidence of Campylobacter spp. infection and high rates among children, Israel. Emerg Infect Dis. 19: 1828–1831. doi: 10.3201/eid1911.120900.

13. Kuwabara S (2004) Guillain-Barré syndrome: epidemiology, pathophysiology and management. Drugs. 64: 597–610.

14. Winer JB (2014) An update in Guillain-barré syndrome. Autoimmune Dis. doi: 10.1155/2014/793024.

15. Mwai HM, William CM, Irving FH, Rushina C, Peter HG, et al. (2012) Bacterial infections in Lilongwe, Malawi: aetiology and antibiotic resistance. BMC Infect Dis. 12: 67.

16. Favaro M, Savini V, Favalli C, Fontana C (2013) A multi-target Real-Time PCR assay for rapid identification of meningitis-associated microorganisms. Mol Biotechnol. 53: 74–79.

17. Sabiiti W, May RC (2012) Mechanisms of infection by the human fungal pathogen Cryptococcus neoformans. Future Microbiol. 7: 1297–1313.

18. Negroni R (2012) Cryptococcosis. Clin Dermatol. 30: 599–609.

19. Tihana B, Harrison TS (2005) Cryptococcal meningitis. Br Med Bull. 72 : 99–118.

20. Li L, Sun G, Liang SJ, Li JJ, Li TY, et al. (2013) Different distribution of HIV-1 subtype and drug resistance were found among treatment naïve individuals in Henan, Guangxi, and Yunnan Province of China. PLoS One. doi: 10.1371/journal.pone.0075777.

21. Lynch JP, Zhanel GG (2009) Streptococcus pneumoniae: epidemiology, risk factors, and strategies for prevention. Semin Respir Crit Care Med. 30: 189–209. doi: 10.1055/s-0029-1202938.

22. Weil OC, Gaillat J (2008) Can the success of pneumococcal conjugate vaccines for the prevention of pneumococcal diseases in children be extrapolated to adults? Vaccine. 32: 2022–6. doi: 10.1016/j.vaccine.2014.02.008.

23. Centers for Disease Control and Prevention (CDC) (2008) Progress in introduction of pneumococcal conjugate vaccine–worldwide, 2000–2008. MMWR Morb Mortal Wkly Rep. 57: 1148–1151.

24. Zar HJ, Madhi SA, Aston SJ, Gordon SB (2013) Pneumonia in low and middle income countries: progress and challenges .Thorax. 68: 1052–1056. doi: 10.1136/thoraxjnl-2013-204247.

25. Gottschalk M, Segura M, Xu J (2007) Streptococcus suis infections in humans: the Chinese experience and the situation in North America. Anim Health Res Rev. 8: 29–45.

26. Pachirat O, Taksinachanekit S, Mootsikapun P, Kerdsin A (2012) Human Streptococcus suis Endocarditis: Echocardiographic Features and Clinical Outcome. Clin Med Insights Cardiol 6: 119–123. doi: 10.4137/CMC.S9793.

27. Wertheim HF, Nghia HD, Taylor W, Schultsz C (2009) Streptococcus suis: an emerging human pathogen. Clin Infect Dis 48: 617–25. doi: 10.1086/596763.

28. Kim SA, Kim DW, Dong BQ, Kim JS, Anh DD, et al. (2012) An expanded age range for meningococcal meningitis: molecular diagnostic evidence from population-based surveillance in Asia. BMC Infect Dis 12: 310. doi: 10.1186/1471-2334-12-310.

29. Abio A, Neal KR, Beck CR (2013) An epidemiological review of changes in meningococcal biology during the last 100 years. Pathog Glob Health 107: 373–380.

30. Panatto D, Amicizia D, Lai PL, Cristina ML, Domnich A, et al. (2013) New versus old meningococcal Group B vaccines: How the new ones may benefit infants & toddlers. Indian J Med Res 138: 835–46.

31. Cai J, Lv H, Lin J, Chen Z, Fang C, et al. (2014) Enterovirus infection in children attending two outpatient clinics in Zhejiang province, China.Med Virol. doi: 10.1002/jmv.23884.

32. Yan Y (2005) Epidemiologic and clinical features of measles and rubella in a rural area in China. J Chin Med Assoc 68(12): 571–577.

33. Liu YX, Feng D, Suo JJ, Xing YB, Liu G, et al. (2009) Clinical characteristics of the autumn-winter type scrub typhus cases in south of Shandong province, northern China. BMC Infect Dis 9: 82. doi: 0.1186/1471-2334-9-82.

34. Feikin DR, Njenga MK, Bigogo G, Aura B, Aol G, et al. (2012) Etiology and Incidence of viral and bacterial acute respiratory illness among older children and adults in rural western Kenya, 2007–2010. PLoS One. doi: 10.1371/journal.pone.0043656.

35. Owusu M, Nguah SB, Boaitey YA, Badu BE, Abubakr AR, et al. (2012) Aetiological agents of cerebrospinal meningitis: a retrospective study from a teaching hospital in Ghana. Ann Clin Microbiol Antimicrob. 11: 28. doi: 10.1186/1476-0711-11-28.

36. Pavić I, Cekinović D, Begovac J, Maretić T, Civljak R, et al. (2013) Cryptococcus neoformans meningoencephalitis in a patient with idiopathic CD4+ T lymphocytopenia. Coll Antropol. 37: 619–623.

37. Jefferies JM, Cooper T, Yam T, Clarke SC (2012) Pseudomonas aeruginosa outbreaks in the neonatal intensive care unit–a systematic review of risk factors and environmental sources. J Med Microbiol. 61: 1052–1061.

38. Murphy CN, Clegg S (2012) Klebsiella pneumoniae and type 3 fimbriae: nosocomial infection, regulation and biofilm formation. Future Microbiol 7: 991–1002.

39. Cornelia T, Adriana M, Miron B (2010) Mortality Risk and Etiologic Spectrum of Community-acquired Pneumonia in Hospitalized Adult Patients. Maedica (Buchar) 5: 258–264.

40. Jafari F, Shokrzadeh L, Hamidian M, Salmanzadeh S, Zali MR (2008) Acute diarrhea due to enteropathogenic bacteria in patients at hospitals in Tehran. Jpn J Infect Dis 61(4): 269–273.

41. Chaisuksant S, Koonsuwan A, Sawanyawisuth K (2013) Appropriateness of obtaining blood cultures in patients with community acquired pneumonia. Southeast Asian J Trop Med Public Health 44: 289–294.

42. Mengistu M, Asrat D, Woldeamanuel Y, Mengistu G (2011) Bacterial and fungal meningitis and antimicrobial susceptibility pattern in Tikur Anbessa University Hospital, Addis Ababa, Ethiopia. Ethiop Med J 49: 349–359.

43. Liu YF, Gao Y, Chen MF, Cao B, Yang XH, et al. (2013) Etiological analysis and predictive diagnostic model building of community-acquired pneumonia in adult outpatients in Beijing, China. BMC Infect Dis 13: 309. doi: 10.1186/1471-2334-13-309.

44. Shibli F, Chazan B, Nitzan O, Flatau E, Edelstein H, et al. (2010) Etiology of community-acquired pneumonia in hospitalized patients in northern Israel. Isr Med Assoc J 12: 477–482.

45. Barr W, Smith A (2014) Acute diarrhea. Am Fam Physician 89: 180–189.

20

Integrating Bacterial and Viral Water Quality Assessment to Predict Swimming-Associated Illness at a Freshwater Beach

Jason W. Marion[1¤a], Cheonghoon Lee[1¤b], Chang Soo Lee[1¤c], Qiuhong Wang[2], Stanley Lemeshow[3], Timothy J. Buckley[1¤d], Linda J. Saif[2], Jiyoung Lee[1,4]*

1 Division of Environmental Health Sciences, College of Public Health, The Ohio State University, Columbus, Ohio, United States of America, 2 Food Animal Health Research Program, Ohio Agricultural Research and Development Center, Department of Veterinary Preventive Medicine, The Ohio State University, Wooster, Ohio, United States of America, 3 Division of Biostatistics, College of Public Health, The Ohio State University, Columbus, Ohio, United States of America, 4 Department of Food Science and Technology, The Ohio State University, Columbus, Ohio, United States of America

Abstract

Background & Objective: Recreational waters impacted by fecal contamination have been linked to gastrointestinal illness in swimmer populations. To date, few epidemiologic studies examine the risk for swimming-related illnesses based upon simultaneous exposure to more than one microbial surrogate (e.g. culturable *E. coli* densities, genetic markers). We addressed this research gap by investigating the association between swimming-related illness frequency and water quality determined from multiple bacterial and viral genetic markers.

Methods: Viral and bacterial genetic marker densities were determined from beach water samples collected over 23 weekend days and were quantified using quantitative polymerase chain reaction (qPCR). These genetic marker data were paired with previously determined human exposure data gathered as part of a cohort study carried out among beach users at East Fork Lake in Ohio, USA in 2009. Using previously unavailable genetic marker data in logistic regression models, single- and multi-marker/multi-water quality indicator approaches for predicting swimming-related illness were evaluated for associations with swimming-associated gastrointestinal illness.

Results: Data pertaining to genetic marker exposure and 8- or 9-day health outcomes were available for a total of 600 healthy susceptible swimmers, and with this population we observed a significant positive association between human adenovirus (HAdV) exposure and diarrhea (odds ratio = 1.6; 95% confidence interval: 1.1–2.3) as well as gastrointestinal illness (OR = 1.5; 95% CI: 1.0–2.2) upon adjusting for culturable *E. coli* densities in multivariable models. No significant associations between bacterial genetic markers and swimming-associated illness were observed.

Conclusions: This study provides evidence that a combined measure of recreational water quality that simultaneously considers both bacterial and viral densities, particularly HAdV, may improve prediction of disease risk than a measure of a single agent in a beach environment likely influenced by nonpoint source human fecal contamination.

Editor: Andrew C. Singer, NERC Centre for Ecology & Hydrology, United Kingdom

Funding: This study was funded by the Public Health Preparedness for Infectious Diseases program (http://phpid.osu.edu) and The Ohio State University Targeted Investment in Excellence program sponsored by the Offices of Academic Affairs, the President, and Research. The human health and exposure data collection effort was funded by the Ohio Water Development Authority. The funders had no role in study design, data collection and analysis, decision to publish, or preparation of the manuscript.

Competing Interests: The authors have declared that no competing interests exist.

* Email: lee.3598@osu.edu

¤a Current address: Department of Environmental Health Science, Eastern Kentucky University, Richmond, Kentucky, United States of America
¤b Current address: Department of Environmental Health and Institute of Health and Environment, Graduate School of Public Health, Seoul National University, Seoul, Korea
¤c Current address: Environmental Biotechnology Research Center, Korea Research Institute of Bioscience and Biotechnology, Yuseong-gu, Daejeon, Korea,
¤d Current address: U.S. Environmental Protection Agency, National Exposure Research Laboratory, Research Triangle Park, North Carolina, United States of America

Introduction

Beach water advisories are issued to discourage human contact (e.g., swimming, wading, etc.) when water is potentially harmful to human health. In the United States, many of these advisories are issued at freshwater beaches when densities of fecal indicator bacteria (*E. coli* or enterococci) are observed or predicted to be in excess of single-day maximum criteria. Prior to November 26,

2012, the U.S. Environmental Protection Agency (USEPA) had established single-day maximum criteria, which were derived from several large epidemiological studies performed in the early 1980s [1]. In 2003, the 1986 *E. coli* criteria were supported by a comprehensive meta-analysis demonstrating *E. coli* was the most consistent indicator for predicting gastrointestinal illness in freshwater [2]. This same study indicated that methods for quantifying *E. coli* were problematic for same-day water quality advisories. The method required 18–24 h incubation and therefore was untimely for communication of risk to susceptible beachgoers [2].

Since the 2003 meta-analysis, several epidemiological studies evaluating associations between illness and more rapid measures of fecal indicators have been performed with an emphasis on genetic markers of bacterial or viral contamination, which have demonstrated the effectiveness of rapidly measured *Enterococcus* via quantitative polymerase chain reaction (qPCR) for predicting human illness at sewage-impacted Great Lakes and marine beaches [3,4]. However, in epidemiology studies on swimmers at non-point source-impacted beaches, associations between qPCR-based bacterial markers and gastrointestinal (GI) illness were not observed [5,6]. A potential reason for the lack of association in both studies could have related to the source of fecal contamination, which was likely dominated by avian sources [7], potentially presenting less risk for swimming-associated gastrointestinal (GI) illness than equivalent amounts of human-associated fecal contamination [8]. The diffuse nature of the source(s) of fecal contamination has been proposed as a possible explanation for the lack of association between bacterial genetic markers and human illness [9–11].

To date, few epidemiological studies on beachgoers have been performed at areas dominated by human-associated non-point source contamination, particularly in freshwater environments. Several peer-reviewed epidemiological studies have evaluated illness associations with human enteric viruses in European recreational waters [12–14] and U.S. waters [6,15,16]. Epidemiological studies pertaining to viruses are highly relevant as viruses are known to have a broad distribution in the aquatic environment [17], and are the most observed etiological agents in disease outbreaks associated with untreated U.S. recreational waters [18]. Recent epidemiological studies on swimmers [9–11] have suggested that viruses were the primary etiologic agents associated with recreational water illnesses based upon relatively short incubation periods following swimming exposure [10,19]. Similarly with regards to incubation periods, among limited-contact recreational users of freshwater in Chicago, Illinois (U.S.A.), most gastrointestinal illnesses generally developed within three days of water exposure [19].

To date, the majority of recreational water-related epidemiological studies have been performed to identify effective single indicators, often bacterial, for practical application among those making beach management decisions. Multiple fecal indicators and multiple genetic markers have been evaluated in recreational waters with respect to their association with each other as well as GI illness frequency among swimmers. There is some inconsistency in the findings of studies that have studied associations (or the lack thereof) between fecal indicator densities and measured pathogen and/or viral levels in freshwater [20] and coastal nvironments [21,22], and legitimate concerns remain regarding the use of single bacterial indicators for predicting and communicating swimming-associated illness risks to the general public [23–25].

To address these knowledge gaps, this study examined previously undescribed samples which were archived during our

prospective cohort study [26] that gathered culture-based *E. coli* and human exposure data. In our 2010 study [26], new GI illnesses among swimmers were associated with increasing culture-based *E. coli* densities at East Fork Lake (Ohio, USA); however, no assessment of associations between genetic marker densities and human health occurred. In 2012, the U.S. Environmental Protection Agency (EPA) emphasized a need for additional evaluation of rapid molecular methods for the timely determination of water quality to protect recreational water users [27]. Building upon this need, we examined associations between GI illness incidence among swimmers exposed to multiple genetic markers targeting both viruses and bacteria in this non-point source human-impacted beach environment. This study presented a unique opportunity to successfully use our historical exposure and health data coupled with our previously unexplored genetic material to do a timely assessment of the effectiveness of viral and bacterial molecular markers for predicting GI illness risk among swimmers who used the East Fork beach in 2009.

Materials and Methods

Overall Approach

The exposure and health data were collected using the prospective cohort study approach adopted by Wade et al. in their epidemiological studies related to recreational water [3,4]. This study builds upon our epidemiological investigations of recreational water-related illnesses by evaluating human illness associations with our recently qPCR-determined densities of bacteria and viruses. In brief, beach water samples, beach water quality data, and beach user exposure/behavior data were collected at East Fork State Park (39.0198° N; 84.1432° W) near Cincinnati, Ohio, U.S.A. Approvals to use this location for water sample collection and beachgoer interviews were kindly provided orally and in writing by Chris Dauner (Park Manager, East Fork State Park), and Dan West (Chief, Ohio Department of Natural Resources, Division of Parks and Recreation). Complete health and exposure data were collected from 891 beachgoers from 278 households. As described in our 2010 study [26], participants reported their health status via a telephone questionnaire after an eight- to nine-day follow-up period. More recently we quantified densities of four viral (human adenovirus (HAdV), human enterovirus (HEntV), and human norovirus genogroup I (HNoV GI) and genogroup II (HNoV GII)) and four bacterial (*E. coli* by *uidA* and 23S, Enterococci by 23S, *Bacteroides-Prevotella* by HuBac) markers from 23 samples collected over 23 weekend days from 2009 using qPCR and paired them with human exposure data.

Ethics Statement

Approvals for the study design, questionnaires, verbal consent procedures, and related materials were obtained from the Institutional Review Board (IRB) at The Ohio State University (IRB Protocol #2009H0107). For this study, adult participants (18 years of age or older) capable of providing verbal consent were welcomed into the study by investigators or key personnel trained and authorized by the university to obtain consent. The written consent waiver permitting verbal consent was granted given the low study risk and because written consent would have required surname information and the gathering of consent documentation in a periodically windy and wet beach environment. Thus, written consent procedures would have increased the likelihood of losing or damaging documentation which would have then included participant surnames that could potentially be matched with telephone numbers and health data. Verbal consent was recorded on the datasheet for each household interviewed. In addition, participants were provided with a card sharing contact information for the principal investigator and the ethics coordinator in the Office of Responsible Research Practices at the university.

Enrollment and Exposure Survey

The East Fork Beach Study [26] recruited beach user households into the study at the beach and interviewed them upon their departure to ascertain information regarding their activities at the beach on that same day. For each household in the study, an adult spokesperson provided investigators with information requested from a standard script. The obtained information was used for classifying exposure status and obtaining information related to potential confounding variables (age, gender, ethnicity, food consumption, source of food/drink, number of beach visits per year, duration of time at the beach, hand hygiene, extent of sand exposure, distance traveled, and number of other beach users). More specifically, individuals were asked whether any household members had: (1) no water contact; (2) waded, played or swam in the water; and/or (3) immersed their head in the water. Questions pertaining to any recent or on-going illnesses were also asked. Individual beach users were dichotomously classified as having or not having each of the above-mentioned exposures as well as any prevalent symptoms of gastrointestinal illness. These exposure data were recently paired with date-specific *E. coli* genetic marker density data to further establish our exposure classification of each beach user.

Health Outcomes Survey

Health outcome data were obtained by Marion et al. [26] in which enrolled households were contacted eight to nine days after their beach visit via telephone. Only adult household members who were at the beach at the time of enrollment were eligible for interview participation. Interviews were conducted using a standard questionnaire inquiring about illness among household members at the beach at the time of enrollment. Reported illnesses were recorded as a yes/no response for a variety of symptoms (e.g., stomach cramps, nausea, diarrhea, vomiting, headache, fever, etc.) for each person who visited the beach. For comparing with other studies, persons were further classified by gastrointestinal illness. Similar to the Wade et al. studies [3,4], persons were defined to have experienced "GI illness" if they were reported to have had any one of the following: nausea, stomach ache or stomach cramps, diarrhea (three or more loose or watery stools in a 24-hour period), or vomiting. With respect to nausea, all persons in this study who reported nausea were considered positive for GI illness. This GI illness definition is slightly different than the Wade et al. studies [3,4], which only included nausea cases into their GI illness definition when the condition interfered with daily activities. In our study, we were unable to make this distinction as we did not ascertain if the nausea interfered with daily activities. Beyond the "GI Illness" definition, using the highly credible gastrointestinal illness (HCGI) definition employed by Colford [5] as "HCGI-1", we likewise coded individuals as positive for HCGI if they were reported to have experienced any of the following: (1) vomiting; (2) diarrhea and fever, (3) stomach-ache and fever, or (4) nausea and fever.

Sample Collection and Water Analysis

Beach water samples used for obtaining genetic marker data were collected on the same day as enrollment and administration of the exposure questionnaire on summer weekends during the time of day generally used for swimming. In total, 91% of samples were collected at the median time of 13:45±3 h. Two samples

(9%) were collected after 16:00 on days when daily swimming attendance was low (n = 4, n = 28) in anticipation of more swimmers late in the day. For each day, 3 L was collected into multiple autoclaved 500 mL bottles (Nalgene, Rochester, NY, USA) and sterile Whirl-Pak bags (Nasco, Fort Atkinson, WI, USA) over 23 weekend days. Samples were collected near the beach center in water with an approximate depth of one meter by sweeping containers 30 cm below the water surface. Within 30 minutes after collection, a 1 L sample aliquot was used for membrane filtration for culturable *E. coli*, a 1 L sample aliquot was temporarily stored (24–48 h) at 4°C and then immediately filtered for bacterial marker analysis, and a 1 L aliquot was stored at −20°C for virus analysis.

E. coli densities were quantified for three separate filtration volumes (20, 50, and 100 mL) for each sample using the culture-based method described in EPA Method 1603 [27] and Marion et al. [26]. Other water quality parameters including temperature, pH, dissolved oxygen, and turbidity were also measured using a YSI 600XL data sonde (Yellow Springs Instruments, Yellow Springs, Ohio, U.S.A.) and a Hach 2100P Turbidimeter (Loveland, Colorado, U.S.A.) as described in Marion et al. [26]. UV index data were obtained from the National Oceanic and Atmospheric Administration [28]. Rainfall, lake stage (surface elevation), and lake inflow data were obtained from the U.S. Army Corps of Engineers [29].

A detailed description of sample preparation, water concentration, and quantification of the bacterial and viral marker densities by qPCR is provided as (**Text S1**), including a description of the primers and probes used in this study (**Table S1**). In brief, samples were filtered to capture bacteria for quantifying the following bacterial markers: *uid*A genes (uidA) and 23S rRNA genes (23S *E. coli*) of *E. coli*, 16S rRNA genes of *Bacteroides-Prevotella* (HuBac), and 23S rRNA genes of *Enterococcus* spp. (23S *Enterococcus*). For concentrating viruses (HEntV, HAdV, HNoV GI, and HNoV GII), membrane filtration was performed using cation (Al^{3+})-coated membranes. DNA or RNA was then extracted from the microbes captured on the membranes using a QIAmp DNA Stool Kit or the RNeasy Mini Kit (Qiagen, Valencia, CA, USA), respectively. RNA extracts for HEntV were amplified by reverse transcription (RT)-PCR and quantified using TaqMan real-time RT-PCR (RT-qPCR) with the QIAGEN OneStep RT-PCR Kit (Qiagen, Valencia, CA, USA). DNA extracts for HAdV and all bacterial markers were amplified by PCR and quantified using a TaqMan-based real-time qPCR system. All RT-qPCR and qPCR reactions except HNoV GI and HNoV GII were carried out in an ABI 48-well StepOne Real Time System (Applied Biosystems, Foster City, CA). RT-qPCR assays for HNoV GI and HNoV GII were carried out with an Eppendorf Mastercycler RealPlex² (Eppendorf, Germany). Quantification of the markers was then determined using standard curves generated by plotting Ct values (y) versus the log gene copy numbers of the target microbes (x) and each limit of detection (LOD) was determined based on the lowest gene copy number from which above 90% of the replicates could be amplified in each qPCR assay. Additionally, with regards to these samples, the presence/absence of qPCR inhibition was previously evaluated for East Fork samples [20] using the Sketa22 qPCR assay as described in Haugland et al. [30].

Data Analysis

The analysis focused on healthy susceptible individuals, and persons who were classified as prevalent or existing cases based upon responses to the enrollment questionnaire were excluded in analyses using incident cases. Logistic regression was employed to evaluate crude associations between genetic marker exposure and new illness among swimmers reporting head immersion. The data for the microbiological terms, including *E. coli* density data, were skewed, accordingly they were log (base 10)-transformed. Prior to log-transforming *E. coli* results, samples with 0 CFU/100 mL were assigned a value of 1 CFU/100 mL. In scatterplots and models containing genetic marker densities, for markers not detected after 45 cycles, densities were assigned a value of half the detection limit in log CFUs per 100 mL or log gene equivalents (GE) per 100 mL for bacterial and viral markers, respectively.

Multivariable logistic regression was used for estimating odds ratios for any GI illness, diarrhea, and HCGI among swimmers and non-swimmers (negative controls) as recommended in observational studies [31] and done by Colford et al. [9] in their beach user health study. The swimmer population was defined as beach users who reported immersing their head in the beach water. Non-swimmers were defined as beach users reporting no water contact or limited water contact that did not include head immersion in the beach water. All swimmers were assumed to have been exposed to the same density of *E. coli* and the various genetic markers observed from the single sample collection for that day. Densities of *E. coli* and the various genetic markers were determined from the single mid-day water sample collection.

The multivariable logistic regression models considered potential confounders and/or modifying influences, including covariates related to demographic, exposure, meteorological, and water quality factors. Since data were obtained from households, for the purpose of statistical analysis, the data were treated as clustered by household [32]. For constructing multivariable models, a backward selection approach was employed whereby covariates were dropped stepwise based on the highest p-value until arriving at the most parsimonious model [32]. The rule of ten events (cases) per covariate was used in logistic regression modeling [33]. Due to the low frequency of HCGI cases, HCGI model construction was limited to only two microbiological terms by relaxing the rule of ten events per covariate [34].

Multivariable logistic regression models were evaluated for fit via the Hosmer-Lemeshow Goodness-of-Fit Test [32] and for model discrimination via the area under the receiver-operating-characteristic curve (AUC) [32]. The modeling efforts and assessments of logistic model fit and discrimination were performed using Stata 11 (Stata Corporation, College Station, TX, USA). A time-series plot was generated with Minitab 16 (Minitab Inc., State College, PA, USA).

Results

Water Quality

Among the 23 weekend water samples collected for qPCR analysis, bacterial markers were more readily detected than viruses (Table 1). HEntV and HAdV were detected in 22% (5/23) and 35% (8/23) of all samples, respectively, whereas, HNoV GI and GII were not detected (0/23). As previously reported [20], qPCR inhibition was not observed in any of the 23 samples. Culturable *E. coli* densities greater than 0 CFU/100 mL were observed in 91% (21/23) of all samples. The time-series plot of culturable *E. coli* and HAdV densities by day (Figure 1) demonstrate the lack of association between the two water quality parameters, which was confirmed by correlation analysis (Spearman's $\rho = 0.147$; $p = 0.503$). Overall, culturable *E. coli* densities exceeded Ohio single-day maximum criteria (>235 CFU/100 mL) in 8.6% (2/23) of our samples; however, no beach advisories were issued by local or state authorities due to their adherence to the one sample per week guideline used by the Ohio Department of Health for

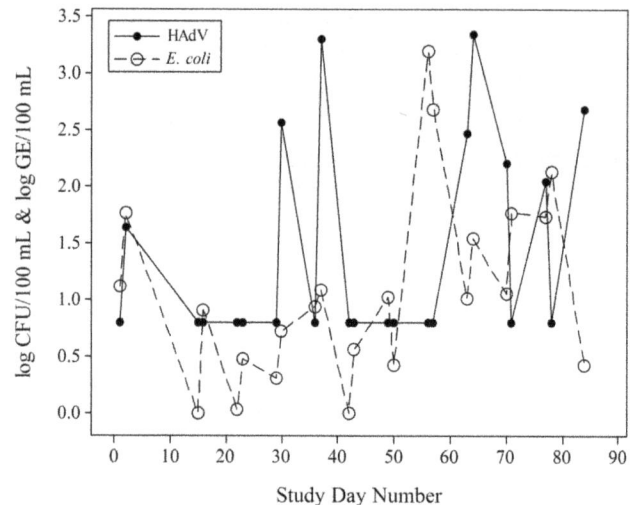

Figure 1. Time series plot for HAdV and *E. coli* densities measured during the 2009 swimming season at the study beach (East Fork Lake, Ohio).

inland waters. Other water quality parameters are summarized in Marion et al. [26].

Study Population

A total of 891 individuals were included in this study (from 278 households). The study population was 93% white, 2.5% black, 1% Hispanic and 3.5% other. The average study participant age was 24 years (median $= 21$ years). Young children (≤ 5 years) represented 13% of the participants on whom data were available. Females were more represented (56%) than males (44%). The population described in this report is a subset of the 965 individuals from 300 households in our previous study [26], which was conducted over 26 weekend days. Genetic marker data were only obtained for 23 of 26 days of the 2009 East Fork Beach Study [26], and accordingly, this study reports the results of the investigation using genetic marker data. The collection of sufficient water for obtaining qPCR data was an additional task added to the previous study on the third sample day.

Among the participants in this study, 618 (69%) individuals reported head immersion in East Fork beach waters. Prevalent GI illness was reported for 18 (2.9%) of these swimmers at enrollment (Table 2). Chronic GI problems were self-reported at enrollment in 9 (50%) of these 18 individuals. All 18 individuals with prevalent GI illness (including chronic GI problems) were excluded from the exposure-related illness models. The prevalence of fever, nausea, and stomach cramping among participants was not ascertained at enrollment.

Water Quality and Human Illness

The qPCR-based densities for bacteria and viruses do not show any significant associations ($p < 0.05$) with HCGI, GI, and diarrhea in single marker models using univariable and multivariable logistic regression when treating marker densities as continuous terms or binary terms in models (Table 3). Among all the continuous terms, HAdV had the strongest association with HCGI (crude OR (cOR) $= 1.6$; 95% CI 0.90–2.9) and diarrhea (adjusted OR (aOR) $= 1.5$; 95% CI 0.98–2.4); however, these associations were not significant but were noteworthy ($p = 0.105$; $p = 0.066$, respectively). When evaluating the association of either HEntV or HAdV detection with HCGI, GI, and diarrhea

Table 1. Microbial water quality measured by various genetic markers and *E. coli* at East Fork Lake, Ohio (N = 23).

Genetic Marker or Fecal Indicator	No. Samples Above LOD[a]	Detection Limit	Median	Range
HAdV (log gene equivalents/100 mL)	8	1.6	BD[b]	BD-3.34
HEntV (log gene equivalents/100 mL)	5	1.9	BD	BD-2.13
uidA (log copies/100 mL)	19	1.5	2.08	1.50-2.49
23S *E. coli* (log copies/100 mL)	19	2.46	2.94	2.46-3.19
HuBac (log copies/100 mL)	18	2.05	3.04	2.05-3.39
23S *Enterococcus* (log copies/100 mL)	17	1.93	2.19	1.93-2.88
E. coli (log CFU/100 mL)	21	ND[c]	1.01	LOD-3.19

[a]Limit of Detection or 0 CFU/100 mL for *E. coli*.
[b]Below Detection.
[c]Not Determined.

incidence, no association was observed ($p>0.05$). The covariates used in the illness models are summarized in **Table S2** and **Table S3**, respectively. The most significant covariate, food consumption at the beach (see **Table S2** and **Table S3**), was used in all genetic marker and *E. coli* models except the HCGI model, as food consumption at the beach was common to all HCGI cases. Beyond food consumption at the beach, specific conductivity and previous 72-hour UV results were the most significant covariates in all of the GI illness models. With respect to the diarrhea illness model, food consumption and previous 72-hour UV data were used as covariates, as they were identified as most significant through the backward elimination approach. In evaluating HCGI models relying on two microbiological terms, the only two-term model achieving significance was a combined model using HAdV and culturable *E. coli* ($p = 0.003$; likelihood ratio test). None of the bacterial markers were significant predictors of HCGI in models using an additional marker.

Using this same bacteria and virus approach for GI illness, we observed a similar association. Since more GI cases were detected than HCGI, the model was able to contain an additional two covariates. In this model, significant ($p<0.05$) or near significant odds ratios ($p = 0.056$) were observed for all covariates in this model (Table 4), including food consumption, specific conductiv-

ity, *E. coli*, and HAdV. Increases in water conductivity were associated with protective effects (aOR<1); whereas, food consumption, increasing HAdV, and increasing *E. coli* were identified as risk factors for GI (aOR>1). The use of two microbial terms was supported in model building as the removal of the HAdV term resulted in significantly lower log-likelihood values for HCGI, GI, and diarrheal models ($p<0.05$), and the two microbial terms had the low p-values throughout the entire backward selection procedure allowing their retention in the model. The final four-term model was evaluated using a negative control group (the non-swimmer group), and no significant associations were observed for any model terms, suggesting no day-effects, and implying a water quality-related association in our exposed group. Lastly, all possible models for predicting GI illness using a single bacterial marker in tandem with either culturable *E. coli* or viral marker levels were developed, and no bacterial markers were associated with illness.

Models constructed for predicting diarrhea using *E. coli* and HAdV preliminarily indicate that HAdV is associated with diarrheal disease incidence as the aOR for HAdV was significant ($p = 0.023$) when adjusting *E. coli* density by including *E. coli* density in the model. Compared to the HCGI and GI models, the diarrheal model provided poor discrimination (AUC <0.70) with

Table 2. Health status among study participants at enrollment and follow-up.

Reported Health Outcomes	Swimmers (n = 618)		Non-Swimmers (n = 274)	
	Health Status at Beach Enrollment (No. (%))	Health Status at Follow-up[a] (No. (%))	Health Status at Beach Enrollment (No. (%))	Health Status at Follow-up[a] (No. (%))
No Reported GI Problems	600 (97)	562 (94)	259 (95)	251 (97)
Any GI Illness	18 (2.9)	38 (6.3)	15 (5.5)	8 (3.1)
Chronic GI Problems	9 (1.5)	ND[b]	8 (2.9)	ND[b]
Diarrhea	6 (0.97)	28 (4.6)	5 (1.8)	8 (3.1)
Fever	ND	10 (1.6)	ND	2 (0.73)
Stomach Cramps	ND	8 (1.2)	ND	8 (1.2)
Nausea + Other GI Illness	ND	7 (1.2)	ND	1 (0.36)
Nausea Only	ND	3 (0.50)	ND	0 (0.00)
Vomiting	6 (0.97)	10 (1.6)	3 (1.1)	1 (0.36)
HCGI	ND	13 (2.2)	267 (97)	1 (0.37)

[a]Health status at telephone follow-up excluding positive cases at enrollment.
Not determined as information was not collected by the questionnaire.

Table 3. Odds ratios for HCGI, GI, and diarrhea associated with exposure to varying levels of various molecular genetic markers and/or fecal indicators at East Fork Lake, Ohio.

Molecular Marker	HCGI		Any GI Illness		Diarrhea	
	cOR[a] (95% CI)	Wald (p)	aOR[b] (95% CI)	Wald (p)	aOR (95% CI)	Wald (p)
HEntV (+)[c]	1.6 (0.34–7.6)	0.552	0.76 (0.21–2.7)	0.674	0.17 (0.02–1.3)	0.081
HAdV (+)	2.1 (0.65–7.1)	0.212	1.3 (0.45–3.5)	0.654	2.2 (0.65–7.6)	0.202
uidA E. coli (+)	1.1 (0.22–5.4)	0.892	0.78 (0.27–2.2)	0.637	0.88 (0.24–3.2)	0.843
23S E. coli (+)	0.69 (0.18–2.7)	0.595	0.78 (0.30–2.0)	0.599	1.1 (0.31–3.8)	0.905
HuBac (+)	1.5 (0.32–7.1)	0.604	1.1 (0.38–3.2)	0.846	0.86 (0.25–2.9)	0.815
23S Enterococcus (+)	0.70 (0.21–2.4)	0.586	0.77 (0.27–2.2)	0.613	0.58 (0.18–1.9)	0.363
Log HAdV	1.6 (0.90–2.9)	0.105	1.2 (0.77–1.9)	0.399	1.5 (0.97–2.4)	0.066
Log uidA E. coli	1.0 (0.38–2.9)	0.927	0.76 (0.38–1.5)	0.442	0.98 (0.34–2.9)	0.974
Log 23S E. coli	0.78 (0.38–1.6)	0.489	0.85 (0.50–1.4)	0.526	1.2 (0.48–3.2)	0.648
Log HuBac	1.5 (0.63–3.7)	0.355	1.1 (0.67–1.8)	0.7	0.78 (0.49–1.2)	0.289
Log 23S Enterococcus	0.96 (0.38–2.4)	0.921	0.89 (0.49–1.6)	0.714	0.67 (0.37–1.2)	0.207

[a]Crude odds ratio.
[b]Adjusted odds ratios, see Table S2 and S3, to see the covariates used for adjustment.
[c](+), Positive detection by qPCR, binary term.

respect to the ability of the model to properly classify diarrhea cases (Table 5). The Goodness-of-Fit test results (Table 5) also demonstrate the GI and HCGI models have better fits, as the p-values for those models are higher, indicating that the modeled results are not significantly different than the observed GI and HCGI results from the health survey.

For considering possible interaction effects, a water quality index was constructed based upon the detection limit of HAdV and the median E. coli density. Table 6 presents the four water quality index values, and the respective E. coli and HAdV densities represented by each water quality index level. When evaluating associations for this model, the reference was set as the

Table 4. Multivariable logistic regression models for predicting new HCGI[a], GI, and diarrhea among swimmers immersing their head and beachgoers not immersing their head in beach water (East Fork Lake, Ohio).

Model & Exposure	Covariate	β	SE_β	Wald (p)	AOR (95% CI)
HCGI Swimmers	Log HAdV (gene equivalents/100 mL)	0.8191	0.2864	0.005	2.3 (1.3–3.9)
	Log E. coli (CFU/100 mL)	1.101	0.3571	0.002	3.0 (1.5–6.1)
	Constant Term	−7.003			
GI Swimmers	Log HAdV (gene equivalents/100 mL)	0.421	0.1978	0.034	1.5 (1.0–2.2)
	Log E. coli (CFU/100 mL)	0.6515	0.2473	0.009	1.9 (1.2–3.1)
	Consumed Food at the Beach	1.543	0.7019	0.029	4.7 (1.2–19)
	Specific Conductivity (µS)	−0.092	0.0477	0.056	0.91 (0.83–1.0)
	Constant Term	19.37			
GI Non-Swimmers	Log HAdV (gene equivalents/100 mL)	0.0788	0.5481	0.886	1.1 (0.37–3.2)
	Log E. coli (CFU/100 mL)	0.2675	0.3346	0.425	1.3 (0.67–2.5)
	Consumed Food at the Beach	0.4254	0.8889	0.633	1.5 (0.26–8.9)
	Specific Conductivity (µS)	0.04	0.0279	0.154	1.0 (0.98–1.1)
	Constant Term	−15.33			
Diarrhea Swimmers	Log HAdV (gene equivalents/100 mL)	0.453	0.1977	0.023	1.6 (1.1–2.3)
	Log E. coli (CFU/100 mL)	0.3275	0.2466	0.186	1.4 (0.85–2.3)
	Constant Term	−4.226			
Diarrhea Non-Swimmers	Log HAdV (gene equivalents/100 mL)	0.0034	0.4905	0.994	1.0 (0.38–2.6)
	Log E. coli (CFU/100 mL)	0.2309	0.336	0.493	1.3 (0.65–2.4)
	Constant Term	−3.735			

[a]A model could not be constructed for HCGI among non-swimmers due to the low sample size resulting in an insufficient number of HCGI cases for model development.

Table 5. Model diagnostics for models from Table 4, pertaining to discrimination (AUC) and model calibration (goodness-of-fit).

Model Name for Swimmers	AUC[a]	Goodness-of-Fit[b] (p)
Multivariable HCGI Model	0.75	0.895
Multivariable GI Model	0.753	0.958
Multivariable Diarrhea Model	0.64	0.206

[a]Area under the receiver-operator-characteristic curve (AUC).
[b]Hosmer-Lemeshow Goodness-of-Fit Test [32].

group of days in which *E. coli* densities were lowest and HAdV was not detected. Here we observe multiple associations with increasing viral and/or bacteria densities and both GI and diarrheal illness incidence. Swimmers with the presumed greatest exposure to *E. coli* and HAdV had the greatest odds of reporting new GI illness (OR = 6.1; 95% CI 1.5–25) compared to swimmers with the least exposure to *E. coli* and HAdV. Exposure to the highest levels of *E. coli* when HAdV levels were low also presented increased GI illness risk (OR = 5.4; 95% CI 1.5–19) compared to those swimmers with low *E. coli* and low HAdV exposure. In the diarrheal illness model, significantly increased odds of diarrhea were only observed in the group who swam on days with elevated *E. coli* and HAdV compared to the reference group (OR = 5.2; 1.3–22). Model discrimination for each model (GI and diarrhea) was evaluated and the AUC values were 0.63 and 0.65, respectively.

Discussion

This prospective cohort study from an inland U.S. beach demonstrates the predictive potential of an integrative, multi-microbial approach for estimating recreational waterborne disease risk from viral and bacterial indicators. The term 'indicator' used here does not imply fecal indicator, but instead refers to 'health-relevant' indicators. Our results showed a positive association between increasing densities of individual health-relevant indicators (HAdV and *E. coli*) and increased odds of GI and HCGI among swimmers at the studied beach. More importantly, the two-indicator model (HAdV and *E. coli*) represented a significant improvement over single health indicator approaches with this data. Although speculative, particularly due to the small sample size of the study, the findings of this two-indicator approach are etiologically plausible as a combined viral + bacterial (ViBac) approach may account for GI and HCGI illness associations with viral and bacterial pathogens. Based upon our cohort study results, we have some reason to speculate that a multiple health-indicator approach may be beneficial for natural recreational waters such as

the East Fork beach, which is part of a watershed comprised of mixed land uses and a high density of septic systems, all of which may promote a more diffuse type of fecal contamination than observed in point-source impacted waters. Within the beach watershed of interest, two municipal wastewater treatment plants (Williamsburg and Bethel WWTPs) and several smaller WWTPs operate, while malfunctioning septic systems are presumed to be a very significant source of contamination [35]. In the East Fork of the Little Miami River watershed, which includes the study beach, the septic system density in sub-catchments has been directly linked to human-associated fecal contamination through the use of human-associated genetic markers [35]. The only Harsha Lake (East Fork Lake) tributary investigated by Peed et al. [35] had the highest mean human-specific marker (HF183) density and the second highest density of septic systems ($41/km^2$) among tributaries investigated suggesting diffuse septic system-associated fecal contamination impacts this beach.

In health studies of swimmers in waters impacted by nonpoint source and/or diffuse fecal contamination, the lack of association between bacteria-based genetic markers and human illness has been observed [5,6,10,16]. Similarly, we did not observe associations between qPCR-based bacterial densities and human illness at our inland freshwater beach. The association of culturable *E. coli* with HCGI and GI was already observed [26], but the lack of association of GI and HCGI with human-specific genetic markers (e.g., HuBac) was unknown in this study population. Two possible reasons for our findings are as follows: (1) transport and fate varies considerably between bacterial genetic markers and viable waterborne pathogens, including viruses; and/or (2) our sample size was not big enough to detect significant associations.

With respect to viruses at the beaches with diffuse contamination, male-specific coliphage density has been associated with HCGI and GI illness in marine studies [5,16]. Similarly, our study observed an association between a virus (HAdV) and GI illness; however, unlike the marine studies, our study did not evaluate

Table 6. Odds ratios for GI and diarrhea associated with exposure to varying levels of HAdV and *E. coli* at East Fork Lake, Ohio.

Water Quality Index	Any GI Illness			Diarrhea		
	Cases/*n* (%)	OR (95% CI)	Wald (p)	Cases/*n* (%)	OR (95% CI)	Wald (p)
Group 1: Low HAdV & Low *E. coli* (HAdV <DL[a], log *E. coli* <1.05)	3/187 (1.6)	Referent		3/189 (1.6)	Referent	
Group 2: Low HAdV & High *E. coli* (HAdV <DL, log *E. coli*>1.05)	16/199 (8.0)	**5.4 (1.5–19)**	**0.011**	9/199 (4.5)	2.9 (0.74–12)	0.126
Group 3: High HAdV & Low *E. coli* (HAdV> DL, log *E. coli* <1.05)	11/126 (8.7)	5.9 (0.88–39)	0.067	9/127 (7.1)	4.7 (0.56–40)	0.153
Group 4: High HAdV & High *E. coli* (HAdV> DL, log *E. coli*>1.05)	8/88 (9.0)	**6.1 (1.5–25)**	**0.011**	7/90 (7.8)	**5.2 (1.3–22)**	**0.023**

[a]Detection Limit.

coliphages, focusing solely on viral pathogens. Like the associations between coliphages and illness [5,16], our finding of HAdV associations with HCGI and GI incidence in the adjusted models [Table 4] preliminarily suggests a possible benefit of using a viral indicator for evaluating recreational water illness risk in certain environments.

Similar to the Colford et al. study [5], human noroviruses (HNoV GI and HNoV GII) were not detected; however, human adenoviruses (HAdV) were detected from eight (35%) samples at East Fork versus one detection in the Colford et al. study [5]. The infrequent detection of HEntV (22%) in our study is not entirely unexpected as enteroviruses have been observed at densities below 1 PFU/100 mL in European waters [36] and have been infrequently detected (9% of samples) elsewhere [37]. These findings are similar to earlier findings from Fleisher et al. [14] that determined positive enterovirus detection (by cell culture) was less likely than negative detection in United Kingdom waters, which was also described as a limitation of the utility of the enterovirus assay for swimming advisory determination. The low detection frequency of viruses coupled with practicality of measurement presents challenges for establishing their use unless monitored in tandem with other indicators of water quality. Their use in a monitoring scheme may complement fecal indicator bacteria which have not effectively predicted viral densities in freshwater and marine environments [17,21,38,39]. Among viruses, adenovirus has shown promise as a potential human-associated marker of fecal contamination, whereby adenovirus presence has been linked to human-associated fecal problems as reflected by human-associated bacterial markers [40,41].

Despite a lack of association between viruses and bacteria, swimming advisories are primarily bacteria-based for practical reasons. Furthermore, there appears to be growing consensus among experts suggesting viruses are responsible for many water-related illnesses [18,19,42]. It is becoming more widely understood that enteric viruses (e.g., noroviruses, rotaviruses) are responsible for a substantial number of GI illnesses among U.S. beach users [18]. With viruses gaining attention and being more frequently measured, approaches for monitoring viruses to support integrative health risk models for water-associated illnesses are meaningful. Viral indicators of GI illness, particularly enteroviruses and bacteriophages, were described as promising predictors in 2003 by Wade et al. [2], but were also described as being limited by the difficulty and time for cultivation and enumeration. Now, with increasing use of molecular approaches such as qPCR, viral detection and enumeration is becoming less difficult and more rapid. In less contaminated or nonpoint source impacted waters, the use of a more commonly detected virus, like HAdV, may serve as an effective viral marker over noroviruses or enteroviruses for beach monitoring, since the detection frequency of adenovirus (36%) has been observed to be much greater than norovirus detection (9%) in European water samples [41,43].

The low detection frequency of norovirus in our samples and elsewhere may involve RNA virus instability, unstable DNA amplification potential from single-stranded RNA, and virus seasonality since the most prevalent human norovirus (GII.4) has clear winter peak seasonality [44] and therefore is less likely to be observed in summer surface waters. Unlike HNoV and HEntV, HAdV is a double-stranded DNA virus presumed to have better stability in environments and greater opportunities for successful detects. Furthermore, adenoviruses are believed to be up to 60 times more resistant to damage from ultraviolet irradiation than RNA viruses [45] likely affording HAdV particles greater integrity and viability leading to more undamaged infectious particles [46]. Given detection frequencies, Wyn-Jones et al. [41] encourages the

consideration of adenovirus over norovirus as a recreational water quality indicator

Accordingly, water quality advisories should be protective for preventing human illness from all potential infectious agents as deemed practical with the available methods. The need for bacteria-based indicators of health risk are warranted, as the historical paradigm supports the notion that individual fecal indicators like *E. coli* and enterococci as well as human-specific markers explain the potential pathogenic bacterial genera (*Shigella, Camplyobacter, Salmonella,* etc.) as well as gastrointestinal illness among swimmers. However, the need for data attempting to address and/or quantify viral-associated human health risks is significant, and some attempt has recently been made using a site-specific quantitative microbial risk assessment (QMRA) for adenovirus illness [47]. Although speculative, virus monitoring may be beneficial in recreational waters where the contamination sources of the aquatic system are complex and impacted by a combination of non-point source human-associated contamination as well as agricultural runoff, as in Kundu et al. [47]. The concept of 'know your beach' appears to be particularly important as it relates to water quality when fecal indicator bacteria are low, and some consideration to broadening the paradigm to include multiple microbiological terms may be warranted with further research, with a particular emphasis on viruses capable of predicting recreational water illnesses more efficiently. Similar approaches demonstrating the value of a holistic design, like our combined virus-bacteria model, for enhancing risk assessments pertaining to water are already gaining attention in microbial source tracking studies using toolbox approaches [22]. Beyond water quality analysis, additional assessments of other known exposures presenting health risks, such as sand quality [48] and hydrology [49] are also recommended to be considered for more holistic beach condition modeling [25]. In this study, our integrative risk model using two microbiological terms, a fecal indicator bacteria and a viral genetic marker, provided a better assessment of human health risk than any single indicator/marker approach with limited data. Additional epidemiological studies using HAdV or other indicators of viral contamination that control for illnesses explained by bacteria are warranted for improving our predictive capability of swimming-related illness as well as our characterization of water quality at inland beaches.

Study Limitations

Future studies with larger populations are needed for drawing less speculative conclusions. The total swimmer population after exclusion is relatively small (n = 600) for rigorous analysis and may be leading us to spurious conclusions. Given the low number of cases presented, model construction was limited to two to four covariates, which therefore limited our ability to adequately assess multiple confounders, interaction effects, and linearity. The cohort study approach used here and in other U.S. studies [1,3,4] also presents several methodological limitations [50] related to potential misclassification of exposure and disease among study participants. We acknowledge a variety of confounders (assessed and not assessed) may be responsible for GI illness cases beyond adverse water quality conditions, such as food consumption at the beach. For example, personal risk perceptions were not measured in this study, which have been linked to self-reported illness among swimmers in other studies [15]. To reduce self-selection bias among swimmers, this study performed modeling comparing swimmers in various exposure groups to a low exposure swimmer group. Exposure misclassification is also relevant, particularly if beach water quality varies significantly throughout each study day which would limit reliable exposure estimates from a single daily sampling effort. Lastly, illness misclassification relying on self-reported information was more likely in this study than in studies using direct follow-up examinations.

Despite this sample size limitation, several constructed models did provide acceptable discrimination (AUC>0.70; Table 5) and acceptable model fit, particularly the HCGI and GI models from Table 4. Although the study presents several limitations, the study likely represents the only prospective epidemiological investigation exploring HAdV associations with recreational water-associated illness at this important beach type (inland lake recreational water). Future studies with larger samples sizes are warranted, particularly in beach environments where fecal contamination is human-associated and from dispersed sources or a mixture of point and dispersed sources.

Conclusions

- No association was observed between exposure to various qPCR-measured bacterial markers and recreational water-associated illness among study participants.
- Increasing levels of qPCR-measured HAdV were associated with increased odds of recreational water-associated gastrointestinal illness among the swimmers.
- Combined measurement of HAdV and culturable *E. coli* densities potentially enhances recreational water illness prediction among swimmers.
- Future studies with larger sample sizes enabling adjustment for additional confounding variables are needed to permit more robust investigations of human illness associations with exposures to HAdV and other viral markers in recreational water environments.

References

1. Dufour A (1984) Health Effects Criteria for Fresh Recreational Waters. U.S. Environmental Protection Agency Report EPA-600-1-84-2004. Cincinnati, OH: U.S. Environmental Protection Agency, Office of Research and Development Available: http://www.epa.gov/nerlcwww/documents/frc.pdf. Accessed 2014 June 19.
2. Wade TJ, Pai N, Eisenberg JN, Colford JMJ (2003) Do U.S. Environmental Protection Agency water quality guidelines for recreational waters prevent gastrointestinal illness? A systematic review and meta-analysis. Environ Health Perspect 111: 1102–1109.
3. Wade TJ, Calderon RL, Sams E, Beach M, Brenner KP, et al. (2006) Rapidly measured indicators of recreational water quality are predictive of swimming-associated gastrointestinal illness. Environ Health Perspect 114 (1): 24–28. doi: 10.1289%2Fehp.8273.
4. Wade TJ, Sams E, Brenner KP, Haugland R, Chem E, et al. (2010) Rapidly measured indicators of recreational water quality and swimming-associated illness at marine beaches: a prospective cohort study. Environmental Health 9:66. doi: 10.1186/1476-069X-9-66.
5. Colford JM, Wade TJ, Schiff KC, Wright CC, Griffith JF, et al. (2007) Water quality indicators and the risk of illness at beaches with nonpoint sources of fecal contamination. Epidemiology . 18 (1), 27–35. doi: 10.1097/01.ede.0000249425.32990.b9.
6. Sinigalliano CD, Fleisher JM, Gidley ML, Solo-Gabriele HM, Shibata T, et al. (2010) Traditional and molecular analyses for fecal indicator bacteria in non-point source recreational marine waters. Water Res 44 (13): 3763–3772. doi: dx.doi.org/10.1016/j.watres.2010.04.026.
7. Gruber SJ, Kay LM, Kolb R, Henry K (2005) Mission Bay bacterial source identification study. Stormwater 6: 40–51.
8. Soller JA, Schoen ME, Bartrand T, Ravenscroft J, Ashbolt NJ (2010) Estimated human health risks from exposure to recreational waters impacted by human and non-human sources of faecal contamination. Water Res 44 (16): 4674–4691. doi: 10.1016/j.watres.2010.06.049.
9. Colford JM, Schiff KC, Griffith JF, Yau V, Arnold BF, et al. (2012) Using rapid indicators for Enterococcus to assess the risk of illness after exposure to urban runoff contaminated marine water. Water Res 46 (7): 2176–2186. doi: 10.1016/j.watres.2012.01.033.
10. Arnold BF, Schiff KC, Griffith JF, Gruber JS, Yau V, et al. (2013) Swimmer illness associated with marine water exposure and water quality indicators: impact of widely used assumptions. Epidemiology 24 (6): 845–853. doi: 10.1097/01.ede.0000434431.06765.4a.
11. Yau VM, Schiff KC, Arnold BF, Griffith JF, Gruber JS, et al. (2014) Effect of submarine discharge on bacterial indicators and swimmer health at Avalon Beach, CA, USA. Water Res 59: 23–36. doi: 10.1016/j.watres.2014.03.050.
12. Fewtrell L, Jones F, Tech B, Kay D, Wyer MD, et al. (1992) Health effects of white-water canoeing. Lancet 339 (8809): 1587–1589. doi:10.1016/0140-6736(92)91843-W.
13. Pike E (1994) Health Effects of Sea Swimming, Phase III – Final Report to the Department of the Environment. WRC Report: DoE 3412/2. Medmenham, U.K. UK: Water Research Center. pp 9–24.
14. Fleisher JM, Kay D, Salmon RL, Jones F, Wyer MD, et al. (1996) Marine waters contaminated with domestic sewage: nonenteric illnesses associated with swimmer exposure in the United Kingdom. Am J Public Health 86 (9): 1228–1234.
15. Fleisher JM, Fleming LE, Solo-Gabriele HM, Kish JK, Sinigalliano D, et al. (2010) The BEACHES Study: health effects and exposures from non-point source microbial contaminants in subtropical recreational marine waters. Int J Epidemiol 39 (5): 1291–1298. doi: 10.1093/ije/dyq084.
16. Abdelzaher AM, Wright ME, Ortega C, Hasan AR, Shibata T, et al. (2011) Daily measures of microbes and human health at a non-point source marine beach. J Water Health 9 (3): 443–457. DOI:10.2166/wh.2011.146Griffen DW, Donaldson KA, Paul JH, Rose JB (2003) Pathogenic human viruses in coastal waters. Clin Microbiol Rev 16 (1): 129–143. doi: 10.1128/CMR.16.1.129-143.2003.
17. Hlavsa MC, Roberts VA, Anderson AR, Hill VR, Kahler AM, et al. (2011) Surveillance for Waterborne Disease Outbreaks and Other Health Events Associated with Recreational Water -United States, 2007-2008. MMWR 60 (ss12): 1–32.
18. Soller JA, Bartrand T, Ashbolt NJ, Ravenscroft J, Wade TJ (2010). Estimating the primary etiologic agents in recreational freshwaters impacted by human sources of fecal contamination. Water Res 44 (16): 4736–4747. doi: 10.1016/j.watres.2010.07.064.
19. Dorevitch S, Pratap P, Wroblewski M, Hryhorczuk DO, Li H, et al. (2012) Health risks of limited-contact water recreation. Environ Health Perspect 120 (2): 192–197. doi: 10.1289/ehp.1103934.
20. Lee CS, Lee C, Marion JW, Wang Q, Saif L, et al. (2014) Occurrence of human enteric viruses at freshwater beaches during swimming season and its link to water inflow. Sci Total Environ 472: 757–766. doi: 10.1016/j.scitotenv.2013.11.088.
21. Noble RT, Fuhrman JA (2001) Enteroviruses detected by reverse transcriptase polymerase chain reaction from the coastal waters of Santa Monica Bay,

California: low correlation to bacterial indicator levels. Hydrobiologia 460: 175–184. doi: 10.1023/A:1013121416891.

22. McQuaig S, Griffith J, Harwood VJ (2012) Association of fecal indicator bacteria with human viruses and microbial source tracking markers at coastal beaches impacted by nonpoint source pollution. Appl Environ Microbiol 78 (18): 6423–6432. doi: 10.1128/AEM.00024-12.

23. Ashbolt NJ, Grabow WOK, Snozzi M (2001) Indicators of microbial water quality. In: Fewtrell L, Bartram J, editors. Water Quality: Guidelines, Standards and Health. London: World Health Organization: pp.289–315.

24. Boehm AB, Ashbolt NJ, Colford JM, Dunbar LE, et al. (2009) A sea of change ahead for recreational water quality criteria. J Water Health 7 (1): 9–20. doi: 10.2166/wh.2009.122.

25. Abdelzaher AM, Solo-Gabriele HM, Phillips MC, Elmir SM, Fleming LE (2013) An alternative approach to water regulations for public health protection at swimming beaches. J. Environ Public Health 2013: 138521. DOI: 10.1155/2013/138521.

26. Marion JW, Lee J, Lemeshow S, Buckley TJ (2010) Association of gastrointestinal illness and recreational water exposure at an inland U.S. beach. Water Res 44 (16): 4796–4804. doi: 10.1016/j.watres.2010.07.065.

27. U.S. Environmental Protection Agency (2002) Method 1603: Escherichia coli (E. coli) in Water by Membrane Filtration Using Modified membrane-Thermotolerant Escherichia coli Agar (Modified mTEC). Office of Water Report EPA-821-R-02-023. Washington D.C. Available: http://www.epa.gov/nerlcwww/documents/1603sp02.pdf. Accessed 2014 June 19.

28. National Oceanic and Atmospheric Administration (2013) Database: UV Index Bulletins Archives. http://www.cpc.ncep.noaa.gov/products/stratosphere/uv_index/uv_archive.shtml. Accessed 2014 June 19.

29. U.S. Army Corps of Engineers, Louisville District (2013) Database: Yearly Lake Reports. http://www.lrl.usace.army.mil/wcds/dlbrpt.htm. Accessed 2014 June 19.

30. Haugland RA, Siefring SC, Wymer LJ, Brenner KP, Dufour AP (2005) Comparison of Enterococcus measurements in freshwater at two recreational beaches by quantitative polymerase chain reaction and membrane filter culture analysis. Water Res 39 (4): 559–568. doi: 10.1016/j.watres.2004.11.011.

31. Lipsitch M, Tchetgen ET, Cohen T (2010) Negative controls: a tool for detecting confounding and bias in observational studies. Epidemiology 21 (3): 383–388. doi: 10.1097/EDE.0b013e3181d61eeb.

32. Hosmer DW, Lemeshow S (2000) Applied logistic regression, 2nd ed. New York: Wiley and Sons. 375 p.

33. Peduzzi P, Concato J, Kemper E, Holford TR, Feinstein AR (1996). A simulation of the number of events per variable in logistic regression analysis. J Clin Epidemiol 49 (12): 1373–1379.

34. Vittinghoff E, McCulloch CE (2007). Relaxing the rule of ten events per variable in logistic and cox regression. Am J Epidemiol 165 (6): 710–718. doi: 10.1093/aje/kwk052.

35. Peed LA, Nietch CT, Kelty CA, Meckes M, Mooney T, et al. (2011) Combining land use information and small stream sampling with PCR-based methods for better characterization of diffuse sources of human fecal pollution. Environ Sci Technol 45 (13): 5652–5659. doi: 10.1021/es2003167.

36. Lodder WJ, de Roda Husman AM (2005) Presence of noroviruses and other enteric viruses in sewage and surface waters in the Netherlands. Appl Environ Microbiol 71 (3): 1453–1461. doi: 10.1128/AEM.71.3.1453-1461.2005.

37. Haramoto E, Katayama H, Oguma K, Ohgaki S (2005) Application of cation-coated filter method to detection of noroviruses, enteroviruses, adenoviruses, and torque teno viruses in the Tamagawa River in Japan. Appl Environ Microbiology 71 (5): 2403–2411. doi: 10.1128/AEM.71.5.2403-2411.2005.

38. Jiang S, Noble R, Chu W (2001) Human adenoviruses and coliphages in urban-runoff impacted coastal waters of Southern California. Appl Environ Microbiol 67 (1): 179–184. doi: 10.1128/AEM.67.1.179-184.2001.

39. Payment P, Lemieux M, Trudel M (1982) Bacteriological and virological analysis of water from four fresh water beaches. Water Res 16 (6): 939–943. doi: 10.1016/0043-1354(82)90026-4.

40. Newton RJ, VandeWalle JL, Borchardt MA, Gorelick MH, McLellan SL (2011) Lachnospiraceae and Bacteroidales alternative fecal indicators reveal chronic human sewage contamination in an urban harbor. Appl Environ Microbiol 77 (19): 6972–6981. doi: 10.1128/AEM.05480-11.

41. Wyn-Jones AP, Carducci A, Cook N, D'Agostino M, Divizia M, et al. (2011) Surveillance of adenoviruses and noroviruses in European recreational waters. Water Res 45 (3): 1025–1038. doi: 10.1016/j.watres.2010.10.015.

42. Sinclair RG, Jones EL, Gerba CP (2009) Viruses in recreational water-borne disease outbreaks: a review. J Appl Microbiol 107 (6): 1769–1780. doi: 10.1111/j.1365-2672.2009.04367.x.

43. Albinana-Gimenez N, Miagostovich MP, Calgua B, Huguet JM, Matia L, et al. 2009. Analysis of adenoviruses and polyomaviruses quantified by qPCR as indicators of water quality in source and drinking-water treatment plants. Water Res 43 (7): 2011–2019. DOI: 10.1016/j.watres.2009.01.025.

44. Leshem E, Wikswo M, Barclay L, Brandt E, Storm W, et al. (2013) Effects and clinical significance of GII.4 Sydney Norovirus, United States, 2012–2013. Emerg Infect Dis 19 (8): 1231–1238. doi: 10.3201/eid1908.130458.

45. Gerba CP, Gramos DM, Nwachuku N (2002) Comparative inactivation of enteroviruses and adenovirus 2 by UV light. Appl Environ Microbiol 68: 5167–5169. doi: 10.1128/AEM.68.10.5167-5169.2002.

46. Fongaro G, Nascimento MA, Rigotto C, Ritterbusch G, da Silva AD, et al. (2013) Evaluation and molecular characterization of human adenovirus in drinking water supplies: viral integrity and viability assays. J Virol 10: 166. doi: 10.1186/1743-422X-10-166.

47. Kundu A, McBride G, Wuertz S (2013) Adenovirus-associated health risks for recreational activities in a multi-use coastal watershed based on site-specific quantitative microbial risk assessment. Water Res 47 (16): 6309–6325. doi: 10.1016/j.watres.2013.08.003.

48. Heaney CD, Sams E, Dufour AP, Brenner KP, Haugland RA, et al. (2012) Fecal indicators in sand, sand contact, and risk of enteric illness among beachgoers. Epidemiol 23 (1): 95–106.

49. Ge Z, Whitman RL, Nevers MB, Phanikumar MS (2012) Wave-induced mass transport affects daily Escherichia coli fluctuations in nearshore water. Environ Sci Technol 46 (4): 2204–2211. doi: 10.1021/es203847n.

50. Fleisher JM, Jones J, Kay D, Stanwell-Smith R, Wyer M, et al. (1993). Water and non-water related risk factors for gastroenteritis among swimmers exposed to sewage-contaminated marine waters. Int J Epidemiol 22 (4): 698–708. doi: 10.1093/ije/22.4.698.

51. Lee C, Agidi S, Marion JW, Lee J (2012) Arcobacter in Lake Erie beach waters: an emerging gastrointestinal pathogen linked with human-associated fecal contamination. Appl and Environ Microbiol 78 (16): 5511–5519. doi: 10.1128/AEM.08009-11.

52. Lee J, Deininger RA (2004) Detection of E. coli in beach water within 1 hour using immunomagnetic separation and ATP bioluminescence. Luminescence 19 (1): 31–36. doi: 10.1002/bio.753.

53. Haramoto E, Katayama H, Oguma K, Ohgaki S (2005) Application of cation-coated filter method to detection of noroviruses, enteroviruses, adenoviruses, and torque teno viruses in the Tamagawa River in Japan. Appl Environ Microbiol 71 (5): 2403–2411. doi: 10.1128%2FAEM.71.5.2403-2411.2005.

54. Monpoeho S, Dehee A, Mignotte B, Schwartzbrod L, Marechal V, et al. (2000) Quantification of enterovirus RNA in sludge samples using single tube real-time RT-PCR. Biotechniques 29 (1): 88–93.

55. Kageyama T, Kojima S, Shinohara M, Uchida K, Fukushi S, et al. (2003) Broadly reactive and highly sensitive assay for Norwalk-like viruses based on real-time quantitative reverse transcription-PCR. J Clin Microbiol 41 (4): 1548–1557. doi: 10.1128/JCM.41.4.1548-1557.2003.

56. Heim A, Ebnet C, Harste G, Pring-Akerblom P (2003) Rapid and quantitative detection of human adenovirus DNA by real-time PCR. J Med Virol 70 (2): 228–239. doi: 10.1002/jmv.10382.

57. Chern EC, Brenner K, Wymer L, Haugland RA (2009) Comparison of fecal indicator bacteria densities in marine recreational waters by QPCR. Water Qual Expo Heath 1 (3–4): 203–214.

58. Chern EC, Siefring S, Paar J, Doolittle M, Haugland RA (2011) Comparison of quantitative PCR assays for Escherichia coli targeting ribosomal RNA and single copy genes. Lett Appl Microbiol 52 (3): 298–306. doi: 10.1111/j.1472-765X.2010.03001.x.

59. Bernhard AE, Field KG (2000) Identification of nonpoint sources of fecal pollution in coastal waters by using host-specific 16S ribosomal DNA genetic markers from fecal anaerobes. Appl Environ Microbiol 66 (4): 1587–1594. doi: 10.1128/AEM.66.4.1587-1594.2000.

60. Okabe S, Okayama N, Savichtcheva O, Ito T (2007) Quantification of host-specific Bacteroides-Prevotella 16S rRNA genetic markers for assessment of fecal pollution in freshwater. Appl Microbiol Biotechnol 74 (4): 890–901. doi: 10.1007/s00253-006-0714-x.

61. Ludwig W, Schleifer KH (2000) How quantitative is quantitative PCR with respect to cell counts? Syst Appl Microbiol 23 (4): 556–562. doi: 10.1016/S0723-2020(00)80030-2.

62. U.S. Environmental Protection Agency (2010) Method A: Enterococci in Water by TaqMan Quantitative Polymerase Chain Reaction (qPCR) Assay. EPA-821-R-10-004. Washington, D.C. Available: http://water.epa.gov/scitech/methods/cwa/bioindicators/upload/rapid1.pdf. Accessed 2014 June 20.

63. Lee CS, Lee J, (2010) Evaluation of new gyrB-based real-time PCR system for the detection of B. fragilis as an indicator of human-specific fecal contamination. J Microbiol Methods 82 (3): 311–318. doi: 10.1016/j.mimet.2010.07.012.

21

Impact of NGO Training and Support Intervention on Diarrhoea Management Practices in a Rural Community of Bangladesh: An Uncontrolled, Single-Arm Trial

Ahmed S. Rahman[1]*, Mohammad Rafiqul Islam[2], Tracey P. Koehlmoos[3], Mohammad Jyoti Raihan[1], Mohammad Mehedi Hasan[1], Tahmeed Ahmed[1], Charles P. Larson[4]

1 Centre for Nutrition and Food Security, International Centre for Diarrhoeal Diseases Research, Bangladesh (icddr,b), Dhaka, Bangladesh, 2 CCEB, School of Medicine and Public Health, University of Newcastle, Newcastle, Australia, 3 Department of Health Administration and Policy, College of Health and Human Services, George Mason University, Fairfax, Virginia, United States of America, 4 Department of Pediatrics, University of British Columbia and Centre for International Child Health, BC Children's Hospital, Vancouver, British Columbia, Canada

Abstract

Purpose/Objective: The evolving Non-Governmental Organization (NGO) sector in Bangladesh provides health services directly, however some NGOs indirectly provide services by working with unlicensed providers. The primary objective of this study was to examine the impact of NGO training of unlicensed providers on diarrhoea management and the scale up of zinc treatment in rural populations.

Methods: An uncontrolled, single-arm trial for a training and support intervention on diarrhoea outcomes was employed in a rural sub-district of Bangladesh during 2008. Two local NGOs and their catchment populations were chosen for the study. The intervention included training of unlicensed health care providers in the management of acute childhood diarrhoea, particularly emphasizing zinc treatment. In addition, community-based promotion of zinc treatment was carried out. Baseline and endline ecologic surveys were carried out in intervention and control villages to document changes in treatments received for diarrhoea in under-five children.

Results: Among surveyed household with an active or recent acute childhood diarrhoea episode, 69% sought help from a health provider. Among these, 62.8% visited an unlicensed private provider. At baseline, 23.9% vs. 22% of control and intervention group children with diarrhoea had received zinc of any type. At endline (6 months later) this had changed to 15.3% vs. 30.2%, respectively. The change in zinc coverage was significantly higher in the intervention villages (p<0.01). Adherence with giving zinc for 10 days or more was significantly higher in the intervention households (9.2% vs. 2.5%; p< 0.01). Child's age, duration of diarrhoea, type of diarrhoea, parental year of schooling as well as oral rehydration solution (ORS) and antibiotic usage were significant predictors of zinc usage.

Conclusion: Training of unlicensed healthcare providers through NGOs increased zinc coverage in the diarrhoea management of under-five children in rural Bangladesh households.

Editor: Susanna Esposito, Fondazione IRCCS Ca' Granda Ospedale Maggiore Policlinico, Università degli Studi di Milano, Italy

Funding: This study was funded by a grant from the Bill & Melinda Gates Foundation (contract # HRN-AA-00-98-00047-00.) The funders had no role in study design, data collection and analysis, decision to publish, or preparation of the manuscript.

Competing Interests: The authors have declared that no competing interests exist.

* Email: ashafiq@icddrb.org

Introduction

Even a decade after into the 21st century and the proven efficacy of oral rehydration salts and zinc therapy, diarrhoea still remains the second leading cause of mortality among under-five children globally [1–4]. It has been estimated that diarrhoea has accounted for about 800,000 out of the total 7.6 million under-five child death globally with the highest contribution from the developing countries [5]. The comparison of 69,000 child death attributed to diarrhoea in Bangladesh in a year [6] to the US child mortality of 300 [7], portrays the ravaging effect of diarrhoea in developing countries. A recent estimate has shown that diarrhoea is responsible for 22% of all under-five child deaths in Africa and 23% in South Asia [6]. Therefore, 'one out of every nine under-5 child death is due to diarrhoea', is a statement bold enough to illustrate the impact of diarrhoea on child mortality. Despite the huge burden of diarrhoea among under-five children, most do not receive appropriate treatment [8]. WHO diarrhoeal management guidelines include treating patients with hypo-osmolar oral rehydrating salt (ORS) and zinc along with recommendation to avoid unnecessary use of pharmacological agents. Continued feeding has also been suggested [9]. Meta-analyses of several randomized controlled trials have confirmed the preventive and prophylactic effects of zinc on diarrhoeal episodes among under-five children [10–12], which complements the WHO guidelines on zinc usage for diarrhoea. It has been estimated that globally, the successful scaling up of zinc treatment for childhood diarrhoea could potentially save 400,000 under-five deaths per year [13]. Antibiotics, on other hand, is indicated in certain types of diarrhoea such as confirmed or suspected cholera, invasive diarrhoea caused by Shigella and E coli. and dysentery induced by other organisms such as Campylobacter spp. [14]. The European Society for Paediatric Gastroenterology, Hepatology and Nutrition (ESPGHAN) has suggested nine components for good diarrhoeal management, which includes, use of oral rehydration solution, use of hypotonic solution (Na 60 mmol/L, glucose 74–111 mmol/L), fast oral rehydration over of the period of 3 to 4 hours followed by normal feeding, avoid using special formula unless justified, avoid using diluted formula unless justified, continued breastfeeding all the time, supplementation with oral rehydration solution and avoid using unnecessary medication [15]. The guideline also stated that more than 8 episodes/day with substantial stool volumes, persistent vomiting, severe underlying disease and age less than 2 months as indications for medical visits for diarrhoeal patients, whereas, telephone consultation is recommended for uncomplicated diarrhoea. As for hospitalization criteria, ESPGHAN recommended the presence of at least one of the following abnormality/condition: shock, severe dehydration (>9% body weight), any neurological abnormalities, intractable or bilious vomiting, ORS treatment failure, failure of caregivers to provide adequate care at home and/or concerns on social/logistic scenario and suspected surgical condition [16]. It is needed to be pointed out that ESPGHAN recommendation for diarrhoeal management does not include zinc therapy, indicating the European population, specifically children may not be zinc deficient like that of many developing nations such as Bangladesh [17]. Bangladesh also do not have a national guideline for child diarrhoeal management, similar to most developing countries. Most hospitals have developed their own protocol which are adopted from WHO guidelines on diarrhoeal management and therefore includes ORS for rehydration, zinc therapy and careful using antibiotics. Additionally, like most of its poor neighbors, Bangladesh do not have a robust health system and telephone consultation as exists in more developed nation, is an usual practice for general practitioners or even visit to qualified doctors is not always possible due to many access barriers especially in lowest rural tier [18]. Under such drawbacks, it is crucial to train and integrate paramedical workforce such as NGO workers in current health system to increase ORS and zinc therapy coverage in the country and provide effective management of diarrhoea to the rural population.

In Bangladesh, following the launch of the national zinc scale-up campaign in late 2006, repeat impact surveys were carried out in order to monitor diarrhoea management practices especially ORS and zinc usage in under-five children [19]. Before the initiation of the mass media campaign, caretakers' awareness of zinc as a treatment for childhood diarrhoea was under 5% in rural areas, however, increased to 55% by 12 months and 75% by 24 months [20]. On the other hand, zinc usage (any amount) as a

treatment of childhood diarrhoea increased from under 5% to 13% during the same time period in rural areas.

Being a low income country, Bangladesh, since its independence in 1971, has been observed to have a pluralistic health system with a large segment of rural population still inclined to seek care from informal health sector providers such as traditional healers, pharmacists and 'village doctors' [21–23]. The fragmented health system also relies heavily on the several hundred or so local and national NGOs who have been playing a significant role in the health sector since the independence of the nation [24]. Under the latest national health, population and nutrition development program strategy of Bangladesh, which follows a sector-wide approach, the role of NGOs are recognized as more pivotal than ever, with increased Government-NGO collaboration [25]. Within the NGO sector, health services is directly provided in the community; however some NGOs also work closely with private sector unlicensed providers who are the preferred source of care seeking in rural communities in Bangladesh for childhood diarrhoea [26]. Involvements of NGOs working through networking with unlicensed providers are therefore a potentially important strategy to be included in the effort to bring zinc treatment of childhood diarrhoea to scale in Bangladesh.

The primary objective of the study was to determine whether a training intervention given to unlicensed health service providers by NGO providers' increases zinc coverage as an adjunct to ORS for the management of childhood diarrhoea in rural communities of Bangladesh.

Materials and Methods

Design and site

The protocol for this trial and supporting CONSORT checklist are available as supporting information; see Checklist S1 and Protocol S1. This uncontrolled, single-arm trial for a training and support intervention on diarrhoea outcomes was employed in a rural sub-district of Bangladesh during 2008. The study was conducted in Sreepur sub-district under Gazipur district of Bangladesh.

Two local NGOs with long working experience on providing health services in the chosen community were selected along with their catchment areas for the purpose of this study. The intervention area included 53 villages having a population of ~95,000 against 49 villages in the control area with a population of ~76,000. The curative health services in these sites were provided by unlicensed (local drug vendors, village practitioners, traditional healers), and licensed government, private or NGO health service providers. A cluster sampling design was employed and the required number of clusters (villages) was randomly selected from the total listed villages in both the intervention and control areas using a random number generating software/calculator. Baseline data was collected during February 2008 and endline data in August 2008.

The study evaluated the effect of intervention primarily on zinc coverage and secondarily on ORS and antibiotic use in childhood diarrhoea through community surveys. The study design was such that the participants (mothers/caretakers) were not aware of the intervention and hence was blinded. A baseline survey was conducted in the intervention and control villages concomitantly with the training of the health service providers in the intervention area and an endline survey around six months following the training. We have hypothesized that greater increased change in zinc coverage for diarrhoea management would be observed in the intervention when compared to control villages six months following the training.

Intervention. The intervention included orientation and training of the unlicensed health care providers (village doctors, drug vendors and traditional healers) regarding zinc treatment in childhood diarrhoea through NGO health care providers. In addition, the NGO conducted community-based promotion of zinc treatment in the intervention villages.

A package of training materials custom designed for the scale up of zinc for young children plus ORS was delivered using a training of the trainers' strategy. The package is described in Table 1.

After the initial training to NGO service providers in the intervention areas, subsequent training was delivered by the NGOs done through quarterly meetings and follow-up sessions with village practitioners throughout the intervention areas. This work was conducted by Sub-Assistant Medical Officers (SAC-MOs). In intervention villages there are at least four SACMOs who have training experience with village practitioners.

Ethical approval

The study was reviewed and approved by the Research Review and Ethical Review Committees of the International Centre for Diarrhoeal Diseases Research, Bangladesh (icddr,b). Informed written consent was obtained in a prescribed form from the caretakers of the enrolled children. The Trial Registration number for this protocol is NCT02143921. It is to be mentioned that due to procedural and institutional reasons, we were only able to register the trial after completing the study.

Sample size estimation

To detect a minimum 50% increase in zinc coverage for childhood diarrhoea in the intervention area with a level of confidence of 0.95, a power of 0.9 and assuming a 1.5 design effect adjustment for clustering, it was estimated 580 cases of childhood diarrhoea per group would be required.

We have randomly selected 28 out of 49 villages from the control NGO's catchment area and 28 out of 53 villages in the intervention NGO's catchment area to meet the sample size requirement during the baseline survey, whereas; 26 and 29 villages respectively were again randomly selected during the endline survey.

Sampling. Baseline and endline data has been collected from all households from the selected villages in both control and intervention areas. Within each village, a central starting point was chosen and door-to-door survey technique of households was implemented for screening and recruiting children with a current or recent episode of diarrhoea (lasting for ≥2 days) within two weeks prior to the survey. Thus, information from all children with diarrhoea in the selected clusters was recorded. However, if more than one child in the household was eligible, one was randomly chosen. The respondents of the survey were the mothers or other caretakers of the identified children of the selected households.

Statistics

Data were entered and verified using SPSS version 10.5 and converted to Stata version 11.5 for all analyses. Data were checked for missing values and recoded to generate new categorical variables using cut-off values. The analyses carried out were both stratified by time of the survey (baseline and endline) and location of residence (intervention and control) and without any stratification. To assess differences in categorical outcomes, chi-square statistical comparisons of proportions with 95% confidence intervals, were calculated. Of particular interest was the identification of disparities in the use of zinc, ORS and antibiotic by area. Age of child, gender, type of diarrhoea, duration of diarrhoea, age of mother, parental year of schooling, parental occupation, type of toilet facility and weekly expenditure on food (own production/purchase) as proxy indicator of financial status were included in the bivariate analysis in order to identify significant predictors of zinc and antibiotic usage. Variables that were significant ($p<0.05$) in bivariate analyses were included in the multiple logistic regression analyses after controlling for area and time in order to assess independent association of the variables with zinc and antibiotic usage. All the analyses were done by taking cluster effect into account using '*svy*' command in Stata.

Results

The survey result shows that at baseline, data of 630 and 612 children were collected from the control and intervention areas with current or recent episode of diarrhoea, whereas; at endline the figure was 650 and 612 children respectively. The trial flow chart is shown in Figure 1. Among the total cases (n = 2504), the most prevalent type of diarrhoea was 'predominantly mucoid' (63.7%) whereas 20.6% cases were 'watery/loose' and 15.7% cases had predominantly bloody diarrhoea. Among all cases, 71% children received ORS during diarrhoeal illness.

Table 1. Training Package for health care providers in the intervention area.

For licensed providers

- Refresher course and up-date on WHO/UNICEF guidelines for treatment of childhood diarrhea
- Training videos (docu-drama)
- Orientation/training materials (zinc babohar nirdeshika)
- Frequently asked questions booklet
- Follow-up support

For unlicensed community health care providers

- Orientation/training materials (flip chart)
- Training videos (docu-drama)
- Zinc commercial (mass media campaign)
- Refresher training and up-date on WHO/UNICEF guidelines for treatment of childhood diarrhea
- Frequently asked questions booklet
- Follow-up support

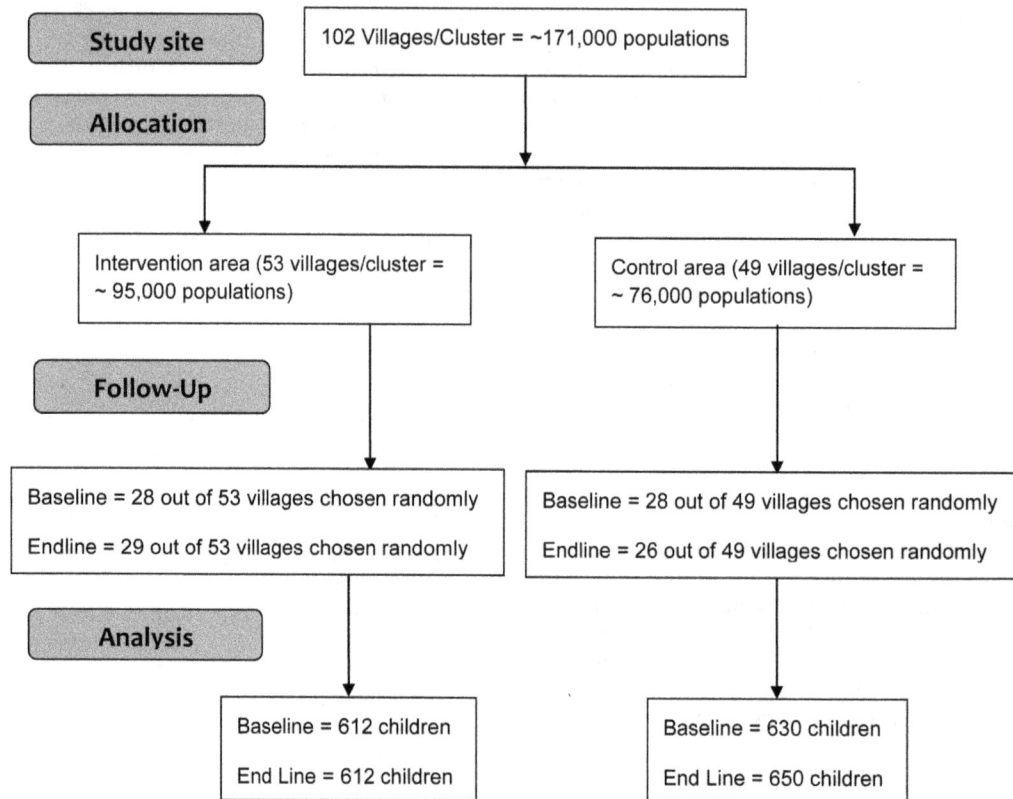

Figure 1. Trial Flowchart.

Descriptive statistics of selected socio-demographic characteristics of households are presented in Table 2. No significant differences were found between control and intervention areas at baseline and endline in terms of age and sex of the study children, age of the mothers and type of toilet facility used by the household. Overall, irrespective of study area and time of the survey, 31% of the children did not seek treatment for diarrhoeal illness from any health service providers (Figure 2). Among the children who did seek treatment from service providers, most of them received treatment from unlicensed (e.g. village doctor, drug vendor, and traditional healers) private providers (68.7%). Almost 16% received treatment from licensed (MBBS) private providers whereas, only 1.6% and 2.1% went to NGO and government facilities respectively to receive treatment for their illness.

Table 3 presents the usage of ORS, zinc and antibiotic usage among children in the control and intervention areas. Compared to control area, ORS usage was significantly higher in the intervention area after 6 months of intervention (65.1 vs. 72.2%, $p<0.01$). Similarly, there was a significant difference in zinc usage between control and intervention areas (15.3% vs. 30.2%; $p<0.01$). After 6 months of intervention, the recommended usage of zinc for 10 days or more in under-5 diarrhoea was significantly higher among children in the intervention area compared to the control area (9.2% vs. 2.5%, $p<0.01$). Compared to the baseline prevalence, antibiotic usage increased more in the intervention area compared to control area at the endline.

Table 4 depicts the results of multiple logistic regression analyses exploring the relationship of potential factors with zinc usage. The older children aged 25–59 months were less likely to use zinc during diarrhoeal illness compared to younger children aged 6–12 months. On the other hand, children with a higher duration (4 to 10+ days) of diarrhoeal illness were more likely to use zinc compared to children with lower duration of illness (1–3 days). The other significant predictors of zinc usage were type of diarrhoea, parental year of schooling as well as ORS and antibiotic usage whereas, age of mother, mother occupation, sex of child, father occupation, type of toilet facility and weekly expenditure on food were insignificant to predict zinc usage.

The results of multiple logistic regression analyses showing significant predictors of antibiotic usage are presented in Table 5. The children aged over 12 months were less likely to use antibiotic during diarrhoeal illness compared to younger children aged 6–12 months. However, children were more likely to use antibiotic who suffered predominately from bloody diarrhoea compared to watery/loose diarrhoea as well as with duration of diarrhoea for 4–9 days compared to 1–3 days. The other significant predictors of antibiotic usage were father's year of schooling, ORS usage and zinc usage.

Discussion

A simple training intervention to unlicensed private providers on diarrhoeal management by local NGOs had significantly increased zinc usage in a rural community compared to nonintervened control area. The study was conducted in 2008 after launching in late 2006 of the national campaign to scale up zinc treatment of childhood diarrhoea in Bangladesh. Two years after the inauguration of zinc program, the national prevalence of zinc usage in under-5 children was 9–13% in rural areas [19]. While in this study, we found that after 6 months of training intervention and community sensitization, zinc usage was

Table 2. Socio-demographic characteristics of the Control and Intervention areas.*

Variable	Baseline		Endline	
	Control Total n = 630	Intervention Total n = 612	Control Total n = 650	Intervention Total n = 612
	%	%	%	%
Age of child in months				
6–12	27.0	23.4	21.2	19.8
13–24	29.1	31.3	25.7	27.3
25–36	18.7	23.2	20.8	18.8
37–59	25.2	22.1	32.3	34.1
Sex of child				
Male	54	52.1	52.9	55.6
Female	46	47.9	47.1	44.4
Age of mother in years				
≤20	15.6	18.6	17.5	20.1
21–25	36.4	40.7	37.1	40.0
26–30	28.1	24.2	28.8	24.8
31–49	19.8	16.2	16.5	14.9
Missing	0.1	0.3	0.1	0.2
Mother's year of schooling				
No education	20.5	13.4	26.8	21.1
1–4 years	18.3	15.7	16.6	12.4
5–9 years	53.3	60.5	47.7	58.8
10–11 years	4.9	5.7	6.2	6.1
> = 12 years	2.9	4.4	2.6	1.3
Missing	0.1	0.3	0.1	0.3
Father's year of schooling				
No education	32.1	24.2	35.7	33.0
1–4 years	14.4	11.2	13.5	11.6
5–9 years	36.0	46.8	33.5	38.9
10–11 years	8.4	8.7	8.9	9.3
> = 12 years	7.3	8.9	8.0	6.5
Don't Know	1.8	0.2	0.3	0.7
Type of toilet facility				
No facility	3.8	5.7	2.8	2.3
Unimproved	65.9	59.2	62.0	59.0
Improved	30.3	35.1	35.2	38.7
Weekly expenditure on food in BDT (Bangladesh Taka)				
< = 500	6.8	4.4	2.0	2.6
501–1000	56.7	46.9	44.2	43.5
1001–1500	25.7	31.5	39.2	34.3
> = 1501	10.8	17.2	14.6	19.6

*Cluster adjusted analyses of all variables.

increased to 30% in the intervention area from the baseline usage of 22% and in the non-intervention area it was reduced to 15% from the baseline usage of 24%. More importantly, the recommended 10 days zinc usage for diarrhoeal management was increased by 7% in the intervention area at the endline. As expected, we demonstrated a significant improvement in ORS usage following the NGO's training intervention to the unlicensed Health Care Providers.

Our finding clearly states the importance of training to the informal health care providers for overall zinc treatment and compliance to 10 days zinc treatment in addition to ORS for childhood diarrhoea management in the rural areas. Rural Bangladesh is facing a shortage of qualified physician (MBBS or above) over a long period of time and the shortage is less likely to be filled in near future [27]. Therefore, most people in the rural communities had to rely on privately owned local drug outlets where unlicensed health care providers such as drug sellers/

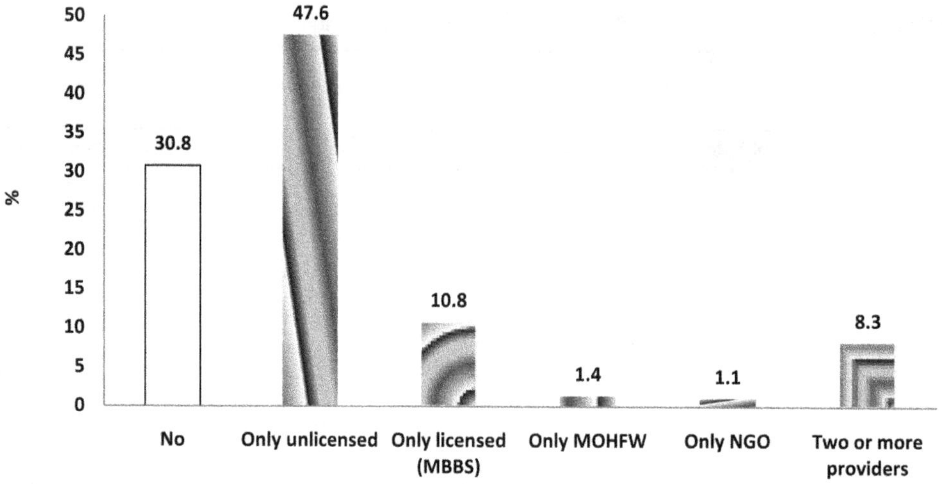

Figure 2. Health seeking behaviour during diarrhoeal illness among children 6–59 months by type of service providers.

vendors and village doctors are providing services. In 2006, Larson CP et al.; reported a dominance of private sector in providing health care delivery for diarrhoeal diseases both in urban and rural communities [26] while unlicensed health care providers remains the first point of privately delivering any health care services in most cases in the rural areas [27]. Training intervention to the unlicensed health care providers and community health workers for improving health is well acknowledged in many developing countries including Bangladesh [28]. Successful training and involvement of these health cadres are now a national policy for tuberculosis control in Bangladesh [29,30].

It can be assumed that there is a difference in knowledge and awareness between unlicensed urban and rural health care providers as well as the urban and rural population. A previous study demonstrates a difference in awareness about zinc treatment for diarrhoeal diseases in children between urban and rural

Table 3. ORS, zinc and antibiotic usage in Control and Intervention areas.*

Variables	Baseline			Endline		
	Control % (95% CI)	Intervention % (95% CI)	p-value	Control % (95% CI)	Intervention % (95% CI)	p-value
ORS usage						
	n=630	n=612		n=650	n=612	
Yes	73.2 (69.1, 77.2)	74.4 (70.3, 78.3)	0.67	65.1 (61.2, 68.9)	72.2 (69, 75.4)	<0.01
Zinc usage of any duration (Tablet or Syrup)						
	n=594	n=608		n=636	n=609	
Yes	23.9 (19.2, 28.7)	22 (17.2, 26.9)	0.57	15.3 (13.1, 17.4)	30.2 (25.2, 35.3)	<0.01
Duration of zinc usage (Tablet or Syrup)						
	n=594	n=608		n=636	n=609	
No use	76.9 (72.2, 81.6)	78.5 (73.7, 83.3)	0.83	84.8 (82.6, 86.9)	69.8 (64.7, 74.8)	<0.01
1–3 day	8.8 (6.7, 10.9)	8.4 (5.7, 11.1)		6.6 (4.8, 8.5)	9.2 (7.1, 11.3)	
4–9 day	11.3 (8.4, 14.2)	9.7 (6.5, 12.9)		6.1 (4.3, 8)	11.8 (8.7, 15)	
≥10 day	3 (1.4, 4.7)	3.5 (1.7, 5.2)		2.5 (0.9, 4.2)	9.2 (6.9, 11.5)	
Duration of zinc usage (Tablet)						
	n=594	n=608		n=636	n=609	
No use	84.5 (80.2, 88.8)	83.9 (79.4, 88.3)	0.78	87.7 (85.6, 89.9)	76.4 (71.8, 80.9)	<0.01
1–3 day	5.7 (3.5, 7.9)	7.1 (4.2, 9.9)		6 (4.7, 7.3)	8.9 (6.7, 11)	
4–9 day	7.6 (4.7, 10.4)	6.6 (3.9, 9.2)		3.9 (2.5, 5.4)	6.9 (4.5, 9.3)	
≥10 day	2.2 (0.9, 3.5)	2.5 (1.2, 3.7)		2.4 (0.8, 3.9)	7.9 (5.4, 10.3)	
Antibiotic usage						
	n=623	n=611		n=639	n=606	
Yes	24.7 (20.5, 28.9)	23.6 (19.2, 27.9)	0.70	28.8 (26.2, 31.4)	36.3 (31.6, 41)	<0.01

*Cluster adjusted analyses of all variable.

Table 4. Predictors of zinc usage in childhood diarrhoea after controlling area and time variation.[*]

Variable[#]	OR (95% CI)	p-value
Age of child in months		
6–12	Reference	
13–24	1.13 (0.86, 1.48)	0.37
25–36	0.74 (0.55, 0.98)	0.04
37–60	0.39 (0.26, 0.59)	<0.01
Type of diarrhoea		
Watery/Loose	Reference	
Predominantly mucoid	0.0.6 (0.47, 0.78)	<0.01
Predominantly bloody	0.65 (0.48, 0.89)	<0.01
Duration of diarrhoea		
1–3 days	Reference	
4–9 days	1.89 (1.49, 2.4)	<0.01
>=10 days	3.76 (2.41, 5.88)	<0.01
Father's year of schooling		
No education	Reference	
1–4 years	0.93 (0.66, 1.3)	0.67
5–9 years	1.07 (0.82, 1.4)	0.62
10–11 years	1.71 (1.16, 2.53)	<0.01
>=12 years	1.03 (0.67, 1.58)	0.9
Mother's year of schooling		
No education	Reference	
1–4 years	1.11 (0.75, 1.66)	0.59
5–9 years	1.55 (1.1, 2.19)	0.01
10–11 years	2.1 (1.34, 3.29)	<0.01
>=12 years	3.36 (1.8, 6.26)	<0.01
ORS usage		
No	Reference	
Yes	5.83 (3.96, 8.61)	<0.01
Antibiotic usage		
No	Reference	
Yes	1.75 (1.35, 2.26)	<0.01

*All analyses were adjusted for cluster effect.
#Variables (age of child, type of diarrhoea, duration of diarrhoea, age of mother, Father's year of schooling, Mother's year of schooling, mother occupation, ORS usage and antibiotic usage) significant (p<0.05) in bivariate analysis (simple logistic regression) were used in multiple logistic regression analyses.

caregivers [20]. Since, the study area is very close to the capital city of the country therefore, it is more likely that the unlicensed health care providers in these areas are privileged for exchanging updated health related information including zinc treatment for diarrhoea in children. Also, the community dwellers are similarly privileged for receiving mass media and other sources of information compared to other rural, remote hard to reach areas. Despite, the above mentioned minor limitations, the findings can be generalized in context of Bangladesh. As the population in Bangladesh is rather homogenous in terms of culture and social characteristics, we do not expect too much variation in statistical findings if any other intervention areas are chosen. It is also to be notified that our study staff has confirmed no report of adverse effect occurred to any participants during the trial period due to the intervention.

We found 12.7% increment in antibiotic usage at endline in the intervention area vs. 4.1% increment in the control area compared

to the baseline usage (23.6% in intervention vs. 24.7% in control area). The rate of antibiotic use was not much different in comparison to national usage of antibiotic for diarrhoeal diseases which was 31 and 36% in female and male children respectively in the rural areas [26]. In this study, the use of antibiotic was higher among younger children and those who were suffering from bloody diarrhoea. However, rational use of antibiotic is indicated in bloody diarrhoea while the reason for higher use of antibiotic in younger children is unclear.

The training intervention repeatedly emphasized that zinc treatment is an adjunct therapy to ORS for the management of childhood diarrhoea. Given this, we observed an increased utilization of ORS in the intervention area (72%) than control area (65%). As illustrated before that the intervention and control areas are rural settings though very close to the capital city and ORS usage in both these areas were comparable to the overall

Table 5. Predictors of antibiotic usage in childhood diarrhoea after controlling area and time variation.*

Variable#	OR (95% CI)	p-value
Age of child in months		
6–12	Reference	
13–24	0.66 (0.48, 0.91)	0.01
25–36	0.69 (0.51, 0.93)	0.02
37–60	0.55 (0.37, 0.84)	<0.01
Type of diarrhoea		
Watery/Loose	Reference	
Predominantly mucoid	1.02 (0.79, 1.3)	0.9
Predominantly bloody	1.79 (1.33, 2.43)	<0.01
Duration of diarrhoea		
1–3 days	Reference	
4–9 days	1.92 (1.58, 2.33)	<0.01
>=10 days	2.78 (1.99, 3.87)	<0.01
Father's year of schooling		
No education	Reference	
1–4 years	1.04 (0.71, 1.51)	0.84
5–9 years	1.43 (1.07, 1.92)	0.02
10–11 years	1.83 (1.24, 2.72)	<0.01
>=12 years	1.62 (1.07, 2.47)	0.02
ORS usage		
No	Reference	
Yes	2.07 (1.64, 2.63)	<0.01
Zinc usage		
No	Reference	
Yes	1.75 (1.36, 2.27)	<0.01

*All analyses were adjusted for cluster effect.
#Variables (age of child, type of diarrhoea, duration of diarrhoea, age of mother, father education, mother education, mother occupation, ORS usage and antibiotic usage) significant (p<0.05) in bivariate analysis (simple logistic regression) were included in multiple logistic regression analyses.

national ORS usage during concurrent time period (52–68%) in rural areas of Bangladesh [19].

Overall, the training intervention to the unlicensed health care providers is very effective in terms of zinc treatment coverage and compliance to 10 days zinc treatment, increasing ORS usage. This training intervention, can be seen as capacity building for non-professionals, who would be able to provide diarrhoeal management for established cases, and for more complicated cases referral would be done to nearest Government Health Care facility, and hence would provide sufficient pace, if scaled-up, to the nation's target to reduce childhood diarrhoeal mortality and morbidity and to achieve Millennium Development Goal (MDG) 4. Nevertheless, training intervention should be critically emphasized on the rational use of antibiotic in diarrhoea in young children.

Conclusions

The study results shows that, a simple inexpensive training intervention for the unlicensed health care providers through NGO network increases the use of zinc for diarrhoea manage-

ment. These efforts therefore need to continue with non-sector (Partnership of NGOs and Private Health Care Providers) provider for successful nationwide zinc scaling up.

Learning

This study will contribute to effort of scaling up zinc by employing an existing network of NGO providers in the training of unlicensed providers.

Acknowledgments

This research was funded by Bill and Melinda Gates Foundation (contract # HRN-AA-00-98-00047-00). icddr,b acknowledges with gratitude the commitment of Bill and Melinda Gates Foundation to its research efforts.

Author Contributions

Conceived and designed the experiments: CPL ASR TPK MRI. Performed the experiments: ASR MRI TPK. Analyzed the data: ASR MRI MJR MMH. Contributed reagents/materials/analysis tools: ASR MRI TPK. Wrote the paper: ASR MRI MJR TA TPK CPL MMH.

References

1. Walker CLF, Perin J, Aryee MJ, Boschi-Pinto C, Black RE (2012) Diarrhoea incidence in low-and middle-income countries in 1990 and 2010: a systematic review. BMC Public Health 12: 220.
2. Bajait C, Thawani V (2011) Role of zinc in pediatric diarrhoea. Indian journal of pharmacology 43: 232.
3. Walker CLF, Black RE (2010) Zinc for the treatment of diarrhoea: effect on diarrhoea morbidity, mortality and incidence of future episodes. International Journal of Epidemiology 39: i63–i69.
4. Wardlaw T, Salama P, Brocklehurst C, Chopra M, Mason E (2010) Diarrhoea: why children are still dying and what can be done. Lancet 375: 870–872.
5. Liu L, Johnson HL, Cousens S, Perin J, Scott S, et al. (2012) Global, regional, and national causes of child mortality: an updated systematic analysis for 2010 with time trends since 2000. The Lancet 379: 2151–2161.
6. Boschi-Pinto C, Velebit L, Shibuya K (2008) Estimating child mortality due to diarrhoea in developing countries. Bulletin of the World Health Organization 86: 710–717.
7. Farthing M, Lindberg G, Dite P (2010) World gastroenterology organisation practice guideline: acute diarrhoea. 2008. Available: http://www.worldgastro enterology. org/assets/downloads/en/pdf/guidelines/01_acute_diarrhoea pdf. Accessed 29.
8. Ahs JW, Tao W, Löfgren J, Forsberg BC (2010) Diarrhoeal Diseases in Low- and Middle-Income Countries: Incidence, Prevention and Management. The Open Infectious Diseases Journal 4: 113–124.
9. WHO U (2004) WHO-UNICEF Joint statement on the clinical management of acute diarrhoea. World Health Assembly Geneva.
10. Bhutta Z, Black R, Brown K, Gardner JM, Gore S, et al. (1999) Prevention of diarrhoea and pneumonia by zinc supplementation in children in developing countries: pooled analysis of randomized controlled trials. The Journal of pediatrics 135: 689–697.
11. Bhutta ZA, Bird SM, Black RE, Brown KH, Gardner JM, et al. (2000) Therapeutic effects of oral zinc in acute and persistent diarrhoea in children in developing countries: pooled analysis of randomized controlled trials. The American journal of clinical nutrition 72: 1516–1522.
12. Lazzerini M, Ronfani L (2008) Oral zinc for treating diarrhoea in children. Cochrane Database Syst Rev 3.
13. Jones G, Steketee RW, Black RE, Bhutta ZA, Morris SS (2003) How many child deaths can we prevent this year? Lancet 362: 65–71.
14. Thapar N, Sanderson IR (2004) Diarrhoea in children: an interface between developing and developed countries. The Lancet 363: 641–653.
15. Szajewska H, Hoekstra JH, Sandhu B (2000) Management of acute gastroenteritis in Europe and the impact of the new recommendations: a multicenter study. Journal of Pediatric Gastroenterology and Nutrition 30: 522–527.
16. Guarino A, Albano F, Ashkenazi S, Gendrel D, Hoekstra JH, et al. (2008) European Society for Paediatric Gastroenterology, Hepatology, and Nutrition/ European Society for Paediatric Infectious Diseases evidence-based guidelines for the management of acute gastroenteritis in children in Europe: executive summary. Journal of pediatric gastroenterology and nutrition 46: 619–621.
17. Ahmed T, Mahfuz M, Ireen S, Ahmed AS, Rahman S, et al. (2012) Nutrition of children and women in Bangladesh: trends and directions for the future. Journal of health, population, and nutrition 30: 1.
18. Parkhurst JO, Rahman SA, Ssengooba F (2006) Overcoming access barriers for facility-based delivery in low-income settings: insights from Bangladesh and Uganda. Journal of health, population, and nutrition 24: 438.
19. Larson CP, Saha UR, Nazrul H (2009) Impact monitoring of the national scale up of zinc treatment for childhood diarrhoea in Bangladesh: repeat ecologic surveys. PLoS medicine 6: e1000175.
20. Larson CP, Koehlmoos TP, Sack DA (2012) Scaling up zinc treatment of childhood diarrhoea in Bangladesh: theoretical and practical considerations guiding the SUZY Project. Health policy and planning 27: 102–114.
21. Ahmed SM (2005) Exploring health-seeking behaviour of disadvantaged populations in rural Bangladesh: Institutionen för folkhälsovetenskap/Department of Public Health Sciences.
22. Ahmed SM, Evans TG, Standing H, Mahmud S (2013) Harnessing pluralism for better health in Bangladesh. The Lancet 382: 1746–1755.
23. Ahmed SM, Hossain MA, Chowdhury MR (2009) Informal sector providers in Bangladesh: how equipped are they to provide rational health care? Health Policy and Planning 24: 467–478.
24. Mercer A, Khan MH, Daulatuzzaman M, Reid J (2004) Effectiveness of an NGO primary health care programme in rural Bangladesh: evidence from the management information system. Health Policy and Planning 19: 187–198.
25. Ministry of Health and Family Welfare B (2011) Health, Population and Nutrition Sector Development Program (2011–2016) Program Implementation Plan. In: Welfare PWMoHaF, editor: Government of the People's Republic of Bangladesh.
26. Larson CP, Saha UR, Islam R, Roy N (2006) Childhood diarrhoea management practices in Bangladesh: private sector dominance and continued inequities in care. International Journal of Epidemiology 35: 1430–1439.
27. Mahmood SS, Iqbal M, Hanifi S, Wahed T, Bhuiya A (2010) Are 'Village Doctors' in Bangladesh a curse or a blessing? BMC international health and human rights 10: 18.
28. Oshiname FO, Brieger WR (1992) Primary care training for patent medicine vendors in rural Nigeria. Social science & medicine 35: 1477–1484.
29. Chowdhury AMR, Chowdhury S, Islam MN, Islam A, Vaughan JP (1997) Control of tuberculosis by community health workers in Bangladesh. The Lancet 350: 169–172.
30. Salim H, Uplekar M, Daru P, Aung M, Declercq E, et al. (2006) Turning liabilities into resources: informal village doctors and tuberculosis control in Bangladesh. Bulletin of the World Health Organization 84: 479–484.

22

Community based Case-Control Study of Rotavirus Gastroenteritis among Young Children during 2008-2010 Reveals Vast Genetic Diversity and Increased Prevalence of G9 Strains in Kolkata

Satarupa Mullick[1], Anupam Mukherjee[1], Santanu Ghosh[1], Gururaja P. Pazhani[1], Dipika Sur[1], Byomkesh Manna[1], James P. Nataro[2], Myron M. Levine[3], Thandavarayan Ramamurthy[1], Mamta Chawla-Sarkar[1]*

1 National Institute of Cholera and Enteric Diseases, Kolkata, India, **2** Department of Paediatrics, University of Virginia, School of Medicine, Charlottesville, Virginia, United States of America, **3** Center for Vaccine Development, University of Maryland, School of Medicine, Baltimore, Maryland, United States of America

Abstract

Background: Group A Rotaviruses are a major etiologic agent of gastroenteritis in infants and young children (<5 years) worldwide. Although rotavirus vaccines have been successfully administered in many countries, in India the introduction of rotavirus vaccine in national immunization program was approved in 2014. Since high disease burden and large number of genetic variants have been reported from low income countries including India, monitoring of rotavirus was initiated prior to implementation of the vaccine in the region.

Methods: A total number of 3,582 stool samples were collected from an urban slum community in Kolkata, among which 1,568 samples were obtained from children of ≤5 years of age, with moderate to severe diarrhoea and 2,014 samples were collected from age-sex matched healthy neighbourhood controls. Rotavirus positive samples were typed by multiplex semi-nested PCR and nucleotide sequencing. Circulating strains were phylogenetically analyzed.

Results: Among 1,568 children with diarrhoea, 395 (25.2%), and among 2,014 asymptomatic children, 42 (2%) were rotavirus positive. G1P[8] was identified as the most common strain (32%) followed by G9P[8] (16.9%), G2P[4] (13.5%) and G9P[4] (10.75%). G12 strains with combinations of P[4], P[6] and P[8] comprised 11.9% of total positive strains. The rest (<10%) were rare and uncommon strains like G1P[4], G1P[6], G2P[8] and animal-like strains G4P[6], G6P[14] and G11P[25]. The 42 rotavirus positive samples from asymptomatic children revealed common genotypes like G1, G2 and G9.

Conclusion: This community based case-control study showed increased predominance of genotype G9 in Kolkata. It also confirmed co-circulation of a large number of genetic variants in the community. Asymptomatic rotavirus positive children though low in number can also be a source of dispersal of infection in the community. This study provides background information to the policy makers for implementation of rotavirus vaccines in this region.

Editor: Ana Paula Arez, Instituto de Higiene e Medicina Tropical, Portugal

Funding: This work was supported by the Bill & Melinda Gates Foundation (grant number 38874). http://www.gatesfoundation.org/. The funder had no role in study design, data collection and analysis, decision to publish, or preparation of the manuscript.

Competing Interests: The authors have declared that no competing interests exist.

* Email: chawlam70@gmail.com

Introduction

Severe gastroenteritis in children below 5 years of age is a major public health problem in humans globally [1]. Worldwide approximately 10.6 million children die before their fifth birthday of which 20% deaths are attributed to diarrhoeal diseases [2]. Although large number of bacterial, viral and parasitic pathogens have been implicated to cause diarrhoea, but Group A rotavirus

(RVA) has been identified to cause severe diarrhoea and approximately 453,000 deaths among children <5 years of age [3–8]. A three year prospective, age stratified, matched case-control study (Global Enteric Multicentre Study or GEMS) was conducted in censused population at four sites in Africa and three in Asia [9] to identify pathogen specific paediatric diarrhoeal disease burden in children aged <5 years. GEMS Study confirmed RVA as the most common pathogens in 0–2 year's age group in sub-Saharan Africa and South Asia [9,57].

The RVA belong to family Reoviridae with a double stranded RNA genome contributing 11 gene segments. Due to segmented genome, genetic reassortments are common among co-circulating strains of human or animal origin [10]. This results in generation of large number of genetic variants for example, currently 27G, 37P, 16I, 9R, 9C, 8M, 16A, 9N, 12T, 14E and 11H genotypes have been identified [11,12]. Six RVA genotypes namely G1, G2, G3, G4, G9 and G12 in combination with P[4], P[6] and P[8] commonly infect humans [13].

To reduce the burden two vaccines namely Rotarix (RV1; monovalent G1P[8]; GlaxoSmithKline Biologicals, Rixensart, Belgium) and RotaTeq (RV5; pentavalent G1, G2, G3, G4,P[8]; Merck Vaccines, Whitehouse Station, NJ, USA) were approved by FDA in 2006. Large scale vaccine trials with Rotarix and RotaTeq have shown high efficacy (~85%) in developed countries of Europe, Australia and USA. Though efficacy is low to moderate (39–72%) in low income countries of Asia and Africa, overall reduction in disease severity as estimated by reduced hospitalization and deaths due to diarrhoea, has been documented [7,16–18]. Another oral live attenuated vaccine Rotavac, which was derived from a neonatal G9P[11] human bovine reassortant strain 116E has been licensed in India recently [14,15].

For introduction of these vaccines in national immunization programme in South Asian countries like India, robust data for estimating rotavirus disease burden was required. Several case-control or cohort studies of enteropathogens associated with childhood diarrhoea have been conducted in various countries with focus on either bacterial or viral aetiologies of diarrhoea [1,19–21]. In India a large number of multistate hospital based studies of rotavirus were conducted [22–29]. In Eastern part of India specially in Kolkata a continuous hospital based monitoring system since 2003–2013 showed a large number of hospitalization (>40%) among children due to rotavirus diarrhoea [30–32]. Unfortunately hospital based studies do not provide the disease incidence rates, thus as an extension of GEMS study, burden of RVA and circulating genotypes of RVA were analyzed. Age matched healthy control children were monitored to estimate the asymptomatic infection rates in community. We also investigated whether there was any unusual strain distribution among controls and diarrhoea cases as well as to identify human animal reassortant strains in the community.

Materials and Methods

Study population, sample collection, and processing

The present study was an extension of Global Enteric Multicenter Study (Project entitled- Diarrhoeal diseases in infants and young children in developing countries), conducted during 2008–2010 [9]. An urban slum community of Kolkata was a study site, where population of <5 years children was 13416 [56,57]. A total number of 3582 stool samples were collected, among which, 1568 samples were obtained from children of ≤5 years of age, with moderate to severe diarrhoea, as well as from the children who were admitted in B. C. Roy Memorial Hospital for Children and Infectious Diseases Hospital in Kolkata, India. A total of 2014 samples were collected from age-sex matched healthy neighbourhood controls in same community. Inclusion criteria for symptomatic children included passing of three or more loose/watery stools within 24 hours and satisfy with at least one of the following criteria for moderate to severe diarrhoea (MSD): 1. Sunken eyes (confirmed by parent/caretaker) as more than normal; 2. Loss of skin turgor defined as an abdominal skin pinch with slow or very

slow (>2 seconds) recoil; 3. Intravenous hydration administered or prescribed; 4. Hospitalization with diarrhoea or dysentery. In asymptomatic control group, children without diarrhoea for the past 7 days were enrolled within maximum of 7 days of index case enrolment [56]. Main objective of this case-control study was, to determine the attributable fraction of diarrhoea due to specific pathogen and then estimated disease burden through Demographic Surveillance System (DSS) in community [9]. The detailed methodology has been described in published article [56]. Stool samples were stored at −70°C for further study.

Ethics Statement

Written informed consent was taken from the parents of the children for participation in this study. Potential controls were randomly selected from the population database and matched to the case by age (±2 months for cases 0–11 months and 11–23 months, and ±4 months for cases 23–59 months), gender, and residence (same or nearby neighbourhood as the case). The study was approved by the Institutional Ethical Committee, National Institute of Cholera and Enteric Diseases, (Reference No. C-48/2008 T&E). This study involved minimal risk to the patients, and did not adversely affect the rights or welfare of the patients.

The stool samples were screened for rotavirus using an enzyme-linked immunoassay (EIA) detecting the VP6 antigen as per the manufacturer's instructions (ELISA ProSpecT Rotavirus kit, Oxoid, Basingstoke, UK) [9].

Viral RNA extraction and genotyping

From the ELISA positive samples, rotavirus double-stranded RNA was extracted from feces by using an automated DNA/RNA extractor (EasyMag, bioMèrieux, Marcy l'Etoile, France). Complementary DNA was synthesized from the extracted viral RNA through reverse transcription in the presence of random hexamers. G and P typing was performed using VP7- and VP4-specific multiplex semi-nested RT-PCRs as described previously [33]. PCR products were purified with a QIAquick PCR purification kit (QiagenGmbH, Hilden, Germany).

Nucleotide sequence and phylogenetic analysis

Nucleotide sequencing was carried out using the ABI Prism Big Dye Terminator Cycle Sequencing Ready Reaction Kit v3.1 (Applied Biosystems, Foster City, California, USA) in an ABI Prism 3730 Genetic Analyzer (PE Applied Biosystems, Foster City, California, USA) as described previously [28]. Nucleotide and protein sequence BLAST search was performed using the National Centre for Biotechnology Information (NCBI, National Institutes of Health, Bethesda, MD) Basic Local Alignment Search Tool (BLAST) server on GenBank database release 143.0 [34]. Pairwise sequence alignments were performed using LALIGN software (EMBnet, Swiss Institute of Bioinformatics, Switzerland), and multiple alignments were done with DDBJ software and CLUSTAL W. Amino acid sequences were deduced using the TRANSEQ software (Transeq Nucleotide to Protein Sequence Conversion Tool, EMBL-EBI, Cambridgeshire, UK). Phylogenetic tree was constructed using the MEGA (Molecular Evolutionary Genetics Analysis) program, version 6. Genetic distances were calculated using the Maximum likelihood method (500 bootstrap replicates) using the MEGA 6 program. According to model testing results, Kimura2 parameter model was selected to construct the phylogenetic dendrograms. Lineage designation for phylogenetic dendrograms of G1, G2, G9 and G12 strains were based on those reported in previous studies [35–38]. Partial nucleotide sequences of VP4 gene and complete nucleotide sequences of VP7 gene of the strains detected during this study

Table 1. Distribution of rotavirus strains genotype at Kolkata, India, during 2008–2010.

P Type	P[4]	P[6]	P[8]	P[14]	P[25]	P-NT	Total
G Type							
G1	10 (2.3)	15 (3.4)	140 (32)	0	0	0	165 (37.8)
G2	59 (13.5)	0	18 (4.1)	0	0	0	77 (17.6)
G4	0	3 (0.68)	0	0	0	0	3 (0.68)
G6	0	0	0	1 (0.22)	0	0	1 (0.22)
G9	47 (10.75)	0	74 (16.9)	0	0	8 (1.8)	129 (29.5)
G11	0	0	0	0	1 (0.22)	0	1 (0.22)
G12	1 (0.22)	26 (5.95)	24 (4.49)	0	0	1 (0.22)	52 (11.9)
G-NT	0	0	0	0	0	9 (2.05)	9 (2.05)
Total	117 (26.8)	44 (10.06)	256 (58.6)	1 (0.22)	1 (0.22)	18 (4.1)	437 (100)

were submitted to the GenBank database under the accession numbers: KM008633–KM008642 (G1 strains); KM008643–KM008652 (G2 strains); KM008653–KM008655 (G4 strains); KM008657–KM008666 (G9 strains); KM008667–KM008675 (G12 strains); KM008676–KM008682 (P[4] strains); KM008683–KM008690 (P[6] strains); KM008691–KM008699 (P[8] strains).

Results

Detection of rotavirus among enrolled children in Kolkata

Among 1568 children (age, ≤5 years) with diarrhoea, 395 (25.2%), and among 2014 asymptomatic children, 42 (2%) were rotavirus ELISA positive. Highest numbers of rotavirus were found in 6–24 months age group children in both case and control population (Figure 1). Detection of rotavirus infection was highest during October to March (Figure 2). G and P typing was done for all 437 samples using multiplex RT-PCR with VP7- and VP4-type specific primers. Among 437 of rotavirus positive samples, only 9 rotavirus positive strains remained untypable for both G and P types. The globally common strain G1P[8] was identified as the most common strain (32%) followed by G9P[8] (16.9%), G2P[4] (13.5%) and G9P[4] (10.75%) (Table 1). G12 strains with combinations of P[4], P[6] and P[8] comprised 11.9% of total positive strains. The rest (<10%) were rare and uncommon strains like G1P[4], G1P[6], G2P[8] and animal-like strains G4P[6], G6P[14] and G11P[25]. Among G types, G1 (37.8%) and G9 (29.5%) strains were most prevalent and comprised 67% of the total strains (Table 1). Among eight G9 and one G12 strain, the P type could not be determined. The 42 RVA positive samples from healthy children revealed similar genotypes like G1, G2 and G9. Most of the uncommon and animal-like rotaviruses were detected from diarrhoea patients, only one unusual strain G6P[14] was detected from an asymptomatic control sample (Table 2).

Analysis of VP7 gene

The VP7 genes of 44 randomly selected rotavirus strains were analyzed following sequencing of the complete ORF (nt 49–nt 1026). Based on nucleotide sequences, phylogenetic dendograms for representative G1 (10/165), G9 (10/129), G2 (10/77), G4 (3/3), G12 (9/52), G6 (1/1) and G11 (1/1) rotaviruses were analyzed with other previously reported representative strains, belonging to the individual G types.

Analysis of G1 strains

G1 rotaviruses exhibited 97–99% nucleotide identities with strains from Australia, Thailand and Japan as well as the previously reported Indian strains (Table 3). Phylogenetic analysis revealed clustering of G1/Kolkata strains with the common G1 strains within lineage I. One strain (Kol-15-10) out of 10 clustered in lineage II (Figure 3A).

Analysis of G2 strains

Comparative analysis of 7 G2 strains showed high sequence identity (98.3–99.6%) with G2 strains of Bangladesh, Thailand, Australia and Italy within lineage IV. But 3 G2 strains, Kol-2-08, Kol-5-08 and Kol-17-08, showed relatively lower nucleotide identity (92–95%) with the lineage IV strains. But according to phylogenetic analysis, all Kolkata G2 strains remain within lineage IV (Figure 3B).

Analysis of G9 strains

G9 was the second highest genotype observed during this study. Most of the G9 strains were found with P[8] and P[4] specificity,

Table 2. Age and type wise distribution of Rotavirus positive Case and Control stool samples (During the year 2008 through 2010).

Age Group	No. Of Collected samples (Case)	No. of Positive samples (Case)	No. of Collected samples (Control)	No. of Positive Samples (Control)
0–6 months	289	64 (22.1%) G1P[8] = 21; G1P[6] = 5; G2P[4] = 20; G2P[8] = 5; G4P[6] = 1; G9P[4] = 3; G9P[8] = 5; G12P[6] = 3; G12P[8] = 1	252	7 (2.8%) G1P[8] = 4; G9P[4] = 1; G9P[8] = 2
6–12 months	434	143 (32.9%) G1P[8] = 32; G1P[4] = 4; G1P[6] = 4; G2P[4] = 15; G2P[8] = 6; G4P[6] = 1; G9P[4] = 21; G9P[8] = 29; G12P[4] = 1; G12P[6] = 15; G12P[8] = 10; G(NT)P[NT] = 5	392	14 (3.5%) G1P[8] = 8; G9P[4] = 3; G6P[14] = 1; G12P[6] = 1; G12P[NT] = 1
12–24 months	572	126 (22%) G1P[8] = 50; G1P[6] = 3; G1P[4] = 2; G2P[4] = 18; G2P[8] = 4; G4P[6] = 1; G9P[4] = 13; G9P[8] = 16; G9P[NT] = 3; G12P[6] = 7; G12P[8] = 5; G(NT)P[NT] = 4	544	12 (2.2%) G1P[8] = 4; G1P[6] = 1; G2P[4] = 1; G2P[8] = 2; G9P[4] = 2; G9P[8] = 2
24–36 months	166	36 (21.7%) G1P[8] = 7; G1P[6] = 2; G1P[4] = 3; G2P[4] = 5; G9P[8] = 5; G9P[NT] = 5; G11P[25] = 1; G12P[8] = 8	497	5 (1%) G1P[8] = 2; G9P[4] = 1; G9P[8] = 2
36–60 months	107	26 (24.2%) G1P[8] = 10; G2P[8] = 1; G9P[4] = 3; G9P[8] = 12	329	4 (1.2%) G1P[8] = 2; G1P[4] = 1; G9P[8] = 1
Total	1568	395 (25.2%)	2014	42 (2%)
0–6 months	289	64 (22.1%) G1P[8] = 21; G1P[6] = 5; G2P[4] = 20; G2P[8] = 5; G4P[6] = 1; G9P[4] = 3; G9P[8] = 5; G12P[6] = 3; G12P[8] = 1	252	7 (2.8%) G1P[8] = 4; G9P[4] = 1; G9P[8] = 2

however a few (1.8%) could not be typed for VP4 gene. Nucleotide and amino acid blast analysis as well as phylogenetic analysis revealed close clustering of Kolkata G9 strains with lineage III G9 strains reported from India, South Korea, Italy and South Africa (Table 3; Figure 4A).

Analysis of G12 strains

G12 strains were found in combination with P[4], P[6] and P[8]. Following nucleotide analysis, all G12 rotaviruses shared maximum identity ($\approx$97%) with G12 strains reported from Bangladesh (Dhaka 12-03), India (mani-485) and Germany (GER172-08) (Table 3). Phylogenetic analysis revealed clustering of current Kolkata G12 strains with lineage III G12 strains (Figure 4B).

Analysis of G4 strains

Only three G4 strains Kol-54-10, Kol-78-10 and Kol-80-10 were identified during the study with P[6] specificity. Preliminary BLAST analysis of VP7 gene of these G4 strains revealed genetic relatedness to porcine G4 strains of China, HeN4 with nucleotide identity of 98% (Table 3). In the phylogenetic dendrogram, also these strains clustered with the porcine strains of China along with porcine-like human G4 strains of India and Vietnam (Figure 5A).

Analysis of G6 and G11 strain

Only one G6 strain RVA/Human-wt/IND/N-1/2009/G6P[14] and one G11 strain RVA/Human-wt/IND/N-38/2009/G11P[25] were identified during this study. The G6 strain N-1/2009, shares 95% nucleotide identity and 97% amino acid

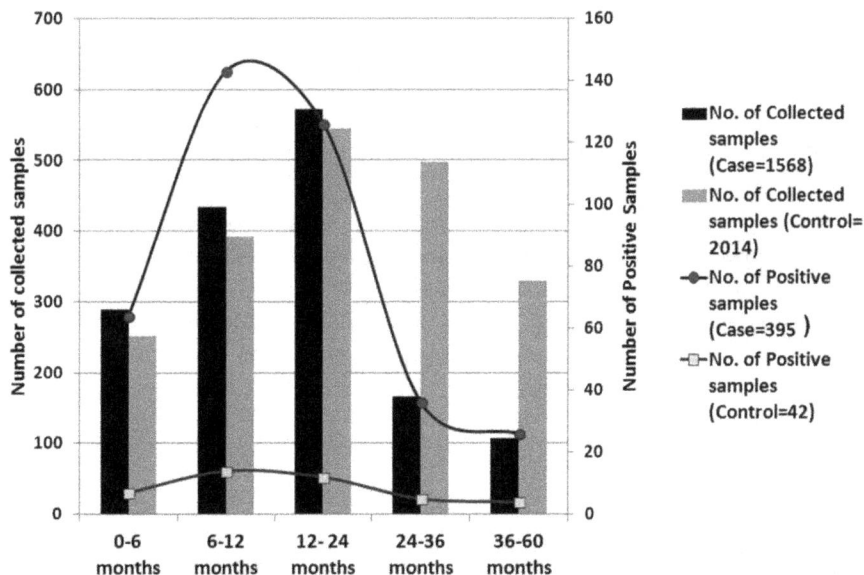

Figure 1. Age distribution. Age –wise distribution of rotavirus-positive Case and Control children (0–5 years) against total collected samples during January 2008 through December 2010.

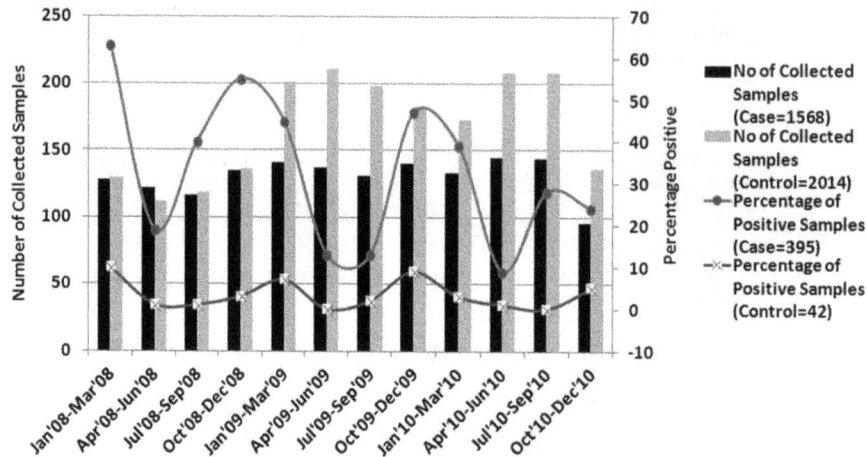

Figure 2. Seasonality of rotavirus in Kolkata. Seasonal distribution of the rotavirus positivity against total collected samples in Case and Control children in an urban slum community in Kolkata, India, during January 2008 through December 2010.

homology with previously reported bovine strain RUBV319 from India [39]. N-1/2009 was found to be in the same cluster with Indian bovine strains and with a caprine strain GO34 from Bangladesh in phylogenetic dendrogram. The G11 strain N-38/2009 showed 98% sequence identity with a porcine-like human strain CRI10795 previously reported from India and 91% nucleotide similarity with a Mexican porcine strain YM. N-38/2009 clustered with porcine-like human G11 strains from Bangladesh, Nepal, India and South Korea [39], all of which were originated from porcine G11 strain YM.

Analysis of VP4 gene

Partial VP4 gene (nt 1–nt 881; VP8* complete ORF 247 aa) sequences of the 26 strains (7 genotype P[4], 8 genotype P[6], and 9 genotype P[8], 1 genotype P[14], 1 genotype P[25] strains) were analyzed.

Analysis of P[4] and P[8] strains

P[4] strains were detected with G1, G2, G9 and G12 genotypes, though majority of P[4] (24%) genotype was associated with G2 and G9. Nucleotide and amino acid sequence analysis revealed that P[4] genotype associated with G2 strains, were more than 97% homologous with common human strains reported from Thailand and India (Table 3). Other P[4] strains, shared of ≈96% nucleotide identity with the human P[4] strains of Japan, Bangladesh, Russia and worldwide (Table 3; Figure 6A). The P[8] rotaviruses commonly associated with G1 genotype, whereas few associated with G9, G2 and G12 also. P[8] associated with G1 strains and one G12 strain, Kol-31-10 exhibited nucleotide identity (96–99%) with RVA strains of India and Bangladesh. Other P[8], associated with G2, G9 and G12 shared 99% nucleotide identity with a G12P[8] strain from Vanderbilt, USA (Table 3; Figure 6B).

Table 3. Diversity of rotavirus genotype and their origin at Kolkata, India, during 2008–2010.

Types	Homology	Origin
Common Types		
G1 (n = 165)	OH2024 (Japan), CMH042 (Thailand), NIV-088325 (India), BA17290 (Brazil), CK20043 (Australia)	Human
G2 (n = 77)	MMC6 (Bangladesh), CMH134 (Thailand), RCH020 (Australia), CK20051 (Australia), PA83/2007 (Italy)	Human
G9 (n = 129)	ISO95 (India), CAU202 (South Korea), 2371WC (South Africa), AV21 (Italy)	Human
G12 (n = 52)	Mani-485 (India), ISO-16 (India), Dhaka12 (Bangladesh), GER172 (Germany), ISO27 (India), VU08-09-6 (USA)	Human
P[4] (n = 117)	CAU209-KK (Thailand), 01076 (Russia), CMH028 (Thailand), Omsk08-464 (Russia), CK20043 (Australia)	Human
P[8] (n = 256)	GRAVP420 (India), VU08-09-39 (Vanderbilt), CAU202 (South Korea), MRC-DPRU1417/2009 (Cameroon)	Human
Uncommon Types		
G4 (n = 3)	HeN4 (China)	Porcine
G6 (n = 1)	RUBV319 (India)	Bovine
G11 (n = 1)	KTM368 (Nepal), YM (Mexico)	Human, Porcine
P[6] (n = 44)	GER172 (Germany), SK277 (Japan), GUB88 (Japan)	Human, Porcine
P[14] (n = 1)	Hun5 (Hungary)	Human
P[25] (n = 1)	Dhaka6 (Bangladesh), KTM368 (Nepal)	Human

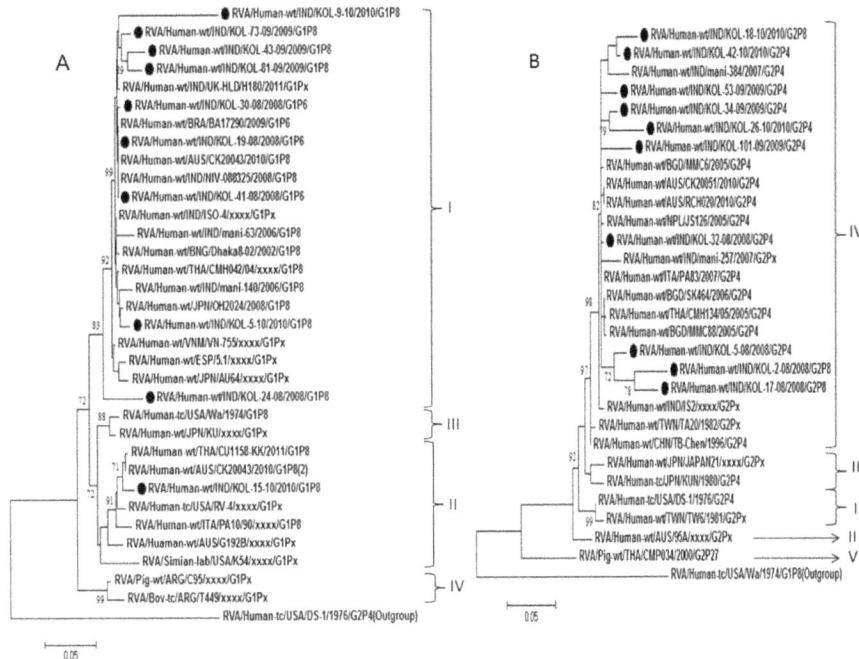

Figure 3. A and B. Phylogenetic trees of the G1 and G2 strains of Kolkata. Phylogenetic trees constructed from the nucleotide sequences of VP7 genes of A. G1; B. G2 strains of Kolkata, isolated during January 2008 through December 2010, with other representative G1 and G2 strains respectively. A. One Kolkata G1 strain showed its relatedness to lineage II G1 strains and the rest G1 strains clustered with lineage I G1 strains. B. All Kolkata G2 strains clustered with lineage IV G2 strains. Scale bar, 0.05 substitutions per nucleotide. Bootstrap values less than 70% are not shown.

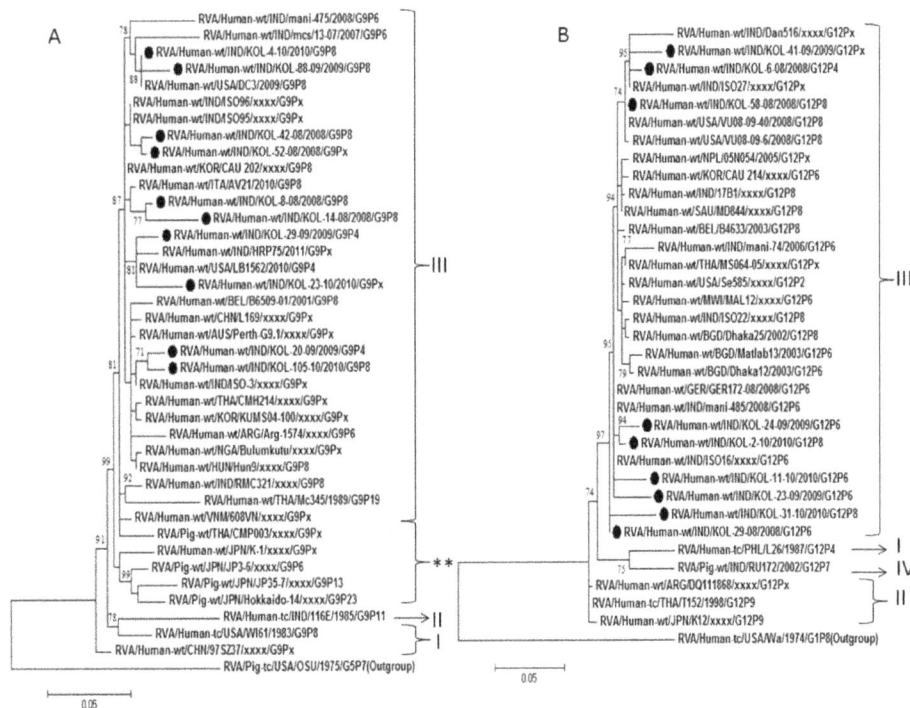

Figure 4. A and B. Phylogenetic trees of the G9 and G12 strains of Kolkata. Phylogenetic trees constructed from the nucleotide sequences of VP7 genes of A. G9; B. G12 strains of Kolkata, isolated during January 2008 through December 2010, with other representative G9 and G12 strains respectively. A. All Kolkata G9 strains showed relatedness to lineage III G9 strains. (**Sub cluster of Japanese and Chinese rotavirus strains). B. All Kolkata G12 strains clustered with lineage III G12 strains. Scale bar, 0.05 substitutions per nucleotide. Bootstrap values less than 70% are not shown.

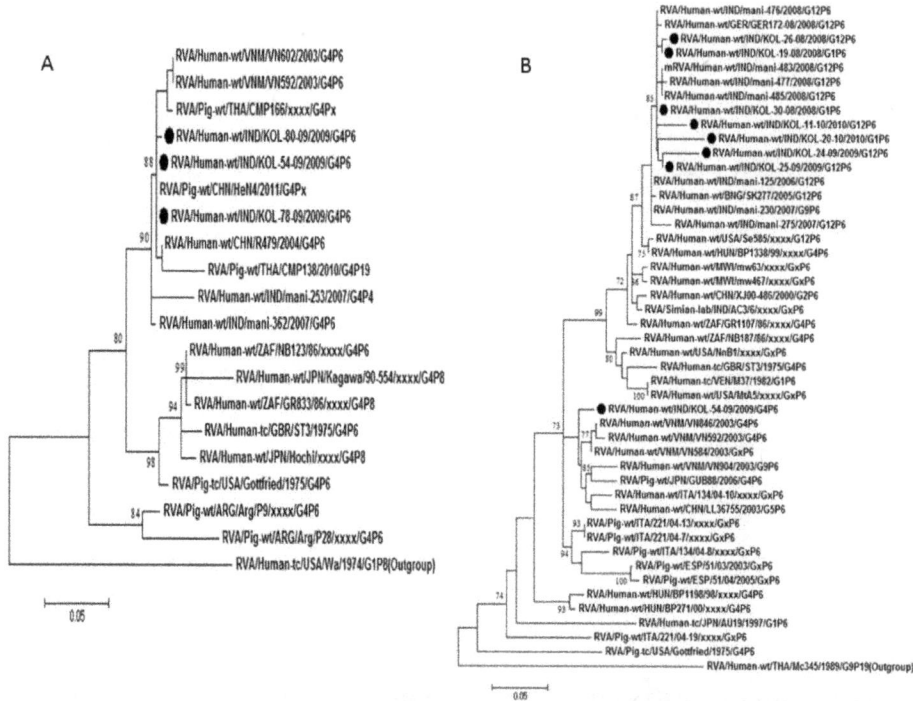

Figure 5. A and B. Phylogenetic trees of the G4 and P[6] strains of Kolkata. Phylogenetic trees constructed from the nucleotide sequences of VP7 genes of A. G4; and VP4 genes of B. P[6] strains of Kolkata, isolated during January 2008 through December 2010, with other representative G4 and P[6] strains respectively. All G4 strains indicated its genetic relatedness with the porcine or porcine-like human G4 strains. Scale bar, 0.05 substitutions per nucleotide. Bootstrap values less than 70% are not shown.

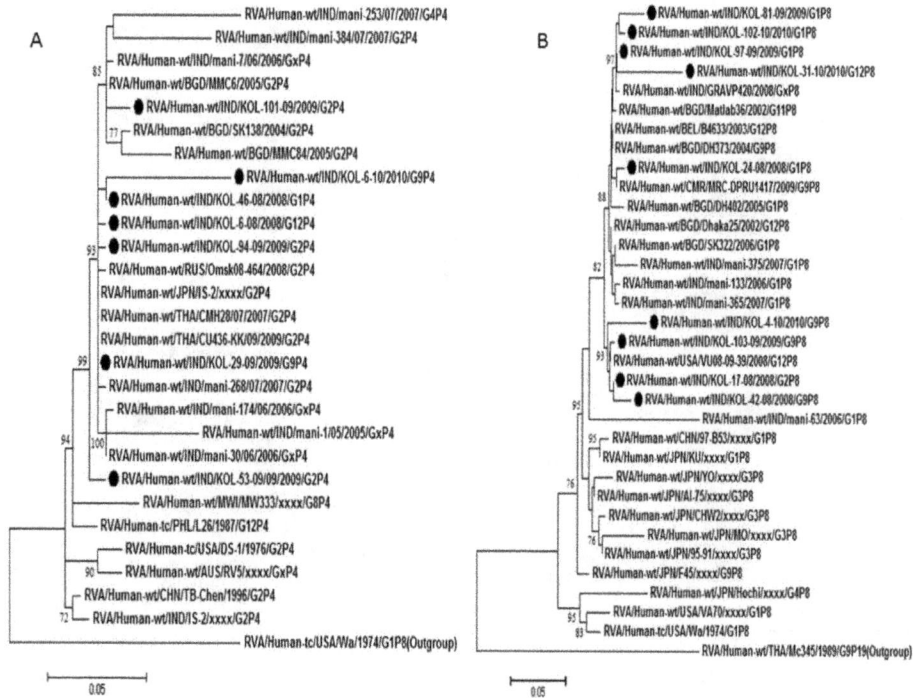

Figure 6. A and B. Phylogenetic trees of the P[4] and P[8] strains of Kolkata. Phylogenetic trees constructed from the nucleotide sequences of VP4 genes of A. P[4]; and B. P[8] strains of Kolkata, isolated during January 2008 through December 2010, with other representative P[4] and P[8] strains respectively. Scale bar, 0.05 substitutions per nucleotide. Bootstrap values less than 70% are not shown.

Analysis of P[6] strains

Eight strains with P[6] genotypes were further analyzed. P[6] strain associated with G4 were 95% nucleotide homolog to the VP4 gene of a Japanese porcine strain GUB88. Other P[6] strains associated with G1 and G12 clustered with other recently emerging porcine-like human P[6] strains from India, Germany, and Japanese porcine strains as shown in phylogenetic tree (Figure 5B).

Analysis of P[14] and P[25] strain

P[14] and P[25] genotypes are very rare. A few of P[14] genotypes are reported in bovine/bovine-like human strains to date from several parts of Europe and India [40–42]. P[25] genotypes are reported previously in Bangladesh, Nepal and India [43,44]. As described previously, P[14] strain detected in this study originated from a bovine strain of India and P[25] strain was found to share its homology with porcine-like human strain KTM368 reported from Nepal [39].

Discussion

Deaths due to rotavirus infection are uncommon in industrialized countries, but rotavirus infection remains an important cause of mortality among young children in the developing countries [45–47]. Due to huge genetic diversity, interspecies transmission, genetic reassortment and recombination, vaccines have not been successful in controlling the infection though vaccination has significant effect on reducing disease severity and hospitalization rates [16].

In developing countries like India where diarrhoea related mortality is high continuous monitoring of the circulating genotypes in the community is required, prior to implementation and evaluation of candidate vaccines. Community based studies are thus important to assess the impact of immunization on the prevalence of common genotypes, emergence of strains that escape immunity and evolution of the genes of wild type rotaviruses as a consequence of immune selective pressure. Inclusion of asymptomatic control children to this study helped to figure out the exact burden and risk factors of rotavirus infection in community, because asymptomatic infections are potential source of dispersal of infection in environment.

During this study, in the year 2008 through 2010, in an urban slum community in Kolkata, India, 25.2% of the children with severe diarrhoea, were detected positive for rotavirus, and 2% of the asymptomatic children were rotavirus positive [9]. As expected percent positivity of rotavirus in community settings (25.2%) is lower compared to ~40%±5% positivity observed in hospital based studies [26,28,30,31,48]. Consistent with previously reported seasonality of RVA infection in India, in this study maximum positivity was observed during October to March (Figure 2) when average temperature remained 21°–23°C [26,28,32]. Similarly age wise distribution revealed maximum rotavirus positive children of 6–24 months old (Figure 1). This is probably due to start of weaning period from 6 months age when child is introduced to semi solid food and infant ready food mixes thus increasing exposure to water and other environmental source of contaminations. We could not found any distinct variation in strain distribution within case and control children. Common strains like G1, G2, G9 and G12 were found within both case and control children (Table 2).

Recent reviews revealed G1P[8], G2P[4], G3P[8] and G4P[8] as the globally important combinations of rotavirus strains detected worldwide [19]. In Kolkata, previous studies during 2003–2007, showed that, in the Eastern part of India, G1 (>50%)

and G2 strains (~23–33%) were dominant, whereas G9 (2–10%) and G12 (8–17%) strains occurred at varied frequency over the period of time (2003–2007) [30,31]. The community based study (2008–2010) showed increasing trend of G9 strains (29.5%) whereas G1 strains (37.8%) were predominant (Table 1). Interestingly the follow up hospital based study in Kolkata during 2011–2013, revealed overall reduction of G1 strains (~16%) and significant increase in G9 strains (~40%) and G2 (~36%) strains [32]. This indicates it was a gradual process of replacement of G1 strains by G9 strains. One of the reasons for the emergence of G9 strains worldwide was that the rare genotypes like the G12 or G9 might escape recognition by the host immune system which recognizes the common G1–G4 genotypes. In addition if complete cross protection is not achieved by current vaccines, RotaTeq (G1–G4 P[8]) and Rotarix (G1P[8]) a selective increase in the prevalence of G9 or other emerging genotypes is possible even though cross protection to other genotypes has been documented [16]. However, in India the increase in G9 strains cannot be attributed to vaccines yet as RVA vaccines have still not been introduced in national immunization program. Due to high incidence of G9 strains in India, efficacy studies on newly licensed G9 based vaccine 116E are being evaluated [15]. Sequence analysis revealed all G9 strains to be similar to lineage III strains reported previously from Asia, Africa and Europe [31,32,53–55]. During previous studies in India G9 strains were commonly observed in combination with P[6] or P[8] [28,31], but during this period almost 10.75% strains belong to G9P[4] genotype. As G9 is normally associated with Wa-like genotype strains and P[4] belongs to Ds-1-like genotype, thus increased occurrence of G9P[4] may be a result of intergenogroup reassortment [58]. Further full genome analysis of these strains is required to understand origin of these G9P[4] strains.

G12 strains have been reported from India, Bangladesh, Brazil, Spain, USA and other countries with varying frequency in association with either P[6] or P[8] genotypes [26,49–52]. G12 strains detected in current study belong to lineage III (Figure 4B) consistent with the previously reported G12 strains worldwide. Other strains like G4, G12, G6, G11 in combination with P[6], P[14], P[25] comprised ~15% of all genotypes (Table 1). Consistent with previous surveillance data from Kolkata, G3 strains were not observed and G4 strains, which were all derived from animal origin (Figure 5A), circulated at very low frequency (~1%).

Systemic case-control study confirms co-circulation of all major genotypes G1, G2, G9, G12, detection of unusual strains, and zoonotic transmissions reflecting the complex epidemiology of group A rotaviruses in India. Such variations may be facilitated by high density population, poor unhygienic conditions, and lack of safe drinking water. Preventive strategies targeting first 2 years of life may accelerate effectiveness in disease control. Continuous longitudinal surveillance programs both before and after introduction of rotavirus vaccine will shed light on the long term efficacy of rotavirus vaccines in India.

Acknowledgments

Satarupa Mullick is supported by Senior Research Fellowship from Indian Council of Medical Research (ICMR), India.

Author Contributions

Conceived and designed the experiments: MCS TR JPN. Performed the experiments: SM AM SG GPP. Analyzed the data: SM BM DS. Contributed reagents/materials/analysis tools: JPN MML. Contributed to the writing of the manuscript: SM MCS. Collected the samples from enrolled children in this study: DS BM. Initial screening of samples: GPP SG.

References

1. Olesen B, Neimann J, Böttiger B, Ethelberg S, Schiellerup P, et al. (2005) Etiology of diarrhoea in young children in Denmark: a case-control study. J Clin Microbiol 43(8): 3636–41.
2. National Collaborating Centre for Women's and Children's Health. (2009) Diarrhoea and Vomiting Caused by Gastroenteritis: Diagnosis, Assessment and Management in Children Younger Than 5 Years. London: RCOG Press; Available from: http://www.nice.org.uk/nicemedia/pdf/CG84FullGuideline.pdf. Accessed March 31, 2012.
3. Akihara S, Phan TG, Nguyen TA, Hansman G, Okitsu S, et al. (2005) Existence of multiple outbreaks of viral gastroenteritis among infants in a day care center in Japan. Arch Virol 150(10): 2061–75.
4. Nair GB, Ramamurthy T, Bhattacharya MK, Krishnan T, Ganguly S, et al. (2010) Emerging trends in the etiology of enteric pathogens as evidenced from an active surveillance of hospitalized diarrhoeal patients in Kolkata, India. Gut Pathog 5; 2(1): 4. doi:10.1186/1757-4749-2-4.
5. Shimizu H, Phan TG, Nishimura S, Okitsu S, Maneekarn N, et al. (2007) An outbreak of adenovirus serotype 41 infection in infants and children with acute gastroenteritis in Maizuru City, Japan. Infect Genet Evol 7(2): 279–84.
6. Lanata CF, Fischer-Walker CL, Olascoaga AC, Torres CX, Aryee MJ, et al. (2013) Global Causes of Diarrhoeal Disease Mortality in Children, 5 Years of Age: A Systematic Review. PLoS One 4; 8(9): e72788. doi:10.1371/journal.pone.0072788.
7. Liu L, Johnson HL, Cousens S, Perin J, Scott S, et al. (2012) Global, regional, and national causes of child mortality: an updated systematic analysis for 2010 with time trends since 2000. Lancet 379: 2151–61.
8. Tate JE, Burton AH, Boschi-Pinto C, Steele AD, Duque J, et al. (2012) WHO-coordinated Global Rotavirus Surveillance Network: 2008 estimate of worldwide rotavirus-associated mortality in children younger than 5 years before the introduction of universal rotavirus vaccination programmes: a systematic review and meta-analysis. Lancet Infect Dis 12(2): 136–41.
9. Kotloff KL, Nataro JP, Blackwelder WC, Nasrin D, Farag TH, et al. (2013) Burden and aetiology of diarrhoeal disease in infants and young children in developing countries (the Global Enteric Multicenter Study, GEMS): a prospective, case-control study. Lancet 382: 209–22.
10. Donato CM, Manuelpillai NM, Cowley D, Roczo-Farkas S, Buttery JP, et al. (2014) Genetic characterization of a novel G3P[14] rotavirus strain causing gastroenteritis in 12year old Australian child. Infect Genet Evol 25: 97–109. doi:10.1016/j.meegid.2014.04.009.
11. Matthijnssens J, Ciarlet M, McDonald SM, Attoui H, Bányai K, et al. (2011) Uniformity of rotavirus strain nomenclature proposed by the Rotavirus Classification Working Group (RCWG). Arch Virol 156: 1397–1413 DOI 10.1007/s00705-011-1006-z.
12. Trojnar E, Sachsenröder J, Twardziok S, Reetz J, Otto PH, et al. (2013) Identification of an avian group A rotavirus containing a novel VP4 gene with a close relationship to those of mammalian rotaviruses. J Gen Virol 94(Pt 1): 136–42. doi:10.1099/vir.0.047381-0.
13. Matthijnssens J, Ciarlet M, Rahman M, Attoui H, Bányai K, et al. (2008) Recommendations for the classification of group A rotaviruses using all 11 genomic RNA segments. Arch Virol 153(8): 1621–9. doi:10.1007/s00705-008-0155.
14. Kumar D, Beach NM, Meng XJ, Hegde NR (2012) Use of PCR-based assays for the detection of the adventitious agent porcine circovirus type 1 (PCV1) in vaccines, and for confirming the identity of cell substrates and viruses used in vaccine production. J Virol Methods 179(1): 201–11. doi:10.1016/j.jviromet.2011.10.017.
15. Bhandari N, Rongsen-Chandola T, Bavdekar A, John J, Antony K, et al. (2014) Efficacy of a monovalent human-bovine (116E) rotavirus vaccine in Indian infants: a randomised, double-blind, placebo-controlled trial. Lancet 11. pii: S0140-6736(13)62630-6. doi:10.1016/S0140-6736(13)62630-6.
16. Matthijnssens J, Nakagomi O, Kirkwood CD, Ciarlet M, Desselberger U, et al. (2012) Group A rotavirus universal mass vaccination: how and to what extent will selective pressure influence prevalence of rotavirus genotypes? Expert Rev Vaccines 11(11): 1347–54. doi:10.1586/erv.12.105.
17. Jiang V, Jiang B, Tate J, Parashar UD, Patel MM, et al. (2010) Performance of rotavirus vaccines in developed and developing countries. Hum Vaccine 6: 532–42.
18. Steele AD, Neuzil KM, Cunliffe NA, Madhi SA, Bos P, et al. (2012) Human rotavirus vaccine Rotarix provides protection against diverse circulating rotavirus strains in African infants: a randomized controlled trial. BMC Infect Dis 12: 213. doi:10.1186/1471-2334-12-213.
19. Kawai K, O'Brien MA, Goveia MG, Mast TC, El Khoury AC (2012) Burden of rotavirus gastroenteritis and distribution of rotavirus strains in Asia: a systematic review. Vaccine 30(7): 1244–54. doi:10.1016/j.vaccine.2011.12.092.
20. Moyo SJ, Blomberg B, Hanevik K, Kommedal O, Vainio K, et al. (2014) Genetic diversity of circulating rotavirus strains in Tanzania prior to the introduction of vaccination. PLoS One 20; 9(5): e97562. doi:10.1371/journal.pone.0097562.
21. Caprioli A, Pezzella C, Morelli R, Giammanco A, Arista S, et al. (1996) Enteropathogens associated with childhood diarrhoea in Italy. The Italian Study Group on Gastrointestinal Infections. Pediatr Infect Dis J 15(10): 876–83.
22. Banerjee I, Ramani S, Primrose B, Iturriza-Gomara M, Gray JJ, et al. (2007) Modification of rotavirus multiplex RT-PCR for the detection of G12 strains based on characterization of emerging G12 rotavirus strains from South India. J Med Virol 79(9): 1413–21.
23. Das BK, Gentsch JR, Cicirello HG, Woods PA, Gupta A, et al. (1994) Characterization of rotavirus strains from newborns in New Delhi, India. J Clin Microbiol 32(7): 1820–2.
24. Das S, Varghese V, Chaudhuri S, Barman P, Kojima K, et al. (2004) Genetic variability of human rotavirus strains isolated from Eastern and Northern India. J Med Virol 72(1): 156–61.
25. Kang G, Kelkar SD, Chitambar SD, Ray P, Naik T (2005) Epidemiological profile of rotaviral infection in India: challenges for the 21st century. J Infect Dis 1; 192 Suppl 1: S120–6.
26. Kang G, Arora R, Chitambar SD, Deshpande J, Gupte MD, et al. (2009) Multicenter, Hospital-Based Surveillance of Rotavirus Disease and Strains among Indian Children Aged <5 Years. The Journal of Infectious Diseases 200: S147–53. DOI:10.1086/605031.
27. Morris SK, Awasthi S, Khera A, Bassani DG, Kang G, et al. (2012) Rotavirus mortality in India: estimates based on a nationally representative survey of diarrhoeal deaths. 2012. Bull World Health Organ 2012; 90: 720–727 | doi:10.2471/BLT.12.101873.
28. Mukherjee A, Chattopadhyay S, Bagchi P, Dutta D, Singh NB, et al. (2010) Surveillance and molecular characterization of rotavirus strains circulating in Manipur, North-Eastern India: Increasing prevalence of emerging G12 strains. Infect Genet Evol 10: 311–320.
29. Chakravarti A, Chauhan MS, Sharma A, Verma V (2010) Distribution of human rotavirus G and P genotypes in a hospital setting from Northern India. Southeast Asian J Trop Med Public Health 41(5): 1145–52.
30. Samajdar S, Varghese V, Barman P, Ghosh S, Mitra U, et al. (2006) Changing pattern of human group A rotaviruses: emergence of G12 as an important pathogen among children in eastern India. J Clin Virol 36(3): 183–8.
31. Samajdar S, Ghosh S, Chawla-Sarkar M, Mitra U, Dutta P, Kobayashi N, et al. (2008) Increase in prevalence of human group A rotavirus G9 strains as an important VP7 genotype among children in eastern India. J Clin Virol 43(3): 334–9. doi:10.1016/j.jcv.2008.07.007.
32. Mullick S, Mandal P, Nayak MK, Ghosh S, De P, et al. (2014) Hospital based Surveillance and Genetic Characterization of Rotavirus strains in Children (< 5 years) with acute gastroenteritis in Kolkata, India, revealed Resurgence of G9 and G2 Genotypes during 2011–2013. http://dx.doi.org/10.1016/j.vaccine.2014.03.018.
33. Taniguchi K, Wakasugi F, Pongsuwanna Y, Urasawa T, Ukae S, et al. (1992) Identification of human and bovine rotavirus serotypes by polymerase chain reaction. Epidemiol Infect 109, 303–12.
34. Schaffer AA, Aravind L, Madden TL, Shavirin S, Spouge JL, et al. (2001) Improving the accuracy of PSI-BLAST protein database searches with composition-based statistics and other refinements. Nucleic Acids Res 29: 2994–3005.
35. Barril P, Martınez L, Giordano M, Masachessi G, Isa M, et al. (2013) Genetic and Antigenic Evolution Profiles of G1 Rotaviruses in Cordoba, Argentina, During a 27-Year Period (1980–2006). Journal of Medical Virology 85: 363–369.
36. Do LP, Nakagomi T, Doan YH, Kitahori Y, Nakagomi O, et al. (2013) Molecular evolution of the VP7 gene of Japanese G2 rotaviruses before vaccine introduction. Arch Virol DOI 10.1007/s00705-013-1804-6.
37. Ghosh S, Varghese V, Samajdar S, Bhattacharya SK, Kobayashi N, et al. (2006) Molecular characterization of a porcine Group A rotavirus strain with G12 genotype specificity. Arch Virol 151: 1329–1344.
38. Matthijnssens J, Heylen E, Zeller M, Rahman M, Lemey P, et al. (2010) Phylodynamic analyses of rotavirus genotypes G9 and G12 underscore their potential for swift global spread. Mol Biol Evol 27: 2431–2436.
39. Mullick S, Mukherjee A, Ghosh S, Pazhani GP, Sur D, et al. (2013) Genomic analysis of human rotavirus strains G6P[14] and G11P[25] isolated from Kolkata in 2009 reveals interspecies transmission and complex reassortment events. Infect Genet Evol 14: 15–21. doi:10.1016/j.meegid.2012.11.010.
40. Iturriza-Gomara M, Dallman T, Ba'nyai K, Bottiger B, Buesa J, et al. (2010) Rotavirus genotypes co-circulating in Europe between 2006 and 2009 as determined by EuroRotaNet, a pan-European collaborative strain surveillance network. Epidemiol. Infect 139(6): 895–909. doi:10.1017/S0950268810001810.
41. Rahman M, De Leener K, Goegebuer T, Wollants E, Van der Donck I, et al. (2003) Genetic characterization of a novel, naturally occurring recombinant human G6P[6] rotavirus. J Clin Microbiol 41 (5), 2088–2095.
42. Matthijnssens J, Potgieter CA, Ciarlet M, Parreño V, Martella V, et al. (2009) Are human P[14] rotavirus strains the result of interspecies transmissions from sheep or other ungulates that belong to the mammalian order Artiodactyla? J Virol 83(7): 2917–29. doi:10.1128/JVI.02246-08.

43. Matthijnssens J, Rahman M, Ciarlet M, Zeller M, Heylen E, et al. (2010) Reassortment of Human Rotavirus Gene Segments into G11 Rotavirus Strains. Emerg Infect Dis 16(4): 625–30.

44. Banerjee I, Iturriza-Gomara M, Rajendran P, Primrose B, Ramani S, et al. (2007) Molecular Characterization of G11P[25] and G3P[3] Human Rotavirus Strains Associated With Asymptomatic Infection in South India. J Med Virol 79(11): 1768–1774.

45. Payne DC, Staat MA, Edwards KM, Szilagyi PG, Gentsch JR, et al. (2008) Active, population-based surveillance for severe rotavirus gastroenteritis in children in the United States. Pediatrics 122(6): 1235–43. doi:10.1542/peds.2007-3378.

46. Forster J, Guarino A, Parez N, Moraga F, Román E, et al. (2009) Hospital-based surveillance to estimate the burden of rotavirus gastroenteritis among European children younger than 5 years of age. Pediatrics 123(3): e393–400. doi:10.1542/peds.2008-2088.

47. Morris SK, Awasthi S, Khera A, Bassani DG, Kang G, et al. (2012) Rotavirus mortality in India: estimates based on a nationally representative survey of diarrhoeal deaths. 2012. Bull World Health Organ 90: 720–727 | doi:10.2471/BLT.12.101873.

48. Paul SK, Kobayashi N, Nagashima S, Ishino M, Watanabe S, et al. (2008) Phylogenetic analysis of rotaviruses with genotypes G1, G2, G9 and G12 in Bangladesh: evidence for a close relationship between rotaviruses from children and adults. Arch Virol 153(11): 1999–2012. doi:10.1007/s00705-008-0212-9.

49. Rahman M, Sultana R, Ahmed G, Nahar S, Hassan ZM, et al. (2007) Prevalence of G2P[4] and G12P[6] rotavirus, Bangladesh. Emerg Infect Dis 13(1): 18–24.

50. Gómez MM, Resque HR, Volotão ED, Rose TL, Figueira Marques da Silva M, et al. (2014) Distinct evolutionary origins of G12P[8] and G12P[9] group A rotavirus strains circulating in Brazil. Infect Genet Evol 18. pii: S1567-1348(14)00129-4. doi:10.1016/j.meegid.2014.04.007.

51. Cilla G, Montes M, Arana A (2014) Rotavirus G12 in Spain: 2004–2006. Enferm Infecc Microbiol Clin 14. pii: S0213-005X(14)00085-8. doi:10.1016/j.eimc.2014.01.012.

52. Mijatovic-Rustempasic S, Teel EN, Kerin TK, Hull JJ, Roy S, et al. (2014) Genetic analysis of G12P[8] rotaviruses detected in the largest U.S. G12 genotype outbreak on record. Infect Genet Evol 21: 214–9. doi:10.1016/j.meegid.2013.11.004.

53. Kiulia NM, Nyaga MM, Seheri ML, Wolfaardt M, van Zyl WB, et al. (2014) Rotavirus G and P types circulating in the eastern region of Kenya: predominance of G9 and emergence of G12 genotypes. Pediatr Infect Dis J 33 Suppl 1: S85–8. doi:10.1097/INF.0000000000000059.

54. Sánchez-Fauquier A, González-Galán V, Arroyo S, Cabornero A, Ruiz-Burruecos A, et al. (2014) Monitoring of children with acute gastroenteritis in Madrid, Spain, during 2010–2011: rotavirus genotype distribution after the vaccines introduction. Enferm Infecc Microbiol Clin 32(5): 280–4. doi:10.1016/j.eimc.2013.07.012.

55. Theamboonlers A, Maiklang O, Thongmee T, Chieochansin T, Vuthitanachot V, et al. (2014) Complete genotype constellation of human rotavirus group A circulating in Thailand, 2008–2011. Infect Genet Evol 21: 295–302. doi:10.1016/j.meegid.2013.11.020.

56. Kotloff KL, Blackwelder WC, Nasrin D, Nataro JP, Farag TH, et al. (2013) The Global Enteric Multicenter Study (GEMS) of diarrhoeal disease in infants and young children in developing countries: epidemiologic and clinical methods of the case/control study. Clin Infect Dis 57(1): 165. doi:10.1093/cid/cis753.

57. Levine MM, Kotloff KL, Nataro JP, Muhsen K (2012) The Global Enteric Multicenter Study (GEMS): impetus, rationale, and genesis. Clin Infect Dis 55 Suppl 4: S215–24. doi:10.1093/cid/cis761.

58. Matthijnssens J, Ciarlet M, Heiman E, Arijs I, Delbeke T, et al. (2008) Full genome-based classification of rotaviruses reveals a common origin between human Wa-like and porcine rotavirus strains and human DS-1-like and bovine rotavirus strains. J Virol. 82: 3204–3219.

23

Escherichia coli STb Enterotoxin Dislodges Claudin-1 from Epithelial Tight Junctions

Hassan Nassour, J. Daniel Dubreuil*

GREMIP, Faculty of Veterinary Medicine, Université de Montréal, Montreal, Quebec, Canada

Abstract

Enterotoxigenic *Escherichia coli* produce various heat-labile and heat-stable enterotoxins. STb is a low molecular weight heat-resistant toxin responsible for diarrhea in farm animals, mainly young pigs. A previous study demonstrated that cells having internalized STb toxin induce epithelial barrier dysfunction through changes in tight junction (TJ) proteins. These modifications contribute probably to the diarrhea observed. To gain insight into the mechanism of increased intestinal permeability following STb exposure we treated human colon cells (T84) with purified STb toxin after which cells were harvested and proteins extracted. Using a 1% Nonidet P-40-containing solution we investigated the distribution of claudin-1, a major structural and functional TJ protein responsible for the epithelium impermeability, between membrane (NP40-insoluble) and the cytoplasmic (NP-40 soluble) location. Using immunoblot and confocal microscopy, we observed that treatment of T84 cell monolayers with STb induced redistribution of claudin-1. After 24 h, cells grown in Ca^{++}-free medium treated with STb showed about 40% more claudin-1 in the cytoplasm compare to the control. Switching from Ca^{++}-free to Ca^{++}-enriched medium (1.8 mM) increased the dislodgement rate of claudin-1 as comparable quantitative delocalization was observed after only 6 h. Medium supplemented with the same concentration of Mg^{++} or Zn^{++} did not affect the dislodgement rate compared to the Ca^{++}-free medium. Using anti-phosphoserine and anti-phosphothreonine antibodies, we observed that the loss of membrane claudin-1 was accompanied by dephosphorylation of this TJ protein. Overall, our findings showed an important redistribution of claudin-1 in cells treated with STb toxin. The loss of phosphorylated TJ membrane claudin-1 is likely to be involved in the increased permeability observed. The mechanisms by which these changes are brought about remain to be elucidated.

Editor: Michael Koval, Emory University School of Medicine, United States of America

Funding: This work was supported by a Natural Sciences and Engineering Council of Canada (NSERC) Discovery Grant (139070). The funders had no role in study design, data collection and analysis, decision to publish, or preparation of the manuscript.

Competing Interests: The authors have declared that no competing interests exist.

* Email: daniel.dubreuil@umontreal.ca

Introduction

Enterotoxigenic *Escherichia coli* (ETEC) represent an important cause of severe diarrhea in newborn animals [1] and diarrhea in humans following the ingestion of contaminated food and water [2]. Expression of both colonization factors and toxins are required for disruption of intestinal fluid homeostasis, leading to diarrhea [3]. ETEC strains are known to produce several types of enterotoxins, including heat-labile enterotoxin (LT), heat-stable enterotoxin a (STa) and heat-stable enterotoxin b (STb) [4]. Enteroaggregative heat-stable toxin 1 (EAST1) was also shown to be produced by ETEC [5,6].

STb, a 48-amino-acid peptide of 5.2 kDa, secreted by ETEC strains is mainly associated with post-weaning diarrhea in piglets [7,8]. *In vivo*, STb binds to its receptor, sulfatide, an acidic glycosphingolipid localized at the surface of intestinal epithelial cells [9]. Then, STb is internalized and stimulates a pertussis toxin-sensitive G protein (Gαi3) [10]. This causes an influx of extracellular calcium ions through a ligand-gated calcium ion channel. The increased intracellular Ca^{++} stimulates protein kinase C (PKC) that phosphorylates and activates the cystic fibrosis transmembrane regulator (CFTR), leading to Cl$^-$ secretion. The calcium increase also activates phospholipases A$_2$ responsible

for the release of arachidonic acid from membrane phospholipids leading to production of prostaglandin E$_2$ (PGE$_2$) and 5-hydroxytryptamine (5-HT) [11,12]. These molecules mediate transport of water and HCO$_3^-$ from enterocytes into the intestinal lumen and prevent Na$^+$ absorption resulting in watery diarrhea [7].

Using immunoblot or enzyme-linked assays, Berberov et al. (2004) demonstrated that EAST-1, LT and STb could be concurrently expressed by porcine ETEC strains [13]. Also, Zhang et al. (2006) observed that only LT-and STb-positive strains caused appreciable diarrhea in 5-days-old pigs [14]. Futher, Erume et al. (2013) results indicated that STb is a more significant contributor to diarrhea for weaned pigs [15]. In the same way, recent data by Loos et al. (2012) suggested a dominant role for STb in small intestinal secretion early after post-weaning infection, as well as in the induced innate immune response through differential regulation of immune mediators like interleukin-1 and interleukin-17 [16].

The intestinal lumen is covered by a uniform single layer of epithelial cells. This epithelial layer serves as an environmental barrier [17]. This barrier comprises a number of transmembrane proteins including, but not limited to, tight junction (TJ) proteins like occludins, claudins, and junctional adhesion molecules (JAMs). TJ-associated proteins includes cytoplasmic peripheral membrane proteins such as ZO-1 and ZO-2 known to be associated with transmembrane proteins that includes occludin and claudin families with the apical perijunction of F-actin ring [18]. The F-actin network forms the cell cytoskeleton [19]. TJs act as a barrier controlling penetration of ions, solutes, and water, through intercellular spaces and act as a fence dividing apical and basolateral domains to compartmentalize the plasma membrane. These characteristics of TJs provide also a barrier to prevent the entry of pathogens and foreign substances from invading and facilitate directional exchanges of material [20]. Besides the cell maintenance TJs are essential to both cellular development and normal barrier function [21].

Although human epithelial cells have incorporated barriers to block microorganisms to gain access to deeper cell layers within tissues, certain pathogens have evolved to exploit and thus control TJs to alter this barrier. These pathogens use an array of tactics to hijack junctional structures to their advantage. Some pathogens use TJ proteins as receptors for attachment and subsequent internalization. Others destroy the TJs thereby providing a gateway to the underlying tissue. For example, pathogens such as enteropathogenic E. coli, serotype O127:H6 [22], enterohemorrhagic E. coli producing a shiga toxin-independent non-bloody diarrhea [23], serotype O157:H7 [24], bacterial toxins such as Clostridium difficile toxins A and B [25], Vibrio cholerae Zonula occludens toxin [26], and E. coli secreted autotransporter toxin [27] disrupt TJs [28].

Many studies on ETEC enterotoxins used T84 human colon cells, a cell line commonly used to study bacterial enterotoxin secretory processes [40]. Kreisberg et al. (2011) observed that LT-producing strains could affect cellular permeability independently of STa production [29]. However, in a study of Nakashima et al. (2013), STa elicited a reduction in TER and causes not only

induction of water secretion but also intestinal barrier dysfunction but did not increase the paracellular permeability to FITC-labelled dextran [30]. For STb toxin, a reduction in TER associated with an increased in paracellular permeability was associated with a marked alteration of F-actin stress fibers [31]. F-actin filament dissolution and condensation were accompanied by redistribution and/or fragmentation of ZO-1, claudin-1, and occludin. Therefore, reduction in TER resistance and paracellular permeability to FITC-labeled dextran is recognized as indices of the decreased integrity of epithelial cells intoxicated with these toxins.

In a recent study, STb toxin generated an increase in cytoplasmically located TJ proteins including claudin-1 [31]. Less phosphorylated claudin-1 is found in the cytoplasm and highly phosphorylated claudin-1 is selectively concentrated at TJs monitored as NP-40-insoluble material [28,32,33]. Detergent insolubility of proteins is considered to indicate their integration into macromolecular phosphorylated complexes such as intercellular junctions [32,34]. Membrane-associated claudin-l is known to be important structural and functional components in maintaining TJ integrity [35].

PKC, a family of serine-threonine kinases, are known to regulate epithelial barrier function. PKC are epithelial calcium-dependent enzymes and appears to regulate both subcellular localization and phosphorylation states of several TJ-associated proteins including claudin-1 [36]. The aim of the present study was to examine the effects of STb on location and phosphorylation state of claudin-1 in T84 intestinal epithelial cells.

Materials and Methods

Culture media, antibodies, and reagents

Dulbecco's modified Eagle medium (DMEM), Ham's F-12 nutrient mixture (F-12), phosphate-buffered saline (PBS; pH 7.4, free of calcium chloride and magnesium chloride), 5% fetal bovine

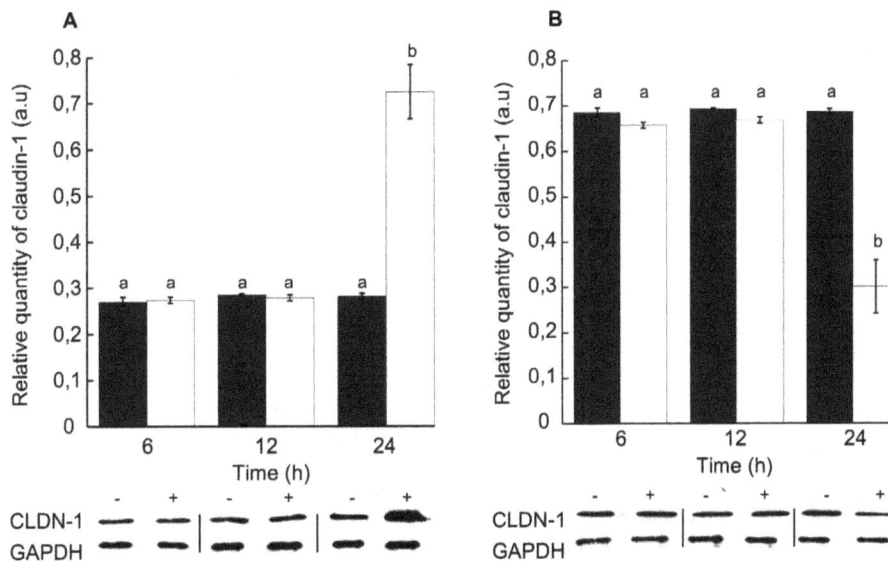

Figure 1. Distribution of claudin-1 in Nonidet P-40-soluble and -insoluble fractions in T84 cell monolayers in response to STb toxin. (A) NP-40-soluble and (B) NP-40-insoluble fractions. Black: untreated cells, white: cells treated with STb for various times. Lower panel: Immunoblot showing claudin-1 and GAPDH used to evaluate their relative amounts. Proteins were separated on a 12% acrylamide SDS-PAGE and immunoblotted with appropriate antibodies. After 24 h, STb treatment induced a loss of claudin-1 in the NP-40-insoluble fraction (membrane location). At the same time, a comparable increase of claudin-1 was observed in the NP-40-soluble fraction (cytoplasm location) (n = 3) (p<0.001). However, no differences were observed between STb-treated and -untreated cell monolayers after 6 or 12 h treatment. CLDN-1: claudin-1; GAPDH: Glyceraldehyde 3-phosphate dehydrogenase. Letters on top of the bars when different indicates a statistical difference between the treatments. The minus and plus signs over the immunoblots indicate respectively that cells were not treated or treated with STb toxin.

Untreated   STb

Claudin-1

F-actin

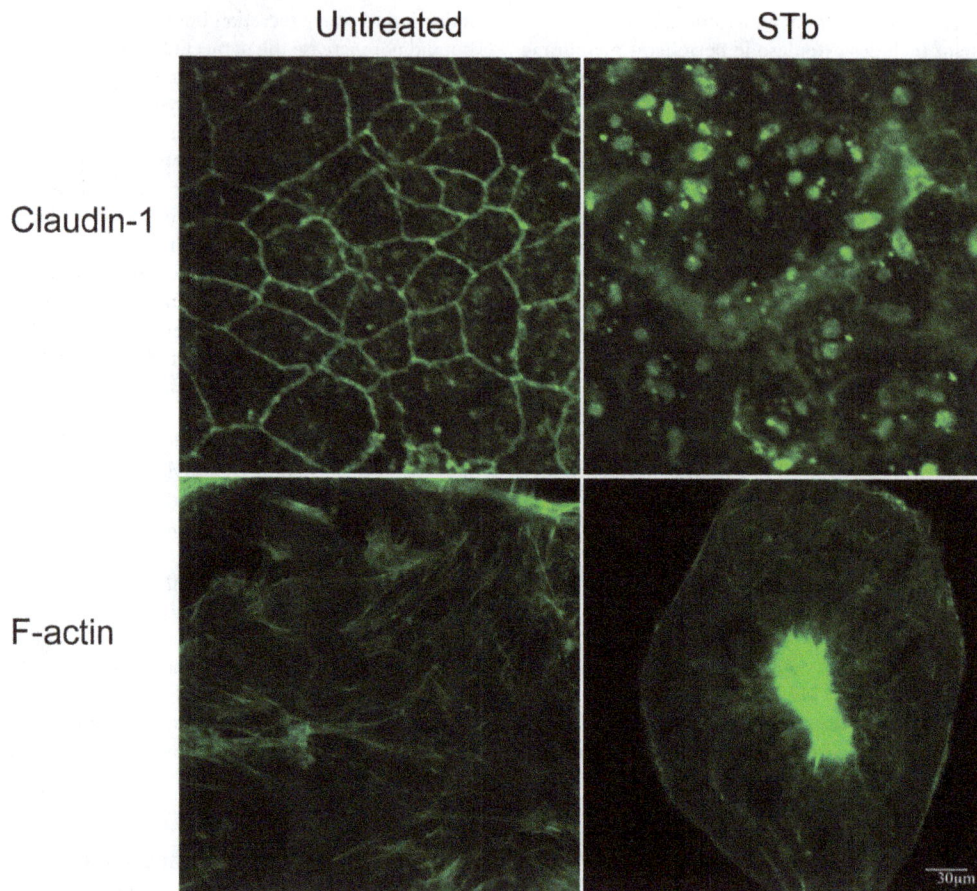

Figure 2. Effect of STb on claudin-1 and F-actin arrangement. After 24 h treatment with STb, T84 cells were fixed, permeabilized, and incubated with anti-claudin-1 antibody. Secondary antibody coupled to Alexa 488 was then added. F-actin was stained using FITC-phalloidin. Untreated cell monolayers stained for claudin-1 showed continuous bands around each cell whereas STb toxin provoked a loss of the "chicken wire" pattern with focal grouping. In untreated cell monolayers, regularly arranged actin filaments around cell contour and as stress fibers were observed. In STb-treated cells, condensation of the F-actin was observed. Three independent experiments were conducted, and representative images are shown ($p < 0.001$). Bar, 30 μm.

serum (FBS), rabbit polyclonal anti-claudin-1, goat anti-rabbit Alexa 488 antibodies, bovine serum albumin (BSA), and DAPI (4′,6-diamidino-2 phenylindole dihydrochloride) were purchased from Invitrogen. FITC-phalloidin and Isopropyl-ß-D-thiogalacto-pyranoside (IPTG) was purchased from Sigma. Factor Xa was from Roche and phenymethanesulfonyl fluoride (PMSF) was from Gibco BRL. Anti-phosphoserine and anti-phosphothreonine antibodies were purchased from Abcam.

Production and STb purification

Recombinant STb toxin was produced as described previously, using a HB101 strain harboring the plasmid pMAL-STb, which codes for the fusion protein MBP-STb [37]. Ampicillin, at a final concentration of 50 mg/ml, was used as the selection agent for bacteria carrying the plasmid pMAL-STb. Bacteria were grown in Rich medium (10 g tryptone, 5 g yeast extract, 5 g NaCl, 2 g dextrose per liter) for 18 h at 37°C in an orbital shaker set at 180 rpm. A volume of 5 ml of an overnight bacterial culture was transferred to 500 ml of fresh Rich medium and returned to the orbital shaker until the absorbance at 600 nm reached 0.5. Then, 0.3 mM IPTG was added to induce the synthesis of the fusion protein. The induction was allowed to proceed for 3 h in the orbital shaker. Cells were harvested by centrifugation at 4,000×g

for 15 min at 4°C. The pellet was gently washed in a volume of 250 ml of 30 mM Tris-HCl (pH 8.0) containing 20% sucrose and 1 mM EDTA. After centrifugation at 8,000×g for 20 min at 4°C, an osmotic shock of bacteria was induced using a solution of 5 mM $MgSO_4$ containing 0.4 mM PMSF and then centrifuged at 7,000 g for 20 min at 4°C. The supernatant containing the fusion protein (MBP-STb) was filter-sterilized using a 0.22-μm-pore-size tangential flow filter (VacuCap; Pall Life Sciences). The fusion protein was affinity-purified at 4°C on a 30 ml amylose column (New England BioLabs) at a flow rate of 0.2 ml/min using a column buffer solution of (10 mM Tris-HCl (pH 7,5), 200 mM NaCl, 1 mM (pH 8.0)). Then, 10 mM of maltose was added to this buffer in order to elute maltose-binding proteins. The eluted proteins were dialyzed against MilliQ water using a 12,000 to 14,000 Da membrane (Spectrum). Dialyzed material was then concentrated using a speed-vac and cleaved using factor Xa enzyme (Roche) in a cleavage buffer consisting of 50 mM Tris-HCl, 100 mM NaCl, and 1 mM $CaCl_2$ (pH 8.0). Using an AKTA-10 purifier system (GE Healthcare), the cleaved material was loaded onto a C_8 reverse-phase column (PerkinElmer) and eluted with a linear gradient of acetonitrile in water solution containing 0.1% trifluoroacetic acid. Using a Nanodrop ND-1000 spectrophotometer (Thermo Scientific), a standard curve of various concentrations of aprotinin (molecular weight of ~6,500)

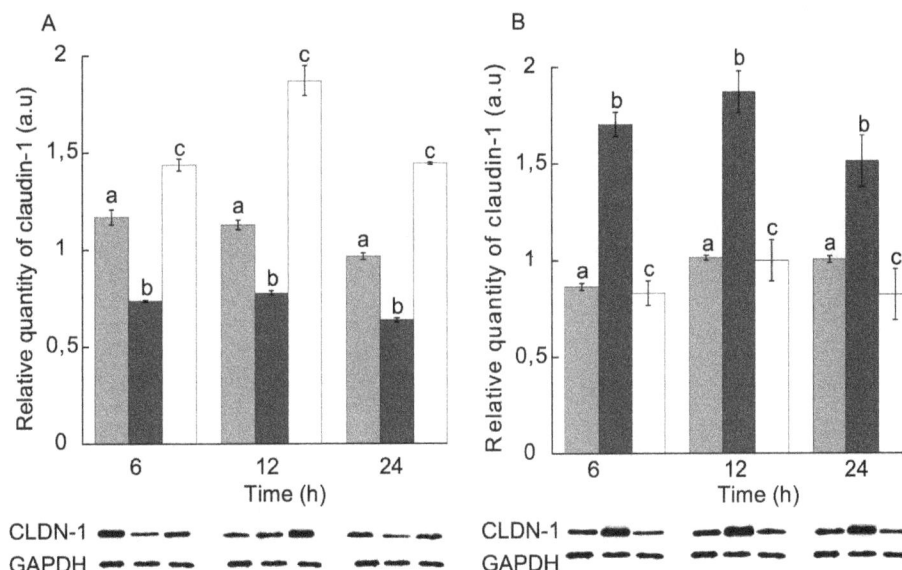

Figure 3. Distribution of claudin-1 in NP-40-soluble and -insoluble fractions in T84 cell monolayers in response to STb toxin after Ca^{++} enrichment. (A) NP-40-soluble and (B) NP-40-insoluble fractions. Gray: calcium-free medium, black: calcium-enriched medium, white: calcium-enriched medium treated with STb. Lower panel: Immunoblot showing claudin-1 and GAPDH used to evaluate their relative amounts. T84 cells were grown in calcium-enriched medium (1.8 mM) for 24 h and treated with STb toxin for 6, 12 or 24 h. Cells were extracted with Nonidet P-40 buffer. In Ca^{++}-enriched medium, the amount of NP-40-insoluble claudin-1 was increased compared to calcium-free condition. Addition of STb toxin provokes dislodgment of NP-40-insoluble claudin-1 to the soluble fraction (n = 3) (p<0.001). CLDN-1: claudin-1; GAPDH: Glyceraldehyde 3-phosphate dehydrogenase. Letters on top of the bars when different indicates a statistical difference between the treatments.

with absorbance at 214 nm was prepared. STb preparations were quantified using the generated standard curve and kept at −20°C until use [38].

Intestinal cell culture and treatments

T84 human colon intestinal epithelial cells, used as a model to study the effects of enterotoxins on TJ proteins [29,30,39–42] were obtained from the American Type Culture Collection. Cells (passage 5 to 18) were maintained in equal volumes of Dulbecco's Modified Eagle Medium (DMEM) and F-12 supplemented with 5% (vol/vol) fetal bovine serum (FBS) (Invitrogen). Cells were grown in T-75 culture flasks (Sarstedt) at 37°C, 5% CO$_2$ in a humidified incubator. Cell viability of T84 cell line was measured using Trypan blue [43]. For maintenance purposes, confluent T84 monolayers were passaged weekly using trypsin-EDTA treatment in phosphate buffered saline (PBS: Invitrogen) free of calcium chloride and magnesium chloride.

For immunofluorescence experiments, T84 cells were seeded, on LabTek 8-well chamber slides (Fisher Scientific), at a density of 150,000 cells/ml and used after 2 days of growth. One hour before treatment with purified STb cell monolayers was washed using PBS and the medium was changed to medium without FBS.

Detergent extraction of cell monolayers

Cell monolayers were grown on tissue culture plates and treated with purified STb (4 nmoles added to 9 ml of cell culture medium) for 0, 6, 12 and 24 h and then subjected to detergent extraction with non-ionic Nonidet P-40 (a non-ionic, non-denaturing detergent) (NP40) according to the method of Sakakibara et al. (1997) [32]. After STb treatment, cells were washed three times with cold PBS, and centrifuged for 10 minutes at 16 000×g. After centrifugation, the cell pellet was lyzed with ice-cold NP-40 buffer (25 mM HEPES/NaOH (pH 7,4), 150 mM NaCl, 4 mM EDTA, 25 mM NaF, 1% NP-40, 1 mM Na$_3$VO$_4$, 1 mM PMSF, 10 μg/

ml leupeptin, 10 μg/ml aprotinin). After centrifugation at 16 000×g, the supertant was collected as the NP40-soluble fraction. The pellet was resuspended in sodium dodecyl sulfate (SDS) lysis buffer (1% SDS, 25 mM HEPES (pH 7.4), 4 mM EDTA, 25 mM NaF) and homogenized. The homogenate was diluted with an appropriate volume of NP40 buffer and the lysate was left for 10 minutes and recentrifuged. The supernatant was collected and used as the NP-40-insoluble fraction.

Gel electrophoresis and immunoblotting

For electrophoresis, equal amounts of total protein within each fraction were loaded onto a polyacrylamide gel. Proteins were dissolved in sample buffer (10% glycerol, 5% β-mercaptoethanol, 3% SDS, 0.0625 M Tris-HCl (pH 6.8), 0.01% bromophenol blue) and heated for 10 minutes at 100°C. Samples were resolved by one-dimensional SDS-PAGE as described by Laemmli (1970) using a 12% gel and the fractioned proteins were electroblotted onto a PVDF membranes (Millipore, 0,45 μm pore size) [44]. After blocking the membrane with 3% milk in PBS containing 0.1% Tween 20 (PBS-T), membranes were incubated with polyclonal antibodies against claudin-1 (1:2000) (Invitrogen), phosphothreonine and phosphoserine (1:2000) (Abcam), washed in PBS-T and further incubated with HRP-conjugated secondary antibodies (1:4000) (Biorad). A liquid substrate system for membranes TM-blue (Sigma) was used to detect the enzymatic activity of the secondary antibody. The density ratio of the specific bands was quantified using ImageJ (National Institutes of Health, Bethesda, MD). Representative blots from multiple experiments (minimum of three) are shown in the figures. Blots were digitally contrasted to preserved relative intensity of specific claudin-1 bands.

Calcium-free	Calcium-enriched	Calcium-enriched/STb

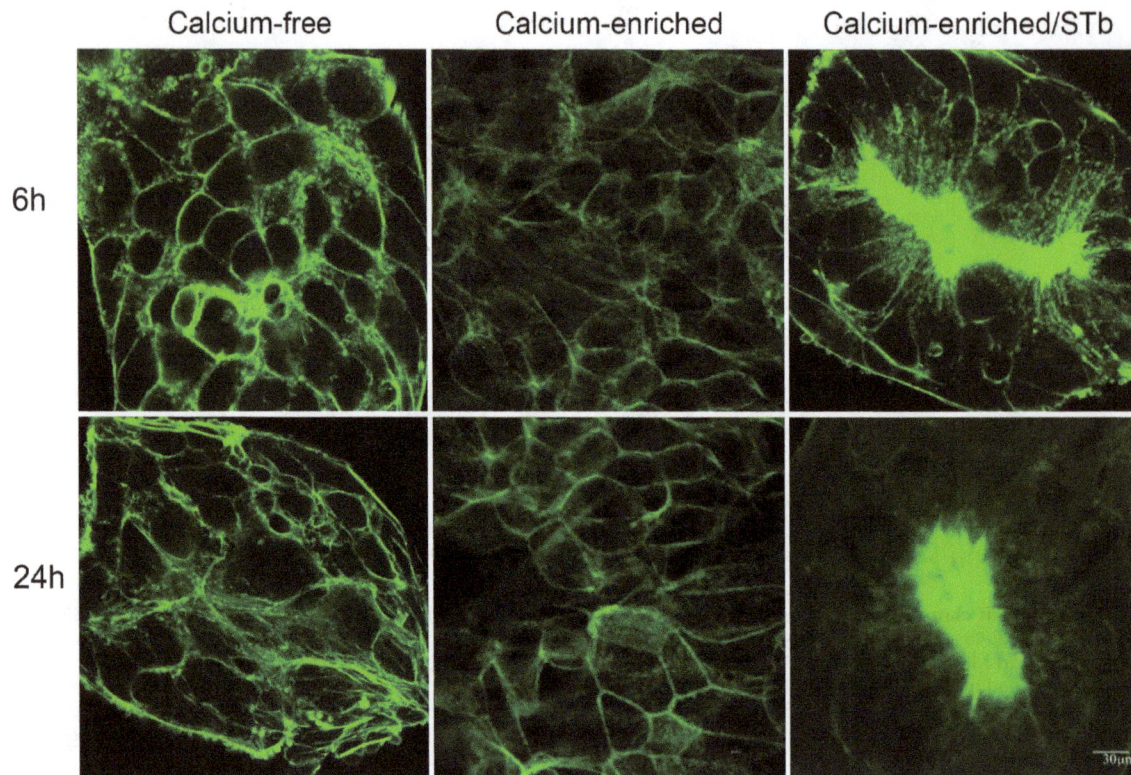

Figure 4. Effect of Ca^{++}-enrichment on the rate of STb toxin activity. Cells grown in calcium-free and calcium-enriched (1.8 mM) media were compared after 6 and 24 h. Confocal microscopy was used to analyze the distribution of actin filaments stained with FITC-phalloidin. Calcium-enriched medium had no visible effect on the actin organization whereas in calcium-enriched medium STb provoked actin condensation after 6 h. In calcium-free medium, actin condensation was observed only after 24 h (Data not shown) Bar, 30 μm.

Cations enrichment studies

T84 cells were grown in calcium-free medium (Dulbecco's Modified Eagle Medium (DMEM), Ham's F-12 nutrient mixture (F-12) with 5% FBS) and then transferred to the calcium-enriched medium (1.8 mM CaCl$_2$) for 24 h and then treated with 4 nmoles of purified STb for 0, 6, 12 and 24 h. Cells were then subjected to detergent extraction, resolved by one-dimensional SDS-PAGE and electrophoretically transferred as described above. The same experiments were done using two others divalent ions, Mg^{++} and Zn^{++}, to assess the specificity of Ca^{++} in the increased rate of claudin-1 dislodgement and actin disorganization.

Immunofluorescence microscopy of actin cytoskeleton and tight junction proteins

For claudin-1 staining, T84 cells were seeded on cover slips at 1×10^5 cells/ml and fixed with 100% ethanol for 20 minutes. Cells were then permeabilized with 1% Triton X-100 in PBS for 10 minutes, soaked in blocking solution (PBS containing 1% BSA) for 1 h, and then incubated with the anti-claudin-1 antibody (1:100) for 1 h in a moist chamber. The samples were washed three times with PBS and then incubated for 1 h with FITC-conjugated goat anti-rabbit IgG (Biorad). Samples were then washed with PBS three times, mounted in PBS containing 1% p-phenylenediamine and 90% glycerol.

For staining of F-actin filaments, cells were washed three times with PBS, permeabilized with 0.1% Triton X-100 for 10 min at room temperature, and blocked with 2% BSA–PBS for 45 min before incubation with fluorescein-phalloidin for 45 min at room temperature [31]. The cell monolayers were washed again three times with PBS. The slides were observed with a confocal microscope (Olympus FV1000IX81) at x40 magnification for claudin-1 and F-actin.

Statistical analyses

For claudin-1 dislodgment study in Ca^{++}-free medium, a linear mixed model was used with treatment as a fixed factor and id (replicated unit) as a random factor to account for the lack of independence among the three samples for each subject. Tukey's post-hoc tests were used to examine the differences between pairs of treatment means.

For divalent-enriched cations experiments, data were transformed using the logarithm base 10 to normalize distributions. A linear mixed model was used with treatment and time as fixed factors and sample id as a random factor. A priori contrasts were performed to compare pairs of means adjusting the alpha level for each comparison using the Bonferroni sequential procedure to maintain the experiment error rate at the nominal value. Statistical analyses were carried out with SAS v.9.3 (Cary, N.C.) and the level of statistical significance was set at 5% throughout.

Results

STb affects the distribution of claudin-1

Since STb toxin was previously shown to increase paracellular permeability [31], we wanted to address whether translocation of TJ proteins was involved in this process. We thus analyzed the time-dependent distribution of claudin-1, a protein with a major

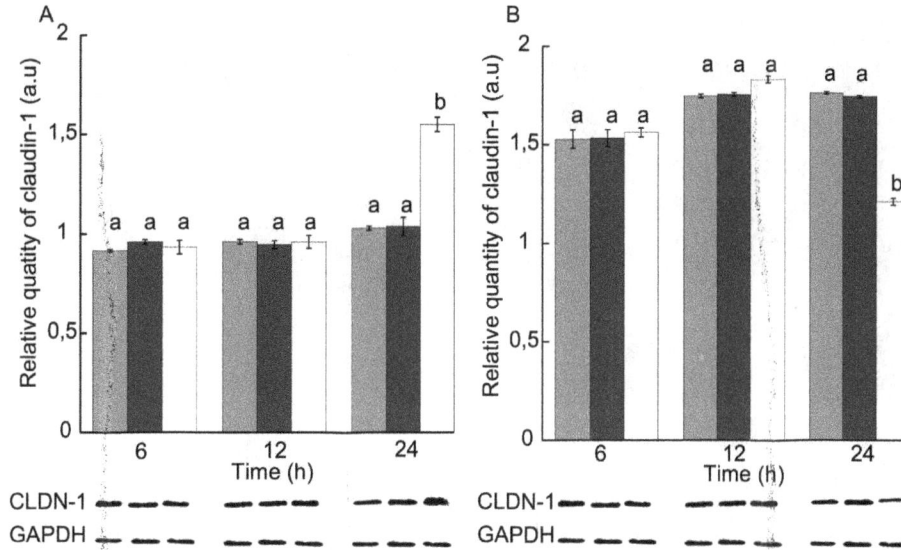

Figure 5. Effect of Mg^{++}-enrichment on claudin-1 displacement rate. (A) NP-40-soluble and (B) NP-40-insoluble fractions. Gray: calcium-free medium, black: Mg^{++}-enriched medium, white: Mg^{++}-enriched medium treated with STb for 6, 12 and 24 h. Lower panel: Immunoblot showing claudin-1 and GAPDH used to evaluate their relative amounts. NP-40 cell extracted proteins were separated on a 12% acrylamide SDS-PAGE and immunoblotted with anti-claudin-1 and anti-GAPDH antibodies. The calcium-free medium was Mg^{++}-enriched (1.8 mM). There was no significant difference in claudin-1 dislogment rate under Mg^{++}-enriched condition compared to calcium-free medium. After 24 h, claudin-1 dislodgement was observed as seen before in calcium-free medium (n = 3) (p<0.001). CLDN-1: claudin-1, GAPDH: Glyceraldehyde 3-phosphate dehydrogenase. Letters on top of the bars when different indicates a statistical difference between the treatments.

role in sealing TJs, between Nonidet P-40-soluble and -insoluble fractions (Fig. 1).

Purified STb toxin (4 nmoles) was added to the apical side of T84 cell monolayers, and incubated for 6, 12 or 24 h. Cell proteins were then extracted with a buffer containing Nonidet P-40 to determine the amount of membrane-associated claudin-1

(NP-40-insoluble) and cytoplasmically located (NP-40-soluble). Extracted proteins were separated on a 12% acrylamide SDS-PAGE and western blotted using an anti-claudin-1 antibody. The relative intensity of claudin-1 protein bands was measured and compared to the intensity of GAPDH, our internal control. The negative control consisted of untreated cell monolayer.

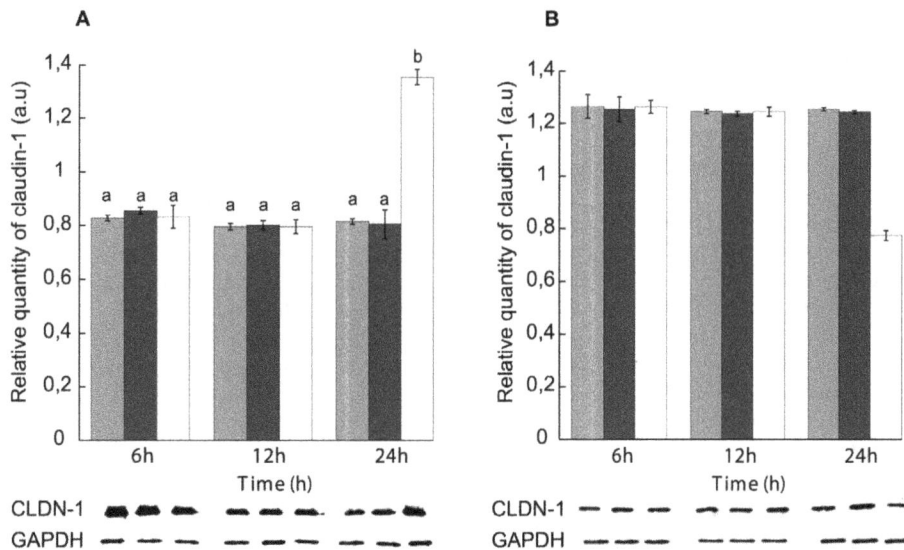

Figure 6. Effect of Zn^{++}-enrichment on claudin-1 displacement rate. (A) NP-40-soluble and (B) NP-40-insoluble fractions. Gray: calcium-free medium, black: Zn^{++}-enriched medium, white: Zn^{++}-enriched medium treated with STb for 6, 12 and 24 h. Lower panel: Immunoblot showing claudin-1 and GAPDH used to evaluate their relative amounts. NP-40 cell extracted proteins were separated on a 12% acrylamide SDS-PAGE and immunoblotted with anti-claudin-1 and anti-GAPDH antibodies. The calcium-free medium was Zn^{++}-enriched (1.8 mM). There was no significant difference in claudin-1 dislogment rate under Zn^{++}-enriched condition compared to calcium-free medium. After 24 h, claudin-1 dislogment was observed as seen before in calcium-free medium (n = 3) (p<0.001). CLDN-1: claudin-1, GAPDH: Glyceraldehyde 3-phosphate dehydrogenase. Letters on top of the bars when different indicates a statistical difference between the treatments.

Calcium-free   Magnesium-enriched   Magnesium-enriched/STb

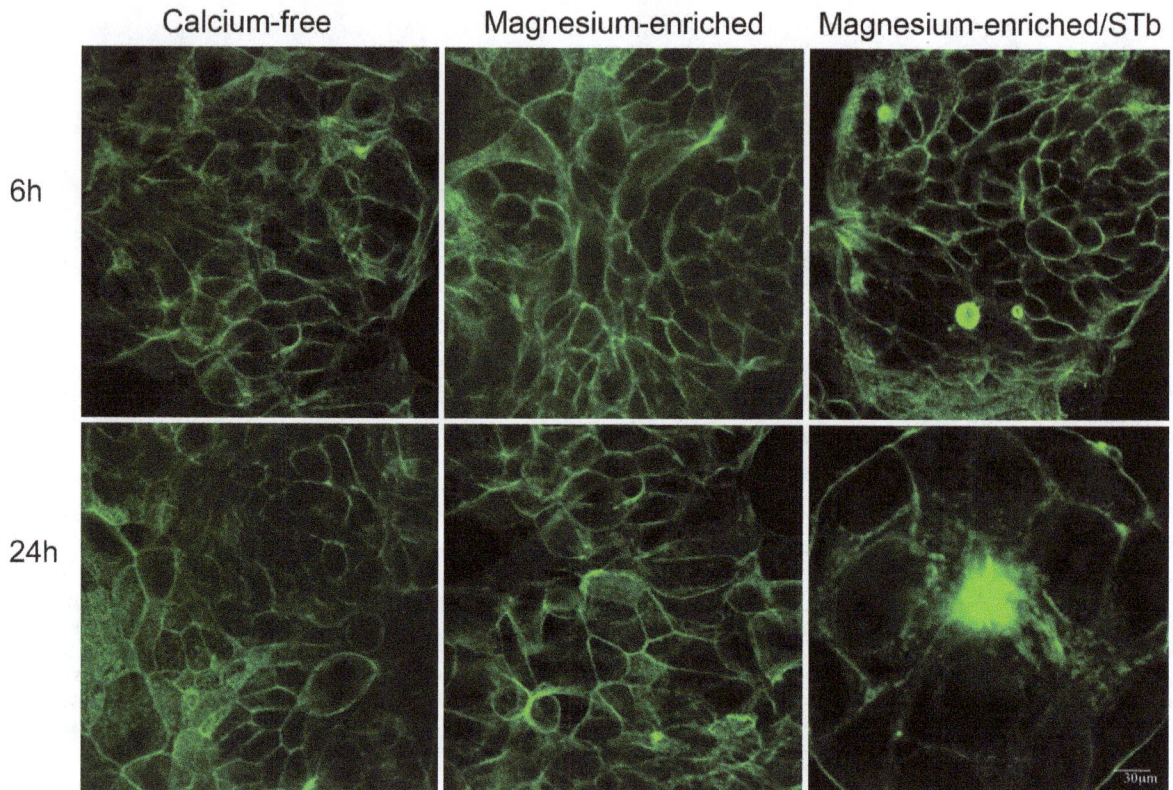

Figure 7. Effect of Mg^{++}-enrichment on the rate of STb toxin activity. Cells grown in calcium-free and magnesium-enriched (1.8 mM) media were compared after 6 and 24 h. Confocal microscopy was used to analyze the distribution of actin filaments stained with FITC-phalloidin. Magnesium-enriched medium had no visible effect on the actin organization whereas in calcium-enriched medium STb provoked actin condensation after 24 h. In calcium-free medium, actin condensation was observed only after 24 h (Data not shown) Bar, 30 μm.

In STb treated cells, we observed, after 24 h, a marked increase in the level of NP-40-soluble claudin-1 and a decrease in NP-40-insoluble claudin-1 (Fig. 1). Densitometric analyses revealed a 40% increase in NP-40-soluble claudin-1 level and a comparable decrease in the NP-40- insoluble level. There were no significant differences in claudin-1 amount between untreated cell monolayers and cell monolayers treated with STb for 6 h or 12 h. After 24 h, the difference in the distribution of claudin-1 was statistically significant compared to the control.

Also, following a 24 h treatment with STb, T84 cell monolayers were fixed, permeabilized, and stained to highlight the F-actin and claudin-1 organization. Using confocal microscopy, untreated T84 cell monolayers showed well-organized F-actin filaments surrounding the cells and as stress fibers and claudin-1 proteins surrounding cell boundaries while STb-treated cell monolayers exhibited a loss of organization and focal grouping of claudin-1 with condensation of F-actin filaments (Fig. 2).

Effect of Ca^{++} on the rate of claudin-1 redistribution

Calcium plays a critical role in the regulation of several cellular processes. As Ca^{++} was previously related to STb toxicity [10] and a calcium enrichment experiment conducted by Sakakibara et al. (1997) revealed that TJ formation was accompanied by an increase in NP-40-insoluble TJ proteins levels including claudin-1 [32], this divalent metal ion was investigated in relation to its possible involvement in claudin-1 distribution.

We thus examined the relation between calcium, STb toxin and NP-40-insoluble claudin-1 level. First, in calcium-free medium in absence of STb, claudin-1 was approximately equally distributed between the NP-40-soluble and -insoluble fractions (Fig. 3A and B; gray bar). However, after calcium enrichment (1.8 mM CaCl$_2$), the bulk of claudin-1 was found in the NP-40-insoluble fraction (Fig. 3B; black bar). Incubation of T84 cells in calcium-enriched medium in presence of STb resulted in a significant dislodgement of claudin-1 observed as an increase in NP-40-soluble claudin-1 (Fig. 3A and B; white bar). For STb-treated cells, in Ca^{++}-enriched medium, changes in the distribution of claudin-1 were apparent after 6 h and were similar after 12 and 24 h (Fig. 3; white bar). Overall, compared to GAPDH, the amount of claudin-1 was similar under the various conditions tested. Only the distribution between membrane and cytoplasmic locations was affected.

To examine how STb in presence of calcium influenced cell morphology, confluent T84 cell monolayers were incubated for 6 h and 24 h. Confocal microscopy analyses indicated that after 6 and 24 h, calcium-enrichment alone had little effect on actin filament organization. In fact, the amount of F-actin detectable at the edges of the cells was lowered. This can be related to the actin rearrangement that is expected when shifting from calcium-free to calcium-enriched medium. Cells grown in calcium-free and calcium-enriched media still showed well-organized F-actin filaments circling each cell as well as stress fibers (Fig. 4; calcium-free and calcium-enriched). However, after 6 h in calcium-enriched medium, STb-treated cell monolayers exhibited disruption of actin filaments surrounding the cells and stress fibers with condensation of F-actin filaments (Fig. 4; calcium-enriched/STb). In calcium-free medium, actin condensation was not observed before 24 h in presence of STb toxin (Data not shown).

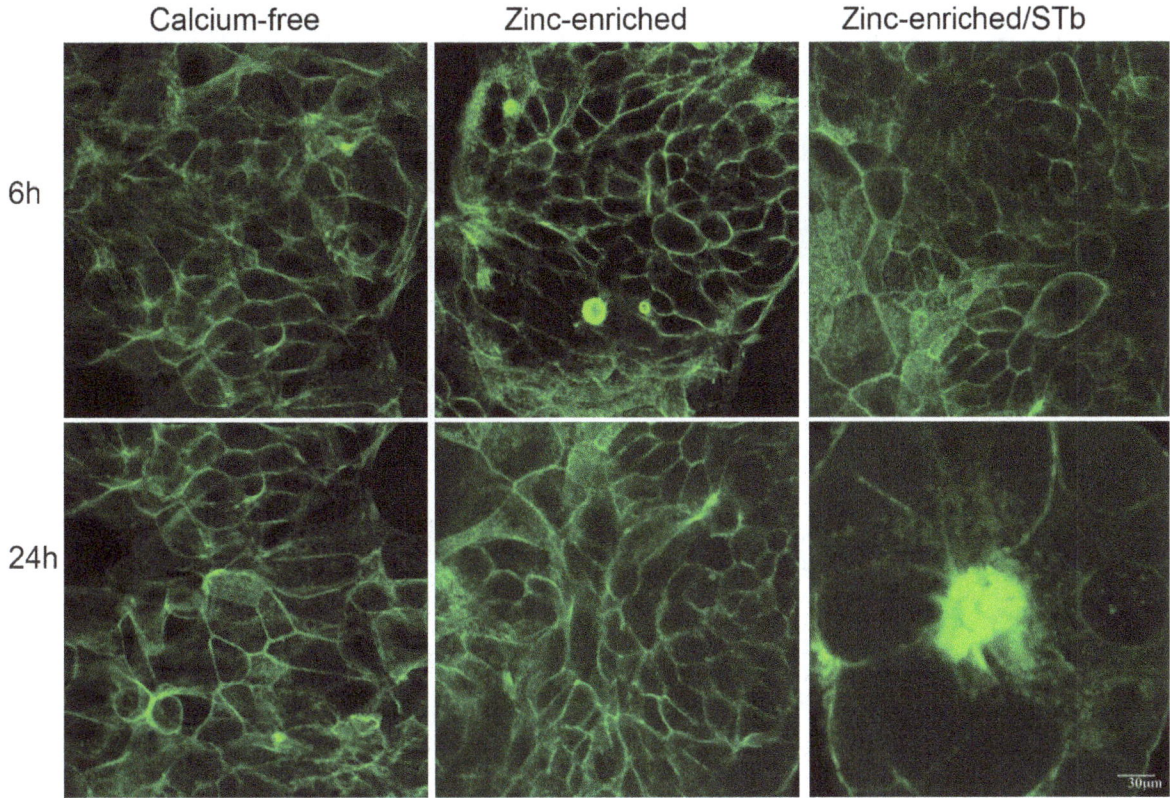

Figure 8. Effect of Zn^{++}-enrichment on the rate of STb toxin activity. Cells grown in calcium-free and zinc-enriched (1.8 mM) media were compared after 6 and 24 h. Confocal microscopy was used to analyze the distribution of actin filaments stained with FITC-phalloidin. Zinc-enriched medium had no visible effect on the actin organization whereas in zinc-enriched medium STb provoked actin condensation after 24 h. In calcium-free medium, actin condensation was observed only after 24 h (Data not shown) Bar, 30 μm.

Effect of Mg^{++} and Zn^{++} enrichment

To assess the specificity of Ca^{++} on the rate of claudin-1 dislodgment and actin condensation, two divalent metal ions, Mg^{++} and Zn^{++} were compared to Ca^{++}. As seen in Figure 5 and 6, the rate in redistribution of NP-40-soluble and -insoluble claudin-1 levels were shown to be Ca^{++} specific as neither Mg^{++} nor Zn^{++} could increase the rate of claudin-1 dislodgement. Nevertheless, changes in claudin-1 location and actin condensation in Mg^{++}- and Zn^{++}- enriched media were observed as described before in calcium-free medium after 24 h (Fig. 7 and 8).

Phosphorylation state of claudin-1

The phosphorylation state of claudin-1 in NP-40-insoluble (membrane location) and -soluble fraction (cytoplasmic location) was studied. For comparison purposes, claudin-1 levels were adjusted, in the various fractions, to the same level as can be observed with anti-claudin-1 (Fig. 9). In untreated T84 cells, threonine phosphorylation was observed in the NP-40-insoluble fraction using anti-phosphothreonine antibodies (Fig. 9B, left panel), while nonphosphorylated threonine was found in the NP-40-soluble fraction (Fig. 9A, left panel). Moreover, the level of phosphothreonine in claudin-1 was reduced in the NP-40-insoluble fraction after 24 h of exposure to STb toxin (Fig. 9B,

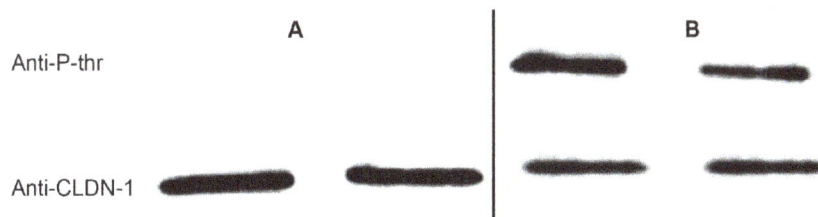

Figure 9. Phosphorylation state of claudin-1 as found in the membrane and cytoplasmic locations. (A) NP-40-soluble and (B) NP-40-insoluble fractions of STb-treated T84 cells. Left panel: untreated, right panel: STb-treated. Cell proteins extracted with NP-40 were migrated on a 12% acrylamide SDS-PAGE and immunoblotted with anti-phosphothreonine (Anti-P-thr). The amount of claudin-1 was adjusted to the same level in the various fractions using the anti-claudin-1 antibodies (anti-CLDN-1). The claudin-1 in NP-40-insoluble fraction is phosphorylated whereas in the NP-40-soluble fraction it is not phosphorylated. The amount of phosphorylated claudin-1 in the NP-40-insoluble was decreased in STb treated cells compared to control (p<0.001).

right panel). Thus, STb toxin induces the dislodgment of claudin-1 from membrane to cytoplasmic location and this change correlated with the observation of non-phosphorylated claudin-1. The same results were observed using an anti-serine antibody (Data not shown).

Discussion

A number of factors can be responsible for epithelial barrier dysfunction, including microbial infection. Enteric pathogens have developed strategies that induce the production of diarrhea in infected hosts, through disruption of intercellular TJs [45,46]. Many studies have indicated that toxins can modulate the epithelial barrier by targeting junctional as well as cytoskeletal cell components and thus for some pathogens the changes facilitates invasion across the mucosal surface [47]. In this study, we investigated effects of STb toxin on claudin-1 location and phosphorylation levels in cultured T84 epithelial cells.

LT and STa toxin were recently shown to cause an increase in the epithelial cell permeability observed as a trans-epithelial resistance (TER) decrease and passage of dextran-FITC by disrupting TJs of T84 cells [30]. We thus compared the cellular NP-40 detergent partitioning and the state of phosphorylation of claudin-1 in epithelial T84 cell line following STb treatment. This cell line display distinct barrier characteristics (i.e., T84 cells form a very tight monolayer with high TER and low permeability to uncharged molecules) [31,33].

We first assessed claudin-1 location in T84 cells by immuno-staining and confocal imaging. Claudin-1 and occludin has been demonstrated before to be apically located sealing the TJs [31,33]. It has also been suggested that claudin-1 contribute to cell adhesion [48]. In our study, claudin-1 was recovered in both the NP-40-soluble and-insoluble fractions of the cell extracts (Fig. 2 a, b). Since the TJ strands are assumed to be resistant to detergent extraction [49], these findings indicates the existence of claudin-1 both as a junctional complex and as a soluble pool of proteins. The distribution of claudin-1 in two distinct subcellular pools had been reported earlier [50].

Mechanisms underlying the perturbation of the epithelial barrier are numerous. Some compounds directly interact with single TJ proteins [51], whereas others disturb barrier function by a general modification of TJ strands [52]. Reorganization of the actin ring also results in loss of tight junction integrity [53]. STb was previously found to affect the actin ring of T84 cells [31]. The authors also reported shortening of the actin filaments and appearance of actin condensation after treatment with STb toxin. This is consistent with our results (Fig. 2) where shortening of the filaments was observed. The lack of reorganization of the actin ring suggests that STb does affect TJs via a change in actin architecture. The relevance of the changes in actin filaments with regard to TJs integrity remains to be established. Claudin-1 interacts with actin through proteins such as ZO-1 and ZO-3 and we have shown in a previous study that the increase in paracellular permeability resulting from STb activity is associated with fragmentation of ZO-1 [31].

The effect of STb on TJ proteins was examined in an attempt to clarify the mechanisms that underlies the observed changes. The loss of claudin-1 from membranes in STb-treated T84 cell monolayers indicates a loss of TJ integrity and therefore changes in barrier properties. Western blotting of T84 cell fractions provided further evidence for a change in subcellular location of the TJ protein claudin-1. The claudin-1 content of the membrane fraction decreased with STb treatment in a time-dependent manner (Fig. 1) while the claudin-1 content of the NP-40-soluble

fraction increased with time, indicating that claudin-1 translocate from the membrane to the cytosol in response to treatment with STb. This shift of claudin-1 into the soluble fraction had been observed in Caco-2 cells following ATP depletion (15, 21).

The observed effect of STb on claudin-1 delocalization is likely contributing to the pathogenesis of ETEC by allowing the passage of electrolytes and water through the paracellular space. As shown in our study, in absence of Ca^{++} this delocalization happened after 24 h but in presence of this metal ion we could observe a similar effect after only 6 h (Figure 3 and 4). Opening of TJs as an early event, we believe, is responsible at least in part for the fluid secretion resulting from STb intoxication. Dreyfus et al. (1993) examined the effect of STb on the internal Ca^{++} concentration of transformed and primary cells of different tissues and animal species. They suggested that STb opens a GTP-binding regulatory protein-linked receptor-operated Ca^{++} channel in the plasma membrane. Beyond these studies, nothing is known of the relation between STb, Ca^{++} and TJ proteins. Our results suggest that STb induces a rapid time-dependent toxicity by translocation of claudin-1 from membrane to a more soluble form.

The increased calcium levels are also thought to regulate phospholipases (A2 and C) that release arachidonic acid from membrane phospholipids, leading to the formation of intestinal secretagogues PGE_2 and 5-HT, which mediate water and electrolyte transport out of intestinal cells [54]. In our study, the important role of calcium was confirmed where by adding the calcium to the culture medium STb increased the rate of disruption of the barrier integrity. Others divalent cations had no significant effect on STb toxicity.

It has been proposed that claudins can be regulated by PKC-mediated phosphorylation, modulating barrier function in the cells [33]. Thus, in Caco-2 cells, inactivation of PKC-Φ reduced phosphorylation of claudin-1 and decreased the membrane to cytosolic distribution of the claudin-1 [55]. In ovarian cancer cells, phorbol ester-mediated PKC activation induced phosphorylation of claudins and decreased barrier function [56], and in human epidermal keratinocytes, formation of TJs was suggested to be regulated by a PKC-induced phosphorylation of claudin-4 [57]. A previous study had shown binding of STb to its receptor is associated with the uptake of Ca^{++} into the cell, activating PKC, which through phosphorylation activates CFTR [58]. Because STb activates PKC and that STb opens a GTP-binding regulatory protein-linked receptor-operated Ca^{++} channel in the plasma membrane [10], we can hypothesize that PKC signalling pathway may be involved in TJs dysfunction as well as cytoskeletal changes. In T84 untreated cells, phosphorylated claudins-1 was found only in NP-40 insoluble fraction, whereas in NP-40 soluble fraction, claudin-1 was not phosphorylated. Since STb induces a major decrease in the apical distribution of claudin-1 and a reduction in the barrier function [31], a change in the phosphorylation state might be the mechanism by which STb acts indirectly.

Acknowledgments

This work was supported by a Discovery grant from the National Research Council of Canada (no. 139070) to J.D.D. The funders had no role in the study design, data collection and analysis, decision to publish, or preparation of the manuscript.

Author Contributions

Conceived and designed the experiments: HN JDD. Performed the experiments: HN. Analyzed the data: HN JDD. Contributed reagents/ materials/analysis tools: HN JDD. Contributed to the writing of the manuscript: HN JDD.

References

1. Nagy B, Fekete PZ (2005) Enterotoxigenic *Escherichia coli* in veterinary medicine. Int J Med Microbiol 295: 443–454.
2. Fleckenstein JM, Hardwidge PR, Munson GP, Rasko DA, Sommerfelt H, et al. (2010) Molecular mechanisms of enterotoxigenic *Escherichia coli* infection. Microbes Infect 12: 89–98.
3. Kaper JB, Nataro JP, Mobley HL (2004) Pathogenic *Escherichia coli*. Nat Rev Microbiol 2: 123–140.
4. Nataro JP, Kaper JB (1998) Diarrheagenic *Escherichia coli*. Clin Microbiol Rev 11: 142–201.
5. Paiva de Sousa C, Dubreuil JD (2001) Distribution and expression of the *astA* gene (EAST1 toxin) in *Escherichia coli* and Salmonella. Int J Med Microbiol 291: 15–20.
6. Savarino SJ, McVeigh A, Watson J, Cravioto A, Molina J, et al. (1996) Enteroaggregative *Escherichia coli* heat-stable enterotoxin is not restricted to enteroaggregative *E. coli*. J Infect Dis 173: 1019–1022.
7. Dubreuil JD (2008) *Escherichia coli* STb toxin and colibacillosis: knowing is half the battle. FEMS Microbiol Lett 278: 137–145.
8. Fairbrother JM, Nadeau E, Gyles CL (2005) *Escherichia coli* in postweaning diarrhea in pigs: an update on bacterial types, pathogenesis, and prevention strategies. Anim Health Res Rev 6: 17–39.
9. Rousset E, Harel J, Dubreuil JD (1998) Sulfatide from the pig jejunum brush border epithelial cell surface is involved in binding of *Escherichia coli* enterotoxin b. Infect Immun 66: 5650–5658.
10. Dreyfus LA, Harville B, Howard DE, Shaban R, Beatty DM, et al. (1993) Calcium influx mediated by the *Escherichia coli* heat-stable enterotoxin B (STB). Proc Natl Acad Sci (U S A) 90: 3202–3206.
11. Harville BA, Dreyfus LA (1995) Involvement of 5-hydroxytryptamine and prostaglandin E2 in the intestinal secretory action of *Escherichia coli* heat-stable enterotoxin B. Infect Immun 63: 745–750.
12. Harville BA, Dreyfus LA (1996) Release of serotonin from RBL-2H3 cells by the *Escherichia coli* peptide toxin STb. Peptides 17: 363–366.
13. Berberov EM, Zhou Y, Francis DH, Scott MA, Kachman SD, et al. (2004) Relative importance of heat-labile enterotoxin in the causation of severe diarrheal disease in the gnotobiotic piglet model by a strain of enterotoxigenic *Escherichia coli* that produces multiple enterotoxins. Infect Immun 72: 3914–3924.
14. Zhang W, Berberov EM, Freeling J, He D, Moxley RA, et al. (2006) Significance of heat-stable and heat-labile enterotoxins in porcine colibacillosis in an additive model for pathogenicity studies. Infect Immun 74: 3107–3114.
15. Erume J, Wijemanne P, Berberov EM, Kachman SD, Oestmann DJ, et al. (2013) Inverse relationship between heat stable enterotoxin-b induced fluid accumulation and adherence of F4ac-positive enterotoxigenic *Escherichia coli* in ligated jejunal loops of F4ab/ac fimbria receptor-positive swine. Vet Microbiol 161: 315–324.
16. Loos M, Geens M, Schauvliege S, Gasthuys F, van der Meulen J, et al. (2012) Role of heat-stable enterotoxins in the induction of early immune responses in piglets after infection with enterotoxigenic *Escherichia coli*. PLoS One 7: e41041.
17. Berkes J, Viswanathan VK, Savkovic SD, Hecht G (2003) Intestinal epithelial responses to enteric pathogens: effects on the tight junction barrier, ion transport, and inflammation. Gut 52: 439–451.
18. Puthenedam M, Williams PH, Lakshmi BS, Balakrishnan A (2007) Modulation of tight junction barrier function by outer membrane proteins of enteropathogenic *Escherichia coli*: role of F-actin and junctional adhesion molecule-1. Cell Biol Int 31: 836–844.
19. Balkovetz DF, Katz J (2003) Bacterial invasion by a paracellular route: divide and conquer. Microbes Infect 5: 613–619.
20. Roselli M, Finamore A, Britti MS, Konstantinov SR, Smidt H, et al. (2007) The novel porcine *Lactobacillus sobrius* strain protects intestinal cells from enterotoxigenic *Escherichia coli* K88 infection and prevents membrane barrier damage. J Nutr 137: 2709–2716.
21. Anderson JM, Balda MS, Fanning AS (1993) The structure and regulation of tight junctions. Curr Opin Cell Biol 5: 772–778.
22. Philpott DJ, McKay DM, Sherman PM, Perdue MH (1996) Infection of T84 cells with enteropathogenic *Escherichia coli* alters barrier and transport functions. Am J Physiol 270: G634–645.
23. Roxas JL, Koutsouris A, Bellmeyer A, Tesfay S, Royan S, et al. (2010) Enterohemorrhagic *E. coli* alters murine intestinal epithelial tight junction protein expression and barrier function in a Shiga toxin independent manner. Lab Invest 90: 1152–1168.
24. Philpott DJ, McKay DM, Mak W, Perdue MH, Sherman PM (1998) Signal transduction pathways involved in enterohemorrhagic *Escherichia coli*-induced alterations in T84 epithelial permeability. Infect Immun 66: 1680–1687.
25. Nusrat A, von Eichel-Streiber C, Turner JR, Verkade P, Madara JL, et al. (2001) *Clostridium difficile* toxins disrupt epithelial barrier function by altering membrane microdomain localization of tight junction proteins. Infect Immun 69: 1329–1336.
26. Schmidt E, Kelly SM, van der Walle CF (2007) Tight junction modulation and biochemical characterisation of the zonula occludens toxin C-and N-termini. FEBS Lett 581: 2974–2980.
27. Guignot J, Chaplais C, Coconnier-Polter MH, Servin AL (2007) The secreted autotransporter toxin, Sat, functions as a virulence factor in Afa/Dr diffusely

28. Suzuki T (2013) Regulation of intestinal epithelial permeability by tight junctions. Cell Mol Life Sci 70: 631–659.
29. Kreisberg RB, Harper J, Strauman MC, Marohn M, Clements JD, et al. (2011) Induction of increased permeability of polarized enterocyte monolayers by enterotoxigenic *Escherichia coli* heat-labile enterotoxin. Am J Trop Med Hyg 84: 451–455.
30. Nakashima R, Kamata Y, Nishikawa Y (2013) Effects of *Escherichia coli* heat-stable enterotoxin and guanylin on the barrier integrity of intestinal epithelial T84 cells. Vet Immunol Immunopathol 152: 78–81.
31. Ngendahayo Mukiza C, Dubreuil JD (2013) *Escherichia coli* heat-stable toxin b impairs intestinal epithelial barrier function by altering tight junction proteins. Infect Immun 81: 2819–2827.
32. Sakakibara A, Furuse M, Saitou M, Ando-Akatsuka Y, Tsukita S (1997) Possible involvement of phosphorylation of occludin in tight junction formation. J Cell Biol 137: 1393–1401.
33. Sjo A, Magnusson KE, Peterson KH (2003) Distinct effects of protein kinase C on the barrier function at different developmental stages. Biosci Rep 23: 87–102.
34. Fujibe M, Chiba H, Kojima T, Soma T, Wada T, et al. (2004) Thr203 of claudin-1, a putative phosphorylation site for MAP kinase, is required to promote the barrier function of tight junctions. Exp Cell Res 295: 36–47.
35. Suzuki H, Kondoh M, Takahashi A, Yagi K (2012) Proof of concept for claudin-targeted drug development. Ann N Y Acad Sci 1258: 65–70.
36. Andreeva AY, Krause E, Muller EC, Blasig IE, Utepbergenov DI (2001) Protein kinase C regulates the phosphorylation and cellular localization of occludin. J Biol Chem 276: 38480–38486.
37. Syed HC, Dubreuil JD (2012) *Escherichia coli* STb toxin induces apoptosis in intestinal epithelial cell lines. Microb Pathog 53: 147–153.
38. Labrie V, Beausoleil HE, Harel J, Dubreuil JD (2001) Binding to sulfatide and enterotoxicity of various *Escherichia coli* STb mutants. Microbiology 147: 3141–3148.
39. Toriano R, Kierbel A, Ramirez MA, Malnic G, Parisi M (2001) Spontaneous water secretion in T84 cells: effects of STa enterotoxin, bumetanide, VIP, forskolin, and A-23187. Am J Physiol Gastrointest Liver Physiol 281: G816–822.
40. Visweswariah SS, Shanthi G, Balganesh TS (1992) Interaction of heat-stable enterotoxins with human colonic (T84) cells: modulation of the activation of guanylyl cyclase. Microb Pathog 12: 209–218.
41. Chao KL, Dreyfus LA (1997) Interaction of *Escherichia coli* heat-stable enterotoxin B with cultured human intestinal epithelial cells. Infect Immun 65: 3209–3217.
42. Strauman MC, Harper JM, Harrington SM, Boll EJ, Nataro JP (2010) Enteroaggregative *Escherichia coli* disrupts epithelial cell tight junctions. Infect Immun 78: 4958–4964.
43. Ricardo R, Phelan K (2008) Counting and determining the viability of cultured cells. J Vis Exp.
44. Laemmli UK (1970) Cleavage of structural proteins during the assembly of the head of bacteriophage T4. Nature 227: 680–685.
45. Viswanathan VK, Koutsouris A, Lukic S, Pilkinton M, Simonovic I, et al. (2004) Comparative analysis of EspF from enteropathogenic and enterohemorrhagic *Escherichia coli* in alteration of epithelial barrier function. Infect Immun 72: 3218–3227.
46. Simonovic I, Arpin M, Koutsouris A, Falk-Krzesinski HJ, Hecht G (2001) Enteropathogenic *Escherichia coli* activates ezrin, which participates in disruption of tight junction barrier function. Infect Immun 69: 5679–5688.
47. Soong G, Parker D, Magargee M, Prince AS (2008) The type III toxins of *Pseudomonas aeruginosa* disrupt epithelial barrier function. J Bacteriol 190: 2814–2821.
48. Kuhn S, Koch M, Nubel T, Ladwein M, Antolovic D, et al. (2007) A complex of EpCAM, claudin-7, CD44 variant isoforms, and tetraspanins promotes colorectal cancer progression. Mol Cancer Res 5: 553–567.
49. Stevenson BR, Anderson JM, Bullivant S (1988) The epithelial tight junction: structure, function and preliminary biochemical characterization. Mol Cell Biochem 83: 129–145.
50. de Oliveira SS, de Oliveira IM, De Souza W, Morgado-Diaz JA (2005) Claudins upregulation in human colorectal cancer. FEBS Lett 579: 6179–6185.
51. Fujita K, Katahira J, Horiguchi Y, Sonoda N, Furuse M, et al. (2000) *Clostridium perfringens* enterotoxin binds to the second extracellular loop of claudin-3, a tight junction integral membrane protein. FEBS Lett 476: 258–261.
52. Krug SM, Fromm M, Gunzel D (2009) Two-path impedance spectroscopy for measuring paracellular and transcellular epithelial resistance. Biophys J 97: 2202–2211.
53. Walsh SV, Hopkins AM, Chen J, Narumiya S, Parkos CA, et al. (2001) Rho kinase regulates tight junction function and is necessary for tight junction assembly in polarized intestinal epithelia. Gastroenterology 121: 566–579.
54. Arriaga YL, Harville BA, Dreyfus LA (1995) Contribution of individual disulfide bonds to biological action of *Escherichia coli* heat-stable enterotoxin B. Infect Immun 63: 4715–4720.
55. Banan A, Zhang LJ, Shaikh M, Fields JZ, Choudhary S, et al. (2005) Theta Isoform of protein kinase C alters barrier function in intestinal epithelium

through modulation of distinct claudin isotypes: a novel mechanism for regulation of permeability. J Pharmacol Exp Ther 313: 962–982.

56. D'Souza T, Indig FE, Morin PJ (2007) Phosphorylation of claudin-4 by PKC-epsilon regulates tight junction barrier function in ovarian cancer cells. Exp Cell Res 313: 3364–3375.

57. Aono S, Hirai Y (2008) Phosphorylation of claudin-4 is required for tight junction formation in a human keratinocyte cell line. Exp Cell Res 314: 3326–3339.

58. Turner SM, Scott-Tucker A, Cooper LM, Henderson IR (2006) Weapons of mass destruction: virulence factors of the global killer enterotoxigenic *Escherichia coli*. FEMS Microbiol Lett 263: 10–20.

24

Dominance of Emerging G9 and G12 Genotypes and Polymorphism of VP7 and VP4 of Rotaviruses from Bhutanese Children with Severe Diarrhea Prior to the Introduction of Vaccine

Sonam Wangchuk[1], Marcelo T. Mitui[2], Kinlay Tshering[3], Takaaki Yahiro[2], Purushotam Bandhari[4], Sangay Zangmo[1], Tshering Dorji[1], Karchung Tshering[1], Takashi Matsumoto[2], Akira Nishizono[2], Kamruddin Ahmed[2,5]*

1 Public Health Laboratory, Department of Public Health, Ministry of Health, Thimphu, Bhutan, 2 Department of Microbiology, Faculty of Medicine, Oita University, Yufu, Japan, 3 Department of Pediatrics, Jigme Dorji Wangchuk National Referral Hospital, Thimphu, Bhutan, 4 Department of Pediatrics, Mongar Regional Referral Hospital, Mongar, Bhutan, 5 Research Promotion Institute, Oita University, Yufu, Japan

Abstract

A prospective study was performed to determine the molecular characteristics of rotaviruses circulating among children aged <5 years in Bhutan. Stool samples were collected from February 2010 through January 2011 from children who attended two tertiary care hospitals in the capital Thimphu and the eastern regional headquarters, Mongar. The samples positive for rotavirus was mainly comprised genotype G1, followed by G12 and G9. The VP7 and VP4 genes of all genotypes clustered mainly with those of neighboring countries, thereby indicating that they shared common ancestral strains. The VP7 gene of Bhutanese G1 strains belonged to lineage 1c, which differed from the lineages of vaccine strains. Mutations were also identified in the VP7 gene of G1 strains, which may be responsible for neutralization escape strains. Furthermore, we found that lineage 4 of P[8] genotype differed antigenically from the vaccine strains, and mutations were identified in Bhutanese strains of lineage 3. The distribution of rotavirus genotypes varies among years, therefore further research is required to determine the distribution of rotavirus strain genotypes in Bhutan.

Editor: Daniela F. Hozbor, Universidad Nacional de La Plata., Argentina

Funding: This study was supported by the Research Funds at the Discretion of the President, Oita University [610000-N5010 and 610000-N5040] to Kamruddin Ahmed. The funders had no role in study design, data collection and analysis, decision to publish, or preparation of the manuscript.

Competing Interests: The authors have declared that no competing interests exist.

* Email: ahmed@oita-u.ac.jp

Introduction

Bhutan is a small landlocked country located between India and China. Part of the population is concentrated in the capital Thimphu, but most are scattered sparsely throughout the country. Diarrhea is a major cause of illness and death in Bhutanese children, and the morbidity rate from diarrhea in <5 years old children is 314.6/1,000 population [1,2], while 13% of deaths are attributable to diarrhea [3]. Approximately 83% of the population have access to safe drinking water and 91% have access to sanitary toilets [1]. A shift from bacterial to possibly viral diarrhea has been observed, although information regarding childhood diarrhea is scarce.

Rotavirus is a major cause of childhood diarrhea throughout the world, and is responsible for 114 million infections and 453,000 child deaths per year [4]. Rotavirus has also been associated with in nondiarrheal diseases [5]. Two rotavirus vaccines are available at present, RotaTeq (Merk & Co. Inc., Whitehouse Station, NJ,

USA) contains G1–4 and P[8] antigens, while the other Rotarix (GlaxoSmithKline Biologicals, Brussels, Belgium) contains G1 and P[8] antigens, and both have been used successfully in several countries [6]. RotaTeq is a live, attenuated vaccine composes of five bovine-human reassortant strains [7]. The monovalent live attenuated Rotarix vaccine is based on the human rotavirus strain RIX 4414 [7]. Worldwide, genotype G1 is dominant, followed by G2–4 and G9, and these genotypes are mainly responsible for rotavirus-related diarrhea [8]. In Bhutan, the genotype distribution is unknown, which has hindered the policy discussion on introduction of rotavirus vaccine by policy makers. Thus, understanding the distribution patterns of circulating genotypes and their relationships with rotaviruses in neighboring countries might facilitate effective rotavirus control in Bhutan by introducing vaccination. Given the level and distribution of the available health services in Bhutan, the introduction of rotavirus vaccine might help to reduce child morbidity, and mortality. However, in contrast to other countries, it would be very challenging for

Bhutan to cope with the possibly undesirable outcomes that might be associated with rotavirus vaccines [9–17], and the environmental monitoring to determine the spread of vaccine-like strains. Thus, a more cautious approach to the introduction of rotavirus vaccine may be appropriate for Bhutan. A cautious approach does not mean that Bhutanese children will be excluded from rotavirus vaccination; it means that policy makers should be aware of the benefit and risk of vaccination. In the present study, we determined the antigenic characteristics of G1 strains, and we performed a phylogenetic analysis of the rotaviruses circulating in Bhutan.

Materials and Methods

Sample collection

This study was undertaken at Jigme Dorji Wangchuk National Referral Hospital (JDWNRH), Thimphu and Mongar Regional Referral Hospital (MRRH), Mongar. This is part of a project to identify the etiology of viral diarrhea in Bhutanese children [18,19]. JDWNRH is the only national reference hospital in the country, and serves the population of Thimphu. MRRH is a regional referral center in the east region, and mainly serves the population of Mongar. Stool samples were collected prospectively from children <5 years attended at the outpatient and inpatient departments of these hospitals with watery diarrhea. A case of diarrhea was defined as three looser than normal stool during a 24 hr period. The samples obtained from JDWNRH were collected between February 2010 and January 2011, while those from Mongar were obtained on April 26, 2010.

Detection of rotavirus, genotyping and electropherotyping

A commercial enzyme-linked immunosorbent assay (Rotaclone, Meridian Diagnostics, Cincinnati, OH, USA) was used to detect rotavirus antigen in stool samples. Genomic RNA was extracted

from the rotavirus positive stool samples using a QIAamp Viral RNA Mini Kit (Qiagen, Hilden, Germany) to determine the G and P types [20]. RNA was extracted with phenol-chloroform-isoamyl alcohol and used to determine the electropherotypes by polyacrylamide gel electrophoresis (PAGE) [21,22].

Nucleotide sequencing and phylogenetic analysis

The nucleotide sequences of the VP7 and VP8* portions of VP4 genes were determined using a BigDye Terminator v3.1 Cycle Sequencing Kit (Applied Biosystems, Gaithersburg, MD, USA). The purified amplicons were sequenced using an ABI3130 Genetic Analyzer (Applied Biosystems). All of the procedures were conducted according to the manufacturer's instructions.

A multiple sequence alignment was performed using CLUSTALW ver. 2 [23]. Phylogenetic analyses were conducted with the neighbor-joining method using MEGA software ver. 5 [24]. The branching patterns were evaluated statistically based on bootstrap analyses of 1,000 replicates. Nucleotide sequences of different strains of rotavirus were obtained from the GenBank.

Ethical statement

This study was approved by the Research Ethics Board of Health, Bhutan (www.health.gov.bt/rebh.php). Informed verbal consent was obtained from the guardians on behalf of the children enrolled in this study. The verbal consent was not recorded. Stool sample collection is a routine work for diarrheal cases and left over samples after routine investigation was used in the present study, besides it is not an invasive procedure, does not cause pain or harm during collection, and is not a life-threatening process therefore written consent was not obtained from the guardians. The ethics board approved the consent procedure.

Results

In total, 44/123 (35.8%) stool samples were positive for rotavirus, and ten electropherotypes, i.e., E1–E10, were detected

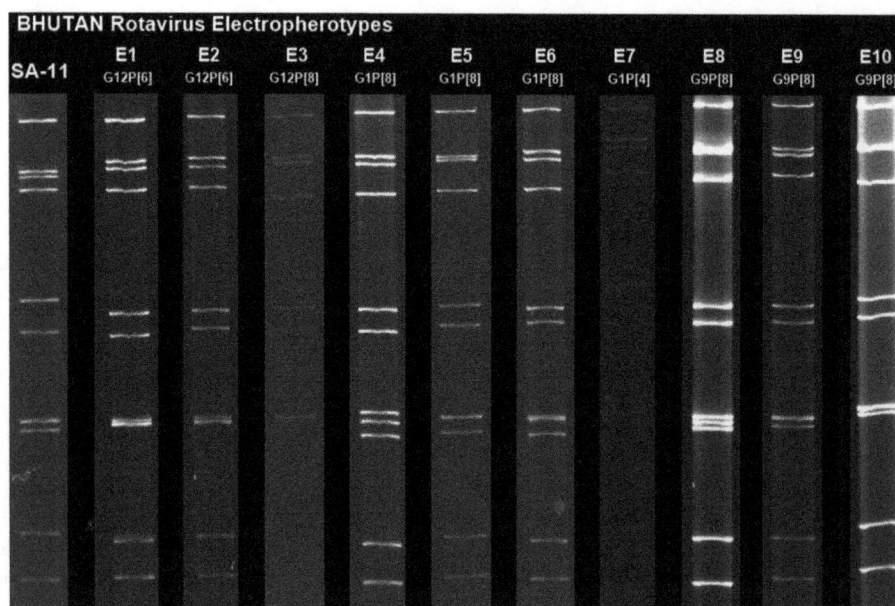

Figure 1. Electropherotypes of rotaviruses identified in Bhutan. On the extreme left, SA-11 indicates the electropherotype of strain Sa-11, which was used as a marker in each electrophoresis run. In total, 10 electropherotypes were identified, E1–E10. The genotype of each electropherotype is shown below the electropherotype. With the exception of E7, the electropherotypes had long patterns. Among five strains from Mongar, three were electropherotype E4, one E10, and one was untypable.

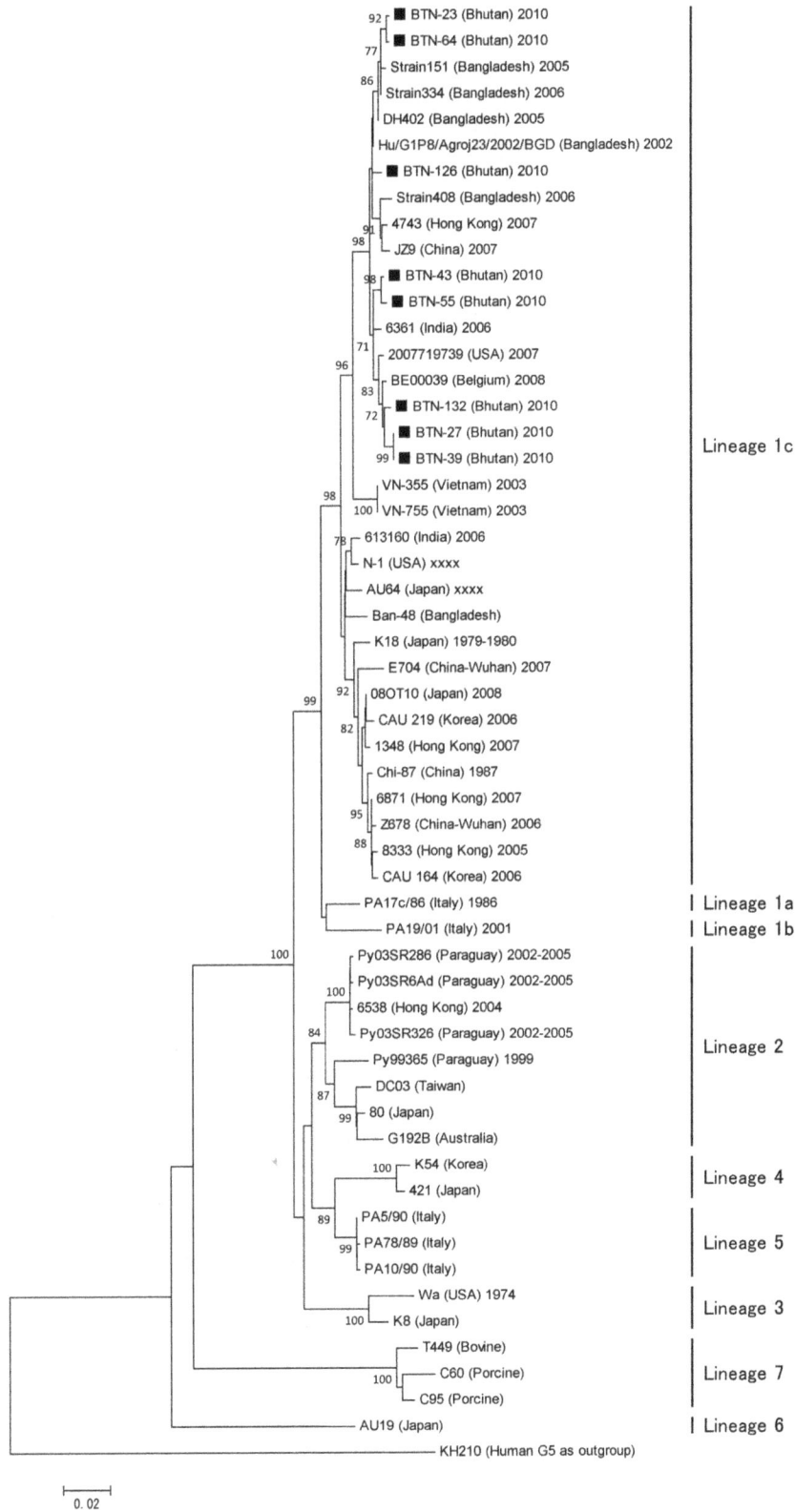

Figure 2. Phylogenetic tree constructed based on the deduced amino acid sequences of the VP7 genes of G1 strains. Bhutanese strains are indicated by black squares, which are followed by the strain numbers. Human rotavirus KH210 (G5) was used as an outgroup. The numbers adjacent to nodes represent the bootstrap values; values <70% have not shown. The scale bar shows the genetic distance, which is expressed as amino acid substitutions per site. The DNA Data Bank of Japan/European Molecular Biology Laboratory/GenBank accessions numbers are: AB905455 (rotavirus strain BTN-23), AB905456 (BTN-64), AB905457 (BTN-55), AB905458 (BTN-126), AB905459 (BTN-43), AB905460 (BTN-132), AB905461 (BTN-27), and AB905462 (BTN-39).

Figure 3. Comparison of the antigenic residues of VP7 present in genotype G1 strains of RotaTeq and Rotarix, and the strains circulating in Bhutan. The respective antigenic epitopes are shown above the residue numbers. The amino acid residues in the Bhutanese strains that differed from those in the vaccine strains are highlighted in blue. The amino acid residues highlighted in yellow indicate that the residue is different from the other vaccine strain and Bhutanese strains.

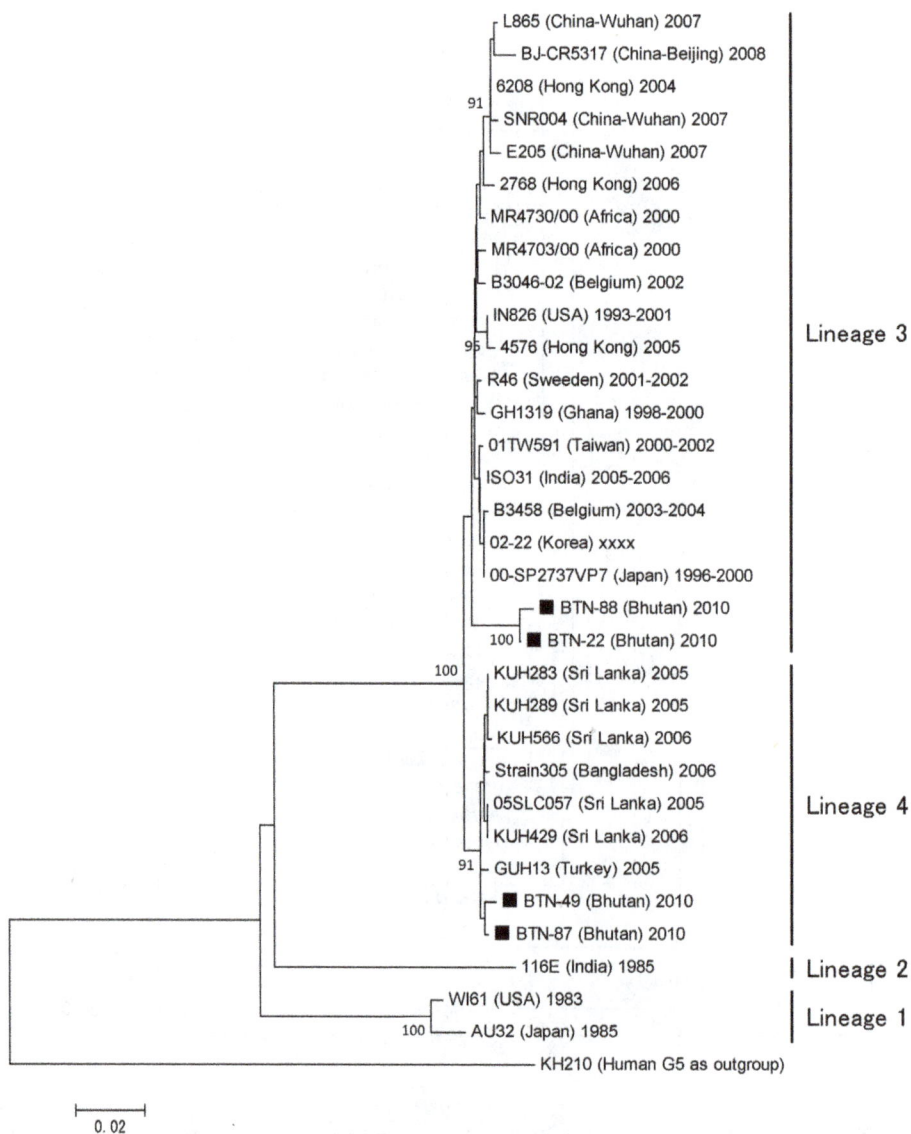

Figure 4. Phylogenetic tree constructed base on the deduced amino acid sequences of the VP7 genes of G9 strains. Bhutanese strains are indicated by black squares, which are followed by the strain numbers. Human rotavirus KH210 (G5) was used as an outgroup. The numbers adjacent to nodes represent the bootstrap values; values <70% are not shown. The scale bar shows the genetic distance, which is expressed as amino acid substitutions per site. The DNA Data Bank of Japan/European Molecular Biology Laboratory/GenBank accessions numbers are: AB905463 (rotavirus strain BTN-22), AB905464 (BTN-49), AB905465 (BTN-87), and AB905466 (BTN-88).

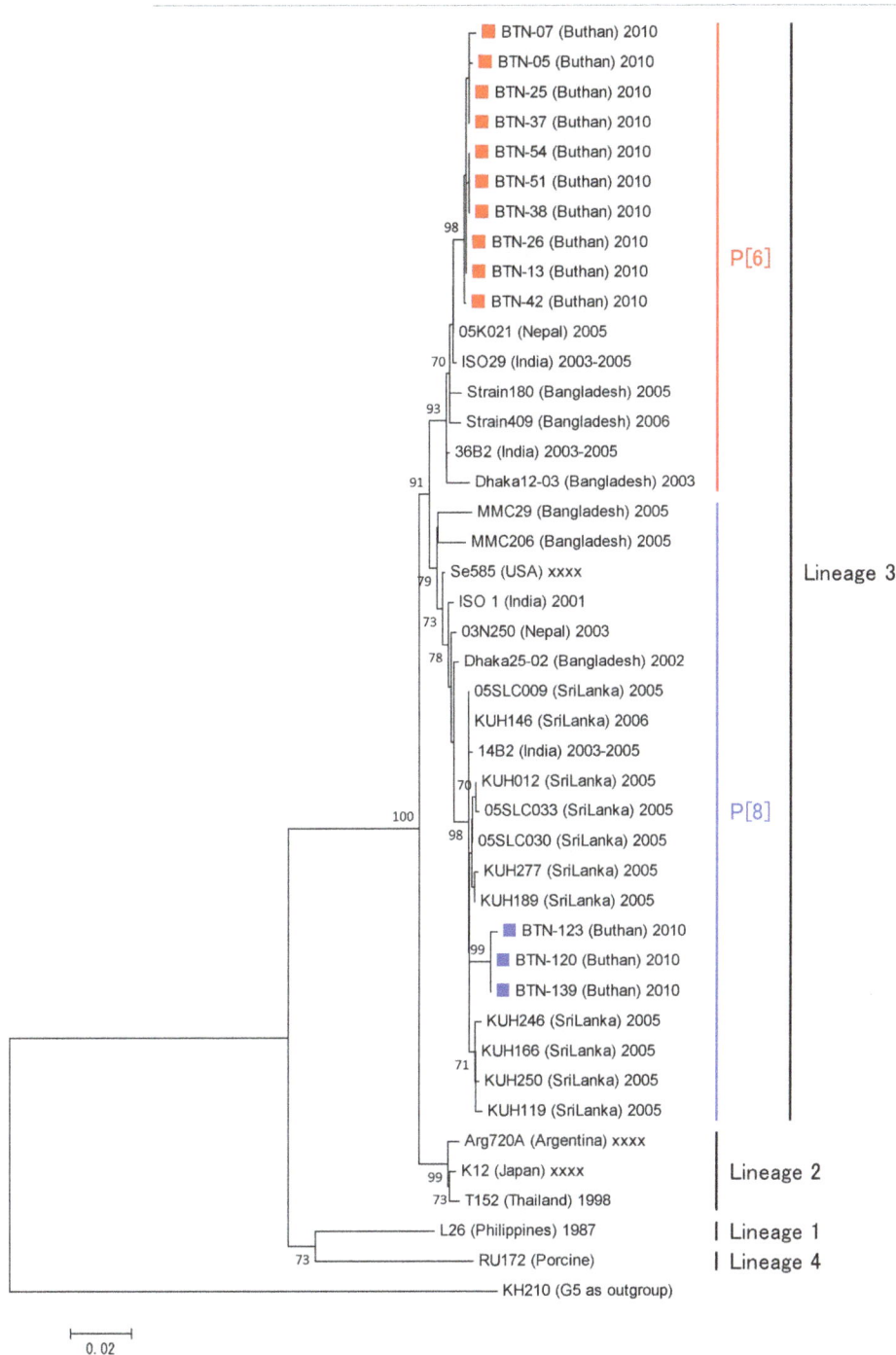

Figure 5. Phylogenetic tree constructed based on the deduced amino acid sequences of the VP7 gene of G12 strains. Bhutanese strains are indicated by black squares, which are followed by the strain numbers. Human rotavirus KH210 (G5) was used as an outgroup. The numbers adjacent to nodes represent the bootstrap values; values<70% are not shown. The scale bar shows the genetic distance, which is expressed as amino acid substitutions per site. The DNA Data Bank of Japan/European Molecular Biology Laboratory/GenBank accessions numbers are: AB905467 (rotavirus strain BTN-05), AB905468 (BTN-07), AB905469 (BTN-13), AB905470 (BTN-25), AB905471 (BTN-26), AB905472 (BTN-37), AB905473 (BTN-38), AB905474 (BTN-42), AB905475 (BTN-51), AB905476 (BTN-54), AB905477 (BTN-120), AB905478 (BTN-123), and AB905479 (BTN-139).

in 38 samples (Figure 1). The frequencies of the G1, G9, and G12 genotypes were 26 (59.1%), five (13.4%), and 13(29.5%), respectively. The relative detection rates for different combinations of G and P genotypes were in the following order: G1P[8] = 21 (47.7%), G12P[6] = 10 (22.7%), G9P[8] = 5 (11.3%), G1P[4] = 5 (11.3%) and G12P[8] = 3 (6.8%).

Of the eight lineages of G1 rotaviruses, the Bhutanese strains belonged to lineage 1c and were closely associated with strains from Bangladesh, India, Belgium, and the USA, thereby indicating that strains similar to Bhutanese G1 clones are also circulating both in the neighboring countries and in distant parts of the world (Figure 2). The phylogenetic analysis indicated that

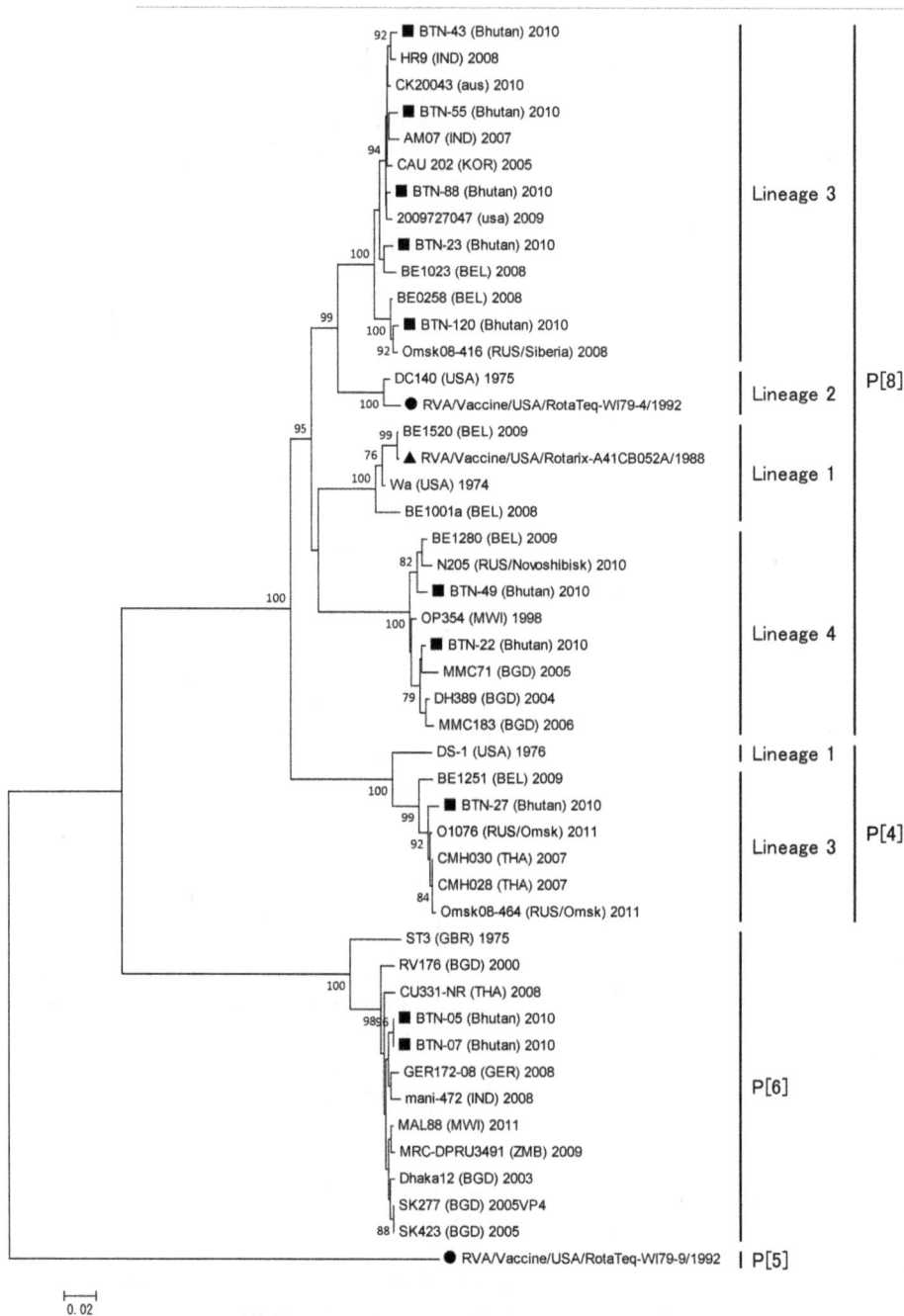

Figure 6. Phylogenetic tree constructed based on the deduced amino acid sequences of the VP8* genes of G1, G9, and G12 strains from Bhutan and global P[8], P[6], P[5], and P[4] strains. The species and country of origin are shown in parentheses after the strain name. The numbers adjacent to node represent the bootstrap values; values<70% are not shown. The scale bar shows the genetic distance, which is expressed as amino acid substitutions per site. The DNA Data Bank of Japan/European Molecular Biology Laboratory/GenBank accessions numbers are: AB905368 (rotavirus strain BTN-05), AB905369 (BTN-07), AB905370 (BTN-120), AB905371 (BTN-23), AB905372 (BTN-88), AB905373 (BTN-49), AB905374 (BTN-22), AB905375 (BTN-27), AB905376 (BTN-43), AB905377 (BTN-55).

Bhutanese G1 possibly originated from a single clone or similar clones before changing via point mutations. The shared nucleotide and amino acid identities of the VP7 gene were 98–100% among Bhutanese G1 strains.

Compared with the VP7 sequences of Rotarix strain RIX4414 [16] and RotaTeq strain W179-9 [25], the Bhutanese G1 strains had 94 and 93% shared amino acid identities. Figure 3 shows the details of the amino acid substitutions. Compared with RotaTeq,

there were amino acid substitutions in 19 residues of all Bhutanese strains, and 11 additional residues were also substituted in some Bhutanese strains. Five of these residues belonged to the 7-1a epitope of the antigenic region [26], where substitutions, in three residues can cause neutralization escape [16], and two of the residues belonged to the 7-2 antigenic region, which is also responsible for neutralization escape. Compared with Rotarix, amino acid substitutions were found in 15 residues of all Bhutanese

									8-3	8-3		8-3	8-3				8-1	8-1	8-1			8-2		8-1	8-1	8-1	8-1	8-1					
Strain	5	19	52	78	99	113	116	120	125	131	141	146	148	150	163	179	183	185	188	190	192	193	195	196	200	217	222	237	245	246	248	255	292
Rotateq	I	H	Y	I	S	N	D	T	N	R	L	S	S	N	K	G	R	I	S	N	A	N	N	D	I	N	N	S	Y	K	A	T	S
Rotarix	I	H	H	N	S	N	D	M	S	S	L	S	S	N	R	G	R	T	S	S	A	N	N	N	T	N	N	P	Y	K	A	I	S
BTN55	I	H	H	T	S	D	D	N	N	R	L	G	S	N	R	G	R	T	S	N	A	N	N	G	T	N	N	S	Y	T	A	T	A
BTN43	I	H	H	T	S	D	D	N	N	R	L	G	S	N	R	G	R	T	S	N	A	N	N	G	T	N	N	S	Y	T	T	T	S
BTN88	I	H	H	T	S	D	D	N	N	R	L	G	S	N	R	G	R	T	S	N	A	N	N	G	T	N	N	S	Y	T	A	T	S
BTN23	I	Y	H	T	S	D	D	N	N	R	L	G	S	N	R	G	R	T	S	N	G	N	N	G	T	N	N	S	Y	T	A	T	S
BTN120	T	Y	H	T	G	N	D	N	N	R	L	G	S	N	K	G	R	T	S	N	A	N	N	G	T	N	N	S	H	K	A	T	S
BTN22	I	Y	H	K	S	D	N	T	S	W	F	G	S	S	R	G	G	V	G	N	S	D	T	S	I	V	Y	S	Y	K	A	I	S
BTN49	I	Y	H	K	S	D	D	T	S	R	F	G	N	S	R	K	G	V	G	N	S	D	T	S	I	V	Y	S	Y	N	A	I	S

Figure 7. Comparison of the antigenic residues in the VP8* head of VP4 from RotaTeq and Rotarix, and strains circulating in Bhutan. The respective antigenic epitopes are shown above the residue numbers. The amino acid residues in Bhutanese strains that differed from those in the vaccine strains are highlighted. The amino acid residues highlighted in yellow indicate that the residue is different from the other vaccine strain and Bhutanese strains. BTN-22 and BTN-49 belong to lineage 4 of genotype P[8].

strains, as well as additional substitutions in 11 other residues in some Bhutanese strains. Four of these residues were located in the 7-1a antigenic region, three of which are responsible for neutralization escape. Only one residue belonged to the 7-2 antigenic region, which is responsible for neutralization escape.

Bhutanese strains belonged to lineages 3 and 4 among the four lineages of G9 rotaviruses (Figure 4). The lineage 3 strains formed an independent cluster, which was closely association with a cluster of strains from Korea, Japan, Belgium, Ghana, India, Taiwan, and Sweden. The lineage 4 strains formed a cluster with strains from Sri Lanka, Turkey, and Bangladesh. The shared nucleotide and amino acid identities of the VP7 gene among the Bhutanese G9 strains were 96–99% and 97–100%, respectively.

Phylogenetic analysis of the G12 strains showed that lineage 3 segregated into two clusters with a bootstrap value of 90%, where one cluster comprised G12P[8] strains and the other comprised G12P[6] strains (Figure 5). The Bhutanese G12P[8] strains clustered with Sri Lankan and Indian strains. The Bhutanese G12P[6] strains clustered with Sri Lankan, Indian, Nepalese, and Bangladeshi strains. The shared nucleotide and amino acid identities of the VP7 gene among the Bhutanese G12 strains were 96–100% and 97–100%, respectively. The shared nucleotide and amino acid identities of the VP7 gene were 99–100% among the Bhutanese G12 P[6] strains. The shared nucleotide and amino acid identities of the VP7 gene were 99–100% among the Bhutanese G12 P[8] strains.

According to the phylogenetic analysis, P[8], P[6], and P[4] of the Bhutanese strains belonged to the globally circulating strains and were closely associated with strains from several different countries, but mainly with those from India and Bangladesh. Bhutanese P[8] belonged to lineages 3 and 4 (Figure 6). The VP8* head of VP4 contains four (8-1 to 8-4) surface-exposed antigenic epitopes, which have been predicted to comprise 25 amino acids [16,27]. All of the Bhutanese P[8] contained G at residues 146, instead of S, which are found in the two vaccine strains. Compared with RotaTeq, there were amino acid substitutions in 6 residues of all Bhutanese strains, and 10 additional residues were also substituted in some Bhutanese strains. Compared with Rotarix, amino acid substitutions were found in 9 residues of all Bhutanese strains, as well as additional substitutions in 9 other residues in some Bhutanese strains. Eleven amino acids of Bhutanese P[8] that belonged to lineage 4 differed from the vaccine strains (Figure 7).

Discussion

The proportion of rotavirus-positive samples detected in Bhutanese children is comparable to that found in neighboring India [28] and Bangladesh [21]. Given the rising cost of health care, the introduction of a rotavirus vaccine might reduce the burden on the health-care system. However, our study demonstrated the high diversity of rotavirus strains in Bhutan, where only the G1, G9, and G12 genotypes are in circulation, which might pose a challenge for the efficacy of rotavirus vaccines. Furthermore, the lower efficacy of rotavirus vaccine in the in low-income countries of Asia and Africa is another challenge [29,30]. The exact cause of this lack of efficacy in low-income countries is largely unknown, but it has been suggested that it may be attributable to the diversity of rotavirus strains, the passage of maternal antibodies to babies via breast-feeding, the presence of other viral agents, and malnutrition [31,32], all of which might be present in Bhutan. The VP7 sequences of Bhutanese G1 strains had low shared amino acid sequence identities with those of Rotarix RIX4414 and RotaTeq strain W179-9 and there were more amino acid differences compared with RotaTeq than with the Rotarix strain. With respect to the amino acid differences that are known to be responsible for generating neutralization escape strains, the Bhutanese strains contained five amino acid differences relative to RotaTeq and four relative to Rotarix. These suggest that Rotarix may be a better choice, although the mechanism responsible for vaccine-induced immunological protection is not clearly understood. Serum and intestinal serotype-specific neutralizing antibodies directed against VP7 and VP4, and virus-specific cytotoxic T lymphocyte induction are responsible for protection, although other proteins may be involved in immune protection against rotavirus [33,34].

The VP4 of Bhutanese strains also differed compared with the vaccine strains. In Rotarix and RotaTeq, P[8] belongs to lineages 1 and 2, respectively, whereas those of the Bhutanese strains belonged to lineages 3 and 4. Lineage 4 of genotype P[8], which is also called OP354-like (P[8]b) VP4, was first detected in Malawi [35], and it has also been detected in India [36], Bangladesh [37], Thailand [38], Vietnam [39], and Finland [40]. Overall, Bhutanese P[8] exhibited divergence compared with the vaccine strains, although there were greater divergences among lineage 4 of the P[8] strains. These results highlight the need to extend this study to the determination of further VP4 nucleotide sequences in more strains from Bhutan to evaluate the differences among the antigenic epitopes.

No previous studies are available, so it is not known whether the dominance of G9 and G12 is attributable to natural fluctuations in rotavirus genotypes or if they represent a unique situation in Bhutan. The emergence of G9 and G12 in Bhutan indicates that no barriers are able to prevent the spread of emerging strains to any corners of the world. According to the phylogenetic analysis, the Bhutanese strains were most closely associated with Indian and Bangladeshi strains, thereby reflecting the close relationships between these countries in terms of commodities and travel. This close association was also found in the two main clusters of G12 strains, which comprised G12P[8] and G12P[6] strains, indicating that the G12 genotype strains circulating in this region are probably derived from two clones. The phylogenetic analysis also showed that Bhutanese P[6] was derived from human strains rather than porcine strains. In the present study, we did not detect any animal derived strains, although >70% of Bhutan is covered with forest and interactions with wild animals are common, particularly via shared water sources that may be contaminated by animal excreta. Thus, further research may be required to detect rotavirus infections caused by animal strains or reassortants.

The detection of 10 different electropherotypes among 38 electropherotyped samples in our study might represent substantial diversity of rotaviruses circulating in Bhutan as compared with Turkey (5/38) [41], Sri Lanka (18/74) [22], Hong Kong (35/432)

[42], and Bangladesh (15/88) [21], respectively. The concentration of populations in urban areas in different parts of the country and their interactions may have generated this high diversity in Bhutan and helped these strains to spread successfully in children. The factors responsible for the high diversity of strains and the unusual genotype distributions found in Bhutan are complex. It is necessary to establish a nationwide surveillance system before introducing rotavirus vaccine into Bhutan. Furthermore, a vaccine trial may be required to evaluate the efficacy in Bhutanese children before selecting a specific vaccine. Both should be considered because of the complex vaccine-induced selection pressure on rotavirus strains.

Author Contributions

Conceived and designed the experiments: SW KA. Performed the experiments: MTM TY SZ TD Kinlay Tshering TM Karchung Tshering PB AN SW KA. Analyzed the data: MTM TY SZ TD Karchung Tshering TM Kinlay Tshering PB AN SW KA. Contributed reagents/materials/analysis tools: MTM TY SZ TD Kinlay Tshering TM Karchung Tshering PB AN SW KA. Contributed to the writing of the manuscript: MTM TY SZ TD Karchung Tshering TM Kinlay Tshering PB AN SW KA. Wrote the initial and final manuscript: SW KA.

References

1. Anonymous (2011) Annual Health Bulletin 2011. Thimphu: Bhutan Health Management Information System, Ministry of Health, Royal Government of Bhutan. 1–135.

2. Anonymous (2006) Results of population and housing census of Bhutan 2005. Thimphu, Bhutan: Office of the Census Commissioner, Langjuphakha, Thimphu, Bhutan. 1–502.

3. Anonymous (2012) Bhutan Maternal, Newborn and Child Survival. Country profile. Available: http://www.childinfo.org. Accessed 2013 January 21.

4. Tate JE, Burton AH, Boschi-Pinto C, Steele AD, Duque J, et al. (2012) 2008 estimate of worldwide rotavirus-associated mortality in children younger than 5 years before the introduction of universal rotavirus vaccination programmes: a systematic review and meta-analysis. Lancet Infect Dis 12: 136–141.

5. Ahmed K, Bozdayi G, Mitui MT, Ahmed S, Kabir L, et al. (2013) Circulating rotaviral RNA in children with rotavirus antigenemia. J Negat Results Biomed 12: 5.

6. Parashar U, Steele D, Neuzil K, Quadros C, Tharmaphornpilas P, et al. (2013) Progress with rotavirus vaccines: summary of the Tenth International Rotavirus Symposium. Expert Rev Vaccines 12: 113–117.

7. Parez N (2008) Rotavirus gastroenteritis: why to back up the development of new vaccines? Comp Immunol Microbiol Infect Dis 31: 253–269.

8. Banyai K, Laszlo B, Duque J, Steele AD, Nelson EA, et al. (2012) Systematic review of regional and temporal trends in global rotavirus strain diversity in the pre rotavirus vaccine era: insights for understanding the impact of rotavirus vaccination programs. Vaccine 30 Suppl 1: A122–130.

9. Gurgel RQ, Cuevas LE, Vieira SC, Barros VC, Fontes PB, et al. (2007) Predominance of rotavirus P[4]G2 in a vaccinated population, Brazil. Emerg Infect Dis 13: 1571–1573.

10. Kirkwood CD, Boniface K, Barnes GL, Bishop RF (2011) Distribution of rotavirus genotypes after introduction of rotavirus vaccines, Rotarix(R) and RotaTeq(R), into the National Immunization Program of Australia. Pediatr Infect Dis J 30: S48–53.

11. Donato CM, Zhang ZA, Donker NC, Kirkwood CD (2014) Characterization of G2P[4] rotavirus strains associated with increased detection in Australian states using the RotaTeq(R) vaccine during the 2010–2011 surveillance period. Infect Genet Evol.

12. Buttery JP, Danchin MH, Lee KJ, Carlin JB, McIntyre PB, et al. (2011) Intussusception following rotavirus vaccine administration: post-marketing surveillance in the National Immunization Program in Australia. Vaccine 29: 3061–3066.

13. Patel MM, Lopez-Collada VR, Bulhoes MM, De Oliveira LH, Bautista Marquez A, et al. (2011) Intussusception risk and health benefits of rotavirus vaccination in Mexico and Brazil. N Engl J Med 364: 2283–2292.

14. Weintraub ES, Baggs J, Duffy J, Vellozzi C, Belongia EA, et al. (2014) Risk of intussusception after monovalent rotavirus vaccination. N Engl J Med 370: 513–519.

15. Yih WK, Lieu TA, Kulldorff M, Martin D, McMahill-Walraven CN, et al. (2014) Intussusception risk after rotavirus vaccination in U.S. infants. N Engl J Med 370: 503–512.

16. Zeller M, Patton JT, Heylen E, De Coster S, Ciarlet M, et al. (2012) Genetic analyses reveal differences in the VP7 and VP4 antigenic epitopes between human rotaviruses circulating in Belgium and rotaviruses in Rotarix and RotaTeq. J Clin Microbiol 50: 966–976.

17. Mandile MG, Esteban LE, Arguelles MH, Mistchenko A, Glikmann G, et al. (2014) Surveillance of group A Rotavirus in Buenos Aires 2008–2011, long lasting circulation of G2P[4] strains possibly linked to massive monovalent vaccination in the region. J Clin Virol 60: 282–289.

18. Yahiro T, Wangchuk S, Tshering K, Bandhari P, Zangmo S, et al. (2014) Novel human bufavirus genotype 3 in children with severe diarrhea, Bhutan. Emerg Infect Dis 20: 1037–1039.

19. Matsumoto T, Wangchuk S, Tshering K, Yahiro T, Zangmo S, et al. (2013) Complete Genome Sequences of Two Astroviruses MLB1 Strains from Bhutanese Children with Diarrhea. Genome Announc 1: e00485–00413.

20. Mitui MT, Chandrasena TN, Chan PK, Rajindrajith S, Nelson EA, et al. (2012) Inaccurate identification of rotavirus genotype G9 as genotype G3 strains due to primer mismatch. Virol J 9: 144.

21. Ahmed K, Ahmed S, Mitui MT, Rahman A, Kabir L, et al. (2010) Molecular characterization of VP7 gene of human rotaviruses from Bangladesh. Virus Genes 40: 347–356.

22. Ahmed K, Batuwanthudawe R, Chandrasena TG, Mitui MT, Rajindrajith S, et al. (2010) Rotavirus infections with multiple emerging genotypes in Sri Lanka. Arch Virol 155: 71–75.

23. Larkin MA, Blackshields G, Brown NP, Chenna R, McGettigan PA, et al. (2007) Clustal W and Clustal X version 2.0. Bioinformatics 23: 2947–2948.

24. Tamura K, Peterson D, Peterson N, Stecher G, Nei M, et al. (2011) MEGA5: molecular evolutionary genetics analysis using maximum likelihood, evolutionary distance, and maximum parsimony methods. Mol Biol Evol 28: 2731–2739.

25. Matthijnssens J, Joelsson DB, Warakomski DJ, Zhou T, Mathis PK, et al. (2010) Molecular and biological characterization of the 5 human-bovine rotavirus (WC3)-based reassortant strains of the pentavalent rotavirus vaccine, RotaTeq. Virology 403: 111–127.

26. Aoki ST, Settembre EC, Trask SD, Greenberg HB, Harrison SC, et al. (2009) Structure of rotavirus outer-layer protein VP7 bound with a neutralizing Fab. Science 324: 1444–1447.

27. Dormitzer PR, Sun ZY, Wagner G, Harrison SC (2002) The rhesus rotavirus VP4 sialic acid binding domain has a galectin fold with a novel carbohydrate binding site. EMBO J 21: 885–897.

28. Mukherjee A, Chattopadhyay S, Bagchi P, Dutta D, Singh NB, et al. (2010) Surveillance and molecular characterization of rotavirus strains circulating in Manipur, north-eastern India: increasing prevalence of emerging G12 strains. Infect Genet Evol 10: 311–320.

29. Armah GE, Sow SO, Breiman RF, Dallas MJ, Tapia MD, et al. (2010) Efficacy of pentavalent rotavirus vaccine against severe rotavirus gastroenteritis in infants in developing countries in sub-Saharan Africa: a randomised, double-blind, placebo-controlled trial. Lancet 376: 606–614.

30. Zaman K, Dang DA, Victor JC, Shin S, Yunus M, et al. (2010) Efficacy of pentavalent rotavirus vaccine against severe rotavirus gastroenteritis in infants in developing countries in Asia: a randomised, double-blind, placebo-controlled trial. Lancet 376: 615–623.

31. Moon SS, Tate JE, Ray P, Dennehy PH, Archary D, et al. (2013) Differential profiles and inhibitory effect on rotavirus vaccines of nonantibody components in breast milk from mothers in developing and developed countries. Pediatr Infect Dis J 32: 863–870.

32. Shin S, Anh DD, Zaman K, Yunus M, Mai le TP, et al. (2012) Immunogenicity of the pentavalent rotavirus vaccine among infants in two developing countries in Asia, Bangladesh and Vietnam. Vaccine 30 Suppl 1: A106–113.

33. Heaton PM, Ciarlet M (2007) Vaccines: the pentavalent rotavirus vaccine: discovery to licensure and beyond. Clin Infect Dis 45: 1618–1624.

34. Ward R (2009) Mechanisms of protection against rotavirus infection and disease. Pediatr Infect Dis J 28: S57–59.

35. Cunliffe NA, Gondwe JS, Graham SM, Thindwa BD, Dove W, et al. (2001) Rotavirus strain diversity in Blantyre, Malawi, from 1997 to 1999. J Clin Microbiol 39: 836–843.

36. Samajdar S, Ghosh S, Dutta D, Chawla-Sarkar M, Kobayashi N, et al. (2008) Human group A rotavirus P[8] Hun9-like and rare OP354-like strains are circulating among diarrhoeic children in Eastern India. Arch Virol 153: 1933–1936.

37. Nagashima S, Kobayashi N, Paul SK, Alam MM, Chawla-Sarkar M, et al. (2009) Characterization of full-length VP4 genes of OP354-like P[8] human rotavirus strains detected in Bangladesh representing a novel P[8] subtype. Arch Virol 154: 1223–1231.

38. Theamboonlers A, Bhattarakosol P, Chongsrisawat V, Sungkapalee T, Wutthirattanakowit N, et al. (2008) Molecular characterization of group A human rotaviruses in Bangkok and Buriram, Thailand during 2004–2006 reveals the predominance of G1P[8], G9P[8] and a rare G3P[19] strain. Virus Genes 36: 289–298.

39. Nguyen TA, Hoang LP, Pham LD, Hoang KT, Okitsu S, et al. (2008) Use of sequence analysis of the VP4 gene to classify recent Vietnamese rotavirus isolates. Clin Microbiol Infect 14: 235–241.

40. Nagashima S, Kobayashi N, Paul SK, Ghosh S, Chawla-Sarkar M, et al. (2010) Identification of P[8]b subtype in OP354-like human rotavirus strains by a modified RT-PCR method. Jpn J Infect Dis 63: 208–211.

41. Bozdayi G, Dogan B, Dalgic B, Bostanci I, Sari S, et al. (2008) Diversity of human rotavirus G9 among children in Turkey. J Med Virol 80: 733–740.

42. Mitui MT, Chan PK, Nelson EA, Leung TF, Nishizono A, et al. (2011) Co-dominance of G1 and emerging G3 rotaviruses in Hong Kong: a three-year surveillance in three major hospitals. J Clin Virol 50: 325–333.

Permissions

All chapters in this book were first published in PLOS ONE, by The Public Library of Science; hereby published with permission under the Creative Commons Attribution License or equivalent. Every chapter published in this book has been scrutinized by our experts. Their significance has been extensively debated. The topics covered herein carry significant findings which will fuel the growth of the discipline. They may even be implemented as practical applications or may be referred to as a beginning point for another development.

The contributors of this book come from diverse backgrounds, making this book a truly international effort. This book will bring forth new frontiers with its revolutionizing research information and detailed analysis of the nascent developments around the world.

We would like to thank all the contributing authors for lending their expertise to make the book truly unique. They have played a crucial role in the development of this book. Without their invaluable contributions this book wouldn't have been possible. They have made vital efforts to compile up to date information on the varied aspects of this subject to make this book a valuable addition to the collection of many professionals and students.

This book was conceptualized with the vision of imparting up-to-date information and advanced data in this field. To ensure the same, a matchless editorial board was set up. Every individual on the board went through rigorous rounds of assessment to prove their worth. After which they invested a large part of their time researching and compiling the most relevant data for our readers.

The editorial board has been involved in producing this book since its inception. They have spent rigorous hours researching and exploring the diverse topics which have resulted in the successful publishing of this book. They have passed on their knowledge of decades through this book. To expedite this challenging task, the publisher supported the team at every step. A small team of assistant editors was also appointed to further simplify the editing procedure and attain best results for the readers.

Apart from the editorial board, the designing team has also invested a significant amount of their time in understanding the subject and creating the most relevant covers. They scrutinized every image to scout for the most suitable representation of the subject and create an appropriate cover for the book.

The publishing team has been an ardent support to the editorial, designing and production team. Their endless efforts to recruit the best for this project, has resulted in the accomplishment of this book. They are a veteran in the field of academics and their pool of knowledge is as vast as their experience in printing. Their expertise and guidance has proved useful at every step. Their uncompromising quality standards have made this book an exceptional effort. Their encouragement from time to time has been an inspiration for everyone.

The publisher and the editorial board hope that this book will prove to be a valuable piece of knowledge for researchers, students, practitioners and scholars across the globe.

List of Contributors

Kyung-Hwan Oh, Su-Mi Jung and Seung-Hak Cho
Division of Enteric Bacterial Infections, Center for Infectious Diseases, Korea National Institute of Health, Osong-eup, Chungcheongbuk-do, Republic of Korea

Dong Wook Kim
Department of Pharmacy, College of Pharmacy, Hanyang University, Ansan, Kyeonggi-do, Republic of Korea

Bissoume Samb-Ba, Catherine Mazenot, Amy Gassama-Sow, Grégory Dubourg, Hervé Richet, Perrine Hugon, Jean-Christophe Lagier, Didier Raoult and Florence Fenollar
Unitéde Recherche sur les Maladies Infectieuses et Tropicales Emergentes (URMITE) UM63, CNRS 7278, IRD 198, INSERM 1095, Aix-Marseille Université, Marseille, France and Dakar, Senegal

Bissoume Samb-Ba and Amy Gassama-Sow
Unitéde Bactériologie Expérimentale, Institut Pasteur de Dakar, Dakar, Senegal

Lisa Hartling, Michele P. Hamm, Donna M. Dryden and Ben Vandermeer
Alberta Research Centre for Health Evidence, Department of Pediatrics, University of Alberta, Edmonton, Alberta, Canada

Ricardo M. Fernandes
Clinical Pharmacology Unit, Faculty of Medicine, Instituto de Medicina Molecular, University of Lisbon, Lisbon, Portugal
Department of Pediatrics, Santa Maria Hospital, Lisbon, Portugal

R. Michele Anholt, Carl S. Ribble and Craig Stephen
Faculty of Veterinary Medicine, University of Calgary, Calgary, Alberta, Canada

John Berezowski
Veterinary Public Health Institute, University of Bern, Bern, Switzerland

Carl S. Ribble and Craig Stephen
Centre for Coastal Health, Nanaimo, British Columbia, Canada

Margaret L. Russell
Community Health Sciences, University of Calgary, Calgary, Alberta, Canada

Chunlan Xu, Rui Sun, Xiangjin Qiao, Xiaoya Shang and Weining Niu
The Key Laboratory for Space Bioscience and Biotechnology, School of Life Sciences, Northwestern Polytechnical University, Xi'an, Shaanxi, China

Youming Wang
Institute of Feed Science, College of Animal Sciences, Zhejiang University, Hangzhou, PR China

Dingfu Xiao, Jianhua He and Maoliang Ran
College of Animal Science and Technology, Hunan Agricultural University, Changsha, China

Yongfei Wang and Zemeng Feng
Research and Development Center, Twins Group Co., Ltd, Nanchang,Jiangxi, China

Gang Liu
Hunan Engineering and Research Center of Animal and Poultry Science and Key Laboratory for Agro-ecological Processes in Subtropical Region, Institute of Subtropical Agriculture, the Chinese Academy of Sciences, Hunan, China

Wei Qiu
Hunan New Wellful Co., LTD, Changsha, Hunan, China

Xionggui Hu
Hunan Institute of Animal and Veterinary Science, Changsha, China

Charles M. Nyachoti
Department of Animal Science, Faculty of Agricultural and Food Sciences, University of Manitoba, Winnipeg, Manitoba, Canada

Sung Woo Kim
Department of Animal Science, North Carolina State University, Raleigh, North Carolina, United States of America

Zhiru Tang
College of Animal Science and Technology, Southwest University, Chongqing, China

Qin Li, Han Yan, Wenting Liu, Hongchao Zhen, Yifan Yang and Bangwei Cao
Department of Oncology, Beijing Friendship Hospital, Capital Medical University, Beijing, China,

Wenting Liu, Hongchao Zhen, Yifan Yang and Bangwei Cao
Beijing Key Laboratory for Precancerous Lesion of Digestive Diseases, Beijing Friendship Hospital, Capital Medical University, Beijing, China
Beijing Digestive Diseases Center, Beijing Friendship Hospital, Capital Medical University, Beijing, China

Tanja Opriessnig and Priscilla F. Gerber
The Roslin Institute and The Royal (Dick) School of Veterinary Studies, University of Edinburgh, Roslin, Midlothian, United Kingdom

Tanja Opriessnig, Chao-Ting Xiao, Jianqiang Zhang and Patrick G. Halbur
Department of Veterinary Diagnostic and Production Animal Medicine, College of Veterinary Medicine, Iowa State University, Ames, Iowa, United States of America

Hiro Takahashi
Graduate School of Horticulture, Chiba University, Matsudo, Chiba, Japan

Hiro Takahashi and Anna Takahashi
Plant Biology Research Center, Chubu University, Kasugai, Aichi, Japan

Hiro Takahashi, Risa Ichinohe, Ayano Doi, Yoko Odaka, Misuzu Okuyama, Hiromi Sakamoto and Teruhiko Yoshida
Division of Genetics, National Cancer Center Research Institute, Tokyo, Japan

Kimie Sai, Yoshiro Saito, Nahoko Kaniwa and Haruhiro Okuda
Division of Medicinal Safety Science, National Institute of Health Sciences, Tokyo, Japan

Yasuhiro Matsumura
Division of Developmental Therapeutics, Research Center for Innovative Oncology, National Cancer Center Hospital East, Kashiwa, Chiba, Japan

Tetsuya Hamaguchi and Yasuhiro Shimada
Gastrointestinal Medical Oncology Division, National Cancer Center Hospital, Tokyo, Japan

Atsushi Ohtsu, Takayuki Yoshino and Toshihiko Doi
Department of Gastrointestinal Oncology, National Cancer Center Hospital East, Kashiwa, Chiba, Japan

Risa Ichinohe and Ayano Doi
Faculty of Horticulture, Chiba University, Matsudo, Chiba, Japan

Nagahiro Saijo
National Cancer Center Hospital East, Kashiwa, Chiba, Japan

Jun-ichi Sawada
Division of Functional Biochemistry and Genomics, National Institute of Health Sciences, Tokyo, Japan

Shuang Zhang, Taiwei Jiao and Min Jiang
Department of Gastroenterology, First Affiliated Hospital of China Medical University, Shenyang, China

Yushuai Chen, Nan Gao and Lili Zhang
Department of Cadre Ward II, First Affiliated Hospital of China Medical University, Shenyang, China

Michael Wilschanski, Montaser Abbasi and Eyal Shteyer
Gastroenterology Unit, Division of Pediatrics, Hadassah Hebrew University Hospital, Jerusalem, Israel

Elias Blanco and Iris Lindberg
Department of Anatomy and Neurobiology, University of Maryland-Baltimore, Baltimore, Maryland, United States of America

Elias Blanco, Michael Yourshaw and Martin G. Martín
Department of Pediatrics, Division of Gastroenterology and Nutrition, Mattel Children's Hospital and the David Geffen School of Medicine, University of California Los Angeles, Los Angeles, California, United States of America

David Zangen
Endocrinology Unit, Division of Pediatrics, Hadassah Hebrew University Hospital, Jerusalem, Israel

Itai Berger
Neurology Unit, Division of Pediatrics, Hadassah Hebrew University Hospital, Jerusalem, Israel

Orit Pappo
Department of Pathology, Hadassah Hebrew University Hospital, Jerusalem, Israel

Benjamin Bar-Oz
Department of Neonatology, Hadassah Hebrew University Hospital, Jerusalem, Israel

Orly Elpeleg
Monique and Jacques Roboh Department of Genetic Research, Hadassah Hebrew University Hospital, Jerusalem, Israel

Ricardo Q. Gurgel, Alda Rodrigues, Robergson R. Ribeiro, Sílvio S. Dolabella, Natanael L. Da Mota and Victor S. Santos
Federal University of Sergipe, Aracaju, Brazil

Alberto De Juan Alvarez and Luis E. Cuevas
Liverpool School of Tropical Medicine, Liverpool, United Kingdom

Miren Iturriza-Gomara and s Nigel A. Cunliffe
Institute of Infection and Global Health, University of Liverpool, Liverpool, United Kingdom

Milinda Lakkam
Institute for Computational and Mathematical Engineering, Stanford University, Stanford, California, United States of America

Stefan Wager
Statistics Department, Stanford University, Stanford, California, United States of America

Paul H. Wise
School of Medicine, Stanford University, Stanford California, United States of America

Lawrence M. Wein
Graduate School of Business, Stanford University, Stanford, California, United States of America

Rosalind Parkes-Ratanshi, Ali Elbireer, Betty Mbambu, Faridah Mayanja, Alex Coutinho and Concepta Merry
Infectious Diseases Institute, Makerere College of Health Sciences, Kampala, Uganda

Ali Elbireer
Johns Hopkins University, School of Medicine, Baltimore, Maryland, United States of America

Concepta Merry
Trinity College Dublin, Dublin, Ireland
Northwestern University, Chicago, Illinois, United States of America

DeAnna C. Bublitz, Patricia C. Wright, Fidisoa T. Rasambainarivo, James B. Bliska and Thomas R. Gillespie
Centre ValBio, Ranomafana, Madagascar

DeAnna C. Bublitz and James B. Bliska
Department of Molecular Genetics and Microbiology, Center for Infectious Diseases, Stony Brook University, Stony Brook, New York, United States of America

Patricia C. Wright
Department of Anthropology, Stony Brook University, Stony Brook, New York, United States of America

Jonathan R. Bodager and Thomas R. Gillespie
Department of Environmental Health, Rollins School of Public Health, Emory University, Atlanta, Georgia, United States of America

Thomas R. Gillespie
Department of Environmental Sciences and Program in Population Biology, Ecology, and Evolution, Emory University, Atlanta, Georgia, United States of America

Alexandra Kleimann, Sermin Toto, Christian K. Eberlein, Stefan Bleich, Helge Frieling and Marcel Sieberer
Department of Psychiatry, Social Psychiatry and Psychotherapy, Hannover Medical School, Hannover, Germany

Jan T. Kielstein
Department of Nephrology and Hypertension, Hannover Medical School, Hannover, Germany

Vittoria Buccigrossi, Gabriella Laudiero, Carla Russo, Erasmo Miele, Morena Sofia and Alfredo Guarino
Department of Translational Medical Science, Section of Pediatrics, University of Naples "Federico II", Naples, Italy

Marina Monini and Franco Maria Ruggeri
Department of Veterinary Public Health & Food Safety, Viral Zoonoses Unit, Istituto Superiore di Sanità Rome – Italy, Rome, Italy

Mohammod Jobayer Chisti, Tahmeed Ahmed, Abu Syed Golam Faruque, Hasan Ashraf, Pradip Kumar Bardhan, Abu S. M. S. B. Shahid, K. M. Shahunja and Mohammed Abdus Salam
International Centre for Diarrhoeal Disease Research, Bangladesh, Dhaka, Bangladesh

Mohammod Jobayer Chisti, Stephen M. Graham and Trevor Duke
Centre for International Child Health, The University of Melbourne Department of Paediatrics and Murdoch Childrens Research Institute, Royal Children's Hospital, Melbourne, Australia

Stephen M. Graham
International Union Against Tuberculosis and Lung Disease, Paris, France

Baiqing Dong
Department of Emergency Response, Guagnxi Zhuang Autonomous Region Health Bureau, Nanning, Guangxi, China

Dabin Liang, Mei Lin, Mingliu Wang, Jun Zeng, Hezhuang Liao, Lingyun Zhou and Jun Huang
Divsion of Bacterial Infectious Disease Control, Guagnxi Zhuang Autonomous Region Center for Disease Prevention and Control, Nanning, Guangxi, China

Xiaolin Wei
School of Public Health and Primary Care, Chinese University of Hong Kong, Hong Kong, China

Guanyang Zou
COMDIS Health Services Delivery Research Consortium, China Program, Nuffield Centre for International Health and Development, University of Leeds, Shenzhen, China

Huaiqi Jing
National Institute for Communicable Disease Control and Prevention, Chinese Center for Disease Control and Prevention, Beijing, China and State Key Laboratory for Infectious Disease Prevention and Control, Collaborative Innovation Center for Diagnosis and Treatment of Infectious Diseases, Beijing, China

Jason W. Marion, Cheonghoon Lee, Chang Soo Lee, Timothy J. Buckley and Jiyoung Lee
Division of Environmental Health Sciences, College of Public Health, The Ohio State University, Columbus, Ohio, United States of America

Qiuhong Wang and Linda J. Saif
Food Animal Health Research Program, Ohio Agricultural Research and Development Center, Department of Veterinary Preventive Medicine, The Ohio State University, Wooster, Ohio, United States of America

Stanley Lemeshow
Division of Biostatistics, College of Public Health, The Ohio State University, Columbus, Ohio, United States of America

Jiyoung Lee
Department of Food Science and Technology, The Ohio State University, Columbus, Ohio, United States of America

Ahmed S. Rahman, Mohammad Jyoti Raihan, Mohammad Mehedi Hasan and Tahmeed Ahmed
Centre for Nutrition and Food Security, International Centre for Diarrhoeal Diseases Research, Bangladesh (icddr,b), Dhaka, Bangladesh

Mohammad Rafiqul Islam
CCEB, School of Medicine and Public Health, University of Newcastle, Newcastle, Australia

Tracey P. Koehlmoos
Department of Health Administration and Policy, College of Health and Human Services, George Mason University, Fairfax, Virginia, United States of America

Charles P. Larson
Department of Pediatrics, University of British Columbia and Centre for International Child Health, BC Children's Hospital, Vancouver, British Columbia, Canada

Satarupa Mullick, Anupam Mukherjee, Santanu Ghosh, Gururaja P. Pazhani, Dipika Sur, Byomkesh Manna, Thandavarayan Ramamurthy and Mamta Chawla-Sarkar
National Institute of Cholera and Enteric Diseases, Kolkata, India

James P. Nataro
Department of Paediatrics, University of Virginia, School of Medicine, Charlottesville, Virginia, United States of America

Myron M. Levine
Center for Vaccine Development, University of Maryland, School of Medicine, Baltimore, Maryland, United States of America

Hassan Nassour, J. Daniel Dubreuil
GREMIP, Faculty of Veterinary Medicine, Université de Montré al, Montreal, Quebec, Canada

Sonam Wangchuk, Sangay Zangmo, Tshering Dorji and Karchung Tshering
Public Health Laboratory, Department of Public Health, Ministry of Health, Thimphu, Bhutan

Marcelo T. Mitui, Takaaki Yahiro, Takashi Matsumoto, Akira Nishizono and Kamruddin Ahmed
Department of Microbiology, Faculty of Medicine, Oita University, Yufu, Japan

Kinlay Tshering
Department of Pediatrics, Jigme Dorji Wangchuk National Referral Hospital, Thimphu, Bhutan

Purushotam Bandhari
Department of Pediatrics, Mongar Regional Referral Hospital, Mongar, Bhutan

Kamruddin Ahmed
Research Promotion Institute, Oita University, Yufu, Japan

Index

www.ingramcontent.com/pod-product-compliance
Lightning Source LLC
Chambersburg PA
CBHW080251230326
41458CB00097B/4265